Wound Care Essentials
PRACTICE PRINCIPLES
SECOND EDITION

Sharon Baranoski, MSN, RN, CWOCN, APN, DAPWCA, FAAN
*Director of Medical Surgical Nursing & The Center for Wound Care and Hyperbaric
Medicine*
Provena Saint Joseph Medical Center
Joliet, Illinois

Elizabeth A. Ayello, PhD, RN, APRN,BC, CWOCN, FAPWCA, FAAN
President
Ayello, Harris & Associates
Copake, New York
Faculty
Excelsior College School of Nursing
Albany, New York
Executive Editor
Journal of the World Council of Enterostomal Therapists
Senior Adviser
The John A. Hartford Institute for Geriatric Nursing
New York
Clinical Associate Editor
Advances in Skin & Wound Care

 Wolters Kluwer | Lippincott Williams & Wilkins
Health
Philadelphia · Baltimore · New York · London
Buenos Aires · Hong Kong · Sydney · Tokyo

STAFF

Executive Publisher
Judith A. Schilling McCann, RN, MSN

Senior Acquisitions Editor
Margaret Zuccarini

Editorial Director
H. Nancy Holmes

Art Director
Mary Ludwicki

Editors
Jennifer A. Kowalak, Julie Munden

Copy Editors
Kimberly Bilotta, Nicholas J. Bilotta,
Jeannine Fielding, Linda Hager

Designer
Matie Anne Patterson

Digital Composition Services
Diane Paluba (manager), Joyce Rossi Biletz,
Donna S. Morris

Associate Manufacturing Manager
Beth J. Welsh

Editorial Assistants
Karen J. Kirk, Jeri O'Shea, Linda K. Ruhf

Indexer
Barbara Hodgson

Cover Photographs
Top to bottom: Necrotic heel pressure ulcer
(Sharon Baranoski), unstageable pressure ulcer
(Elizabeth Ayello), venous leg ulcer (Harold Brem),
abdominal dehiscence (Sharon Baranoski), diabetic
ulcer with wound track completely through toe
(James McGuire)

WCE2010807

Library of Congress Cataloging-in-Publication Data

Baranoski, Sharon.
   Wound care essentials : practice principles / Sharon Baranoski, Elizabeth A. Ayello. — 2nd ed.
      p. ; cm.
   Includes bibliographical references and index.
    1. Wounds and injuries—Patients—Care—Handbooks, manuals, etc. 2. Wounds and injuries—Nursing—Handbooks, manuals, etc. 3. Wound healing—Handbooks, manuals, etc. I. Ayello, Elizabeth A. II. Title.
    [DNLM: 1. Wounds and Injuries—therapy. 2. Wound Healing. WO 700 B225w 2008]
   RD94.B374 2008
   617.1—dc22
ISBN-13: 978-1-58255-469-3 (alk. paper)
ISBN-10: 1-58255-469-2 (alk. paper)   2007018677

Wound Care Essentials
PRACTICE PRINCIPLES
SECOND EDITION

Contents

PART ONE
Wound care concepts

Color illustrations • following page 242

PART TWO
Wound classifications and management strategies

Contributors and consultants

Contributors

Mona Baharestani, PhD, ANP, CWOCN, FACCWS
Director, Wound Healing
Long Island Jewish Medical Center
Schneider Children's Hospital
New Hyde Park, N.Y.

Christine Barkauskas, RN, BA, CWOCN, APN
Certified WOC Nurse
Silver Cross Hospital
Joliet, Ill.

Dan R. Berlowitz, MD, MPh
Director, Center for Health Quality,
Outcomes and Economic Research
Professor of Public Health and Medicine
Bedford VA Hospital
Boston University School of Public Health

Joyce M. Black, PhD, RN, CPSN, CWCN, FAPWCA
Associate Professor
University of Nebraska Medical Center,
College of Nursing
Omaha

Steven B. Black, MD, FACS
Director of Wound Healing
Nebraska Medical Center
Omaha

Harold Brem, MD, FACS
Associate Professor of Surgery
Division of Plastic Surgery
College of Physicians and Surgeons
Columbia University
New York

David M. Brienza, PhD
Professor
University of Pittsburgh
Department of Rehabilitation Science and
Technology, Department of Bioengi-
neering
McGowan Institute for Regenerative
Medicine

Gregory Brown, RN, ET
Surgical Case Manager
Dallas Veterans Medical Center

Janet E. Cuddigan, PhD, RN, CWCN, CCCN
Assistant Professor and Interim Chair of
Adult Health and Illness Department
University of Nebraska Medical Center,
College of Nursing
Omaha

Linda Dallam, MS, APRN,BC, CWCN, GNP
Nurse Practitioner
Pain Management Team
Department of Anesthesiology
Montefiore Medical Center
Bronx, N.Y.

Tami De Araujo, MD, FAAD
Voluntary Assistant Professor
Department of Dermatology and Cutaneous
Surgery
University of Miami Miller School of
Medicine

Rita A. Frantz, PhD, RN, CWCN, FAAN
Professor and Chair, Systems and Practice
Nursing
College of Nursing
The University of Iowa
Iowa City

Linda Galvan, RN, BSN, CWOCN, APN
Certified Wound, Ostomy & Continence
Nurse
The Center for Wound Care and Hyperbaric
Medicine
Provena Saint Joseph Medical Center
Joliet, Ill.

Susan L. Garber, MA, OTR, FAOTA, FACRM
Professor
Department of Physical Medicine and
Rehabilitation
Baylor College of Medicine
Houston

Susan Gardner, PhD, RN, CWCN
Assistant Professor
The University of Iowa
Iowa City

Mary Jo Geyer, PT, PhD, FCCWS, CLT-LANA, C.Ped
Assistant Professor
Chatham University
Pittsburgh

Keith Harding, MB, ChB, MRCGP, FRCS
Head, Department of Wound Healing
Cardiff University
Wales, United Kingdom

Vanessa Jones, MSc, RN, NDN, RCNT, PGCE
Senior Lecturer/Course Director
Department of Wound Healing
Cardiff University
Wales, United Kingdom

Robert S. Kirsner, MD, PhD
Professor & Vice Chairman
Department of Dermatology & Cutaneous
    Surgery
University of Miami Miller School of
    Medicine

Carl A. Kirton, RN, ACRN. APRN,BC, MA
*Administrative Director and Nurse
    Practitioner*
North General Hospital
New York
Clinical Associate Professor
College of Nursing, New York University
President
Association of Nurses in AIDS Care

Ronald A. Kline, MD, FACS, FAHA
Chief, Division of Vascular Surgery
Carondelet, St. Joseph's Hospital
Medical Director
Center for Advanced Wound Care
St. Joseph's Hospital
Medical Director for Wound Care
Kindred Hospital
Co-Director
Arizona EndoVascular Center
Tucson

Steven P. Knowlton, JD, RN
Managing Attorney, Locks Law Firm, PLLC
Nyack, N.Y.

Diane K. Langemo, PhD, RN, FAAN
President, Langemo & Associates
*Adjunct Professor and Fritz Distinguished
    Professor Emeritus*
University of North Dakota College of
    Nursing
Grand Forks

Lawrence A. Lavery, DPM, MPh
Professor of Surgery
Scott and White Hospital & Texas A&M
    University Health Science Center College
    of Medicine
Temple

Courtney H. Lyder, ND, GNP, FAAN
*Professor and Chair, Department of Acute
    and Specialty Care*
University of Virginia Medical Center
University of Virginia School of Nursing
Charlottesville

James McGuire, DPM, PT, CPed, CWS, FAFWCA
*Chairman, Department of Podiatric Medicine
    and Orthopedics*
*Director, Leonard Abrams Center for
    Advanced Wound Healing*
Temple University School of Podiatric
    Medicine
Philadelphia

Andrea McIntosh, RN, BSN, CWOCN, APN
Manager, Wound Healing & Treatment Center & WOCN Department
Silver Cross Hospital
Joliet, Ill.

Mary Ellen Posthauer, RD, CD, LD
Consultant Dietitian
Supreme Care West
Long Term Facilities
Evansville, Ind.

Pamela Scarborough, PT, MS, CDE, CWS, FACCWS
Director of Education
PARKS Institute
Wimberley, Tex.

Gregory Schultz, PhD
Professor, Obstetrics & Gynecology and Biochemistry
University of Florida
Gainesville

R. Gary Sibbald, BSc, MD, FRCPC (Med)(Derm), FAPWCA, MEd,
Professor of Public Health Sciences and Medicine
Director of Dermatology Day Care and Medical Education
Chair 3rd meeting of the World Union of Wound Healing Societies, Toronto, June 4th-8th 2008
University of Toronto, Women's College Hospital
Ontario, Canada

Mary Y. Sieggreen, MSN, APRN,BC, CVN
Nurse Practitioner, Vascular Surgery
Clinical Nurse Specialist, Wound Care
Harper University Hospital, Detroit Medical Center
Associate Clinical Professor
Wayne State University
Detroit

Stephen Sprigle, PhD, PT
Associate Professor
Georgia Institute of Technology
Atlanta

Joyce Stechmiller, ARNP, PhD, CS
Associate Professor and Chair of the Department of Adult and Elderly Nursing
University of Florida
Gainesville

David R. Thomas, MD, FACP, AGSF, GSAF
Professor of Medicine
Division of Geriatric Medicine
Saint Louis University School of Medicine

Marjana Tomic-Canic, PhD, RN
Director, Tissue Repair Laboratory; Associate Scientist
Hospital for Special Surgery of the Weill Cornell Medical College
New York

Terry Allen Treadwell, MD, FACS
Medical Director
Institute for Advanced Wound Care
Montgomery, Ala.

Angela Colette Willis, RN, CWS, CDE
Staff Nurse
Wound Healing Program
The Mount Sinai Medical Center
New York

Karen Zulkowski, DNS, RN, CWS
Associate Professor
College of Nursing
Montana State University
Bozeman

Consultants

Barbara Bohanan, RN, WOCN, CWCN
Vice President of Education
Medical Multiplex, Inc.
Louisville, Ky.

Phyllis A. Bonham, PhD, RN, CWOCN
Director, Wound Care Education Program,
*   Clinical Assistant Professor*
College of Nursing, Medical University of
    South Carolina
Charleston

Kathy E. Davis, MSN, RN, CWOCN
Assistant Professor of Nursing
Gordon College
Barnesville, Ga.

Rose Miller, RN, MAS
Registered Nurse
Dr. Steven R. Miller and Associates
Grosse Pointe, Michigan

Kodzo Pongo, RN, PhD
Staff RN
Howe Developmental Center
Tinley Park, Ill.

Barbara Pieper, PhD, RN
Professor/Nurse Practitioner
Wayne State University
Detroit

Catherine Rogers, APRN, BC, CWCN, CWS
Program Manager and Advanced Practice
Wound Care Clinic, Swedish American
    Hospital
Rockford, Ill.

Donna Scemons, MSN, RN, FNP, CNS, CWOCN
President
Healthcare Systems, Inc.
Castaic, Calif.

Frances E. Schuda, MSN, RN, CWOCN, CNDLTC,
NHA, DAPWCA
Assistant Administrator, Director of Nursing
Parkhouse, Providence Pointe
Royersford, Pa.

Patricia A. Slachta, PhD, APRN,BC, CWOCN
Clinical Nurse Specialist, Wound, Skin, and
*   Ostomy*
Medical University of South Carolina
Medical University Hospital Authority
Charleston

Deidre D. Wipke-Tevis, RN, PhD
Associate Professor
MU Sinclair School of Nursing
University of Missouri-Columbia

Kathy Wright, RN, MS, CWOCN, APRN
Clinical Director, Nanticoke Wound Care
*   and Hyperbaric Center*
Nanticoke Health Services
Seaford, Del.

Foreword

When I was asked to write the foreword for the first edition of *Wound Care Essentials: Practice Principles*, I complied as a favor to my good friends Elizabeth Ayello and Sharon Baranoski. My enthusiasm for the project was ignited only after I reviewed the galleys for that edition and discovered it to be a unique combination of the state of the science and the state of the art of wound care. The book greatly exceeded the ordinary in terms of the wide variety of topics covered and the exceptional thoroughness of that coverage.

After the galleys for the second edition arrived, I leafed through the chapters with great curiosity and anticipation. It was hard for me to believe that the first edition could be improved upon—but it has been! Of course, the new edition has retained and updated all of the content from the first edition—from legal aspects of wound care to sickle cell ulcer management strategies—that elevated the book above the ordinary. In addition to the typical content on wound infection, support surfaces for wound beds, and common chronic wounds, the new edition includes not-so-typical content that discusses wound bioburden, seating support surfaces, and atypical wounds.

All the chapters, references, and tables in the second edition of *Wound Care Essentials: Practice Principles* have been revised with the latest theory and practice information, and great attention has been paid to evidence that emerged since the first edition was published. The expert chapter authors have been chosen from a wider variety of disciplines and represent a good balance of researchers and clinicians.

The second edition has several notable updates and additions. Portions of the book have been reorganized to give the flow of information a more intuitive feel. The editors and authors have used several strategies to allow for a more thorough treatment of certain topics. For example, a chapter from the first edition that covered both arterial and venous wounds was split into separate chapters and expanded to reflect the complexity of wound healing in these situations. In other instances, specific content was targeted for expansion, so that this edition contains more information on skin conditions, such as xerosis and pruritus, and on the important role of nutrition in wound healing.

I'm excited that new content has been added on surgical wound care, palliative care, and wound care in pediatric patients and bariatric patients. These topics are fairly new to standard texts on wound care and to general offerings at conferences, but they aren't new to clinicians who have been coping with problems in these areas for a long time, unassisted by peers or wound care experts.

Finally, the look and feel of the textbook are pleasing and useful. The formatting helps to emphasize key points and keep the reader focused on the information being presented. "Practice points" throughout the text help the reader grasp the most salient messages in a given passage. The number of full-color photos has been doubled, to more fully illustrate various issues in wound care.

Samuel Johnson once said, "Knowledge is of two kinds. We know a subject ourselves, or we know where we can find information on it." In this book, the novice and the expert alike can find the information needed in order to be truly knowledgeable. It's a rare text that can please both scientist and clinician, but this one does it well!

Barbara Braden, PhD, RN, FAAN
Dean, University College
Creighton University
Omaha, Nebr.

Preface

Thank you dear colleagues for your enthusiastic support of *Wound Care Essentials*! Your response to our book was beyond our expectations. We were delighted to have contributed to the wound care literature with this practical compilation of the essential knowledge needed for today's clinicians. We were honored that our first edition was chosen by our peers as an *American Journal of Nursing* Book of the year in 2004 and printed in Portuguese as *O Essencial Sobre O Tratamento De Feridas Principios Practicos*.

We are thrilled to know that our book hasn't sat on a shelf unused. Many of you shared how helpful our book is whether in studying for certification, writing policies and procedures or, most of all, in your daily patient care. Making a difference in the lives of patients and their families is our continued dream. Your comments and encouragement to continue our efforts gave us the impetus to write this second edition.

We have retained the original vision of the book, which was to share what we learned in the trenches of patient care. We have married it with our experience in education because we hold dearly the belief that excellence in practice depends upon excellence in education. Our book continues to combine all that we have learned from our patients, colleagues, research, literature, industry, seminars, and educational programs into one concise wound care source.

We are doubly honored to create a new edition filled with more chapters, photos, and practical information to guide you in the care of your patients. All chapters have been thoroughly reviewed and updated with the most current information available at the time of writing. One of the things you'll notice about this second edition is that we've added several new chapters and sections, which include palliative care, neonatal/pediatrics, and bariatrics. Some content has been reorganized; for example our vascular chapter is now two dynamic chapters on venous and arterial disease. As requested, we've increased the number of color pictures to the maximum that space would allow.

Once again we had a great group of writers. We are grateful that most of our authors were able to contribute to this edition. We are also honored to welcome several new colleagues to share their expertise with you. We are delighted that once again Barbara Braden has written our foreword! Without the willingness of these wound care experts to share their time, knowledge, and expertise, this book wouldn't be a reality. Thank you all for being part of this second edition.

Just as in practice, teamwork is important in publishing. We are saddened by the passing our mentor and dear friend, Roberta Abruzzese. Dr. Abruzzese was instrumental in guiding us in our writing and education careers. We will miss her greatly.

It takes a village to write a book! The diligent editing, meticulous attention to detail, understanding, and flexibility from our Lippincott Williams & Wilkins, Wolters Kluwer Health team made it a much less tenacious and threatening experience. We are grateful to the LWW-WKH staff who worked behind the scenes on our behalf. We may not know all of you personally, but your efforts are evident in the book and much appreciated. Thank you to Margaret Zuccarini, Susan Rainey, Nancy Holmes, and Jennifer Kowalak for your guidance and support in making it the second time around.

To our readers, we hope the pages will be tattered and torn from use and that it doesn't sit on your bookshelf. We enjoy thinking about the places our book might be on any given day and in which lab coats it might be traveling around in a health care facility.

For we both believe the old adage "Knowledge is important, but what you *do* with the knowledge is *more important*."

Sharon and Elizabeth

Dedication

Wound Care Essentials: Practice Principles, Second Edition, took almost 1½ years to write. It was a true labor of dedication, commitment, and desire to give you, our readers, an excellent resource to use when caring for patients.

To my family (Jim, Jim Jr., Deborah, Jeff, and J.R.) who gave me the space to write this book and gave me the emotional support to persevere through a challenging personal year. To my husband Jim, your love and never-ending confidence in me is so appreciated—words can't express how much I value you as my "never-ending partner."

To my co-editor, Elizabeth A. Ayello, a very special friend. Albert Schweitzer said "Sometimes our light goes out but is blown into flame by another human being. Each of us owes deepest thanks to those who have rekindled this light." Elizabeth, thanks for keeping my light rekindled with your love, support, and *can do* attitude.

And finally to my Mom, your spirit is with me every day. I sure do miss you. This one's for you.

Sharon

"Family is everything."

To my mom Phyllis who, throughout her lifetime, often said these words. They grow ever so more meaningful with each passing day. Since the first edition of this book, so many more important people, both friends and family, in my life have passed away and joined you and Bert.

Thanks also to Roberta, who taught me the power of words, and my dad Tony, who as a professional musician taught me that "when words leave off, music begins." Dad, the wound care conferences just don't seem the same without you! I miss all of you! Your everlasting guidance and love along with those who are still here, gave me the strength to continue writing this second edition.

To my dear brothers Bob and Ron and their families. Your love and support have nurtured me always. Thank you for planning parties and family gatherings around my hectic schedule

To Stephen, Florence, Russ, Aunt Betty, Aunt Ann, and their families. Thank you for showing me that caring comes in many ways

To Katie, Ron, and family. There is no one else like you. As William James said, "Wherever you are, it is your own friends that make your world."

To Teddy and David, for knowing just when to call.

To Carl, Sheila, Vinny, Courtney, Harold, Gary, Steve, Bob, Paula, Larry, and Janet, for always "being there" for me. Your presence in my life has made a difference.

To Cara, Mike, Lori, Eric, and their families. Thank you for reminding me how important it is to stop and take time to share holidays with friends.

To Sharon. With challenges and losses in our personal lives, this one has been difficult, but as Mark Twain said, "Grief can take care of itself, but to get the full value of joy you must have somebody to divide it with." Thank you for letting me share with you the happiness of this book.

To my darling daughters — Sarah, your courage in overcoming whatever challenges life may give you has inspired me to persevere, and Wendy, our newest health care professional, your kindness, talents, achievements, and promise remind me daily to be future-focused.

To my husband, A. Scott, with love always. Thank you for your understanding and patience and for enduring long weekends alone while I was in Chicago writing at Sharon's home. Now it is time to celebrate; let's dance!

E.A.A

Part One

Wound care concepts

CHAPTER 1

Quality of life and ethical issues

Mona Mylene Baharestani, PhD, ANP, CWOCN, FCCWS, FAPWCA

OBJECTIVES

After completing this chapter, you'll be able to:

- describe how wounds and those afflicted by wounds are viewed

- identify quality-of-life impact on patients with wounds and their caregivers

- describe ethical dilemmas confronted in wound care

- identify issues and challenges faced by caregivers of patients with wounds

- describe strategies aimed at meeting the needs of patients with wounds and their caregivers.

Treating the patient as well as the wound

The practice of wound healing is undergoing revolutionary change as research unlocks the mysteries of the complex processes of tissue degradation, regeneration, and repair. Research has also given birth to many new wound-healing technologies, including tissue-engineered skin, matrix metalloproteinase modulation, topical growth factors, negative pressure, normothermia, and slow-release antimicrobial therapies. Such therapies are now within the armamentarium of wound-care practitioners, making possible the healing of previously recalcitrant wounds.

But faster, more efficient healing is only one element of providing advanced wound care as wounds affect different patients on different levels. Indeed, wounds bring financial, psychological, and social implications to the patient that must also be addressed. Yet, in our fast-paced, stressful clinical practices, do we encourage the patient to disavow his wounds?[1] Do we acknowledge the profound life changes and day-to-day challenges faced by chronic wound sufferers?[2] Do we perpetuate patients' fear, shame, and isolation?[1] Do we give patients and their families and caregivers the impression that "wound care is a dehumanizing and reductionist specialty"?[3]

Assessing the meaning and significance of the wound to the patient and his caregiver should be as routine as assessing wound size and the percentage of granulation and necrotic tissue, but is it? Hyland et al.[4] report that patients spend an average of 1.5 to 2 hours per day thinking about their leg ulcers. Do we know what the patient is thinking? Do we ever ask? The answer to the question "What impact has your wound had on your quality of life?" posed by a caring and concerned practitioner provides valuable insight into the patient's experience and needs, while also setting the stage for mutual goal identification and treatment planning.

Beyond possession of knowledge in basic science, anatomy, pathophysiology, wound-care dressings, drugs, and technologies, advanced wound-care practitioners must be able to deliver care in a compassionate manner, sensitive to the unique impact wounds have on quality of life.

How are wounds viewed?

A wound is defined as a disruption of the integrity and function of tissues in the body. The state of having a wound infers an imperfection, an insult resulting in a physical and emotional vulnerability.[5] Wounds and their management are described within a variety of personal, philosophical, and socioeconomic paradigms. (See *Emotional impact of wounds*.)

How are patients with wounds viewed?

Given the negative image by which wounds are viewed, it isn't surprising that patients with wounds are sometimes considered unattractive, imperfect, vulnerable, a nuisance to others and, in some cases, even repulsive.[5-8] Health care professionals, in particular, often blame patients and caregivers for the development and recalcitrance of pressure ulcers and venous ulcers, as the following comments reveal.

"When I have a pressure ulcer, health care professionals ask, 'What happened?' This makes me feel ashamed because I was unable to prevent the pressure ulcer. Why is it that other complications of quadriplegia don't carry this type of stigma? Nobody makes me feel guilty when I have a urinary tract infection."[1]

A 79-year-old caregiver for her bedridden, paralyzed 83-year-old spouse states, "I thought it was nothing." (Referring to nine pressure ulcers.) "The plastic surgeon was

> ## Emotional impact of wounds
>
> In addition to the dangers associated with wounds and the physical discomfort they often bring, wounds have an emotional effect on the patient, caregivers, family, friends, and strangers he may encounter. Even health care professionals aren't immune to an emotional response to a patient's wound.
> Wounds are typically perceived as:
> - a betrayal of one's own body
> - appalling, disgusting, repulsive
> - haunting, scary, associated with horror movies
> - nuisance, time-consuming, costly
> - smelly
> - unpleasant, uncomfortable.
> - The patient's own perception of his wound may include such feelings as:
> - embarrassment, humiliation
> - guilt, shame
> - needing bandages to "hide the evidence" (that is, of imperfection).

quite angry about the sores, asking why I waited so long to bring him to the hospital. I was just dumbfounded. I felt so bad, I said, I just thought it was a sore that would just heal up. I feel so guilty that I didn't do the right thing."[9] According to Charles [10], patients often feel that they are "relegated to a low priority in terms of medical understanding and delivery of service." Lack of explanation regarding what procedures will entail, results of diagnostic testing, and treatment options and prognosis often results in anger, frustration, resentment, and distrust on the part of patients and their families toward health care professionals.[10-13]

Wounds on the face, neck, and hands are obviously the most difficult to conceal, not only from others, but also from the patient's own view. The emotional trauma experienced by facial disfigurement requires long periods of adjustment.[14] In fact, one study reports that 30% to 40% of adult burn patients with facial scarring experienced severe psychological problems up to 2 years after discharge from rehabilitation.[15]

For those with visible wounds, even a walk down the street may seen daunting.[16] According to Partridge,[16] disfiguring wounds on the face create a painful double bind of "extreme self-consciousness and self-imposed social isolation." Bernstein[17] describes a "social death" among facially disfigured patients. Social death occurs as the patient's self-consciousness about being in public increases, ties with family and friends are severed and, ultimately, all social interactions cease. Without positive social reinforcement, the patient's self-esteem and self-confidence vanish.[17]

PRACTICE POINT

Wounds that are hidden under clothing or beneath dressings may spare patients from strangers' stares but can still cause emotional pain when exposed to family members and health care personnel.

Feelings of shame, embarrassment, powerlessness, and fear can be overpowering for patients during physical examinations. Therefore, as health care practitioners, we must be especially aware of the way we touch and dress wounds as well as our posturing and distance from the patient.[16] Partridge[16] emphasizes that we must pay particular attention to the unspoken word conveyed by our communication triangle (from the eyes to the chin).

Quality of life

Unquestionably, wounds have varying effects on the quality of life of those afflicted and on their caregivers. To explore the impact further requires a definition of this complex, multifactorial construct.

Quality of life is a vague and ethereal concept that reflects a patient's perspective on life satisfaction in a variety of situations.[18,19] In an attempt to narrow down the all-encompassing term "quality of life," the term "health-related quality of life" (HRqol) was first used in the late 1980s.[20] In Price's[20] view, "health-related quality of life is defined

as the impact of disease and treatment on disability and daily living, or as a patient-based focus on the impact of a perceived health state on the ability to lead a fulfilling life."

Franks and Moffatt[21] add, "The state of ill health may be defined as feelings of pain and discomfort or change in usual functioning and feeling. This is key to the concept of health-related quality of life since it's the patient's own sense of well-being which is important, not the clinician's opinion of [the patient's] clinical status."

Schipper et al.[22] describe the four domains of quality of life as physical and occupational function, psychological state, social interaction, and somatic sensation, with some theorists adding a financial component.

Physical and occupational function

In separate studies by Brod's[23] and Ribu & Wahl[24], which examined the impact of lower extremity ulcers on patients with diabetes, participants reported feeling drained and fatigued due to sleep disturbances and the high energy expenditure required for mobility. Additionally, antibiotic-related adverse effects of nausea, fatigue, and general malaise were considerable.[23] In Brod's[23] sample, 50% of patients (N = 14) had to retire early or lost their jobs because of an ulcer. Even patients who were still employed experienced decreased productivity, lost time from work due to health care appointments, and lost career opportunities.[23]

In a study of 21 patients with diabetic foot ulcers by Ashford, McGee, and Kinmond[25], 79% of patients reported an inability to maintain employment secondary to decreased mobility and fear of someone inadvertently treading on their affected foot. In another study, all patients interviewed felt that the leg ulcer limited their work capacity, with 50% adding that their jobs required standing most of their shift.[26] In that same study, 42% of patients identified the leg ulcer as a key factor in their decision to stop working. Even for younger patients, leg ulceration was correlated with time lost from work and job loss, ultimately affecting finances.[26]

Marked restrictions in activities of daily living (ADLs) among those with leg ulcers are also reported in many studies, including those by Hyland et al.,[4] Brod,[23] Phillips et al.,[26] and Walshe.[27] In a study consisting of 88 patients with chronic leg ulcers, 75% reported difficulty performing basic housework.[28] Yet another study by Hyland et al.[4] demonstrated that of 50 patients with leg ulcers, 50% had problems getting on and off a bus and 30% had trouble climbing steps.

In terms of changing one's own clothing and bathing, pain, leg edema, fatigue, and bulky dressings can make such simple acts frustrating, if not impossible.[23,27,28] Phillips et al.[26] conducted personal interviews of 73 patients with leg ulcers; of those patients, 81% described their mobility and ability to carry out ADLs as adversely affected by their ulcer, with edema being the dominant factor.

Psychological function

Multiple factors affect the psychological response to having a wound or caring for a loved one with a wound. (See *Factors affecting patient response to wounds*.)

Etiology

According to Magnan,[29] a patient's psychological response to a wound may correlate closely with *how* he was wounded. Indeed, imagine the terrifying flashbacks the patient and family caregivers may feel upon viewing open amputation wounds sustained after motor vehicle accidents or burn wounds exposed during whirlpool treatments or the extreme emotions and fears elicited when gangrenous limbs from peripheral vascular disease or necrotic pressure ulcers that extend to the bone are exposed.

PRACTICE POINT

Each dressing change draws attention to the wounded body part and its associated pain, but it also serves as a reminder of the circumstance or disease that resulted in the injury and engenders fears about the future.[29]

Preparedness

From the onset of hospital, rehabilitation, and home care admission, health care profes-

---

Factors affecting patient response to wounds

Factors that shape a patient's emotional response to his wound include:
- age
- coping patterns
- etiology
- gender
- healing outcomes
  - expectation of healing
  - time to healing
  - acute versus chronic
- impact on activities of daily living
- meaning, significance
- odor, leakage
- pain
- preparedness
- response of others
- social supports
- spirituality
- visibility.

---

sionals plan for a patient's discharge by preparing patients and caregivers for independence. But are we sensitive to the patient's psychological and emotional readiness to deal with his wound? To that end, the patient and his family may need to relinquish control to the health care provider.[1] The reality is that some patients can't cope with their physical wounds because they're simultaneously struggling with deep, emotional wounds. This point is illustrated by one patients' remarks: "It took everything I had to deal with the reality of having to spend the rest of my life as a quadriplegic" ... "When I have an ulcer (referring to a pressure ulcer), I don't want to see it. I feel like I am in hell and to survive I must separate myself from the wound." ... "I fear the sight of the ulcer."[1]

Visibility

As discussed previously, the visibility, severity, and circumstances under which wounding occurred can dramatically affect the patient's acceptance of the wound into his changed body image. For some, the wounded body part becomes objectified as though it does not belong to them.[30]

Response of others

Not only is it difficult for patients to view their own wounds, but it is hard for patients to be rebuked by others at the sight of their wounds. Acceptance, pity, dismay, fear, repulsion, and avoidance are the gamut of responses displayed by others to wounds and to those who have been wounded. This can dramatically affect a patient's emotional response to his wound and his self-esteem. For patients who must endure the displeasing stares of others to their bandaged wounds, a wound clinic may be the only place where they can receive positive energy and reinforcement.[30]

Pain

Physical pain associated with wounds is one of the areas in which health care professionals are least attentive. Krasner[31] describes pain "as one of those experiences of being that often confounds our understanding, sometimes we may actually flee from facing it." Yet pain is a major factor affecting the HRqol of those with wounds, as we'll see in the section discussing somatic sensation (pain).

Malodor and leakage

The impact of malodor from a fungating breast wound, a necrotic pressure ulcer, or a draining and infected venous leg ulcer can be emotionally and psychologically devastating. A patient may try in vain to mask wound malodor with perfumes and colognes. Their self-image can be crushed by feelings of shame and disgust. The patient may say that the wound's malodor makes them feel dirty, and may apologize to others about the malodor. Some patients may even limit their social encounters due to fear of offending others. Unfortunately, friends and family members may add to these feelings of isolation by avoiding the patient because of the wound's malodor.

Roe et al.[28] reported increased anxiety and depression scores, lower life satisfaction, and decreased social contacts among those with malodorous leg ulcers. Similarly, leakage of highly exudative wounds on to clothing and bed linens can lead to feelings of embarrassment and inhibited sexuality and intimacy.[32-34] As women attempt to conceal bulky, saturated dressings with pants, long skirts or baggy clothing, they become stripped of their feminity.[11,35,36] For palliative care patients and their families, malodor, heavy exudate and bleeding may further heighten the daily misery of uncontrollable disease.[33,34]

Healing outcomes

For patients and their caregivers, just hearing that there's hope of healing, that improvement will occur, and that the pain, malodor, and restrictions will one day be gone or lessened can make the situation easier to bear.[6,27]

In clinical practice, the three questions most frequently posed by patients and caregivers are:

- Will this wound heal?
- How long will it take to heal?
- Will the treatment cause pain?

Among patients with chronic leg ulcers and high recurrence rates, healing potential is often viewed with pessimism.[27] In interviews of 73 patients with leg ulcers by Phillips et al.,[26] only 3% felt their ulcers would ever heal. This uncertainty toward healing is often echoed by health care professionals.[27] Chase and colleagues[30] explain how whole healing from an acute illness for a healthy person has a positive connotation of health and restoration, whereas it may not be the same for those with a chronic illness, such as venous insufficiency ulcers. Indeed, patients describe the healing process as ever present, requiring constant vigilance and need for health care follow up.[30] For patients with chronic ulcers, there are also limitations in mobility, activity, bathing, dressing, and working.[30] This may leave patients feeling powerless, spending more time caring for their ulcers than for themselves.[30] The uncontrolled nature of the condition often leads to a lack of ownership and a 'who cares' attitude.[30] In a sense, freedom is gone and the threat of ulcer recurrence (and possible amputation) is ever present.[30]

Time to healing
Lack of a known time scale for healing is a common complaint from patients, leading to increased frustration, depression, and restricted ADLs by those with leg ulcers,[4,27] pressure ulcers,[37] and other types of wounds. Krasner's[38] phenomenological study examined the impact of painful, venous ulcers on HRqol and identified frustration as the major theme. In this study, patients suffering with leg ulcers from 2 months through 7 years reported their frustration as stemming from slow healing rates, lower limb swelling, infection, and the formation of new ulcers.[14,38] Other frustrations were related to years of multiple unsuccessful treatments, inadequacy of care from health care professionals, or self-blame for the lack of healing.[38]

Although many patients desire wound healing, there are others who use their wounds to get attention or continue health care benefits. Although it's obvious that most patients desire wound healing, we would be remiss to not ask our patients about their specific goals in relation to their wounds. Wientjes[39] identifies four common behavioral attitudes exhibited by patients whose wounds heal:

• sets attainable goals (for example, to return to work, attend child's wedding)
• receptive to learning
• compliant with treatment
• curious; willingness to see the wound and actively participate in care.

As mentioned earlier, many patients are eager to strive for a goal of wound healing. However, according to Myss,[40] "assuming that everyone wants to heal is both misleading and potentially dangerous. Illness can, for instance, become a powerful way to get attention a patient might not otherwise receive." For some, there can be a manipulative value to keeping a wound, a figurative "street value or social currency." Defining oneself by the wound is an attitude described by Myss as "woundology."[40] For these patients, staying wounded provides benefits, such as continued nursing visits, Meals On Wheels,[28] home health aide services, an excuse to remain unemployed, and continued attention by family and health care professionals.[39]

Acute versus chronic
Some wounds heal quickly and uneventfully, whereas others are present for years or even a lifetime. But are these wounds similarly perceived by those afflicted? Do coping styles vary based on wound chronicity?

Expanding on the works of Parsons,[41] O'Flynn[42] postulates that following an acute minor wound event, the wound and its treatment become the immediate focus of the patient and his family. Viewing his wound as deviant, the patient is eclipsed by the wound and readily assumes the role of "sick person." Individual roles and responsibilities are overshadowed and interrupted (to an extent) by the patient's pain and incapacity.[42] During the healing and coping phase the individual continues to be the "patient." Once healing is achieved, however, the individual re-emerges, and normality is regained as good health and quality of life are restored.[42]

How a person reacts emotionally to a wound changes as the circumstances surrounding the wound differ. For example, trauma patients experience extreme emotions and employ various defense mechanisms, such as suppression, regression, denial, distraction, magical thinking, or rationalization.[43] According to Lenehan,[44] the severe injuries endured may open floodgates of suppressed, intense emotions and disturbed images of self. As a result, the patient may present with a rather shallow or blunted affect or "ego constriction" in an attempt to conserve psychological energy.[44] An inner battle occurs between anger, depression, and fear as the patient asks himself, "Will I be treated differently?" and "Will anyone care for me in light of disability and disfigurement?"[44]

Conversely, Phillips et al.,[26] Price and Harding,[45] and Walshe[27] report that patients with chronic wounds cope with the impaired mobility, pain, and sleep disturbances by the process of normalization. Coping with chronic wounds, according to Dewar and Morse,[46] is accomplished by adaptation, or the untenable process of silent acceptance. Interestingly, Price and Harding[45] found that those who suffered from venous leg ulcers longer than 24 months rated themselves as having less pain and better general health than those with ulcers of less than 24 months.

Neil and Munjas [2] conducted a phenomenological study of 10 patients with chronic nonhealing wounds, in which two patterns and six themes emerged. The two identified patterns were contending with the wound and staying home or staying back.[2]

Contending with the wound includes four themes:
• being in pain
• contending with exudate and odor—issues that can cause significant distress, social isolation, and embarrassment
• losing sleep
• noticing; that is, the first time the patient noticed the wound wasn't improving, and other people noticing and caring for the wound.

The second constitutive pattern, staying home or staying back, includes the two themes of isolation and trouble walking. Isolation stems from the patient's fear of going out and acquiring infection and being housebound secondary to immobility (for example, having to stay in bed or with the affected leg elevated). Trouble walking stems from pain or loss of function secondary to the wound. For these participants "the wound becomes the focus of their lives as it makes them immobile or makes walking difficult."[2]

Contrary to other authors who described feelings of normalization among those with chronic wounds, Neil and Munjas[2] found that "chronic wound participants 'became their wound.' The wound is all encompassing. The participant constantly hopes that their wound will get better so that they can resume their former wound-free life. With each passing year, or if the wound worsens despite therapy, hope and compliance may fade."

Bietz[12] conducted a phenomenological study of 16 patients living with chronic wounds and reported similar findings as Neil & Munjas. The themes identified were:
• adapting and maladapting
• altered sleeping habits
• changes in eating patterns
• contending with chronic illness
• dealing with the wound

• explaining causes of wounds
• healing and recuperating
• living and aging
• living with pain
• losing mobility
• meaning and significance of wound
• receiving care.

To better understand how a patient's HRqol is affected, what his goals are, and how we can best assist him, we must first gain insight into the meaning and significance that the wound holds for the patient. As one patient aptly states, "True understanding doesn't occur unless we share our strengths, fears, and weakness."[1]

Painful venous ulcers have been described as "the literal breakdown of the skin and the figurative breakdown of the embodied self."[48] Pressure ulcer formation has been described by family caregivers as a, (unfortunately) normal thing to happen to the bedridden[9] and as "truly the worst thing that can happen" by those directly afflicted.[1]

As described in this section, the psychological effects of a wound are deeply ingrained in the patient as a whole. No matter if the wound is acute or chronic, it is on the mind of the patient at all times. In other words, living with a chronic wound reshapes every aspect of one's life, leaving one subordinate to the wound, the associated pain and, with every dressing change, tension and worry as to how the wound will look…will it be deeper, infected or gangrenous?[32, 47]

Impact on activities of daily living

Physical, somatic, financial, and medical restrictions can result in limitations on a patient's ability to engage in ADLs, further impacting on the psychological and emotional ramifications of the wound experience. Hopkins and colleagues [49] describe how pressure ulcers can produce a such a restricted life. In their phenological study, patients' described how pain from the wound restricted their desire to move and turn or reposition themselves.

Coping patterns

Breaches in the skin, as with other types of loss, can illicit the process of grieving.

Although most patients transcend the continuum from denial, depression, anger, and bargaining to ultimate acceptance, some may become frozen at a certain point or even exhibit regressional behavior about their wound. Walshe's[27] phenomenological study examining what it's like to live with a venous leg ulcer from the elderly patient's perspective identifies four major coping strategies.
• Coping by comparison—by comparing himself to others with ulcerations, the patient experiences normalization; by comparing himself to patients with other illnesses (such as stroke), the patient feels more fortunate.
• Feeling healthy—despite the leg ulcerations and the associated debilitating symptoms and restrictions, the patient feels otherwise healthy.
• Altering expectation—the patient reports having reached a point of acceptance, viewing the ulcer as a part of the aging process.
• Being positive—the patient describes himself as lucky and dismisses the symptoms as "not bad at all."[27]

Spirituality
The power of prayer, hope, and support of a patient's religious beliefs can't be underestimated in providing emotional strength.

Social supports
Many patients with wounds feel pushed to the "side-lines"[24] seeing a shrinking of their social circle as pain, fears, and physical restrictions increase. The patient with a wound may experience guilt about friends having to change their activities to accommodate his limitations, and may therefore further limit social interaction.[23] As discussed earlier, malodor, leakage, and wound visibility may also result in decreased social contact. For some patients, overdependence for physical, emotional, and psychological strength may fall on a single caregiver, usually a spouse.

Hopkins et al [49] studied the impact of pressure ulcers on not only the patient but also on the caregiver and found feelings to be conflicted. These feelings were expressed as the burden the pressure ulcer, and its subsequent care, places on the caregiver, as well as the feelings of uselessness on the part of the patient receiving the care. Conversely, however, several patients commented that without family support, things would be worse.[49]

Age
It appears that the younger the wound patient is may adversely affect his psychological state of mind, For instance, a study by Phillips et al.[26] found that younger patients exhibited greater negativity related to their leg ulcers and greater problems with mobility ($p < 0.001$) than older patients. Older patients proved more effective in coping with or adapting to their limitations and disability.[26] Franks and Moffatt[50] reported similar findings.

In a cross-sectional study using the Nottingham Health Profile (NHP) and age- and sex-matched normal scores of 758 patients with leg ulcers, younger males were found to experience the greatest negative impact on HRqol.[50] Among those with diabetes and lower extremity ulcers, Brod[23] reported that older patients were less effected in the social, employment, and familial arenas. Conversely, in a study measuring HRqol in 63 patients with chronic leg ulcers, age wasn't statistically significant.[45]

Gender
There's great debate in the literature as to the impact of gender on HRqol in those with wounds. Lindholm et al.[51] report that males have significantly poorer HRqol than females in the areas of pain and physical mobility. Additionally, when compared to the normative scores for males in the areas of sleep disturbance, emotional reaction, and social isolation, males with leg ulcers exhibited increased scores.[51] Price and Harding[45] found poorer HRqol scores in women in the domains of vitality and physical and social functioning. A database of 758 patients with leg ulcers similarly reports women to have a poorer HRqol than males.[21]

But, as Franks and Moffatt[50] point out, in studies of the general population, women score worse on HRqol than males, especially in older age groups. Therefore, the poorer scores among women with leg ulcers may not be directly related to the ulcer.

Social interaction

Limitations in social interactions among those with wounds may stem from the following:

• impaired mobility secondary to pain, causing many patients to become essentially housebound[4,27,28,49]

• treatment restrictions, such as the need to stay on bed rest for pressure ulcer management [37,52,53]; leg elevation for edema control, and the need to be homebound to receive skilled home care nursing services

• need for an isolation room secondary to neutropenia or multi-drug resistant infection, resulting in increased feelings of loneliness, powerlessness and social abandonment[53]

• avoidance of social activities where crowds, children, or pets might be encountered, out of fear of injuring the wound site or creating new ulcers [4,27]

• fatigue from disrupted sleep and adverse effects of antibiotics [28,37]

• embarrassment from odor, [49] leakage, and wound visibility

• need to rely on others and assistive devices[23]

• additional time required to perform dressing changes [4,23]

• difficulty maintaining appearance because shoes and clothing no longer fit over bulky dressings.[4,28]

Patients with wounds may be forced to make significant life changes and find satisfaction in new activities.[48] The ability to participate in such activities as enjoying a sauna, bicycling, running, swimming, or tennis is eliminated because of bulky dressings and compression wraps.

Although health care professionals encourage and recognize the value of social interaction to a patient's psychological and emotional function, do we not simultaneously blame patients or label them as nonadherent when they come to our offices with worsening of their edema and deterioration of their leg and foot ulcers secondary to being out and trying to enjoy life?

PRACTICE POINT

As health care professionals, we must not only acknowledge, but also creatively work with the patient in the challenge of balancing physical wound healing with psychological and emotional healing.

Listen to the words of a patient describing the difficulties of maintaining bed rest to heal his pressure ulcer: "I can remember lying in the hospital ... looking at the paint on the wall. And I could tell you how many little bubbles were in that particular spot. I memorized them to keep from going mad."[37]

Somatic sensation

According to Schipper et al.,[22] the domain of somatic sensation "encompasses unpleasant physical feelings that may detract from someone's quality of life, such as pain." Regardless of the underlying cause of pain, it's one of the most feared sensations in life,[55] and is the most compelling reason that individuals seek out health care.[56] And, although the threshold of pain varies from patient to patient, making it undeniably subjective, it's an area that's too often neglected in wound care.[56,57]

The devastating impact of painful wounds on all aspects of a patient's HRqol has been the subject of recent numerous studies,[2,21,26,27,37,38,48,49,54,55] although incorporation of findings into clinical practice has been slow to follow.

Patients have described pain as the worst thing about having a leg ulcer,[27,55,58] with the "first daily act of weight bearing as the most severe pain they experience."[58] The unrelenting, unpredictable nature of the pain frequently makes patients feel like they aren't in control, [27] but rather the ulcer and its manifestations rule them.[35,47] Leg elevation often makes the burning, stabbing, drilling, throbbing pain worse.[59] Sleep is frequently disrupted by pain,[58] and pain medication is often ineffective.[27] Among those with venous ulcers, pain is often described in three distinct locations: within the ulcer, around the ulcer, and elsewhere in the leg.[58] Additionally, pain for many is felt to be an early warning sign of new ulcers forming or of impending infection.[11]

Krasner's[48] qualitative phenomenological study of 14 patients with painful venous ulcers identifies 8 key themes. (See *Painful venous leg ulcers: Key themes.*)

Participants in Krasner's[48] study vividly described the pain as "the worst thing I have ever gone through in my life" ... "like someone is sticking pins in you all the time" ... "absolute murder." Pain was described as even worse when the leg was more edematous and during infection. Pain during and after debridement was considered the most intense pain experienced by patients, bringing on a cycle of pain and fear that left many depressed. In a phenomenological study by Langemo et al.,[37] pain is described as "getting a knife and really digging in there good and hard" and "stinging." Yet, despite the pain, suffering, and limitations brought on by these ulcers, patients tried to view the pain as an expected (albeit unwanted) occurrence and to "carry on despite the pain."[48]

The duration of pain is also described as an issue most of the time, even during and after closure.[37,52] Indeed, in a Heideggenan phenomenological pilot study, Hopkins et al[49] found endless pain to be one of the three major themes in their sample of 8 pressure ulcer patients. And, among 32 patients with stage III and IV pressure ulcers, Szor and Bourguignon[60] found that 88% experienced pain with dressing changes, although dressings used were consistent with principles of moist healing. Furthermore, 84% of the participants reported pain at rest, and 18% described the pain as horrible or excruciating.[60] Among patients with granulating postoperative pilonidal cyst excision and abdominal wounds, Price and colleagues[61] described pain as negatively impacting patient's sleeping patterns and appetite.

Despite the prevalence and intensity of pain among those with wounds, however, Roe et al.[62] found that 55% of community nurses don't include pain as a part of their assessment. Ayello and colleagues[63] found that among patients with chronic wounds in an outpatient clinic, those with pressure ulcers were least likely to be assessed for pain as compared to patients with vascular or neuropathic ulcers. Walshe[27] and Hollinworth and Collier[64] report that patients' descriptions of pain are often devalued and dismissed. In studies by Hollinworth[65] and Dallam et al.[53], pain medications were seldom administered to manage pain associated with dressing changes, despite the fact that

Painful venous leg ulcers: Key themes

Krasner[35] identifies eight key themes in patients with painful venous leg ulcers:
- Being unable to stand
- Expecting pain with the ulcer
- Experiencing pain caused by swelling
- Feeling frustrated
- Having to make life changes
- Interfering with the job
- Starting the pain all over again with painful debridements
- Trying to find satisfaction in new activities

81% of registered nurses report that patients experience the most pain with dressing changes.[62] Similarly, Szor and Bourguignon[60] reported a mere 6% of patients received medication for pressure ulcer pain.

Among patients with diabetic foot ulcers, Ashford and colleagues[25] found that 50% of patients experienced pain during dressing changes, when supine, and during ambulatory attempts. However, Ribu and Wahl[24] conducted a study that found patients with diabetic foot ulcers fear analgesic dependency.

Pieper and colleagues[66] study of 32 patients with a history of I.V. drug abuse and chronic venous ulcers found that those with larger wounds reported a significantly higher pain intensity than those with smaller wounds.

In patients with malignant fungating wounds, pain was related to nerve or blood vessel damage, exposed dermal nerve endings, or nerve damage resulting in neuropathic pain.[34]

In an attempt to capture nurses' stories about coping with patients' pressure ulcer pain, Krasner[31] conducted a phenomenological study of 42 nurses, identifying three patterns and eight themes:
- Nursing expertly includes the ability to recognize, validate, attend to, acknowledge, and caringly empathize with the patient in pain.
- Denying the pain includes assuming it doesn't exist or failing to hear the patient's complaints or cries. This was described as an

effective coping mechanism for the health care professional, assisting them in avoiding feelings of failure but obviously at severe detriment to the patient.

• Confronting the challenge of pain occurs when the health care professional must come to terms with his own feelings of frustration. Negative feelings associated with wound care include anger, helplessness, hopelessness, being upset about performing a procedure that will cause pain, and experiencing pain along with the patient. Perhaps we must, as Krasner[31] states, "take a step back and make a special effort to understand the nearness of the near." By "being with" the patient we may gain insight into the meaning that the pain experience holds for the patient.[31]

In examinations of the impact of leg ulcer clinics on HRqol, a study of 57 patients found 88% with pain at baseline; after 8 weeks of 4-layer compression therapy this fell to 60%.[67] Even more significantly, in another sample of 185 patients, 78% reported pain prior to entering a community leg ulcer clinic; after 12 weeks of 4-layer compression therapy this dropped to 22%.[68]

Financial impact

Time lost from work, missed career opportunities, decreased productivity on the job secondary to pain, early retirement, and loss of a job are just a few of the financial stressors affecting the HRqol of the patient with a wound. Too often, patients are faced with having to choose between compliance with medical management (such as keeping one's leg elevated or remaining non-weight bearing) and keeping their job. How does a truck driver, a cashier, or a health care professional keep his leg elevated and still perform his job? How do wound patients pay their mortgages, pay the bills, and feed their families? What happens when a wound patient loses his health care coverage after losing his job? According to Charles[10], the financial sequelae of a chronic wound is the societal inheritance of a person who was a positive contributor to one who becomes dependent upon it.

Beyond occupational stressors and dilemmas, patients may also incur additional out-of-pocket expenses for transportation, parking, telephone bills for medical follow-up, home health aide services, dressing supplies not covered by insurance, and drug costs if they have no prescription plan. Those who have no insurance but don't qualify for public assistance may be forced to tap into their savings or refinance their homes. To illustrate this point, listen to the words of wives caring for their bedridden husbands with full-thickness pressure ulcers.

"...all these medical supplies you need to treat these bedsores. I think in the past 2 months, I've spent close to $300 out of my pocket and you're on a fixed income." ... "Thirty-five dollars per month for the hospital bed and $10 for the chair. I paid with our Social Security checks and his pension. Also there were bills and food...not much was left...He had a pension and I used to put that aside and we had to live on my Social Security which was $302."[69] Concerns about finances may be linked to the health care insurance system in the patient's country. For example, finances was not raised as an issue for the pressure ulcer study in Europe by Hopkins et al.[49]

Additional expenses may also be incurred for home modifications, such as wheelchair ramps.

Additionally, patients with diabetic foot ulcers face the ongoing challenge of affording correctly fitted footwear as their feet are constantly undergoing change with episodes of edema related to diuretics, infection, and the amount of dressing material required. Health care professionals, rather than simply dismissing patients as nonadherent, should show empathy, acknowledging access and financial hardships faced by patients and partner with their patients in addressing these issues.[2,24]

Ethical dilemmas in wound care

No other wound type is fraught with as much ethical dispute as pressure ulcers. Despite major technological breakthroughs in wound healing, the area of pressure ulceration continues to be the "scarlet letter of poor care."[9] Pressure ulcers are considered an individual and institutional embarrassment, a point of frustration, failure, and a marker of inferior care rendered.[9] Great expense is incurred in "hiding the ulcer." As Moss and La Puma[70] state, "to hide ugly aesthetics and to unknowingly deny the conditions that contribute to pressure ulcer development, our clinical response may be to cover up or remove the sore, using dressings, skin grafts, myocutaneous flaps, disarticulations, amputations, and hemicorporectomies." But what right do we have as health care providers to make such decisions? What gives us the right to exhaust our patients' finances and subject them and their families to spending their lives undergoing aggressive procedures? Decisions for care, and the degree of aggressiveness or lack thereof, must be consistent with the patient's overall physiological status, as well as the patient's and family's "goals of restoration, of function, prolongation of life, or only provision of comfort."[71]

It's important to remember that HRqol is the *patient's* perception of well-being, not your opinion of their clinical status. [19] Finding out what the patient wants and what his goals are is paramount. [72] Acknowledging this, clinicians must partner with patients and their families in making short- and long-term treatment decisions, regardless of wound etiology. According to Beitz[73], quality wound care is defined by:
• doing the right things right, which may seem basic, but is influenced by multiple variables
• the legal community (inadvertently)
• practice guidelines and standards of care designed by health care providers
• the person receiving it and the person perceiving it.

Using general systems theory, Beitz[73] suggests that barriers to quality wound care fall into three general levels: individual, group, and societal.

Individual barriers

Individual barriers to quality wound care include:
• deleterious life-style habits, such as drug use, homelessness, or lack of attention to skin hygiene
• fiscal restraints, such as limited health care coverage and limited savings

• lack of a knowledge regarding preventive measures[73]
• poor health accountability, such as smoking, abusing alcohol, and overeating.

Group barriers

Group barriers to quality wound care include:
• fiscal restraints, resulting in limited home care visits and reimbursement under prospective payment, leading to increased demands placed on family members
• inadequate knowledge of basic wound care on the part of the caregiver
• lack of meaningful organizational partnerships (Although seamless delivery of health care is desired, continuity from acute care to long-term care and home care remains inadequate.)
• lack of well-disseminated, valid wound care guidelines, algorithms, and decision trees [73]
• poor quality improvement processes, wherein data may be collected, but outcomes are inadequately analyzed and acted upon.

Societal barriers

Societal barriers to quality wound care include:
• fiscal restraints[73]
• lack of focus on population-based outcomes (An outcomes-based perspective is critical in a fiscally restrained environment. Considering that some patients with chronic wounds won't heal, appropriate goals should be identified and an ethical rationing of resources established.)
• lack of national wound care benchmarks
• national nursing and faculty shortage.

Possible solutions

Systemic solutions to the delivery of cost-efficient, effective chronic wound care as identified by Bietz[73] include:
• access to innovative electronic communication, such as telehealth, image transmissions, less expensive video conferencing, and timely consultation with distant caregivers
• acknowledgement that increasing wound care-related litigation should serve as a much needed impetus for securing funding for pre-

vention, improved communication, and protocol development
• alternate sites of care such as mobile wound care units
• establishment of a sense of 'collective worry' and concern by health care professionals, patients, family caregivers, and legislatures regarding chronic wound care and the resources consumed
• health care renaissance, which focuses on collaboration and a transdisciplinary approach to disease prevention and health promotion[73]
• innovative wound care treatments
• new perspective on health, which focuses on promotion and disease prevention
• partnerships between businesses, industry, health care, and academia
• recognition of limited resources
• use of alternative health care providers possessing the critical combination of population-based thinking, outcomes assessment, and educational and fiscal abilities.

Transitioning to health promotion

In a climate of decreased hospital stays, managed care, and prospective payment with decreased allowances for home visits and supplies, moral and ethical conflicts for community health care nurses abound.[74] In fact, community health care nurses' focus has had to change from disease prevention and health promotion to the provision of acute care.[74] Documentation of care, limited visits, supply purchasing, and whether the wound care prognosis will better focus on long-term management or short-term cure are ethical concerns and financial realities faced by community care nurses on a daily basis.[74] Community-based ethical concerns in wound care include:[74]
• what kind of wound care is most safe, efficacious, and cost-effective?
• what kind of wound care can be performed at home by trained family members?
• what is the most cost-effective source of wound care supplies?

The new economy is forcing autonomy on vulnerable and often frail elderly patients and

family members as never before.[74] Too often, patients and family caregivers are quickly labeled as nonadherent without regard to underlying issues such as:[74]
• confusion over what supplies are needed from medical supply companies
• lack of knowledge
• lack of money to pay for costly drugs, supplies, transportation, office-visit co-pays and insurance deductibles
• lack of sufficient hospital discharge planning.

In a time of limited health care dollars, which patients have access to all available resources, regardless of cost, to close their chronic or complex wounds? We're already seeing the ramifications of the 'health care cost blindness' described by Bell[74], where if too much money is spent on some patient's supplies, money will ultimately not be available for others. Will only those with financial means, youth, better health, and more quantifiable productive years be the limited recipients? What choices will be available for elderly patients, those with chronic diseases, and those receiving palliative care? Who will provide care, for how long, and with what resources? Will patients' and their families' concerns, choices, and wishes be heard and acknowledged?

In caring for patients with wounds a strong patient/provider relationship is critical.[75] Patients want to be seen, to be heard, and to be known.[75] According to Scherwitz and Rountree[75], the two essential components to healing are the joining between a provider devoted to healing and to the relationship and the allowance of a patient's rights to choose regarding the healing process.

Issues and challenges for caregivers

For the family member, the only prerequisite to becoming a caregiver is willingness to take on the role. However, most often, family members are untrained and unprepared for this role.[9] Along with the patient, family caregivers also have to deal with their own varying levels of grief. Caregivers' grief is further affected by the patient's overall status, the circumstances leading to the wounded state, and the patient's response to the wound. They also deal with the increased stress and strain of family tension and receive the brunt of the patient's anger and frustration.[23]

As the patient struggles with fears of burdening others, social isolation, loss of control and independence, possible disfigurement, and rejection, the caregiver also struggles. Fears commonly voiced by family caregivers include damaging the wound from a lack of knowledge; development of new wounds; wound recurrence; need for amputation, re-hospitalization, ER visits, or surgery; disfigurement; reaction of others; possible disability; and fear that the wound may never heal.

Spouses may sleep apart out of fear of dislodging I.V. lines and wound drainage tubes.[76] Living, dining, and bedrooms may become filled with boxes of antibiotics, I.V. and wound dressing supplies, serving as constant reminders of the patient and families' wounded state, an uncertain future, and dwindling resources. [76] The privacy once enjoyed by families is visibly shaken with visits now by medical supply representatives, home care nurses, and possibly care aides.[76]

A recurring fear among caregivers is that they themselves might become ill or disabled and unable to provide care.[9,23] Family caregivers are often dealing with disrupted sleep secondary to worrying about the patient and responding to the patient's restlessness. [9,23]A general lack of attention to their own health, progressive fatigue, decreased appetite, and decreased nutritional intake may occur as all attention is focused on the patient.[9,23]

Caregivers often find their social circle decreasing as they spend increased time providing care. [23] Even time taken for respite may be fraught with feelings of guilt. Emotionally, caregivers may experience deep feelings of fear and loss—fear of losing their loved one, fear of losing the relationship and, possible, death—as they witness a loved one's bedridden or increasingly debilitated state. Reminiscing about how things used to be may be all that some caregivers have to pull them through. Elderly caregiving spouses usually pursue nursing home placement only as a last resort, holding true to their vows of "till death do us part."[9]

Family caregivers also experience financial struggles owing to increased out-of-pocket expenses, decreased productivity in the workplace, unpaid days off due to used vacation and personal time, forced early retirement, and potential job loss. [23] Among elderly caregivers, frustration and confusion regarding reimbursement for needed wound care supplies and drugs and the inability to afford private help in the home are compounded by their meager funds from Social Security and pension checks. [23]

Summary

Having a wound or caring for a loved one with a wound can affect multiple facets of a patient's life, possibly unleashing unprecedented fears and vulnerabilities.

 PRACTICE POINT

If we as health care professionals are to help our patients with wounds and their family caregivers, we need to "...stay connected with our patients; listen, attend ("be with") and comfort; and use a gentler hand."[31]

In each patient and family caregiver encounter, we as health care professionals should ask ourselves "Do we care enough about the patient's perspective to bear the costs involved to ensure that each person feels that they are being treated as a person?"[77] "Do our actions show that we care?" It is our job as health care professionals to care for the whole patient, including the psychological, emotional, and financial issues related to his wound care.

Show what you know

1. *Those afflicted with wounds are often viewed as:*

   A. pleasant and comfortable.
   B. pain-free.
   C. appalling and repulsive.
   D. attractive.

ANSWER: C. Those with wounds are often viewed as appalling and repulsive.

2. *Which of the following is one of the four domains of quality of life as identified by Schipper et al [18]?*

A. Pain-free
B. Financial freedom
C. Religious expression
D. Somatic sensation

ANSWER: D. In addition to physical and occupation function, psychological state, and social interaction, somatic sensation is identified as a domain of quality of life.

3. *Wound assessment is commonly lacking in the area of:*

A. size.
B. odor.
C. drainage.
D. pain.

ANSWER: D. Assessment of pain is commonly lacking in wound assessment; size, odor, and drainage are usually assessed.

4. *Quality of life treatment decisions should be based on the:*

A. patient's perception of well-being.
B. nurses' perceptions of well-being.
C. family's perception of well-being.
D. physicians' perceptions of well-being.

ANSWER: A. The patient's perceptions of well-being should direct quality of life treatment decisions.

References

1. van Rijswijk, L., and Gottlieb, D. "Like a Terrorist," *Ostomy/Wound Management* 46(5):25-26, May 2000.
2. Neil, J.A., and Munjas, B.A. "Living with a Chronic Wound: The Voices of Sufferers," *Ostomy/Wound Manage-ment* 46(5):28-38, May 2000.
3. Harding, K. "Complete Patient Care," *Journal of Wound Care* 4(6):253, June 1995.
4. Hyland, M.E., et al. "Quality of Life of Leg Ulcer Patients: Questionnaire and Preliminary Findings," *Journal of Wound Care* 3(6):294-298, June 1994.
5. van Rijswijk, L. "The Language of Wounds," in *Chronic Wound Care: A Clinical Sourcebook for Health Care Professionals*, 3rd ed. Edited by Krasner, D.L., et al. Wayne, Pa.: HMP Communications, 2001.
6. Anderson, R.C., and Maksud, D.P. "Psychological Adjustments to Reconstructive Surgery," *Nursing Clinics of North America* 29(4):711-24, December 1994.
7. Faugier, J. "On Being Wounded," *Senior Nurse* 8(1):18, January 1988.
8. Hopkins, S. "Psychological Aspect of Wound Healing," *Nursing Times Plus* 97(48):57-58, 2001.
9. Baharestani, M.M. "The Lived Experience of Wives Caring for their Frail, Home-bound, Elderly Husbands with Pressure Ulcers," *Advances in Wound Care* 7(3):40-52, May 1994.
10. Charles, H. "Living With a Leg Ulcer," *Journal of Community Nursing* 9(7):22-24, 1995.
11. Hyde, C., et al. "Older Women's Experience of Living With Chronic Leg Ulceration," *International Journal of Nursing Practice* 5(4):189-98, 1999.
12. Beitz, J.M. "The Lived Experience of Having a Chronic Wound: A Phenomenological Study," *Dermatology Nursing* 17(4):272-305, 2005.
13. Hollinworth, H., and Hawkins J. "Teaching Nurses Psychological Support of Patients with Wounds," *British Journal of Nursing* 11(20):S8-18, 2002.
14. Knudson-Cooper, M. "Adjustment to Visible Stigma: The Case of the Severely Burned," *Social Science Medicine* 15B:31, 1981.
15. Wallace, L., and Lees, J. "A Psychological Follow-up Study of Adult Patients Discharged from a British Burns Unit," *Burns* 14:39, 1988.
16. Partridge, J. "The Psychological Effects of Facial Disfigurement," *Journal of Wound Care* 2:168-71, May 1993.
17. Bernstein, N. *Emotional Care of the Facially Disfigured.* Boston: Little, Brown & Co., 1976.
18. Campbell, A., et al. *The Quality of American Life: Perceptions, Evaluations and Satisfaction.* New York: Russell Sage, 1976.
19. Price, P. "Quality of Life," in *Chronic Wound Care: A Clinical Source Book for Health Care Professionals*, 3rd ed. Edited by Krasner, D.L., et al. Wayne, Pa.: HMP Communications, 2001.
20. Price, P. "Defining and Measuring Quality of Life," *Journal of Wound Care* 5(3):139-40, March 1996.
21. Franks, P.J., and Moffatt, C.J. "Quality of Life Issues in Patients with Chronic Wounds," *Wounds* 10(suppl E):1E-11E, September-October 1998.
22. Schipper, H., et al. "Quality of Life Studies: Definitions and Conceptual Issues," in *Quality of Life and Pharmacoeconomics in Clinical Trials*, 2nd ed. Edited by Spilker, B. Philadelphia: Lippincott-Raven, 1996.
23. Brod, M. "Quality of Life Issues in Patients with Diabetes and Lower Extremity Ulcers: Patients and Caregivers," *Quality of Life Research* 7(4):365-72, May 1998.
24. Ribu L., et al. "Living with a Diabetic Foot Ulcer: A Life of Fear, Restrictions and Pain," *Ostomy/Wound Management* 50(2):57-67, 2004.
25. Ashford R.L., et al. "Perception of quality of life by patients with diabetic foot ulcers," *The Diabetic Foot* 3(4):150-55, 2000.
26. Phillips, T., et al. "A Study of the Impact of Leg Ulcers on Quality of Life: Financial, Social and Psychological Implications," *Journal of American Academy of Dermatology* 31(1):49-53, July 1994.
27. Walshe, C. "Living with a Venous Leg Ulcer: A Descriptive Study of Patients' Experiences," *Journal of Advanced Nursing* 22(6):1092-100, December 1995.
28. Roe, B., et al. "Patient's Perceptions of Chronic Leg Ulcers," in *Leg Ulcers: Nursing Management: A Research Based Guide.* Edited by Cullum, N., and Roe, B. Harrow, U.K.: Scutari Press, 1995.
29. Magnan, M.A. "Psychological Considerations for Patients with Acute Wounds," *Critical Care Nursing Clinics of North America* 8(2):183-93, June 1996.
30. Chase S.K., Melloni M., Savage A. "Forever Healing: The Lived Experience of Venous Ulcer Disease," *Journal of Vascular Nursing* 15(2):73-77, 1997.
31. Krasner, D. "Using a Gentler Hand: Reflections on Patients with Pressure Ulcers who Experience Pain," *Ostomy/ Wound Management* 42(3):20-29, April 1996.
32. Bland M. "Challenging the Myths: The Lived Experience of Chronic Leg Ulcer," *Nursing Praxis in New Zealand* 10(1):73-78, 1995.

33. Price E. "The stigma of smel," *Nursing Times* 92(20):70,72, 1996.

34. Naylor W.A. "A Guide to Wound Management in Palliative Care," *International Journal of Palliative Nursing* 11(11):572-79, 2005.

35. Rich A., McLachlan L. "How Living with a Leg Ulcer Affects People's Daily Life: A Nurse-led Study," *Journal of Wound Care* 12(2):51-54, 2003.

36. Neil J.A. "The Stigma Scale: Measuring Body Image and the Skin," *Dermatology Nursing* 12(1):32-36, 2000.

37. Langemo, D.K., et al. "The Lived Experience of Having a Pressure Ulcer: A Qualitative Analysis," *Advances in Skin & Wound Care* 13(5):225-35, September/October 2000.

38. Krasner, D. "Painful Venous Ulcers: Themes and Stories about their Impact on Quality of Life," *Ostomy/Wound Management* 44(9):38-49, September 1998.

39. Wientjes, K.A. "Mind-body Techniques in Wound Healing," *Ostomy/Wound Management* 48(11):62-67, November 2002.

40. Myss, C. *Why People Don't Heal and How They Can.* New York: Three Rivers Press, 1997.

41. Parsons, T. "The Sick Role and the Role of the Physician Reconsidered," *MMFQ/ Health & Society* 53(3):257-78, Summer 1975.

42. O'Flynn, L. "The Impact of Minor Acute Wounds on Quality of Life," *Journal of Wound Care* 9(7):337-40, July 2000.

43. Schnaper, N. "The Psychological Implications of Severe Trauma: Emotional Sequelae to Unconsciousness," *Journal of Trauma* 15(2):94-98, February 1975.

44. Lenehan, G.P. "Emotional Impact of Trauma," *Nursing Clinics of North America* 21(4):729-40, December 1986.

45. Price, P., and Harding, K. "Measuring Health-related Quality of Life in Patients with Chronic Leg Ulcers," *Wounds* 8(3):91-94, May-June 1996.

46. Dewar, A.L., and Morse, J.M. "Unbearable Incidents: Failure to Endure the Experience of Illness," *Journal of Advanced Nursing* 22(5):957-64, November 1995.

47. Ebbeskog, B., Eckman, S.L. "Elderly Person's Experience of Living with Venous Leg Ulcers: Living in a Dialectal Relationship Between Freedom and Imprisonment," *Scandanavian Journal of Caring Science* 15:235-43, 2001.

48. Krasner, D. "Painful Venous Ulcers: Themes and Stories about Living with the Pain and Suffering," *Journal of Wound, Ostomy, and Continence Nursing* 25(3):158-68, May 1998.

49. Hopkins, A. et al . "Patient Stories of Living with a Pressure Ulcer," *Journal of Advanced Nursing* 56(4)345-53, November 2006.

50. Franks, P.J., and Moffatt, C.J. "Who Suffers Most from Leg Ulceration?" *Journal of Wound Care* 7(8):383-85, September 1998.

51. Lindholm, C., et al. "Quality of Life in Chronic Leg Ulcer Patients," *Acta Dermato-Venereologica* 73(6):440-43, December 1993.

52. Fox, C. "Living with a Pressure Ulcer: A Descrptive Study of Patient's Experiences," *Wound Care* 7(6 Suppl):10,12,14,16,20,22, 2002.

53. Laurent, C. "Beating Bedtime Blues," *Nursing Times* 95(11):61-64, 1999.

54. Dallam, L, et al. "Pressure Ulcer Pain: Assessment and Quantification," *Journal of Wound, Ostomy, and Continence Nursing* 22(5):211-18, September 1995.

55. Hamer, C., and Cullum, N.A. "Patients' Perceptions of Chronic Leg Ulcers," *Journal of Wound Care* 3(2):99-101,1994.

56. Shukla, D., et al. "Pain in Acute and Chronic Wounds," *Ostomy/Wound Management* 51(11):47-51, November 2005.

57. Price, P. "A Holistic Approach to Wound Care," *WOUNDS* 17(3):55-57, March 2005.

58. Goncalves, M.L., et al. "Pain in Chronic Leg Ulcers," *Journal of Wound, Ostomy, Continence Nursing* 31(5):275-283, 2004.

59. Hofman, D., et al. "Pain in Venous Ulcers," *Journal of Wound Care* 6(5):222-24, May 1997.

60. Szor, J.K., and Bourguignon, C. "Description of Pressure Ulcer Pain at Rest and at Dressing Change," *Journal of Wound, Ostomy, and Continence Nursing* 26(3):115-20, May 1999.

61. Price, P.E., et al "Measuring Quality of Life in Patients With Granulating Wounds," *Journal of Wound Care* 3(1):49-50, 1994.

62. Roe, B.H., et al. "Assessment, Prevention and Treatment of Chronic Leg Ulcers in the Community: Report of a Survey," *Journal of Clinical Nursing* 2(5):299-306, September 1993.

63. Ayello EA., Wexler, SS, Harris, WS. "Is pressure ulcer pain being assessed?" (in review)

64. Hollinworth, H. and Collier, M. "Nurses' Views About Pain and Trauma at Dressing Changes: Results of a National Survey," *Journal of Wound Care* 9(8):369-373, 2000.

65. Hollinworth, H. "Nurses' Assessment and Management of Pain at Wound Dressing Changes," *Journal of Wound Care* 4(2):77-83, 1995.

66. Pieper, B , Szczepaniak, K., and Templin, T. "Psychosocial Adjustment, Coping, and Quality of Life in Persons With Venous Ulcers and a History of Intravenous Drug Use," 27(4):227-239, 2000.

67. Liew, I.H., et al. "Do Leg Ulcer Clinics Improve Patients' Quality of Life?" *Journal of Wound Care* 9(9):423-26, October 2000.

68. Franks, P.J., et al. "Community Leg Ulcer Clinics: Effects on Quality of Life," *Phlebology* 9:83-86, 1994.

69. Baharestani, M.M. "The Lived Experience of Wives Caring for their Homebound Elderly Husbands with Pressure Ulcers: A Phenomenological Investigation" (doctoral dissertation, Adelphi University, 1993). Dissertation Abstracts International (No. 9416018), 1993.

70. Moss, R.J., and La Puma, J. "The Ethics of Pressure Sore Prevention and Treatment in the Elderly: A Practical Approach," *Journal of the American Geriatric Society* 39(9):905-8, September 1991.

71. La Puma, J. "The Ethics of Pressure Ulcers," *Decubitus* 4(2):43-44, May 1991.

72 Schank, JE. "Whose Goal of Care is it? A Colostomy Patient with a Peristomal Lesion of Uncertain Etiology," Journal of the World Council of Enterostomal Therapist 27(3): July-September 2007.

73. Beitz J.M. "Overcoming Barriers to Quality Wound Care: A Systems Perspective," *Ostomy/Wound Management* 47(3):56-64, March 2001.

74. Bell, S.E. "Community Health Nursing, Wound Care, and....Ethics?," *Journal of Wound, Ostomy, Continence Nursing* 30(5):259-65, 2003.

75. Scherwitz, L.W., Rountree, R., and Delevitt, P. "Wound Caring is More Than Wound Care: The Provider as a Partner,"*Ostomy/Wound Management* 43(9):42-46, 48, 50, October 1997.

76. Pittman, J. "The Chronic Wound and the Family," *Ostomy/Wound Management* 49(2):38-46, 2003.

77. Price, P. "Health-related Quality of Life and the Patient's Perspective," *Journal of Wound Care* 7(7):365-66, July 1998.

CHAPTER 2

Regulation and wound care

Courtney H. Lyder, ND
Dan R. Berlowitz, MD, MPH

OBJECTIVES

After completing this chapter, you'll be able to:

- discuss the significance of the U.S. Centers for Medicare and Medicaid Services

- discuss reimbursement issues related to hospitals, skilled nursing facilities, home health agencies, and managed care

- identify quality improvement efforts

- describe essential wound documentation required for reimbursement.

Role of regulation in health care

Regulations are a pervasive feature of our American health care system, and not surprisingly, significantly impact on the delivery of wound care. Quite often, regulations and what's reimbursed determines who receives wound care and the level of wound care that's delivered. Thus, knowledge about the regulations that impact wound care in their specific practice setting are essential if clinicians are to provide optimum care.

Although many clinicians may view the current regulatory environment as burdensome and unnecessary, it's essential to recognize the important purpose that regulations fulfill. Quite simply, regulations are the mechanism through which government may promote its interest in the general welfare of society. Experience has demonstrated that government cannot rely solely on conventional market forces, such as the laws of supply and demand, to guide the use of resources to provide optimal care. These market forces, in the absence of the guiding hand of regulations, are often insufficient to ensure that health care resources are distributed equitably. In the case of wound care, the goal of current regulations is to ensure access to high quality wound care, particularly for vulnerable populations such as the elderly and nursing home residents. Wound-care regulations must be viewed from the perspective of how well they are achieving this goal.

At least four different types of regulatory instruments are available to the government to help achieve this goal. Government regulations may rely on subsidies or direct payments to providers; they may involve entry restrictions such as licensure and accreditations that seek to limit the ability to offer a particular service; they could use rate or price-setting controls that determine reimbursements for care provided; or they could involve quality controls that seek to improve the care that is provided. Of these different potential mechanisms, the latter two are clearly the major regulatory instruments used in wound care today and will be the focus of this chapter. Specifically, we describe the major regulatory organization involved in wound care—the Centers for Medicare and Medicaid Services (CMS)—provide an overview of how wound care is being reimbursed by CMS, and describe their efforts at improving the quality of wound care.

Centers for Medicare and Medicaid Services

The CMS is a federal agency within the U.S. Department of Health and Human Services. Prior to July 1, 2001, it was called the Health Care Financing Administration (HCFA). CMS administers the Medicare and Medicaid programs—two national health care programs that benefit about 75 million Americans. Moreover, because CMS provides the states with 50% of their finances for health care costs, the states must comply with federal regulations. CMS also regulates all laboratory testing (except research) performed on humans in the United States.

Both the Medicare and Medicaid programs are administered through federal statutes that determine beneficiary requirements, what's covered, payment fees and schedules, and survey processes of clinical settings (such as skilled nursing facilities or home health agencies). Both programs have a wide variance on coverage, eligibility, and payment fees and schedules. Thus, it's important for the clinician to know what's covered and the level of reimbursement prior to developing a treatment plan with the patient. Since CMS remains the largest health insurance agency, many private insurance companies will provide coverage at similar levels.

Medicare

The Medicare program was developed in 1965 by the federal government.[1] In order to qualify for Medicare benefits, a person must be age 65 or older, have approved disabilities under age 65, or have end-stage renal disease.

In 2005, Medicare provided coverage to 42.5 million people, spending $330 billion on benefits.[2] These benefit payments are funded from two trust funds—the Hospital Insurance (HI) trust fund and the Supplementary Medical Insurance (SMI) trust fund. Most often these are referred to as Medicare Part A and Medicare Part B, respectively.[2]

The HI trust fund pays for a portion of the costs of inpatient hospital services and related care. Those services include critical access hospitals (small facilities that give limited outpatient and inpatient services to people in rural areas), skilled nursing facilities, hospice care, and some home health care services. The HI trust fund is primarily financed through payroll taxes, plus a relatively small amount of interest, income taxes on Social Security benefits, and other revenues.

The SMI trust fund pays for a portion of the costs of physicians' services, outpatient hospital services, and other related medical and health services. The current premium for Medicare Part B is $58.70 per month. However, in some cases this amount may be higher if the person doesn't choose Medicare Part B when they first become eligible at age 65. In addition, as of 2006, the SMI trust fund pays for private prescription drug insurance plans to provide drug coverage under Part D of the program. The separate Part B and Part D accounts in the SMI trust fund are financed through general revenues, beneficiary premiums, and interest income and, in the case of Part D, special payments from the States.

By combining both payment sources, the total expenditures from the HI and SMI trust funds are projected to increase at a significant pace in the absence of further reforms. Total Medicare expenditures are estimated to be 3.2 % of gross domestic product (GDP) in 2006, reaching 11% in 2008.[2] These increases reflect growth in medical prices and the volume and intensity of services. In addition, the retirement and aging of the "baby boom" generation will also increase expenditure growth rates for Medicare. Indeed, Medicare has become the second most expensive entitlement program next to Social Security in the U.S.

The Medicare + Choice program was authorized by the Balanced Budget Act of 1997.[3] In this program, the beneficiary has the traditional Medicare Part A and Part B, but they may also select Medicare managed care plans (such as Health Maintenance Organizations [HMOs] or Perspective Payment Organizations [PPOs] or Medicare Private Fee-for-Service plans). Medicare + Choice plans provide care under contract to Medicare. They may provide benefits like coordination of care or reducing out-of-pocket expenses. Some plans may also offer additional benefits, such as prescription drugs.

In January 2006, CMS introduced a prescription drug benefit for all Medicare beneficiaries independent of income, health status, and prescription drug usage,[4] Medicare Part D. There are a range of plan options available, so the beneficiaries have multiple options for coverage. Moreover, persons can add drug coverage to the traditional Medicare plan through a "stand alone" prescription drug plan or through a Medicare Advantage plan, which include an HMO or PPO, that typically provides more benefits at a significantly lower cost through a network of doctors and hospitals. Presently, no wound care products are covered under this benefit.

Medicaid

The Medicaid program was developed in 1965 as a jointly funded cooperative venture between the federal and state governments to assist states in the provision of adequate medical care to eligible people.[5] Medicaid is the largest program providing medical and health-related services to America's poorest people. Within broad national guidelines provided by the federal government, each of the states:
- administers its own program
- determines the type, amount, duration, and scope of services
- establishes its own eligibility standards
- sets the rate of payment for services.

Thus, the Medicaid program varies considerably from state to state, as well as within each state over time. This wide variance also affects what's covered in wound care. For example, the number of times a wound can be debrided (and that is reimbursed) differs by state.

Reimbursement across health care settings

Reimbursement directly impacts how clinicians deliver care. Increasingly, third-party payer sources (Medicare, Medicaid, health maintenance organizations) are examining where their money is going and whether they're getting the most from providers on behalf of their beneficiaries. Thus, third-party payers are requiring more documentation regarding patient outcomes to justify payment. Clinicians who can document comprehensive and accurate assessments of wounds and outcomes of their interventions are in a stronger position to obtain and maintain coverage.

Wound care that's evidence-based should always be the goal of clinicians. However, they're increasingly being challenged to provide optimum wound care dependent on health care setting and third-party payer. This section reviews various health care settings and how wound care products and services are reimbursed by CMS.

Hospitals

Hospitals are reimbursed at a predetermined, fixed rate for each discharge under the prospective payment system (PPS). The payment amount for a particular service is derived based on the classification system of that service. For hospitals, wound care products, devices, and support surfaces are included in the amount. Because the PPS is based on an adjusted average payment rate, some cases will receive payments in excess of cost (less than the billed charges), whereas others will receive payment that's less than cost.[6] The system is designed to give hospitals the incentive to manage operations more efficiently by evaluating those areas in which increased efficiencies can be instituted without affecting the quality of care and by treating a mix of patients to balance cost and payments.

Coverage under the surgical dressings benefit

To have the cost of dressings reimbursed under the Medicare/Medicaid surgical dressings benefit, the following criteria must be met:

- The dressings are medically necessary for the treatment of a wound caused by, or treated by, a surgical procedure.
- The dressings are medically necessary when debridement of a wound is medically necessary.

In certain situations, dressings aren't covered under the surgical dressings benefit, including those for:

- drainage from a cutaneous fistula which has not been caused by or treated by a surgical procedure
- first-degree burn
- stage I pressure ulcer
- wounds caused by trauma that don't require surgical closure or debridement (such as skin tears and abrasions)
- venipuncture or arterial puncture site other than the site of an indwelling catheter or needle.

Examples of dressing classifications that are covered under the surgical dressing benefit include:

- foam dressings
- gauze
- nonimpregnated and impregnated dressings
- hydrocolloids
- alginates
- composites
- Hydrogels.

Rehabilitation hospitals and units and long-term-care facilities (defined as those with an average length of stay of at least 25 days) are excluded from PPS. Instead, they're paid on a reasonable-cost basis, subject to per-discharge limits.[6] They're also paid depending on hospital-specific contracts and different payer sources. Note that CMS doesn't recognize subacute status; rather, subacute facilities are governed by the skilled nursing facility regulations.

Hospital outpatient centers
The Balanced Budget Act of 1997 provided authority for CMS to develop a PPS under Medicare for hospital outpatient services. The new outpatient PPS took effect in August 2000.[7] All services paid under this PPS are called Ambulatory Payment Classifications (APCs). A payment rate is established for each APC, depending on the services provided. Services in each APC are similar clinically and in terms of the resources they require. Currently, there are approximately 500 APCs. Hospitals may be paid for more than one APC per encounter. A coinsurance amount is initially calculated for each APC

based on 20% of the national median charge for services in the APCs. The coinsurance amount for an APC doesn't change until the amount becomes 20% of the total APC payment. It should be noted that the total APC payment and the portion paid as coinsurance amounts are adjusted to reflect geographic wage variations using the hospital wage index and assuming that the portion of the payment/coinsurance that's attributable to labor is 60%.

The surgical dressings benefit covers primary and secondary dressings in outpatient acute care clinic settings (for example, a hospital outpatient wound center) and physician offices.[8] (See *Coverage under the surgical dressings benefit*.)

Skilled nursing facilities
A patient who is eligible for Medicare will receive Medicare Part A for up to 100 days per benefit period in a skilled nursing facility (SNF).[8] The patient must satisfy specific rules in order to qualify for this benefit. These rules include the following:

- Beneficiary is admitted to SNF or to the SNF level of care in a swing-bed hospital

within 30 days after the date of hospital discharge.
• Beneficiary must have been in a hospital receiving inpatient hospital services for at least 3 consecutive days (counting the day of admission, but not the day of discharge).
• Beneficiary requires skilled nursing care by or under the supervision of a registered nurse; or requires physical, occupational, or speech therapy that could only be provided in an inpatient setting.
• Services are needed on a daily basis.
• Skilled services are required for the same or related health problem that resulted in the hospitalization.

After the SNF accepts a patient with Medicare Part A, all routine, ancillary, and capital-related costs are covered in the PPS. Thus, wound care supplies, therapies, and support surfaces are included in the PPS per diem rate. The Balanced Budget Act (BBA) of 1997 modified how payments were made for Medicare SNF services.[8] After July 1, 1998, SNFs were no longer paid on a reasonable cost basis or through low volume prospectively determined rates, but rather on the basis of a PPS. The PPS payment rates are adjusted for case mix and geographic variation (urban versus rural) in wages. It also covers all costs of furnishing covered SNF services. The SNF isn't permitted to bill under Medicare Part B until the 100 days are in effect.[9]

All SNFs participating in Medicare and Medicaid must also comply with federal and state regulations. In November 2004, CMS released its revised interpretative guidance on pressure ulcers (F-314).[10] This 40-page document is used by both federal and state surveyors to determine the SNF compliance with F-314. It also provides the SNFs with evidence-based approaches to prevent and treat pressure ulcers. If the SNF is found to be noncompliant with the pressure ulcer regulation, they can receive civil money penalties which currently range from $500 to $10,000/day or CMS and State can withhold payments and close the facility due to system-wide eminent danger of residents. Additional regulations that contain skin or wound regulations are F-309, which could be sited for all other ulcers beyond pressure ulcers; and F-315 (urinary incontinence), which addresses

the need to protect the skin from the effects of the incontinence.

Resident assessment Instrument

After a person is admitted to the SNF, an assessment using the Resident Assessment Instrument (RAI) must be completed. The RAI includes the Minimum Data Set (MDS 2.0), Resident Assessment Protocols (RAPs), and utilization guidelines. The MDS is a 400-item assessment form that attempts to identify functional capacity of residents in SNFS.[11] Based on the MDS section, further assessments are triggered by RAPs, which assess common clinical problems found in SNFs, such as pressure ulcers and urinary incontinence. RAPs also have utilization guidelines that assist the health care team in planning the overall care of the resident. The comprehensive RAI is completed annually, with quarterly MDS assessments (less comprehensive) completed between the annual date. The SNF is required to do another RAI if the resident's health status changes significantly. Only pressure and stasis ulcers are clearly delineated on the MDS 2.0 version; all other ulcers are grouped in the "other" category. Section M of the MDS assesses ulcers from staging, type of ulcer (pressure or stasis), other skin lesions, skin treatments, and foot problems. Presently, the CMS is working on revising the MDS with a 3.0 version to eliminate the confusion of Section M that requires staging of all chronic ulcers.

The RAI is a very useful instrument to plan the care of SNF residents. It's also linked to payment. All Medicare Part A is linked to the RAI and, in some states, Medicaid payments are solely based on completion of the MDS. Since 1998, SNFs are required to complete and transmit MDS data to the designated state agency for all residents as a condition of participation in the Medicare and Medicaid programs.

Resource utilization groups

Based on the MDS, each resident is assigned to one of 44 resource utilization groups (RUGs).[12] RUGs are clusters of nursing home residents based on resident characteristics that explain resource use.[13] RUG rates are

computed separately for urban and rural areas, and a portion of the total rate is adjusted to reflect labor market conditions in each SNF's location. The daily rate for each RUG is calculated using the sum of three components:
- a fixed amount for routine services (such as room and board, linens, and administrative services)
- a variable amount for the expected intensity of therapy services
- a variable amount reflecting the intensity of nursing care patients are expected to require.

Because of RUGs, it's essential for the SNF to complete the MDS correctly. The SNF must pay close attention to all health problems of the resident because the more intensive the care required, the higher the daily rate. Moreover, completing the MDS accurately and in a timely manner will help to ensure correct payments. If a SNF doesn't complete the MDS in a timely manner, they receive a default payment, which is usually significantly lower, or they may not receive payment at all.

The majority of SNFs accept the Medicaid program as the major payer for residents. Like Medicare, most state Medicaid programs pay a per diem rate for SNF services. If Medicaid is paying for SNF services and the resident has Medicare Part B, some wound products (such as dressings and negative pressure wound therapy) may be covered.

Home health agencies

The Balanced Budget Act of 1997 called for the development and implementation of a PPS for Medicare home health services. In October 1, 2000, home health PPS was implemented.[14] (See *Qualifying for home health benefits*.)

OASIS

The process of quality wound management begins on admission. Suggested components of a quality program are assessment (including risk assessment and intervention), documentation and wound measurement, case manager report and collaboration, protocols and physician orders, ulcer care, management

---

Qualifying for home health benefits

A patient who is Medicare-eligible can also receive Medicare home health services. To qualify for this benefit, the patient must satisfy the following criteria:
- The patient's physician must first determine that medical care is needed in the home and thus generate a care plan.
- The patient must need at least one of the following:
  - intermittent physical therapy
  - intermittent skilled nursing care
  - intermittent speech/language therapy.
- The patient must be classified as homebound according to the condition for participation in Medicare.

---

of tissue loads, nutrition, and outcomes tracking.[15]

When it's determined that a Medicare patient can receive home health services, the Outcome and Assessment Information Set (OASIS) must be completed. OASIS is a group of comprehensive assessments that form the basis for delivering care to the patient, as well as for measuring patient outcomes for purposes of outcome-based quality improvement. Revisions to the OASIS tool were introduced in late 2002, resulting in a 25% reduction in dataset questions. The new tool also drops 45 items from follow-up assessments, establishes a patient data tracking sheet, and eliminates two collection timepoints. Additional changes are pending approval by CMS.

Major items on the OASIS include sociodemographic, environmental, support system, health status, and functional status. Based on these assessments, a care plan can be generated. The OASIS document specifically classifies stasis ulcers, surgical wounds, and pressure ulcers. [16]

Payment for home health services is directly linked to the completion of OASIS. A case-mix is also applied to calculate reimbursement. Hence, the case-mix involves 20 data points to assess three factors within the case-mix: clinical severity, functional status, and service utilization. The system has created 80 home health resource groups (HHRGs).[17] Patients are grouped into the HHRGs based on the OASIS.

Medicare pays home health agencies for each covered 60-day episode of care,[14] and a patient can receive an unlimited number of medically necessary episodes of care. Payments cover skilled nursing and home health aide visits, covered therapy, medical social services, and routine and nonroutine supplies. For each 60-day episode, the payment system can range from about $1,100 to $5,900, depending on the HHRG, with adjustments to reflect area wage differences.[17]

Home health agencies are required to electronically transmit OASIS data to the State system. Improper completion of OASIS can lead to significantly low payments or no payments at all. Thus, accurate assessments and charting is essential for recouping payments. Some authors[15,18,19,20] have described innovative ways of teaching staff and assuring their competency in completing OASIS.

PRACTICE POINT

Accurate completion of OASIS by clinicians is essential. If you don't answer the questions appropriately, accurately, and completely, your facility won't receive the money and will lose reimbursement.

Durable medical equipment carriers

Implementation of the Medicare program (for instance, eligibility requirements and payments) in home care is handled by numerous insurance companies that are subcontracted by CMS. In 1993, CMS contracted four carriers to process claims for durable medical equipment, prosthetics, orthotics, and supplies (DMEPOS) under Medicare Part B.[21] CMS divided the country into four regions, with each region having its own DME regional carrier (DMERC). The Healthcare Common Procedure Coding System (HCPCS), an alpha-numeric code used to identify coding categories not included in the American Medical Association's CPT-4 codes are usually used with DMEPOS.[22]

In January 2006, CMS eliminated fiscal intermediaries who processed Medicare claims (Medicare Part A only) and carriers (Medicare Part B only).[23] They also eliminated the DMERCs. In January 2006, CMS awarded four specialty contractors through a competitive bidding process. The new Durable Medical Equipment Medicare Administrative Contractors (DME MACs) will be responsible for handling the administration of Medicare claims from suppliers of DMEPOS. The benefit of the new system is a more streamlined process between the beneficiary and the supplier. The DME MACs will serve as the point of contact for all Medicare suppliers, whereas beneficiaries can register their claims-related questions to Beneficiary Contact Centers. The four DME MACS and corresponding states are:

• *AdminaStar Federal,* serving Illinois, Indiana, Kentucky, Michigan, Minnesota, Ohio, and Wisconsin

• *National Heritage Insurance Company,* serving Connecticut, Delaware, District of Columbia, Maine, Maryland, Massachusetts, New Hampshire, New Jersey, New York, Pennsylvania, Rhode Island, and Vermont

• *Noridian Administrative Services,* serving Alaska, American Samoa, Arizona, California, Guam, Hawaii, Idaho, Iowa, Kansas, Missouri, Montana, Nebraska, Nevada, North Dakota, Northern Mariana Islands, Oregon, South Dakota, Utah, Washington, and Wyoming

• *Palmetto Government Benefits Administrator,* serving Alabama, Arkansas, Colorado, Florida, Georgia, Louisiana, Mississippi, New Mexico, North Carolina, Oklahoma, Puerto Rico, South Carolina, Tennessee, Texas, U.S. Virgin Islands, Virginia, and West Virginia.

DME MACs clearly define medical coverage policies. The beneficiary usually pays the first $100.00 for covered medical services annually. Once that has been met, the beneficiary pays 20% of the Medicare-approved amount for services or supplies. If services weren't provided on assignment, then the beneficiary pays for more of the Medicare coinsurance plus certain charges above the Medicare-approved amount.

Medicare Part B also provides coverage for negative pressure wound therapy (NPWT) pumps.[24] In order for a NPWT pump and supplies to be covered, the patient must have a chronic stage III or IV pressure ulcer, neuropathic ulcer, venous or arterial insufficiency ulcer, or a chronic (at least 30 days) ulcer of mixed etiology. Extensive documentation is required prior to a DME MAC approving coverage for NPWT. Thus, it's important to review the coverage policy prior to applying for coverage. (*Note:* In 2007 CMS is proposing to pilot competitive bidding for NPWT with sole source contracts, thus decreasing provider choice in NPWT.[25])

Support surfaces are also covered under Medicare Part B.[26-28] The CMS has divided support surfaces into three categories for reimbursement purposes.

• Group 1 devices are those support surfaces that are static and don't require electricity. Static devices include air, foam (convoluted and solid), gel, and water overlay or mattresses.

• Group 2 devices are powered by electricity or pump and are considered dynamic in nature. These devices include alternating and low-air-loss mattresses.

• Group 3 devices are also considered dynamic in nature. This classification comprises only air-fluidized beds.

Specific criteria must be met before Medicare will reimburse for support surfaces; therefore, it's essential to review the policy before applying for coverage.

Managed care

Manage Care Organizations (MCOs) were developed to provide health services while controlling costs. They combine the responsibility for paying for a defined set of health services with an active program to control the costs associated with providing those services, while at the same time attempting to control the quality of and access to those services. The health benefits, which usually range from acute care services to dental/vision are usually clearly identified as well as the payment, co-payment, and deductibles that are required for a specific health procedure (e.g. compression therapy for chronic venous insufficiency ulcer). Moreover, the MCO usually receives a fixed sum of money to pay for the benefits in the plans for the defined population of enrollees. Typically, this fixed sum is constructed through premiums paid by the enrollees, capitation payments made on behalf of the enrollees from a third party, or both. There's a wide variance of MCOs and services they provide for patients with wounds.

Providing wound care in a complex reimbursement environment

The challenge of providing quality wound care can be magnified when the patient moves from one health care sector to another. That's why it's imperative as wound care professionals to understand some of the nuances of the reimbursement agency. A good illustration would be a Medicare beneficiary who was discharged home with a pressure ulcer that had 100% eschar covering the surface. In this scenario, the home care agency would receive no reimbursement for providing wound care until the eschar was removed. However, if the same Medicare beneficiary was discharged to a SNF, the nursing home could receive full payment for the pressure ulcer with 100% eschar. This reimbursement schism can make providing quality wound care extremely challenging.

Quality improvement efforts

Regulations related to reimbursements are tightly integrated with efforts in quality assessment and improvement. Indeed, care that's found not to meet quality standards may not be reimbursed. Even appropriate care may not be reimbursed if the condition being treated is the result of a medical error. Moreover, claims for reimbursements for substandard care could be viewed as fraudulent and result in criminal penalties. However, CMS doesn't rely solely on such punitive methods and various other initiatives exist—most of these efforts center on pressure ulcers and may serve as a model for other wounds.

Measuring quality of care

Measurements of quality are viewed as central to ensuring quality of care. If you don't measure it, you can't improve it. There are a variety of methods by which quality measurement can be used to improve care, and different health care settings employ different approaches. Facilitating such quality measurement is the wealth of data available in existing databases, such as MDS and OASIS, that provide a wealth of patient-specific information, which reflects processes and outcomes of care.

First, quality measurement is being used to empower consumers of health care. The assumption is that patients and their families, if given information on quality, will select those providers offering the best care. Such information then needs to be made available to patients in a timely fashion. Further, providers need to proactively improve their care to attract patients. This approach is exemplified by the Nursing Home Compare website maintained by CMS.[29] Prevalence rates of pressure ulcers, both for high- and low-risk patients, are calculated from MDS and described for nearly every nursing home in the country. These rates are presented along with national and state-wide rates to permit easy comparisons. Whether this approach will indeed be successful in improving care, however, remains uncertain.[30]

Quality measures are also being used in quality improvement activities. The systematic use of such data can aid in the identification of quality-of-care problems and help determine the nature of these problems.[31] Nearly all health care provider organizations are involved in continuous quality improvement activities, with varying levels of implementation into clinical practice. A central component of such activities is feedback on performance. Indeed, demonstration projects have suggested that providing home care agencies with performance feedback, a process known as Outcome-Based Quality Improvement, does result in reduced rates of hospitalization. Thus, CMS uses OASIS to calculate risk-adjusted rates of pressure ul-

cers, and not only posts them on a website, but encourages home care agencies to use the data as part of their internal quality improvement program.

Finally, quality measures may help to focus more detailed analyses of the care provided to individual patients. For example, the Agency for Healthcare Research and Quality (AHRQ), as part of its patient safety initiative, has developed a set of indicators based on hospital discharge data. Among the indicators is one for the presence of a pressure ulcer. Patients flagged by the indicator may undergo a more detailed review of the care processes associated with the development and treatment of the pressure ulcer. In nursing homes, state survey agencies are required to conduct annual unannounced surveys at SNFs to determine compliance with federal regulations regarding quality of care. A major focus of these surveys is an evaluation of pressure ulcer prevention and treatment practices and whether it's compliant with care as specified in the Federal Tag 314 (F-314). Cases reviewed are often identified based on the MDS quality indicators.

Improving quality of care

CMS also actively promotes quality improvement activities directed towards Medicare beneficiaries. The primary mechanism for this is through the Quality Improvement Organizations (QIOs), formerly known as Peer Review Organizations (PROs).[32] PROs initially relied on an "inspect and detect" approach to quality assessment in which medical record reviews would identify problems and be linked to interventions to correct substandard care. The approach was adversarial, penalties for substandard care could be harsh, and few improvements in quality of care could be documented.

In 1992, the Health Care Quality Improvement Initiative significantly changed the role of PROs. Rather than individual case reviews, PROs were to focus now on patterns of care. National guidelines, rather than local criteria, were to be used in evaluating quality of care. Most importantly, PROs were to work collaboratively with providers to improve health care delivery. Recognizing this new emphasis on quality improvement, PROs were renamed QIOs in 2001.

QIOs have since developed initiatives in diverse clinical areas and settings. In wound care, most of these efforts have again centered on pressure ulcers. In New York, tool kits have been developed where hospitals can assess and improve their pressure ulcer prevention and treatment practices. In nursing homes, QIOs from three states developed a strategy to train nursing home teams in quality improvement methods and proper pressure ulcer care. This training was reinforced through the use of outside mentors who regularly met with the teams. As a result of these initiatives and interventions, key processes of care dramatically improved. [33] Such training of nursing homes in quality improvement activities has since expanded to other states.

Pay 4 performance

In support of improving quality throughout health settings, CMS has begun a series of pilot projects aimed at improving quality, while protecting patients and providing cost-effective care, called Pay 4 performance (P4P).[34] This bold federal initiative is predicated on effective pay-for-performance initiatives in collaboration with providers and other stakeholders, to ensure that valid quality measures are used, that providers aren't being pulled in conflicting directions, and that providers have support for achieving actual improvement. Numerous organization are collaborating with CMS on this initiative. Some of the national organizations involved in P4P include the National Quality Forum (NQF), the Joint Commission of the Accreditation of Health Care Organizations (JCAHO), the National Committee for Quality Assurance (NCQA), the Agency for Health Care Research and Quality (AHRQ), the American Medical Association (AMA), and many others.

Given that each health care sector (hospital, nursing home, etc.) confronts different health issues, core measures will be developed for each sector. For example, wound healing may not be an appropriate quality measure for hospitals, but it may be an ideal quality measure in nursing homes and home health, given their high incidence and prevalence of wounds.

Essential wound documentation

For essential wound care documentation, include the following:
- Change in clinical status or wound healing progress
- Characteristics of the wound, including:
  - depth
  - exudate amount
  - length
  - pain
  - tissue type
  - width
- Education of patient and caregivers
- Local wound care
- Minimum Data Set (MDS 2.0) per schedule in the skilled nursing facility
- Moisture management
- Nutritional status
- Outcome and Assessment Information Set (OASIS) per schedule in home health care
- Pressure-reducing support surfaces (both bed and chair)
- Regular assessment and reassessment of the wound (such as daily or weekly)
- Repositioning and turning schedules
- Routine skin assessment and care

Documentation

Comprehensive documentation is the critical foundation for successful reimbursement of services and products. Indeed, regulatory agencies, independent of health care setting, set forth the requisite documentation for reimbursement, and their requirements for documentation should always be carefully reviewed prior to applying for coverage. Lastly, thorough documentation justifies the medical necessity of services and products and should reflect the care required in the prevention or treatment of wounds. (See *Essential wound documentation*.)

Summary

Regulatory agencies play a major role in wound care. With the increasing need to evaluate the cost-effectiveness of wound care, regulatory agencies will most likely impose further regulations. Increasing regulation will lead to greater complexity in obtaining and maintaining reimbursements. Thus, the key to providing optimum wound care will depend on good documentation that clearly articulates the need for services and products and clearly identifies assessment of the patient, interventions instituted, and outcomes achieved. When this is accomplished, the patient, provider, and regulatory agency benefit.

Show what you know

1. *Medicare Part B is a federal program that:*

 A. supports state programs to provide services and products to the poor.
 B. reimburses hospitals for wound care services.
 C. reimburses for selected wound services and products in skilled nursing facilities and home health agencies.
 D. doesn't require copayment from beneficiary.

ANSWER: C. A is incorrect because it refers to the Medicaid program, which is a collaboration between the federal and state governments to deliver care. B is incorrect because Medicare Part A is for inpatient hospital costs. D is incorrect because Medicare Part B requires the beneficiary to pay a 20% copayment.

2. *For which one of the following health care settings is completion of OASIS required?*

 A. Hospitals
 B. Home health agencies
 C. Hospital outpatient centers
 D. Skilled nursing facilities

ANSWER: B. OASIS is only used by home health agencies to assess patients and determine reimbursement.

3. *Which one of the following criteria must a patient with a wound meet in order to qualify for skilled nursing facility care?*

 A. Skilled services must be required for the same or related health problem that resulted in the hospitalization.
 B. Beneficiary must be in the hospital for 2 consecutive days.
 C. Services are needed once per week.

 D. Beneficiary must be admitted to the SNF within 90 days of admission to the hospital.

ANSWER: A. B is incorrect because the beneficiary must spend 3 consecutive days in the hospital. C is incorrect because skilled nursing services must be needed on a daily basis. D is incorrect because the beneficiary must be admitted within 30 days of hospitalization.

4. *Which of the following approaches is not being used by CMS to improve the quality of care?*

 A. Empower consumers to select high quality providers through the provision of information on performance.
 B. Increase payments to providers of better care.
 C. Develop computer reminders on when to turn patients.
 D. Work with providers through regional quality improvement organizations.

ANSWER: C. A is incorrect because data on performance of hospitals, nursing homes, and health agencies is readily available on the CMS web site. B is incorrect as there is tremendous interest at CMS to reward providers of high-quality care, known as pay-for-performance. D is incorrect because QIOs are now emphasizing working with providers to improve care rather than just detecting episodes of poor care.

References

1. www.cms.hhs.gov/History/
2. www.cms.hhs.gov/apps/media/press/release.asp?Counter=1846
3. www.medicare.gov/Choices/Overview.asp
4. www.cms.hhs.gov/hillnotifications/downloads/124PartDTransitionDemoFactSheet.pdf
5. www.cms.hhs.gov/medicaid
6. www.cms.hhs.gov/providers/hipps/default.asp
7. www.cms.hhs.gov/regulation/hopps
8. www.umd.nycpic.com/rev21_ch17-1_dressings_psc.html
9. www.cms.hhs.gov/providers/snfpp/default.asp
10. www.cms.hhs.gov/transmittals/downloads/R4SOM.pdf
11. www.cms.hhs.gov/medicaid/mds20/default.asp
12. Fries, B.E., et al. "Refining a Case-mix Measure for Nursing Homes: Resource Utilization Groups (RUG-III)," *Medical Care* 32(7):668-85, July 1994.
13. Rantz, M.J., et al. "The Minimum Data Set: No Longer Just for Clinical Assessment," *Annals of Long Term Care* 7(9):354-60, September 1999.
14. www.cms.hhs.gov/providers/hhapps/default.asp
15. Johnston, P.J. "Wound Competencies and OASIS-One Organization's Plan," *The Remington Report* 10(3), 5-10, May-June, 2002.
16. www.cms.hhs.gov/oasis/hhoview.asp
17. www.cms.hhs.gov/medlearn/hh0201b1v2.pdf
18. Wright, K., and Powell, L. "Wound Competencies and OASIS-One Organization's Plan," *Caring Magazine* XXI(6):10-13, June 2002.
19. Cullen, B., and Parry, G. "Wound Competencies and OASIS-One Organization's Plan," *Caring Magazine* XXI(6):14-16, June 2002.

20. Everman, R., and Ferrell, J. "Wound Care Case Management Influences Better Patient Outcomes," *The Remington Report* 10(3):36-37, May-June 2002.
21. www.umd.nycpic.com/aboutdme.html
22. www.tricenturion.com/content/hcpcs.cfm
23. www.cms.hhs.gov/MedicareContractingReform/ Downloads/mac_jurisdiction_facts.pdf
24. www.umd.nycpic.com/rev22_ch14-31_negative_pressure_psc.html
25. www.cms.hhs.gov/quarterlyproviderupdates/ downloads/cms1270p.pdf
26. www.umd.nycpic.com/rev22_ch14-22_group1_psc.html
27. www.umd.nycpic.com/rev22_ch14-23_group2_psc.html
28. www.umd.nycpic.com/ch14-24_group3_psc.html
29. Harris, Y., and Clauser, S.B. "Achieving Improvement Through Nursing Home Quality Measurement," *Health Care Financing Review* 23(4): 5-18, 2002
30. Mukamel, D.B., and Spector, W.B. "Quality Report Cards and Nursing Home Quality," *Gerontologist* 43(special issue II):58-66, 2003.
31. Karon, S.L., and Zimmerman, D.R. "Using Indicators to Structure Quality Improvement Initiatives in Long-term Care," *Quality Management in Health Care* 4(3): 54-66, 1996.
32. www.cms.hhs.gov/apps/media/press/release.asp? Counter=1343
33. Baier, R.R., et al. "Quality Improvement for Pressure Ulcer Care in the Nursing Home Setting: The Northeast Pressure Ulcer Project," *Journal of the American Medical Director's Association* 4(6):291-301, November-December 2003.
34. www.cms.hhs.gov/apps/media/press/release.asp%3F Counter%3D1343

CHAPTER 3

Legal aspects of wound care

Steven P. Knowlton, JD, RN
Gregory Brown, RN, BBA, BSN, CWOCN

OBJECTIVES

After completing this chapter, you'll be able to:

* identify and describe the major litigation players and their roles in a lawsuit

* define the four elements of a malpractice claim

* describe the general rules for proper wound care charting

* identify and describe the ways the medical record, standards, or guidelines can be used in a malpractice case

* state documentation practices that predispose the medical record to legal risks

* describe strategies to improve consistency and accuracy of medical record documentation that minimize potential litigation risk.

The current climate

In recent years, the concept of patients as "consumers of health care" has risen to the forefront. Rather than blindly trusting clinicians, the consumer-patients of today are better educated and more aware of health care issues and more willing to make use of legal resources when treatment goes awry. Although wound care generates no more litigation than many areas of health care practice, and arguably less than some others, the threat of litigation still affects the way clinicians approach the delivery of care.

Clinicians need to protect themselves while ensuring evidence-based, high-quality care to their consumer-patients. This chapter sets forth basic legal principles and suggests practice strategies that protect clinicians *and* advance patient care.

Litigation

Over the course of human history, it became apparent that some nonviolent means of settling disputes must be developed. The law and the legal process, including litigation, were and continue to be one of civilized society's experiments at achieving nonviolent resolutions to disputes. The success of this experiment is itself the source of much dispute, to which no resolution (nonviolent or otherwise) is currently in sight.

Contrary to television and film portrayals, the real-life litigation process is arduous and time-consuming. While fictitious television and film lawsuits resolve in a matter of weeks or months, usually ending with a dramatic trial resulting in a stunning jury verdict, most real-life cases take years to get through the legal system. In some jurisdictions with crowded dockets, they can take as long as 5 years to resolve. Those that require appeals can take considerably more time before all issues are finally put to rest. Trials (dramatic or not) are few and far between, as nearly all lawsuits are settled before trial. When trials do happen, they're usually slow-moving, uninteresting affairs that tax the patience and attention of jurors. Litigants expecting "Perry Mason" moments from their attorneys are sure to be disappointed and, as anyone who has ever served on jury duty knows, closing arguments by attorneys are never, ever over in the 5 minutes before the final commercial.

Despite the difficulties and drawbacks, the litigation process does afford citizens an impartial forum for dispute resolution grounded in the law. And the law, as Plato stated, is "a pledge that citizens of a state will do justice to one another."

The discussion in this chapter is limited to *civil litigation;* that is, litigation in which citizens have a dispute with each other—rather than *criminal litigation,* in which the state or a government seeks to prosecute a party for the violation of law. There are significant differences between the two forms of litigation (standards of proof, for example). The remedy sought in civil litigation is monetary damages. In contrast, only the prosecuting state or government may seek to deprive the alleged lawbreaker of his liberty by incarceration.

How is a medical malpractice lawsuit born?

Litigation begins the moment a person believes he has been wronged by another and seeks the advice and counsel of an attorney in an effort to "right the wrong" or "get justice." During the initial interview between the prospective client and the attorney, the attorney makes a number of preliminary judgments usually based solely on the client's presentation:

• Is this the type of case the attorney is capable of handling? Does it fall within his expertise and practice experience? Does the attorney have the time to handle the matter?
• Is the client's story credible?
• Will the client make a good witness?
• Are the damages, if proven, sufficient to warrant entering into the litigation process?
• Is there a party responsible (liable) for the client's injuries?
• How likely is it that both liability and damages can be proven?
• Are there any glaring problems or difficulties with the case?

If the answers to these questions are satisfactory and the client wishes to retain the attorney, a lawsuit has then been conceived.

Before filing the legal documents that start the litigation process in a medical malpractice case, most attorneys perform an intensive investigation in order to definitively answer questions concerning liability and damages. Medical records and other information must be obtained and examined by an expert to determine whether a malpractice claim can be made, information related to the identities of potential defendants must be analyzed, and strategic legal issues related to jurisdiction (which court can the case be brought in) must be thought through. If after this investigation the attorney still believes the case has merit, legal papers starting the actual lawsuit will be filed, and a lawsuit will be born. (See *Players in the litigation process,* page 32.)

The pretrial litigation process

The pretrial litigation process consists of several steps: complaint and answer, discovery, and motion practice.

Complaint and answer
The initial legal paper that gives rise to a lawsuit is called the *complaint*. While procedural requirements vary between jurisdictions, generally the complaint is a document that sets out the claims made by the plaintiff against the defendant, the basis of the jurisdiction of the court, the legal theories under which the

Players in the litigation process

The litigation process is initiated and enacted by people with a dispute to resolve and those whose task it is to aid in resolving that dispute.

The parties

The principal parties involved in litigation are the *litigants*—the individuals on either side of the dispute. The *plaintiff* is the person who initiates the lawsuit and who claims he has suffered injury due to the actions of another. A lawsuit may be filed by multiple plaintiffs.

The plaintiff sues the *defendant*—the person or organization alleged to have injured the plaintiff by his or its actions. In most cases the parties are individuals, but parties can be corporations, companies, partnerships, government agencies or, in some cases, governments themselves.

The judge

The *judge* is an individual, usually an attorney, who has been appointed or elected to oversee lawsuits on behalf of the state or government under whose jurisdiction the lawsuit is brought. The judge acts as referee during the pretrial phase of the case and decides legal issues that arise as the lawsuit progresses toward trial. In a trial, the judge's responsibility is *to interpret the law.*

The jury

The *jury* is a panel of citizens chosen by the attorneys for the litigants to hear evidence in the case and render a decision or verdict. The jury's responsibility is *to determine the facts* in a trial. It's up to the jury to decide whether the plaintiff and his attorney proved their case, thereby rendering a decision about the defendant's liability and the amount of damages the defendant should pay to the plaintiff.

---

plaintiff is making the claims, and in some jurisdictions, the amount of damages claimed.

The defendant must then file an *answer* within the permitted time that responds on a count-by-count basis to the plaintiff's complaint and which, depending again on jurisdictional rules, may also include claims against the plaintiff. These two basic *pleadings* initiate the formal lawsuit.

Discovery

Discovery is the process by which the parties find out the facts about each other, about the incidents that have given rise to the claims of malpractice alleged by the plaintiff, and the defenses to those claims asserted by the defendant. In order to obtain discovery, the law has provided discovery devices—procedural mechanisms by which the parties ask for and receive information. Demands are routinely made for documents and other tangible items related to the lawsuit's claims, for statements made by the parties to others, and for witnesses to the incidents. Then, pretrial testimony (*deposition*) is taken of the parties to the lawsuit. This testimony, while out of court, is sworn testimony transcribed by a certified court reporter and can be used for any purpose in the lawsuit, including for purposes of *impeachment*—the demonstrating of prior untruthful or inaccurate testimony, or a challenge to the credibility of a witness—at trial.

Finally, *expert discovery*—information about the opinions of experts retained by the parties—is usually permitted. Experts are individuals accepted by the court to assist the finder of fact—the jury—in understanding issues that commonly fall outside of the experience of the typical juror. In medical malpractice cases, as you will read later, the plaintiff must prove that there was a deviation from the standard of care that resulted in an injury. Expert testimony related to the field of medicine, treatments, and standards of care at issue in the case is usually essential to successfully meet proof requirements for each element of a malpractice claim brought by a plaintiff. Likewise, the defense of such claims nearly always mandates opposing expert testimony—in essence, an explanation by a credentialed individual supporting the actions taken by the defendant from which the claim of malpractice stems.

Motion practice

Disputes over discovery often arise in the context of a lawsuit and those disputes that can't be resolved by the parties require court intervention. Formal resolution of these disputes usually requires an application to the court—a *motion*—setting forth the dispute and the position of the party making the application (the moving party, or *movant*) and requesting certain *relief* or results to be *ordered* by the court. Naturally, this requires a response from the other party—the *opposition*—that sets out the reasons why the court shouldn't grant the relief requested.

Some motions can be decided by the court *on the papers*, that is, without a formal oral presentation (*oral argument*) by the parties before the judge is assigned. More complicated motions, especially those seeking to eliminate or modify legal claims, almost always require argument before the presiding judge or court.

The trial

While the vast majority of lawsuits settle sometime before trial ("out-of-court settlements"), some cases do proceed to trial. Medical malpractice trials are almost without exception jury trials. Once it's determined that settlement isn't an option, a trial date is set and the attorneys begin to prepare. In federal jurisdictions and many state courts, litigants are required to prepare pretrial statements and submissions. They also disclose exhibit lists (materials and documents the attorneys anticipate they will use at trial). Furthermore, they designate deposition testimony to be read or, if the testimony was videotaped, to be shown at trial. The pretrial submission and disclosure process helps to ensure that the trial is as fair as possible and eliminates the possibility of "trial by ambush"—thus, the "Perry Mason" moments of

television and film renown are relatively few and far between.

On the day of the trial, the attorneys for the parties proceed with jury selection. Each attorney tries to select jurors that he believes will decide in favor of (*find for*) his client. Procedurally, the jury selection process varies widely by jurisdiction. In some courts, the trial judge will take an active role by questioning the jurors. The fight over selection is then left to the attorneys. Other jurisdictions permit the attorneys to question jurors directly without court supervision and the trial judge becomes involved only when a dispute arises. As you can imagine, jury selection in a jurisdiction with strong judicial control is a much briefer process than in those jurisdictions where the attorneys are left to their own devices. No matter what the individual procedure, once the jury is chosen (*empanelled*), the trial begins.

At trial, the parties each give opening statements, one of the two times in the entire trial that the attorneys are permitted to speak directly to the jurors. After opening statements, the plaintiff's attorney states the plaintiff's case. Because the burden of proof is on the plaintiff, the plaintiff's attorney goes first. After the plaintiff's direct case is finished, the plaintiff "rests," and the defendant's attorney presents the defendant's case. The *direct case* consists of factual testimony from witnesses (the plaintiff and others) as well as expert testimony, deposition testimony, and demonstrative evidence, such as charts, medical records, graphs, photographs, and drawings.

The opposing party has the right to cross-examine each witness after the direct examination, and then redirect examination and re-cross-examination may follow as necessary. After all the evidence has been presented by both sides, the parties make closing statements (*summations*), which is the last time the attorneys are permitted to speak directly to the jurors.

Once summations are completed, the judge then instructs the jurors on the appropriate law that they're to apply to the facts of the case. Remember that the jury is the *finder of fact*—it determines what happened, when it happened, who did it, where it happened, and how it happened—and the judge is the *interpreter of the law.* After the jurors receive the judge's instructions, they leave the courtroom and begin deliberations.

Every trial attorney hopes to be lucky enough to serve on a jury that goes to deliberations. For trial lawyers, understanding what happens inside the jury room during deliberations is the Holy Grail of trial practice. In jurisdictions that permit attorneys to interview jurors after verdict, attorneys often spend many hours with the jurors who are willing to discuss the case in order to determine what did—and what didn't—work during the trial. It's often surprising to find that what the lawyer thought was of prime importance wasn't so important to the jury. The jury room in our legal system is sacrosanct, and, no matter how it happens, the jury will eventually arrive at a verdict that will be delivered to the parties in open court. Once the verdict is read and the jury excused, the trial is over.

Appeals

Each jurisdiction has an appellate process, of which the litigants may take advantage. Depending on the jurisdiction, appeals may add years (and many dollars) to the resolution of claims and lawsuits.

Legal elements of a malpractice claim

A medical malpractice claim is made up of four distinct elements, each of which must be proven to the applicable standard of proof in the jurisdiction of the case. The usual standard of proof for civil cases is a *preponderance of the evidence.* The preponderance standard can be best described as a set of scales that represent the plaintiff on one side and the defendant on the other, which are evenly balanced at the start. In a trial, the party that wins is the scale that dips lower at the end. In other words, in order to prevail, plaintiffs need to show by only 50.0000001%—just a bit more than one-half—that they've proven each of the elements that make up a malpractice claim.

The four general elements that make up a malpractice claim are:
• existence of a duty owed to the plaintiff by the defendant
• breach of that duty
• injury that's causally related to that breach of duty
• damages recognized as law.

Duty

In general, there's no duty to protect a person endangered by the actions or omissions of another if there's no special relationship between the two persons. The patient-physician relationship is the basis for the claim of duty between the plaintiff-patient and the defendant-health care professional in medical malpractice cases because that relationship permits the patient to rely upon the physician's knowledge, expertise, and skill in treatment. Thus, the allegations of medical negligence arise within the course of that professional relationship. Translating that definition into health care terms, some examples of a duty may be the obligation of a health care practitioner to give patients care that's:
• consistent with level of experience, education, and training
• permitted under the applicable state practice act
• authorized or permitted under the policies and procedures of the institution that are applicable to the position.

PRACTICE POINT

Duty: In negligence cases, *duty* may be defined as obligation, to which the law will give recognition and effect, to conform to a particular standard of conduct toward another. The word *duty* is used throughout the Restatement of Torts to denote the fact that the actor is required to conduct himself in a particular manner at the risk that if he doesn't do so, he becomes subject to liability to another to whom the duty is owed for any injury sustained by such other, of which that actor's conduct is a legal cause. (Restatement, Second, Torts, Section 4.)[1]

Breach of duty

In addition to proving the existence of a duty, the plaintiff must also prove the defendant breached that duty. Breach of duty can be by either commission, omission, or both. Most often, to establish this element of the claim, the plaintiff in a medical malpractice case must also show that the defendant health care practitioner deviated from an accepted standard of care or treatment. The practitioner isn't required to provide the highest degree of care, but only the level and type of care rendered by the average practitioner. What the standard of care is, and whether and how it was deviated from, must be established for the jury, and this is most often the province of expert testimony.

Breach of duty in the health care setting may be illustrated in the following ways:
• failure to give care within the applicable practice act
• failure to perform professional duties with the degree of skill mandated by the applicable practice act
• failure to provide care for which the circumstance of the patient's condition warrants.

 PRACTICE POINT

Breach: The failure to meet an obligation to another person that's owed to that person; the breaking or violating of a law, right, obligation, engagement, or duty by either commission, omission, or both.[1]

Injury causally related to a breach of duty

In a medical malpractice case, proof of an injury isn't enough unless that injury can be causally linked to a breach of duty by a health care practitioner. That breach of duty is then considered the proximate cause. Without the breach of duty, the injury wouldn't have occurred. (See *Proving proximate cause.*)

Proximate cause in the health care setting can be illustrated by the following examples:

Proving proximate cause

While standards of proof related to proximate cause may vary among jurisdictions, one of two questions is almost always used to determine this issue:
• Was the health care practitioner's negligent conduct a "substantial factor" in causing the injury?
• Would the injury not have happened if the health care practitioner hadn't been negligent?

• fractured hip due to a fall because of failure to raise the siderails of the bed
• decreased total protein due to failure to provide nutrition (either failure to provide actual nourishment or failure to call consult)
• osteomyelitis resulting in limb amputation for failure to call infectious disease consult and provide antibiotic therapy.

 PRACTICE POINT

Proximate cause: That which, in a natural and continuous sequence, unbroken by any efficient intervening cause, produces injury, and without which the result wouldn't have occurred and without which the accident couldn't have happened, if the injury be one which might be reasonable anticipated or foreseen as a natural consequence of the wrongful act.[1]

Damages

Finally the fourth element that makes up a malpractice claim is damages. A health care practitioner may be held liable for damages when the jury finds that the practitioner deviated from the applicable standard of care in treating the plaintiff-patient and as a result, caused injury resulting in legally recognized damages. In most jurisdictions, a plaintiff may recover for proven monetary losses (lost wages and unreimbursed medical expenses) and for pain and suffering that result from the proven injury. As noted previously, it's the jury—the finder of fact—that sets the monetary award to the plaintiff.

PRACTICE POINT

Damage: Loss, injury, or deterioration caused by the negligence, design, or accident of one person or another, in respect of the latter's person or property.

Damages: A pecuniary compensation or indemnity, which may be recovered in the courts by any person who has suffered loss, detriment, or injury, whether to his person, property, or rights, through the unlawful act or omission or negligence of another.[1]

As we have shown, in order for a plaintiff to prevail in a medical malpractice claim all four of the elements discussed above must be satisfied. Three of four won't do. They must score perfectly on all four to prevail before a jury.

The medical record in litigation

The medical record is arguably the single most important piece of evidence in a medical malpractice case. It serves as a crucial tool for the delivery of science-based care. It's also:
- a legal document
- a communication tool
- the supporting basis for treatment decisions and modifications
- one of the primary tools for the evaluation of treatment modalities.

At one time or another in the education of a health care practitioner, whatever the specialty or discipline, this directive is taught: "If it wasn't written down, it didn't happen." Nowhere does this statement ring more true than in a medical malpractice case. (See *Effects of incomplete charting.*) Before we consider the role documentation plays in the medical-legal world, let's first consider for a moment how important the medical record is in the care and treatment of patients.

Communication tool

The medical record is the primary method of communication between members of the health care team. Oral report and rounding are essential communication devices, but it's impractical and unrealistic to expect that every health care team member be present during report or rounds. Such disciplines as physical therapy, occupational therapy, and respiratory therapy are rarely present for report or rounds. The myriad medical specialists available to the primary physician (infectious disease consultants, for example) are also rarely present during rounds, yet it's imperative for the delivery of good science-based care that every health care team member have the most current and up-to-date patient information. The medical record is the only way to accomplish this. It's available 24 hours per day to any practitioner who can utilize it to stay informed about the patient's progress.

Treatment evaluation and support

Documenting patient treatment outcomes and responses in the medical record is a key method for evaluating treatment modalities and therapies. The typical patient with pressure ulcers will undergo an extended course of treatment that will change over the course of time. In order to establish a basis for treatment and modification, there must be well-documented observations and evaluations of the patient. Upon initiation of treatment, careful observation and documentation of the patient's condition is critical in order to establish a baseline for initial treatment and care and to measure treatment against. Without a carefully documented record, treatment, evaluation, patient outcomes, and treatment modifications are impossible to justify—in court or at the bedside. (See *General documentation guidelines,* page 38.)

PRACTICE POINT

Accurate and complete patient outcomes and responses to treatment and care must be documented in the record, as they're the basis for care decisions and legal defense.

Legal aspects of wound documentation

Wound assessments are some of the most detailed and time-consuming documentation a health care provider will perform. Radiologists can view internal organs with a variety of internal imaging techniques and generate detailed, consistent reports. A wealth of laboratory values are also available to monitor internal organ system functions. Wounds, however, are not yet amenable to sophisticated imaging techniques and many accepted laboratory values cannot monitor their healing objectively. Wound assessment and documentation is still mostly a subjective, visual, pen-and-paper exercise that requires a good base of knowledge to perform accurately. Wound assessment and monitoring is typically left to the staff nurse or wound specialist. Wounds require an intricate, multi-faceted assessment of their many attributes. (See chapter 6, Wound assessment and documentation.) Different levels of knowledge among caregivers can result in inaccurate, inconsistent, and erroneous wound documentation. Multiple areas of documentation for wound issues can make quick access to this information difficult. Multiple wounds on one patient adds even more of a documentation burden. Such complexity can lead to inconsistent documentation—and treatment—and may leave a provider or facility open to legal liability.

The medical record serves several purposes. First and foremost it is a communication tool that allows real-time coordination of care by multiple disciplines. It also acts as a historical record to determine the efficacy of past interventions that guides future care. The medical record is also a factual record utilized in lawsuits to determine the quality of care rendered, the occurrence of physical harm, and other legal issues. (See *Red flags in documentation,* page 39.) Most state nursing and medical boards and federal regulatory agencies require "timely and accurate" documentation of findings in the medical record. Due to the wide range of specialty care areas and ever-changing rules, regulations, and laws, state and federal boards offer little guidance on *how* to meet this documentation

Effects of incomplete charting

What happens when charting is incomplete? In addition to providing a poor medical record of a patient's care to help jog the practitioner's memory if a lawsuit occurs, it can create other problems. Competent attorneys can create havoc when gaps exist in the record. Nothing makes proving the plaintiff's case easier than such gaps, especially near or around the time of the alleged malpractice if the claim revolves around a single incident. If the claim concerns a continuous or extended course of treatment, the absence of documentation related to treatment outcomes, observations, and the basis for the treatment is strong evidence of negligence. Where the record contains gaps, you can be certain that the plaintiff's attorney will be happy to suggest to a jury what happened during those undocumented times, and those suggestions won't be of benefit to the health care facility or the individual practitioner.

standard. It's left to the individual facility or provider to determine the appropriate standards. The absence of standards has resulted in a wide range of documentation practices.

The following recommendations are suggested by the authors to improve the consistency and documentation of care for pressure ulcers, acute and chronic wounds, or any other untoward event that occurs while a patient is under care. These recommendations are not designed to promulgate or establish a particular standard of care for wound documentation, but rather to make providers aware of the common difficulties that may occur with wound documentation and to propose solutions.

General documentation guidelines

Listed here are some general rules for documentation that serve your patient's needs and can help in the defense of a lawsuit.

- Be thorough—record the date and time for each entry.
- Be accurate—use units of measure instead of estimates (for example, "patient had a 6-oz cup of ice chips" instead of "patient had some ice chips").
- Be factual—think of yourself as a newspaper reporter and answer the following questions: who, what, when, where, why, and how.
- Be objective—record only the facts. Remember that you're communicating information that others will rely on. If your patient is to benefit from your professional training, judgment, and observational skills, your colleagues must have objective, factual information to rely upon.
- Write legibly—print if necessary.
- Only use approved abbreviations.
- Make contemporaneous entries—finish your documentation before you leave work for the day. Don't add notations days later unless your facility permits such additions—and even then, adhere strictly to your facility's policy governing such additions.
- Be truthful—don't fake, misrepresent, exaggerate, or misstate the facts in the medical record.
- Most importantly, don't assign blame. While it's important to relate the facts completely and accurately, assigning blame in the medical record is fodder for malpractice actions and does nothing to advance the care of your patients.

The flow of information

To find the latest laboratory value in a chart you go to the lab section. To find the latest chest X-ray result you go to the radiology section. To find the latest wound description you go to…? Wound documentation is often found scattered throughout the chart in activity of daily living (ADL) forms, nursing assessments, narrative notes, wound assessment forms, and many other sections. The organization and composition of the medical record in any given facility often evolves over the years with no real appreciation for how one would look at the chart globally. This is especially true of nursing documentation forms as they are added to and modified over time. In such situations duplication of information becomes increasingly common. Consistent documentation by nursing staff then becomes much more difficult to provide and to review at a later date.

In order to evaluate the effectiveness of the medical record as a communication tool, one should critically examine from an outsider's perspective just how information flows within the record. A medico-legal reviewer attempting to determine if care was accurately and consistently provided can sometimes be stymied by a poorly structured chart whose organization makes sense to the facility—yet to no one else. If information cannot be readily found it will often be ignored. If the appropriate form or the proper location in the chart cannot be easily found, certain information may not be documented. If wound care documentation can take place in multiple areas of the chart it may be documented multiple times—or not at all because of the uncertainty as to where the information should be properly entered. The medical record is a documentation system. If documentation is inconsistent , a systems approach may be applied in order to evaluate and improve the structure and flow of documentation, rather than actually getting staff to just "document more."

Admission assessment

Both the medical and nursing admission assessment provide a "snapshot" of the patient's status at the time of admission. The admission assessment is an area where one cannot over-document. The more informa-

Red flags in documentation

Certain elements in a medical record can serve as red flags that catch the attention of the plaintiff's attorney. When documenting information about the patient with a wound, try to avoid the following errors.

Findings that don't add up

Make sure the information you're documenting is as accurate as possible. Questions may be raised if the assessment findings don't logically support the resulting diagnosis. This list shows assessment findings that were documented for a patient with a stage III pressure ulcer on his coccyx; note that they don't lead one to believe that a stage III pressure ulcer should have developed.

- Braden score = 17 (mild risk)
- Ambulates well
- Bed-to-chair transfer with assistance
- Continent when on a toileting schedule
- Fair appetite
- Medical diagnoses: diet-controlled diabetes, hypertension, arthritis, benign prostatic hyperplasia

Documentation that's too good to be true

The second entry in this sample chart shows a dramatic, yet highly unlikely, improvement in the patient's ulcer, especially considering his rapid decompensation 5 days later. Describe wounds as accurately as possible. Read the previous notes so that you can precisely chart how the wound is progressing.

6/5/07 Stage IV pressure ulcer to sacrum, 6 x 7 cm, 3 cm deep, 4 cm tunneling at 8 o'clock, 65% necrotic tissue in base, foul-smelling gray drainage, alginate dressing QOD.

6/9/07 Sacrum ulcer improved, 2 x 2 x 1 cm, 100% granulation tissue, minimal serous drainage.

6/14/07 Unresponsive, BP 60/40, HR 156, Temp 102.4°F, MD called, Sent to ER.

Inconsistencies within the record

Documentation within the medical record should provide a consistent picture of the patient. As this example illustrates, three different forms in the record give three different pictures of the patient. Which is a jury to believe?

Monthly summary: Skin remains intact. Turned Q 2 hours while in bed. Up in chair for 1 hour Q day. Eating 75% to 100% of meals. Fed by staff. Hydration maintained.

Flow sheets: Turned every 4 to 6 hours. Eating 25% of meals. 7-lb weight loss in last month. Intake 500 to 700 cc per 24 hours.

Nurse's notes: Stage III ulcer on coccyx. Hydrocolloid intact. In chair 0900 to 1500 daily.

Courtesy of J. Cuddigan, PHD, RN, CWCN.

---

tion that's documented about the patient at the time of admission the better informed the health care team is, and thus decisions can be made based on the best information available. Discovery and description of any lesion during admission assessment is critical in determining the course of care and, in a lawsuit, the ultimate liability of any wounds that develop or deteriorate during the patient's stay. Preexisting lesions should be carefully and thoroughly documented as to size, loca-

tion, and characteristics. A detailed description of the wound is more important than an actual wound diagnosis during admission assessment. The chart should reflect what interventions were taken and who was notified of the existence of the wound and any other findings.

A general rule often heard in nursing and wound care circles is that any pressure ulcer that develops after 24 hours of admission is considered to be acquired at the facility rather than inherited. However, the definition of deep tissue injury (a deep tissue bruise under intact skin that may ultimately evolve to a full-thickness lesion), as established in 2005 by the National Pressure Ulcer Advisory Panel (NPUAP), makes this general rule difficult to defend. For example, the patient may be admitted with an inconspicuous looking bruise in the sacral area or other bony prominence that ultimately evolves into a full-thickness pressure ulcer. The process of tissue ischemia and necrosis can take several days to become visible to the naked eye when all that was observed and documented on admission was a sacral bruise. Therefore, nursing and medical staff should be made aware of this new NPUAP definition[2] and incorporate it into their assessments. (For more information, see chapter 13, Pressure ulcers).

Because pressure ulcers are a frequent reason for litigation in health care they will be highlighted as a key exemplar in the remainder of this chapter.

Pressure ulcer risk assessment

A pressure ulcer risk assessment can include any validated scale, such as the Braden or Norton scale. Risk scales are tools that quantify such risk factors associated with pressure ulcer development as nutrition, moisture and mobility, among others. A pressure ulcer risk assessment scale can provide detailed insight into the care needs of the patient far beyond skin protection. The frequency of risk assessment is open to debate and is primarily based on the guidelines or custom of the individual nursing unit.

Ideally, every patient admitted to a health care facility should have a risk assessment upon admission to identify individuals at risk for pressure ulcer development. Individuals at risk should then have routine follow-up assessments during their stay. A risk assessment is also recommended when the patient is transferred to another unit or whenever there is a significant change in the condition. The RN admission and daily assessment is a logical chart area in which to document risk assessment. The most important aspect with any risk assessment scale is: What is done with the information? Validated risk assessment tools are powerful and accurate predic-

tors of pressure ulcer development but are useless if the information they provide is not acted upon. Each risk factor is ideally suited as an individual plan to prevent, mitigate, or improve a decline in the level of functioning.

Pressure ulcer development

Sometimes the underlying problems that result in the development of pressure ulcer's can be managed, healed, or avoided altogether. In other instances the disease burden can be so great that they will occur or fail to heal despite the best of care. Indeed, CMS recognizes that pressure ulcers are unavoidable if the facility had 1) evaluated the resident's clinical condition and pressure ulcer risk factors, 2) defined and implemented interventions that are consistent with resident needs, goals, and recognized standards of practice, 3) monitored and evaluated the impact of the interventions, and 4) revised the approaches as appropriate.[3] Any documentation system regarding pressure ulcer prevention should be able to clearly and efficiently outline this criteria.

Nursing units where the disease burden of patients is extremely high include intensive care units (ICUs), long-term care units, and hospice. For ICU patients, frequent and consistent monitoring should be performed on the high-risk areas of the sacrum, heel and trochanter, and the occipital area. The authors frequently find in chart reviews that dynamic, pressure distributing mattresses are obtained *after* the development of a pressure ulcer. While this may be a logical and justifiable escalation of care and intervention for a general medical-surgical population, it's important that special emphasis be placed on these high-risk populations.

The infamous "Turn Q 2" check box

Many nursing patient-care flow sheets have "Turn Q 2" (turn every 2 hours) on their checklist of pressure ulcer prevention strategies. The presence or lack of a check in this box on these flow sheets is often used by attorneys to undermine or paint a negative picture of the quality and consistency of care delivered by nursing staff. The origins of the requirement to reposition patients every 2 hours for pressure ulcer prevention are obscure and not well-grounded in science. The 1994 Agency for Health Care Policy and Research (AHCPR) guidelines specifically recommended repositioning every 2 hours.[4] Such an absolute time requirement for repositioning or other interventions does not permit individual clinical judgment. Patient care should be based on the dynamic evaluation of a patient's status by qualified personnel and not a single, fixed point. Some patients may require more frequent repositioning, some less due the presence of a pressure-distributing mattress or the need for uninterrupted sleep. Some may be unable to turn due to critical illness. Some may have undergone diagnostic procedures, thereby precluding staff from attending to them every 2 hours. There are simply too many variables that determine when and how a patient is positioned to require a rigid timetable that likely bears little or no resemblance to the patient's actual needs..

The authors recommend removing the "Turn Q 2" check box from nursing forms, admission order templates, pressure ulcer prevention orders, and other areas. The check box could be replaced with a statement such as "reposition according to patient needs determined by pressure ulcer risk assessment" or some other language determined to better meet patient care needs and risk-management requirements for proper documentation. We note, however, that this more flexible standard requires a more rigorous approach to documentation of the actions taken by health care personnel. Many staff members are accustomed to the check-off system and may fail to adequately document interventions without such a system. Management should consider training and monitoring to assure compliance with documentation standards. This new method connects the risk assessment to the intervention and allows much more flexibility for staff to deliver timely and effective care rather than basing care on a single number.

Discovery of a pressure ulcer

The initial discovery of a pressure ulcer is typically documented in the nursing narrative note section. Any ongoing assessments (and actions, including notification of appropriate medical personnel) should then be documented per facility policy in a wound care form, ADL form or narrative notes, but preferably in just one place in the chart for easy access. The response to the discovery of the lesion is just as critical as documenting the lesion itself. Documentation should include: what immediate interventions were taken; who was notified (the charge nurse, the oncoming staff, the physician, the wound care specialist, or the family); what topical care was provided to the lesion (ointments or creams, hydrocolloids or other dressings); actions that were taken to minimize further damage (an air mattress, heel suspension boots, lowering the head of bed, repositioning, and other interventions). Such documentation demonstrates that your facility has a system in place to act quickly and appropriately to changes in the patient's condition.

Correct identification of the lesion

The etiology of the lesion must be correctly identified in order to provide the most appropriate and effective care. Examine the wound for yourself, review the patient's medical history, make your own judgment, and if it differs with others discuss your concerns with the team. When in doubt about the etiology or progress of a wound don't make a speculation in the chart, just document what you observed. Remember, objective description beats subjective guessing every time.

Differentiating between a pressure ulcer or ischemic ulcer in the lower extremity can be particularly difficult. For example, is the development a wound on the lateral aspect of the foot in a person with peripheral vascular disease the result of pressure or arterial insufficiency? The argument could be that "but for" the pressure, the lesion would not have occurred. The counterargument could be that "but for" the arterial insufficiency, the tissue could have easily tolerated the pressure exerted on the foot. Objective data is required to solve this dispute. In this case, formal vascular laboratory studies are needed to determine the extent of ischemia and the avoidability of such lesions. Most chronic wounds have distinctive locations, sizes, and presentations and can be easily differentiated by trained personnel. However, some wounds will defy easy categorization or diagnosis. All lesions require as much objective data as possible to establish the correct diagnosis and appropriate care plan.

Notification and participation of the physician

The patient's primary physician must be notified of any untoward event in a timely manner, including development of a pressure ulcer or other wounds. Good practice requires documentation of when the physician was notified, the response to the notification, any orders given, and the plan for examination and follow-up. Physicians must also meet the standard care (what a reasonable and prudent provider would do in a same or similar situation) when managing a patient's wound. In facilities with an active wound care department the routine management of the lesion is often handed to staff by the primary physician. The physician typically signs verbal orders that are written by these specialties. This allows interdisciplinary care, and provides maximum potential to heal or mitigate the wound. This does not, however, relieve the physician of the responsibility to monitor the condition of the wound.

Physicians should arrange to examine the wound on a routine basis, have a good understanding of the rationale behind the wound care orders being signed, and be involved in consulting other specialties as needed to maximize healing. Physicians should take the lead in notifying the patient's family about the development of any lesion, just as they would any other negative event that occurred under their care. Pressure ulcers are symptoms of underlying medical, physical, and psychosocial problems. They are therefore a multidisciplinary issue involving nursing, nutrition, social work, physical therapy—and medicine— among many other specialties.

Notifying the patient and family

Prompt and thorough notification of the patient and family of any new wound or other adverse event is critical to ensure full understanding and participation in care. Full disclosure of all facts related to the development of the wound should be provided: When was it discovered? How was it discovered? What interventions were being taken to prevent the wound? What interventions are being taken now? Give plenty of time for the information to be absorbed and allow for questions.

Many in the lay community believe that pressure ulcers or "bedsores" are the result of negligence. An initial negative reaction to an adverse event is to be expected, but prompt and full disclosure of the situation will go a long way toward minimizing lingering doubts and suspicions about the adequacy of care in your facility. When discussing the situation with the patient and family use explanations, not excuses. While the patient's health status may have played a significant role in the development of the adverse event (for example, a pressure ulcer, dehisced surgical incision, or other chronic wound) it is probably best not to dwell on this topic initially as it may be interpreted by family members as "blaming the patient." Follow-up conversations and briefings with the patient and family may serve as a better time to discuss the realistic goals of healing, once they digest the initial information and the effects of the care plan are better known.

The patient and family should also be educated that new wounds, especially pressure ulcers, are likely to look worse before they look better. A deep tissue injury (DTI) may look rather innocent to the family as a simple deep bruise with maybe a little torn skin. The DTI may evolve through a course that can include tissue ischemia, tissue necrosis, necrotic tissue separation (sloughing), and even ultimate cavitation or ulceration. Lay persons could easily and incorrectly construe such a change in the wound as substandard care. Advance preparation and setting expectations will reduce the shock of seeing a wound go through this natural process. Any conversations with family members and their response to the information should be promptly documented.

Ongoing wound documentation

Wound documentation places a significant burden on the health care provider due to the intricate nature of wound assessments. One way to ease this burden is to use logical, well-structured wound documentation forms or computer templates. Check boxes or drop-down lists are recommended for efficient documentation and to limit erroneous entries. Wound assessment forms can be structured in many different ways and will almost always improve the accuracy and consistency of documentation. Such forms can be created easily with word-processing or spreadsheet software. A glossary of terms should also be developed for the more obscure terminology used on the wound care form. Drop-down menus, forms, and check boxes however, are no substitute for narrative nursing assessments when required, and space must be provided in the medical record for such notes as needed.

Frequency of assessment will depend on the wound type, its phase of healing, the resources available to the wound care specialist, and other factors. CMS recommends a weekly thorough assessment with daily monitoring of the dressing and wound to assess for complications in long-term care patients.[3] Weekly assessments by a wound specialist allow subtle changes to be noticed that would ordinarily be missed with more frequent inspection. Daily monitoring can be noted in either the narrative notes, treatment sheets, or on a wound assessment form per facility policy, but preferably in just one location for ease of reference. Wound documentation should be consistent and concise. Frequent brief, but thorough, notes indicate consistent care.

Wound photography...or wound imaging?

Wound photography has become more popular with the advent of inexpensive, quality digital cameras. Two national organizations have positions statements about the use of wound photography in wound care.[5,6] What is the rationale behind wound photography? Is it for assessment and diagnosis or just an attempt to mitigate legal liability? Consider *wound imaging* as an assessment and diagnostic tool just like an X-ray or magnetic resonance imaging (MRI). If thought of in this manner, wound imaging might be obtained routinely and consistently (per your facility policy and procedure) as with any other assessment and diagnostic imaging. A series of

wound images will allow for more efficient and informed interventions and may assist in a legal defense should one become necessary. This regular, methodical approach is in contrast to taking one or two photographs during an inpatient stay to "cover ourselves legally"; taking this approach often backfires. What would any individual, and especially a juror, react more positively to: A series of detailed photographs showing progress of the wound or one or two photographs taken at odd intervals throughout the patient's stay? One reveals consistency; the other does not.

Wound imaging supplements—but does not replace—the need for written documentation. Each image should have accompanying text discussing what is observed in the photograph. This is similar to obtaining a radiologist report after medical imaging. Consent for non-invasive medical imaging is rarely required and the same should also be true for wound imaging as long as the patient cannot be readily identified. Management should clear the consent issue with legal counsel and risk managers.

Collaboration, coordination, and communication

Collaboration, coordination, and communication of all specialty services is essential in maximizing the potential for wound healing. Documentation of "the three Cs" may also demonstrate to the medico-legal expert—and ultimately to a jury—that coordinated, interdisciplinary care was provided consistently. Most facilities with a wound care team have policies that specify consultation for certain types of lesions. Many Wound, Ostomy, and Continence (WOC) nurses provide both consult services and hands-on care at their facility. If the WOC nurse acts in a consultant role she should examine how consults by other facility services are structured and document in a similar manner. Consultants not only provide recommendations or establish a care plan but they also educate other providers on their specialty and the rationale for their recommendations.

Wound care services are also provided by physical therapist in many facilities. As with WOC nurses, consults ideally should be based on the format at their facility and include a care plan and follow-up. Adequate follow-up by either a WOC or staff nurses should be ensured prior to the patient being discharged from physical therapy services. In addition, consults to plastic surgery, vascular surgery, or other surgical specialties are also part of interdisciplinary care. Because there are wide variations in approaches to chronic wound care by these specialties, disagreements can arise. Therefore, consistent documentation of communication among the specialties will resolve any differences and is an indicator of quality, interdisciplinary care.

Policies and procedures: normative or positive?

Policies and procedures (P&Ps) establish standards of care within the facility. In any legal proceeding, P&Ps will be scrutinized and compared to the care that is documented in the chart. P&Ps are typically divided into two types of philosophies: normative and positive. A normative P&P describes what care *can* realistically and consistently be provided. A positive P&P describes what care *should* ideally be provided. P&Ps with a positive, ideal focus can cause great trouble in legal proceedings because they set unrealistic and unattainable goals that often exceed a reasonable standard of care.[7]

When establishing P&Ps in your facility, avoid using absolute terms like "will" and "must" and specifying exact time frames for routine nursing interventions unless absolutely necessary. For example, a P&P that states "All patients will have a Braden PU Risk Assessment every Tuesday and Friday" sets an unrealistic expectation. By missing 1 day or doing the assessment on a Saturday is a violation of your own standard of care. Rewording the P&P to read "All bedfast or chairfast patients should have a Braden PU Risk Assessment twice a week" gives nursing staff more leeway in their care and documentation. In a lawsuit, "violations" of P&Ps are not always a liability in the defense of such actions. Departures that are explained by and supported by science-based care—and that are fully and completely documented contemporaneously—can often be used to the advantage of the defense. Sometimes P&Ps must spell out exactly when and where something will or must be done, but mostly they should focus on guiding and educating staff members rather than enforcing strict rules and timelines for care.

Pressure ulcer prevention and treatment[4] practices have undergone significant revisions and changes since the first AHCPR guidelines were released 13 years ago. Guidelines from the Wound, Ostomy and Continence Nurses Society (WOCN) in 2003 and CMS in 2004 incorporate the latest research and recommendations.[3,8] The CMS guidelines in particular are thorough, complete and easy to read by a wider range of health care providers. While developed for long-term care, they are easily adaptable to acute care and other settings and provide comprehensive education and guidance while avoiding "absolute" terminology. Incorporation of these WOCN or CMS guidelines into your P&Ps indicates that your facility is up-to-date on the latest changes that impact pressure ulcer care. In addition to these guidelines, P&Ps should also include new information from seminars or studies or new types of dressings and therapies, without having to extensively revise a policy or procedure.

Discharge—to home or another facility

The patient and caregiver should have adequate resources to manage the wound upon discharge to the home or another facility.[7] Documentation of this coordination should include teaching strategies and the patient/caregiver response to them, consults to social work or home care, and any equipment or supplies sent home with the patient. Ensure the patient has adequate follow-up for medical and wound issues.

The discharge assessment should be a thorough and complete "snapshot" of the patient before leaving your facility. As with the admission assessment, you cannot over-document in this area. Thoroughly assess and document any wounds and the condition of high-risk pressure ulcer areas. Document any communication with the receiving facility. Alert the receiving facility to any wounds and describe them in detail. The medical discharge summary typically does not go into significant detail about wound therapy, and thus the onus for this communication is placed on nursing. List all previous and current wound therapies, which will avoid wasted time in trying therapies that have already yielded little or no results. List all previous and current preventative measures and equipment, for example, air mattresses, seat cushions, and heel protectors.

Summary

The patient's chart is an important legal document because it provides the written record of the care provided. It also serves as a means of communication among health care professionals about the patient's responses to care. Completeness and accuracy of documentation is essential not only for good patient care but is the basis for mounting a defense in the event of legal action. Make your entries in the patient's record legible, thorough, professional, and factual. Ensure that all information is correct and accurate.

Consistent documentation is a reflection of the quality, interdisciplinary care provided to an individual. Chronic wounds are often symptoms of many underlying medical, physical, and psychosocial problems. Documentation of these multiple issues requires a well-structured documentation system. Ensure your documentation system allows health care providers to consistently and concisely communicate and access their findings. Policies and procedures should be updated as new research and practices appear. The documentation system should incorporate and reflect these new practices. Such interventions will maximize communication among the interdisciplinary team and help to improve patient outcomes.[7]

Show what you know

1. *In a medical malpractice trial, what's the role of the jury and the judge?*

   A. Interpreter of the law; finder of fact
   B. Finder of fact; finder of fact and interpreter of the law
   C. Finder of fact; interpreter of the law
   D. Both judge and jury find fact and interpret the law

ANSWER: C. The jury determines who, what, when, why, where, and how—in other words, what happened. The judge interprets the law by instructing the jury about the law to be applied to the facts as it has determined them. The other options are incorrect.

2. *At trial, how many of the four elements of a medical malpractice claim must a defendant convince a jury that the plaintiff has failed to prove in order to successfully defend against a claim of medical malpractice?*

   A. One
   B. Two
   C. Three
   D. Four

ANSWER: D. The plaintiff must prove all four elements in order to prevail at trial.

3. *The medical record is:*

   A. a communication tool.
   B. destroyed after 1 year.
   C. a tool to communicate opinions related to a patient's care.
   D. an optional part of health care.

ANSWER A. Opinions related to patient care aren't proper entries in a medical record. The medical record is a communication tool between practitioners, and is best used for the transmittal of factual information. The other options are incorrect.

4. *Which one of the following statements about standards of care, practice guidelines, and policies and procedures is FALSE?*

   A. They should be reviewed at regular intervals but never amended.
   B. They should be reviewed at regular intervals and amended to reflect new information and research.
   C. They should be based on research and practice experience.
   D. They should be patient-outcome oriented and quantifiable.

ANSWER: A. Standards must be reviewed and amended to reflect the latest research and practice experience in a treatment area. Standards based on practice experience only and not supported by research may not survive judicial scrutiny at trial, and don't offer the patient the best care.

5. *Given the new definition and understanding of deep tissue injury (DTI) from NPUAP, a deep bruise looking area on an immobile patient's sacrum that was not documented on admission but appears 24 hours later would:*

   A. be classified as an acute medical wound.
   B. be documented as a stage IV pressure ulcer.
   C. have occurred prior to admission.
   D. be documented as a stage III pressure ulcer.

ANSWER: C. DTI damage may occur days before it is visibility evident on the patient. The other options are incorrect.

6. *Which one of the following exemplifies the best way to document frequency of turning a patient in the medical record?*

A. A 2-hour check box
B. Regular turning q 2 hour
C. Q 4-hour turning
D. Individualized turning schedule based on patient assessment q 4-hour turning

ANSWER: D. An individualized turning schedule based on patient assessment q 4-hour turning is the best way to document the frequency of turning in the medical record. The other options are incorrect because they are rigid and inflexible and do not allow for individualized patient care. Too many variables can impact repositioning to mandate an absolute time frame for all patients.

7. *Normative policies and procedures describe care that can be:*

A. realistically and consistently provided.
B. used for normal staffing situations only.
C. ideally strived for.
D. exceeded to achieve magnet status.

ANSWER: A. Normative policies and procedures describe care that can be realistically and consistently provided. The other options are incorrect. Answer B is the definition of a positive P&P; C, policies are not based on staffing ratios; and D, has nothing to do with normative policies.

References

1. *Black's Law Dictionary*, 5th ed. New York: West Publishing Company, 1979.
2. *2007 Pressure Ulcer Staging Definition.* www.npuap.org. Accessed May 2007.
3. Centers for Medicare and Medicaid Services (CMS) Tag F-314. *Pressure Ulcers. Revised guidance for surveyors in long term care.* Issued November 12, 2004. Available at: http// new.cms.hhs.gov/manuals/download/som107ap_pp_guidelines_ltcf.pdf. Accessed December 2006.
4. Bergstrom, N., et al. *Treatment of Pressure Ulcers.* Clinical Practice Guideline. No. 15 AHCPR No. 95-0652. Rockville, MD: Agency for Health Care Policy and Research; December 1994.
5. National Pressure Ulcer Advisory Panel Photography FAQ. Available at http://www.npuap.org. DOCS/PhotographyFaq.doc. Accessed December 2006.
6. Wound, Ostomy and Continence Nurses Society. Professional Practice Series. Photography in Wound Documentation. Available at http://www.wocn.org/publication/posstate/pdf/photo position.pdf. Accessed December 2006.
7. Brown, G. "Wound Documentation: Managing Risk," *Adv Skin Wound Care* 19(3):155-65, March 2006.
8. Wound Ostomy and Continence Nurses Society. Guideline for Prevention and Management of Pressure Ulcers. Glenview, IL. Wound Ostomy and Continence Nurses Society, Vol 2. 2003.

CHAPTER 4

Skin: An essential organ

Sharon Baranoski, MSN, RN, CWOCN, DAPWCA, APN
Elizabeth Ayello, PhD, RN, APNBC, CWOCN, FAPWCA, FAAN
Marjana Tomic-Canic, PhD, RN

OBJECTIVES

After completing this chapter, you'll be able to:

- discuss the different layers of the skin

- state the functions of the skin

- list skin changes associated with the aging process

- differentiate between a skin and wound assessment

- describe risk factors and treatments for skin tears

- identify and classify common skin conditions.

Skin anatomy and physiology

Human skin is composed of two distinct layers: the epidermis, the outermost layer; and the dermis, the innermost layer. (See *Layers of the skin,* page 48.) The dermal-epidermal junction, commonly referred to as the basement membrane zone (BMZ), separates the two layers. Under the dermis lies a layer of loose connective tissue, called subcutaneous tissue, or hypodermis. (See *Skin layer functions,* page 49.)

The epidermis is a thin, avascular layer that regenerates itself every 4 to 6 weeks. It's divided into four layers or strata (presented in order from the outermost layer inward). (See *Layers of the epidermis,* page 50.)

- *Stratum corneum*—consists of dead keratinocyte cells; flakes and sheds; is easily removed during bathing activities and more efficiently by scrubbing the surface of the skin.
- *Stratum granulosum*—also contains Langerhans cells in addition to keratinocytes.[1]
- *Stratum spinosum*—contains keratinocytes and Langerhans cells.
- *Stratum basale or germinativum*—single layer of epidermal cells (keratinocytes); contains melanocytes; can regenerate.

A fifth layer, the *stratum lucidum,* lies between the stratum corneum and the stratum granulosum. This packed translucent line of cells is found only on the palms and soles and not seen in thin skin.

The epidermis is composed of keratinocyte cells. Basal keratinocytes (stratum basale) have the capacity to divide, giving rise to

Layers of the skin

Two distinct layers of skin, the epidermis and dermis, lie above a layer of subcutaneous fatty tissue (also called the hypodermis). The dermal-epidermal junction (also called the basement membrane zone) lies between the dermis and epidermis.

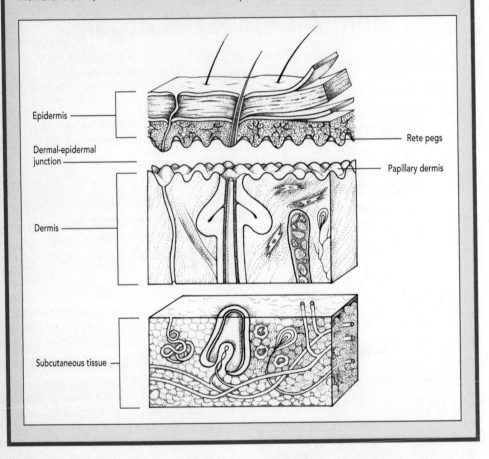

Epidermis

Dermal-epidermal junction

Dermis

Subcutaneous tissue

Rete pegs

Papillary dermis

suprabasal layers of epidermis. Once basal keratinocytes leave the stratum basale, they start the process of differentiation, during which they die. This process involves making insoluble proteins and their crosslink which, along with lipids and membrane components, form the insoluble, horny stratum corneum layer.[2,3,4,5] In order to maintain the barrier, keratinocytes have the capacity to completely regenerate the epidermis. If damaged (such as wounded, burned, exposed to UV light or chemicals) keratinocytes, in order to repair the damage, change their biology. Instead of differentiating, they become "activated," and start to divide rapidly and, in the case of a wound, they migrate over the gap to repair the damage.[3] They also signal to other neighboring cell types, such as fibroblasts, Langerhans cells, and melanocytes, that the skin barrier is compromised and that they're needed to help repair the damage. Once the damage is repaired, the keratinocytes cease their activation and resume their normal differentiation process.[6]

The BMZ divides the epidermis from the dermis. It contains fibronectin (an adhesive glycoprotein), type IV collagen (a nonfiber forming collagen), heparin sulfate proteogly-

Skin layer functions

The chart below shows characteristics and general functions of each layer of the skin.

Skin layer	Characteristics	General function
Epidermis	• Outer layer of skin • Consists of five layers (or strata): corneum, lucidum, granulosum, spinosum, and basale (or germinativum) • Repairs and regenerates itself every 28 days	• Protective barrier • Organization of cell content • Synthesis of vitamin D and cytokines • Division and mobilization of cells • Maintaining contact with dermis • Pigmentation (contains melanocytes) • Allergen recognition (contains Langerhans cells) • Differentiates into hair, nails, sweat glands, and sebaceous glands
Dermis	• Consists of two layers—papillary dermis and reticular dermis—composed of collagen, reticulum, and elastin fibers • Contains a network of nerve endings, blood vessels, lymphatics, capillaries, sweat and sebaceous glands, and hair follicles	• Supports structure • Mechanical strength • Supplies nutrition • Resists shearing forces • Inflammatory response
Subcutaneous tissue (hypodermis)	• Composed of adipose and connective tissue • Contains major blood vessels, nerves, and lymphatic vessels	• Attaches to underlying structure • Thermal insulation • Storage of calories (energy) • Controls body shape • Mechanical "shock absorber"

can, and glycosaminoglycan.[7] The BMZ has an irregular surface—called rete ridges or pegs—projecting downward from the epidermis that interlocks with the upward projections of the dermis. The two interlocking sides resemble the two sides of a waffle iron coming together. This structure anchors the epidermis to the dermis, preventing it from sliding back and forth. As skin ages, the basement membrane flattens, and the area of contact between the epidermis and dermis is decreased by 50%, thus increasing the risk of skin injury by traumatic, accidental separation of the epidermis from the dermis. (See *Effects of aging on the BMZ,* page 50.)

The dermis is an essential part of the skin and is commonly referred to as the "true skin."[8] As the second layer, it's the thickest layer and is composed of many cells. The major proteins found in this layer are collagen and elastin, which are synthesized and secreted by fibroblasts; collagen forms up to 30% of the volume or 70% of the dry weight of the dermis.[7-9] The dermis is a matrix that serves to support the epidermis. It's divided into two areas, the papillary dermis and the reticular dermis.[7]

• The *papillary dermis* is composed of collagen and reticular fibers. Its distinct, unique pattern allows fingerprint identification for each individual. It contains capillaries for skin nourishment and pain touch receptors (pacinian corpuscles and Meissner's corpuscles).

• The *reticular dermis* is composed of collagen bundles that anchor the skin to the subcutaneous tissue. Sweat glands, hair follicles,

Layers of the epidermis

The epidermis consists of five layers, as illustrated below.

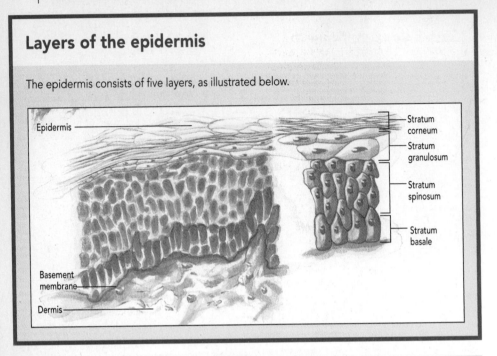

Epidermis

Stratum corneum

Stratum granulosum

Stratum spinosum

Stratum basale

Basement membrane

Dermis

Effects of aging on the BMZ

The illustrations below show the effects of aging on the basement membrane zone (BMZ). Specifically, the basement membrane flattens, reducing the area of contact between the epidermis and the dermis by 50%.

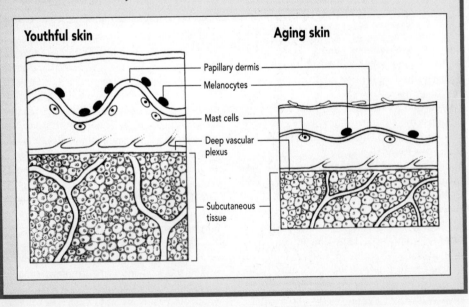

Youthful skin

Aging skin

Papillary dermis

Melanocytes

Mast cells

Deep vascular plexus

Subcutaneous tissue

nerves, and blood vessels can be found in this layer.

The main function of the dermis is to provide tensile strength, support, moisture retention, and blood and oxygen to the skin.[8] It protects the underlying muscles, bones, and organs. The dermis also contains the sebaceous glands that secrete sebum, a substance rich in oil that lubricates the skin. Furthermore, it also contains hair follicles that are the source of multipotent stem cells, which have the capacity to restore the epidermis.[6]

The subcutaneous tissue, or hypodermis, attaches the dermis to underlying structures. Its function is to promote an ongoing blood supply to the dermis for regeneration. It's primarily composed of adipose tissue, which provides a cushion between skin layers, muscles, and bones. It promotes skin mobility, molds body contours, and insulates the body.

Skin function

Skin is an important organ whose diverse functions are not always appreciated. (See *Skin functions.*) The largest external organ, the skin weighs, in adults, between 6 and 8 lb (2.7 to 3.6 kg) and covers over 20 ft^2 (1.9 m^2). Skin thickness varies from 0.5 mm to 6 mm according to its location on the body; for example, skin can be as thin as $\frac{1}{50}''$ on the eyelids and as thick as $\frac{1}{3}''$ on the palms and soles, where greater protection is needed. The skin receives one-third of the body's circulating blood volume—an oversupply of blood compared to its metabolic needs.

The normal range of skin pH is 4 to 6.5 in healthy people.[10,11] This "acid mantle" helps to maintain a normal skin flora by serving as a protective barrier against bacterial and fungal infections. It also supports the formation and maturation of epidermal lipids and assists in maintaining their protective barrier function. The acid mantle also provides indirect protection against invasion by microorganisms and protection against alkaline substances.[10] If the acid mantle loses its acidity, the skin becomes more prone to damage and infection. Frequent use of soap products and overwashing can alter the stratum corneum and its ability to serve as a protective barrier. Alternatively, several skin conditions can *increase* the skin's surface pH, including eczema, contact dermatitis, atopic dermatitis, and dry skin.[12,13] Systemic diseases may also increase the skin's surface pH, such as in diabetes, chronic renal failure, and cerebrovascular disease.[14]

The skin's major functions are protection, sensation, thermoregulation, excretion, metabolism, and communication.[15] Skin protects the body by serving as a barrier from invasion by organisms such as bacteria. Because staphylococcal species (such as *Staphylococcus aureus* or *Staphylococcus epidermis*) tolerate salt, they are present in large numbers as resident bacteria on the skin.[15,16] Another organism found on the skin is yeast, which is commonly found on the trunk and ears and as fungus between the toes.[15,16] In addition, skin makes its own antimicrobial peptides called defensins.[17,18]

Sensation is a key function of the skin. Areas that are most sensitive to touch have a greater number of nerve endings.[16] These include the lips, nipples, and fingertips. In humans, the fingertips are the most sensitive touch organ and enable us to correctly identify objects by touch (stereognosis) rather than by sight. Many tactile corpuscles lie at the base of hair follicles, and shaving reduces the tactile sensibility of that skin area. In hairless body regions, the tactile corpuscles are called Meissner's corpuscles.[16] Pleasurable, firm touching sensations, such as from a massage or hugs of affection, are transmitted via the

Skin functions

Functions of the skin include:
- protection from:
  - fluid and electrolyte loss
  - mechanical injury
  - ultraviolet injury
  - pathogens
- temperature regulation
- fluid and electrolyte balance
- metabolism
- sensation
- synthesis
- communication.

skin as they generate nerve transmissions through these tactile corpuscles.

Itch is one of the alarm sensations of the skin and serves as a defense mechanism. Chemicals that are released after skin injury may promote the inflammatory process and can also induce itch or pain. Itch and pain are in close regulatory relationship—for example, central pain inhibition may enhance the act of itching, while also inhibiting the act of itching.[19]

Somatic pain (from the outer body surfaces and framework) is also communicated through the skin. Superficial (acute) pain to a local area is usually transmitted by very rapid nerve impulses by A-delta fibers[16] and tends to be sharp, but ceases when the pain stimulus stops. Deep (chronic) pain impulses are transmitted slowly over the smaller, thinly myelinated C fibers. In contrast, this type of pain tends to spread over a more diffuse area, lasts for longer periods of time, and remains even after the pain stimulus is gone.[16] As a sign of possible skin injury, pressure also serves as a protective warning sensation.

Temperature regulation and fluid and electrolyte balance are achieved in part by the skin. Thermoregulation is controlled by the hypothalamus in response to internal core body temperature. Peripheral temperature receptors in the skin assist in this process called *temperature homeostasis*.[20] By losing a copious amount of water—for example, sweating—through the skin, lungs, and buccal mucosa, homeostasis of body temperature is maintained. Skin temperature is controlled by the dilatation or constriction of skin blood vessels. When body core temperature rises, the body will attempt to reduce its temperature by releasing heat from the skin. This is accomplished by sending a chemical signal to increase blood flow in the skin from vasodilation, thus increasing skin temperature.

PRACTICE POINT

Increased temperature → Skin blood vessel vasodilation → Heat loss from epidermis → Body maintains temperature homeostasis.

In contrast, the opposite occurs when the body's core temperature is reduced; the chemical signal causes decreased blood flow from vasoconstriction, thus lowering the skin's temperature.[20,21]

PRACTICE POINT

Decreased temperature → Skin blood vessel vasoconstriction → Heat conservation → Body maintains temperature homeostasis.

The skin also aids in the excretion of end products of cell metabolism and prevents excessive loss of fluid. Other important functions of the skin include its manufacturing ability and immune functions.[22] For example, when exposed to ultraviolet light, the skin can synthesize vitamin D.[23] And, although the skin's hypersensitivity responses in allergic reactions are commonly seen, the skin's role in immune function isn't always fully appreciated. Indeed, Langerhans cells and tissue macrophages, which play an important role in digesting bacteria, as well as mast cells, which are needed to provide proper immune system functioning, are all present in the skin.[1,7,15]

Skin integrity and aging skin

Alteration in skin integrity is a clinical practice issue in every continuum of care. Because normal skin changes occur with aging, elderly people are especially vulnerable to alterations in skin integrity.[24] (See *Hallmarks of aging skin*.) As skin ages, the epidermis gradually thins. The dermal-epidermal junction flattens and dermal papillae and epidermal rete pegs are effaced, making the skin more susceptible to mild mechanical trauma. Decreases in the number of sweat glands and their output explains some of the dry skin seen in elderly people.[25] The ability to retain moisture is decreased in aging skin due to diminished amounts of dermal proteins, which causes oncotic pressure shifts and diminished fluid homeostasis, thereby putting elderly patients at risk for dehydration. Because soap increases the skin's pH to an alkaline level, using emollient soap and bathing every other day, instead of every day, can decrease the incidence of skin injury, such as skin tears, in elderly patients.[10]

An elderly person's skin is more easily stretched due to a decrease in elastin fibers.[25] Because of the thinning of the epidermal layer, the skin becomes a less-effective barrier against water loss, bruising, and infection, accompanied by impaired thermal regulation, decreased tactile sensitivity, and decreased pain perception.[25-27] Due to a decreased amount of dermal proteins, the blood vessels become thinner and more fragile, thereby leading to a type of hemorrhaging known as senile purpura. According to Selden and colleagues,[28] the pathophysiology of skin tears parallels that of senile purpura.

Age-related changes in the dermis are numerous, but the most striking is the approximately 20% loss in dermal thickness that probably accounts for the paper-thin appearance of aging skin.[25] This decrease in dermal cells and proportional reduction in collagen fibers, blood vessels, nerve endings, and collagen leads to altered or reduced sensation, thermoregulation, rigidity, moisture retention, and sagging skin. The decrease of differentiation and formation of the stratum corneum is also detected in aging skin. However, in spite of age-related skin changes, elderly patients usually heal sufficiently after injury.

The subcutaneous fat below the dermis consists primarily of adipose tissue and provides mechanical protection and insulation. Its loss during aging results in parallel reductions in these protective functions. Subcutaneous tissue undergoes site-specific atrophy in such areas as the face, dorsal aspect of the hands, shins, and plantar aspects of the foot, increasing the energy absorbed by the skin when trauma occurs to these areas.[28] A decrease in pain perception may make elderly people more vulnerable to traumatic environmental insults such as wearing tight shoes, stepping on an object, or hitting legs on the side of a chair. Aging skin is also less able to manufacture vitamin D when exposed to ultraviolet sunlight.[25] The number of Langerhans cells and mast cells diminishes in aging skin, translating into decreased immune function.[25,28]

Medications also have adverse affects on the skin's immune function. For example, steroids cause a thinning of the epidermis.[29]

Hallmarks of aging skin

The following changes in skin can occur due to the normal aging process.

Decreased
- Dermal thickness, causing thinning of the skin (especially over the legs and forearms)
- Fatty layers (leaving the bony prominences less protected)
- Collagen and elastin fibers (leaving the elastin unable to recoil)
- Size of rete ridges (making the basement membrane flatter, which allows the epidermis and dermis to separate more easily, increasing the risk for injury such as a skin tear)
- Sensation and metabolism
- Sweat glands (leading to dry skin)
- Subcutaneous tissue (leading to less padded protection over bony prominences)
- Circulation (leaving the elderly patient more prone to heat stroke)

Increased
- Time for epidermal regeneration (leading to slower healing)
- Damage to skin from the sun

Skin assessment vs. wound assessment

Although not always given the priority in clinical practice, the skin or integumentary system should be part of the routine head-to-toe assessment of all patients.[30] A skin assessment should include an actual observation of the entire body. It differs from a wound assessment in that a skin assessment looks at the patient's entire body and not just open wounds.

Lacking consensus in the literature as to what constitutes a minimal skin assessment, the Centers for Medicare and Medicaid Services nevertheless recommend the following five parameters as a minimal skin assessment in long-term care settings: temperature,

Elements of a basic skin assessment

To perform a basic skin assessment you must, at a minimum, assess its temperature, color, moisture, turgor, and integrity.

Temperature
- Normally warm to the touch
- Warmer than normal could signal inflammation
- Cooler than normal could signal poor vascularization

Color
- Intensity: paleness may be an indicator of poor circulation
- Normal color tones: light ivory to deep brown, yellow to olive, or light pink to dark, ruddy pink
- Hyperpigmentation or hypopigmentation reflect variations in melanin deposits or blood flow

Moisture
- Dry or moist to touch
- Hyperkeratosis (flaking, scales)
- Eczema (endogenous or exogenous)
- Dermatitis, psoriasis, rashes
- Edema

Turgor
- Normally returns to its original state quickly
- Slow return to its original shape (dehydration or effect of aging)

Integrity
- No open areas
- Type of skin injury (Use the appropriate classification system to identify and record injury type.)

color, moisture, turgor, and intact skin or presence of open areas.[31,32,33] (See *Elements of a basic skin assessment*.) However, some patients may require more comprehensive as-sessment, which would include looking for and documenting any lesions, scars, bruising, or hemosiderin deposits. (See *Elements of a comprehensive skin assessment*.)

Once skin integrity is lost and the epidermis is no longer intact, a thorough wound assessment with documentation is required. (See chapter 6, Wound assessment and documentation, for more information.) The first step is to identify the type or etiology of the wounded skin—for example, differentiate a skin tear from a pressure ulcer. Next, a wound assessment should minimally describe the following characteristics: location, size, exudate, and type of tissue. Remember the phrase frequently heard in wound care, "Look at the whole patient, not just the hole in the patient."

Implications for practice

Alterations in skin integrity, perhaps due to skin trauma or other skin conditions, may cause undue pain and suffering to patients. Health care professionals should have up-to-date information about prevention techniques, the appropriate use of dressings and tapes and, most importantly, the prevention of skin integrity injuries.

Skin trauma
Skin tears

Skin tears, sometimes called *skin* or *epidermal skin stripping injuries*, are a clinical challenge, especially among older patients.[34] A skin tear is a traumatic wound occurring principally on the extremities of older adults. Skin tears are a result of friction alone or shearing and friction forces that separate the epidermis from the dermis (partial-thickness wound) or that separate both the epidermis and the dermis from underlying structures (full-thickness wound).[35]

Maintaining skin integrity in patients who have frail skin first requires awareness of the severity of the problem. In addition, in the case of injury and tear, documenting and reporting such occurrences is of utmost importance and may save lives because early detection halts progression. The friction and shear

Elements of a comprehensive skin assessment

Consider the following criteria when performing a comprehensive skin assessment.

Inspection
- Normally smooth, slightly moist, and same general tone throughout
- Tone depends on patient's melanocytes—skin pigmentation continuum can vary from light ivory, deep brown, black, yellow to olive, light pink to dark ruddy pink, or red
- Pigmentation can exhibit:
  - pallor: mucosa, conjunctivae
  - cyanosis: nail beds, conjunctivae, oral mucosa
  - jaundice: sclerae, palate, palms
  - hyperpigmentation: increased (Results from variation in melanin deposits or blood flow; palpate for skin temperature and for edema over these areas to assess circulation.)
  - hypopigmentation: decreased vascular/venous patterns, usually symmetric
  - scars and bruises for location, color, length, and width

Palpation
- Moisture: perspiration
- Edema: extremities, sacrum, eyes
- Tenderness
- Turgor, elasticity
- Texture

Olfaction
- Normal body odor
- Absence of pungent odor
- May indicate presence of bacteria or infection
- Poor hygiene

Observation of hair and nails
- Hair
  - Hirsutism: excessive body hair
  - Alopecia: hair loss
- Nails (can reflect the patient's overall health)
  - Color, shape, contour
  - Clubbing, texture, thickness

Skin alterations
- Previous scars
- Graft sites
- Healed ulcer sites

that may occur with turning or lifting an elderly patient can injure the skin. Ambulating or transferring patients may also present a problem if they bump into objects, such as chairs, beds, or tables. Removing adhesive dressings or tape can shear delicate skin. However, skin stripping is a potential problem for any person regardless of age when adhesive dressings or tape is incorrectly removed or vulnerable skin isn't adequately protected. Despite the frequency with which skin tears are seen in practice, the literature contains limited information about these wounds.

Prevalence

Skin tears are common in elderly patients. It's reported that long-term care residents have at least two skin tears per year. Hanson and colleagues report a prevalence of 6.3% and 6.4% in two different rural nursing homes.[36] In another study[37] skin tear incidence was reported as an average of 18 skin tears per month.

Skin tears occur most commonly in the upper extremities.[36,38] In a retrospective study, almost one-half were found to have occurred without any apparent cause. When the cause is known, approximately one-quarter resulted from wheelchair injuries, and one-quarter were caused by accidentally bumping into objects. Transfers and falls accounted for 18% and 12.4%, respectively.[38]

Although nearly 70% to 80% of skin tears occur on the arms and hands,[35,36] these wounds may occur on other areas of the body as well. Skin tears that occur on the back and buttocks are commonly mistaken for stage II pressure ulcers. Pressure may be a related cause

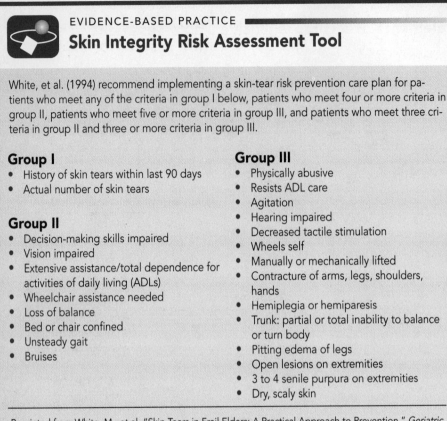

EVIDENCE-BASED PRACTICE
Skin Integrity Risk Assessment Tool

White, et al. (1994) recommend implementing a skin-tear risk prevention care plan for patients who meet any of the criteria in group I below, patients who meet four or more criteria in group II, patients who meet five or more criteria in group III, and patients who meet three criteria in group II and three or more criteria in group III.

Group I
- History of skin tears within last 90 days
- Actual number of skin tears

Group II
- Decision-making skills impaired
- Vision impaired
- Extensive assistance/total dependence for activities of daily living (ADLs)
- Wheelchair assistance needed
- Loss of balance
- Bed or chair confined
- Unsteady gait
- Bruises

Group III
- Physically abusive
- Resists ADL care
- Agitation
- Hearing impaired
- Decreased tactile stimulation
- Wheels self
- Manually or mechanically lifted
- Contracture of arms, legs, shoulders, hands
- Hemiplegia or hemiparesis
- Trunk: partial or total inability to balance or turn body
- Pitting edema of legs
- Open lesions on extremities
- 3 to 4 senile purpura on extremities
- Dry, scaly skin

Reprinted from White, M., et al. "Skin Tears in Frail Elders: A Practical Approach to Prevention," *Geriatric Nursing* 15(2):95-99, March-April 1994, © 1994 Mosby, with permission from Elsevier.

in skin tears, but the etiology of skin tears differs from that of pressure ulcers.[28] Skin tears need to be documented as separate occurrences and not grouped into pressure ulcer categories. (See chapter 13, Pressure ulcers.)

Risk factors
According to a retrospective review by White and colleagues,[39] the patients most at risk for sustaining skin tears are those requiring total care for all activities of daily living. These patients frequently experience skin tears resulting from routine activities, such as bathing, changing clothing, or being repositioned or transferred. Independent ambulatory residents sustained the second highest number of skin tears, primarily on the lower extremities. Many of these patients had edema, purpura, or ecchymosis. Slightly impaired residents made up the third highest risk category.

These patients sustained injury from hitting stationary equipment or furniture as well as the reasons just described in the dependent and independent ambulatory patients.[39]

Prevention protocols
Little has been written about the prevention of skin tears. However, a skin integrity risk assessment tool with three groups of patients at risk for skin tears was developed by White and colleagues in 1994.[39] (See *Skin Integrity Risk Assessment Tool.*) This tool can be used to identify patients at risk for skin tears.

Common-sense protocols gleaned from the literature could prevent many skin injuries. If the patient is at risk, consider these preventive measures:
- Encourage your colleagues and the patient's family members to use proper positioning, turning, lifting, and transferring.

EVIDENCE-BASED PRACTICE

Payne-Martin classification system for skin tears

This classification system augments documentation and allows for better tracking of outcomes of care for patients with skin tears.

Category I: Skin tears without tissue loss

A. Linear type—Epidermis and dermis pulled apart as if an incision has been made.
B. Flap type—Epidermal flap completely covers the dermis to within 1 mm of the wound margin.

Category II: Skin tears with partial tissue loss

A. Scant tissue loss type—25% or less of the epidermal flap lost.
B. Moderate to large tissue type—More than 25% of the epidermal flap lost.

Category III: Skin tears with complete tissue loss

Adapted with permission from Payne, R.L., and Martin, M.L. "Defining and Classifying Skin Tears: Need for a Common Language," *Ostomy/Wound Management* 39(5):16-20, 22-24, 26, June 1993.

• Promote the use of long sleeves and pants to add a layer of protection.
• Secure padding to bed rails, wheelchair arm and leg supports, and any other equipment that may be used.
• Use paper tape or nonadherent dressings on frail skin. Always remove these products gently to prevent skin injury.
• Use skin sealants, thin hydrocolloids, or foam dressings to protect vulnerable skin from adhering tapes and dressings.
• Use stockinettes, gauze wrap, or a similar type of wrap to secure dressings and drains.
• Use pillows and blankets to support dangling arms and legs.
• Move and turn the patient with a lift sheet.
• Minimize the use of soap and alcohol solvents; consider the use of waterless cleansers.
• Avoid scrubbing skin when bathing.
• Pat skin dry rather than rubbing it dry.
• Apply a moisturizing agent to dry skin.
• Provide a well-lit environment to prevent falls.
• Educate staff on the importance of gentle care.

Research has shown that skin tears can be reduced in nursing homes when skin care protocols are used.[36,37,40] Skin tears in a long-term care facility declined from 23.5% to 3.5% with the implementation of a no-rinse, one-step, bed bath protocol rather than soap and water.[40] Skin tears were significantly decreased in two different rural nursing homes when skin care protocols were introduced. Hanson and colleagues found that skin tear prevalence was reduced from 6.3% to 1.4% in nursing home A and 6.4% to 3.3% in nursing home B.[36] By educating staff and implementing the above-mentioned skin care protocols, skin tears were reduced from a monthly average of 18 to 11.[37]

Classification

The initial classification system for skin tears evolved in the late 1980s, thanks to the research of Regina Payne and Marie Martin.[41] This pilot research study led to the development of the Payne-Martin Classification for Skin Tears.[33] This useful tool provides health care professionals with a method to enhance documentation and track outcomes of care in the assessment of skin tears. Several researchers have used this new taxonomy in their studies as tool validation continues.

According to the revised 1993 Payne-Martin Skin Tear Classification System, the system is divided into three categories based on whether tissue is lost in the skin tear.[35] (See *Payne-Martin classification system for skin tears.*)

Xerosis

This photo depicts xerosis—also know as *dry skin*—of the foot.

Management

The management or treatment of skin tears varies according to institution, and indeed, little has been published as to what are the preferred treatments for skin tears. However, the basic goals of care should aim to control bleeding, prevent infection, control pain, restore skin integrity, and promote patient comfort.[35] Many types of skin and wound care products are used to promote a healing environment. In fact, a review of the literature reveals that these methods are used to treat skin tears[32, 42-44]: petrolatum ointment and nonadherent dressings; hydrogels, Telfa, and collagen dressings, foams, and transparent films; and hydrocolloids and adhesive strips. In one case study, changing a skin tear treatment plan from antibiotic ointment and gauze dressing to a sodium carboxymethlcellulose dressing covered with a nonadherent secondary dressing and a gauze wrap was effective.[45] Skin tear healing time was reduced to 30.16 days (SD +26.19) compared to 39.07 days (SD +38.26) prior to implementation of a skin care protocol using skin protectants on the dry skin of the upper extremities of nursing home residents.[36]

Skin conditions

Although there are many skin conditions that warrant attention in clinical practice, two leading skin conditions in elderly people, xerosis and pruritus, aren't always given the importance and priority they deserve. These seemingly minor skin problems cause the skin to dry, itch, and crack and, without effective recognition and intervention, the skin continues to deteriorate, leading to more chronic skin conditions including fissures, infection, and cellulitis. Because there are many other skin conditions that are beyond the focus of this chapter, the authors recommend consulting the dermatology literature.

PRACTICE POINT

Skin assessments are required in all health care settings.

Xerosis

Xerosis is the medical term for dry skin.[46] In xerosis, the skin appears dry, scaly, and flaky. (See *Xerosis*.) Although there is a xerosis scale, it's not widely used in clinical practice. Clinicians generally classify xerosis as mild, moderate, and severe. (See *Xerosis terminology*.)

The term xerosis has no particular diagnostic implication. Xerosis can be caused by environmental factors or a symptom of an underlying disease. For this reason, a patient's complaint of "dry" skin needs to be explored further. Skin exposure to a dry environment, such as central heating, wind, temperature extremes, or air conditioning, can all lead to xerosis.

The goal in treating xerosis is to protect the skin from excessive transdermal water loss and return the natural moisturizing factors to the stratum corneum. This is best accomplished by using moisturizing agents that contain lipids—an essential component in forming an impervious barrier, or seal, on the stratum corneum, thus preventing further water loss. (See *Moisturizer functions and ingredients*.) As water is retained, the skin surface is flattened, and scaling is reduced.[46]

Management
Cleansing
Instruct the patient to:
• avoid long baths (less than 15 minutes) or consider showering instead
• bathe every other day rather than daily
• use tepid water rather than hot water

Xerosis terminology

Mild	Moderate	Severe

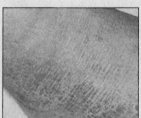 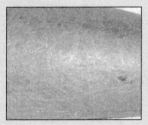 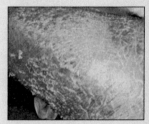

Dry skin with minimal flaking
Treatment: Hydrate the skin
using a moisturizing agent
frequently.

Dry skin with scaling fish-like
appearance that's easily
rubbed off skin surface
Treatment: Use an exfoliat-
ing emollient moisturizing
agent.

Cracking, parched appear-
ance of skin that resembles
dry earth
Treatment: Use moisturizer
with urea, AHA, or lactic acid
to exfoliate calloused dry
skin.

• use pH-balanced soaps (4.0 to 6.5), avoid excessive use of deodorant soaps, and rinse well
• avoid vigorously using a washcloth to clean the skin
• pat or blot the skin, rather than rubbing with a towel, so some water is left on the skin
• apply moisturizers *immediately* after bathing or showering.

Environmental
Instruct the patient to:
• use a humidifier during the winter months when central heating is being used
• drink plenty of water
• wear a sunscreen with a sun protection factor (SPF) of 15 or higher that contains a moisturizer
• use non-fragrant laundry detergents, fabric softeners, and products.

Hydration
Instruct the patient to:
• use moisturizers, applying frequently, using correct gentle application technique for specific product (check product directions on how to use), and implementing fall safety

Moisturizer functions and ingredients

Moisturizer functions
• *Humectants* promote water retention within the stratum corneum.
• *Occlusives* minimize water loss to the external environment.
• *Emollients* contribute to stratum corneum hydration.

Moisturizer ingredients (main types)
• Humectants
  – glycerin
  – urea
  – hydroxy acids (lactic aid)
  – propylene glycol
  – emollients
  – protein rejuvenators
• Occlusives and emollients
  – petrolatum
  – mineral oil
  – lanolin

Itch-scratch-itch cycle

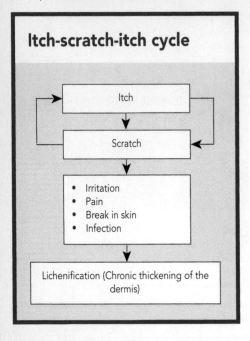

occurrence of lichenification. (See *Itch-scratch-itch cycle.*)

Pruritus

Pruritus is the medical term for itchy skin and is a common symptom for several diseases. Therefore, taking a detailed history aids in determining if the cause is from such an underlying disease or if it's just untreated xerosis. For example, pruritus may be a symptom of renal or liver disease, scabies, or dry skin from aging. (See *Pruritus.*) Helping patients understand the itch-scratch-itch cycle and their own behavioral pattern is important to successful management. Treating the person with pruritus incorporates many of the elements listed in Xerosis, page 14. (See *Treatment plan for pruritus.*)

Summary

The skin is the largest organ of the body and commonly the most forgotten. Skin is exposed daily to environmental irritants and chemicals as well as physical and mechanical injury, any of which may lead to impaired skin integrity. This chapter provided an overview of skin structure and criteria for a skin assessment versus a wound assessment. Identification and classification of skin tears as an exemplar for acute traumatic skin injury was also presented, which includes skin tear risk factors and prevention opportunities, as well as treatment strategies. The importance of identifying two common skin conditions, specifically xerosis and pruritus, and the role of breaking the itch-scratch-itch cycle and the use of moisturizers in their treatment, was also highlighted.

precautions because bathing surfaces may be slippery if using bath oils.

PRACTICE POINT

Stop the Xerosis Cycle!
- Dry skin (xerosis)
- Pruritus
- Scratching

Because many moisturizers dissipate after 3 to 4 hours, these authors recommend using long-lasting moisturizers to cool, soothe, and restore barrier function. The goal is to break the itch-scratch-itch cycle, which happens because dry skin is often itchy, causing patients to scratch their skin. In turn, excessive scratching can ultimately lead to a break in the skin. Once the skin barrier is broken, it becomes a portal of entry for bacteria, which can lead to infection. This repetitive scratching causes chronic thickening of the dermis known as lichenification. Therefore, prompt identification of the itch-scratch-itch cycle as well as teaching the patient about skin damage (from scratching) is extremely important in helping the skin to heal and reducing the

Show what you know

1. While bathing a patient, you notice some flakes of skin on the washcloth. Which layer of the skin is this?

    A. Stratum granulosum
    B. Stratum spinosum
    C. Stratum lucidum
    D. Stratum corneum

Pruritus

Pruritus is frequently seen in the following conditions and diseases:
- Brain tumor
- Biliary cirrhosis
- Diabetes mellitus
- Drugs
- Idiopathic (has no diagnostic cause)
- Liver disease
- Malignancies (especially in prevalent Hodgkin's where one-third of patients may have itching lasting up to 1 year)
- Multiple sclerosis
- Polycythemia (itch occurs after a hot bath)
- Psychological (anxiety disorders)
- Renal failure
- Senile pruritus (idiopathic pruritus in the elderly)
- Thyroid disorders (improves with treatment)
- Topical infections

Adapted with permission from Tomic-Canic, M. "Keratinocyte Cross-Talks in Wounds." *Wounds* 17:S3-S6, 2005.

Treatment plan for pruritus

- Manage the underlying disease that causes the pruritus.
- Use topical emollients and bathing strategies as outlined in the xerosis care plan.
- Implement behavior modification (stopping scratching and break the itch-scratch-itch cycle).
- Keep nails short.
- Wear gloves at night to decrease skin damage.
- Use cotton sheets, which may be more soothing to itchy skin.
- Help the patient avoid wearing clothing that can irritate the skin, such as wool or other "scratchy" fabrics.
- Limit the indiscriminate use of topical steroids and antihistamines as their effectiveness needs further investigation.[26]

Adapted with permission from Gilhar, A., et al. "Ageing of Human Epidermis: The Role of Apoptosis, Fas and Telomerase," *Br J Dermatol* 150:56-63, 2004.

ANSWER: D. The cells of the stratum corneum can shed and look like flakes during routine cleaning activities such as bathing.

2. *Which one of the following is a normal function of the skin?*

    A. Synthesis of vitamin K
    B. Elimination of carbon dioxide
    C. Regulation of glucose levels by the Langerhans cells
    D. Thermal regulation by skin blood flow dilation or constriction

ANSWER: D. Upon stimulus from the hypothalamus, skin blood vessels will either vasoconstrict (heat needs to be conserved to elevate temperature) or vasodilate (heat needs to be eliminated to lower temperature) depending upon specific needs. Skin can synthesize vitamin D, not vitamin K. Carbon dioxide is eliminated via the lungs. Glucose levels are regulated by the islets of Langerhans in the pancreas, not the Langerhans cells in the skin.

3. *What is the role of keratinocytes in skin?*

    A. Differentiation
    B. Cross-talk to fibroblasts
    C. Participating in BMZ
    D. Maintenance and repair of the barrier

ANSWER: D. The entire biology of keratinocytes is dedicated to barrier formation and its maintenance.

4. Which one of the following is NOT considered part of a routine skin assessment?

A. Color
B. Turgor
C. Temperature
D. Ankle-brachial index (ABI)

ANSWER: D. ABI is a test used for peripheral vascular disease; it does not tell you about skin assessment. Answers A, B, and C should all be part of a skin assessment.

5. Which one of the following patients is most at risk for skin tear injury?

A. A 22-year-old male postoperative for an inguinal hernia repair
B. A 37-year-old male with a fractured humerus
C. A 64-year-old female 3 days postcataract extraction
D. A 72-year-old female with rheumatoid arthritis on steroid therapy

ANSWER: D. A 72-year-old female is the oldest, least mobile, and receiving steroids, which are known to further cause thinning of the skin, so her skin is at highest risk.

6. A partial-thickness skin tear with less than 25% of the epidermal flap loss using the Payne-Martin method would be classified as:

A. category I.
B. category II.
C. category III.
D. category IV.

ANSWER: B. Answers A and C are incorrect, and the Payne-Martin classification system contains no category IV.

7. Which of the following interventions for a resident in a long-term care facility with a skin tear on the lower right leg should you question?

A. Clean the patient daily using detergent.
B. Pad the wheelchair arm and leg supports.
C. Apply a nonadherent dressing to the skin tear.
D. Encourage the patient to wear soft, fleece-lined pants.

ANSWER: A. Nonemollient soaps should be used instead of detergent, which dries the skin. The literature suggests that routine every-other-day bathing for elderly people is adequate (unless the skin is soiled) and can reduce skin tear injury.

8. Which one of the following should be included in the care plan of a person with xerosis?

A. Have the patient shower daily.
B. Use a deodorant soap.
C. Dry the skin completely with vigorous rubbing.
D. Apply an emollient immediately after bathing.

ANSWER: D. Emollient moisturizers are a cornerstone in the treatment of xerosis. Answer A is incorrect because daily cleaning of the skin either by showering or bathing is not recommended as it further dries the skin. Answer B is incorrect because a low pH soap needs to be used as deodorant soaps have a high pH that makes the skin alkaline. Answer C is incorrect because rubbing can irritate dry skin.

9. Which of the following best defines pruritus?

A. Multiple blisters on the skin
B. Traumatic open area on the skin
C. Itchy skin
D. Weepy skin

ANSWER: C. Pruritus is the medical term for itchy skin.

References

1. Koch, S., et al. "Skin Homing of Langerhans Cell Precursors: Adhesion, Chemotaxis, and Migration," *J Allergy Clin Immunol* 117:163-68, 2006.
2. Blumenberg, M., and Tomic-Canic, M. "Human Epidermal Keratinocyte: Keratinization Processes," *EXS* 78:1-29, 1997.
3. Freedberg, I.M., et al. "Keratins and the Keratinocyte Activation Cycle," *J Invest Dermatol* 116:633-40, 2001.
4. Tomic-Canic, M., et al. "Epidermal Repair and the Chronic Wound," in *The Epidermis in Wound Healing*. Edited by Rovee, D.T., and Maibach, H.I. Boca Raton, Fla.: CRC Press LLC. 25-57, 2004.
5. Tomic-Canic, M. "Keratinocyte Cross-Talks in Wounds," *Wounds* 17:S3-6, 2005.
6. Morasso, M.I., and Tomic-Canic, M. "Epidermal Stem Cells: The Cradle of Epidermal Determination, Differentiation and Wound Healing," *Biol Cell* 97:173-83, 2005.
7. Habif, T.P. *Clinical Dermatology: A Color Guide to Diagnosis and Therapy*. Philadelphia: Mosby, 2004.
8. Kanitakis, J. "Anatomy, Histology and Immunohistochemistry of Normal Human Skin," *Eur J Dermatol* 12:390-99; quiz 400, 2002.
9. Eckes, B., and Krieg, T. "Regulation of Connective Tissue Homeostasis in the Skin by Mechanical Forces," *Clin Exp Rheumatol* 22:S73-76, 2004.
10. Yosipovitch, G., and Hu, J. "The Importance of Skin pH," *Skin and Aging* 11:88-93, 2003.
11. Waller, J.M., and Maibach, H.I. "Age and Skin Structure and Function, A Quantitative Approach (I): Blood Flow, pH, Thickness, and Ultrasound Echogenicity," Skin Res Technol 11:221-35, 2005.
12. Rippke, F., et al. "Stratum Corneum pH in Atopic Dermatitis: Impact on Skin Barrier Function and Colonization with *Staphylococcus Aureus*," *Am J Clin Dermatol* 5:217-23, 2004.
13. Yilmaz, E., and Borchert, H.H. "Effect of Lipid-Containing, Positively Charged Nanoemulsions on Skin Hydration, Elasticity and Erythema-An In Vivo Study," *Int J Pharm* 307:232-38, 2006.
14. Kurabayashi, H., et al. "Inhibiting Bacteria and Skin pH in Hemiplegia: Effects of Washing Hands with Acidic Mineral Water," *Am J Phys Med Rehabili* 81:40-46, 2002.

15. Damjanov, I. *Pathology for the Health-Related Professions.* Philadelphia: W.B. Saunders, 2000.

16. Hughes, E., and Van Onselen, J. *Dermatology Nursing: A Practical Guide.* London: Churchill Livingstone, Inc, 2001.

17. Bardan, A., et al. "Antimicrobial Peptides and the Skin," *Expert Opin Biol Ther* 4:543-49, 2004.

18. Niyonsaba, F., and Ogawa, H. "Protective Roles of the Skin Against Infection: Implication of Naturally Occurring Human Antimicrobial Agents Beta-Defensins, Cathelicidin LL-37 and Lysozyme," *J Dermatol Sci* 40:157-68, 2005.

19. Stante, M., et al. "Itch, Pain, and Metaesthetic Sensation," *Dermatol Ther* 18:308-13, 2005.

20. Charkoudian, N. "Skin Blood Flow in Adult Human Thermoregulation: How It Works, When It Does Not, and Why," *Mayo Clin Proc* 78:603-12, 2003.

21. Minson, C.T. "Hypoxic Regulation of Blood Flow in Humans. Skin Blood Flow and Temperature Regulation," *Adv Exp Med Biol* 543:249-62, 2003.

22. Kupper, T.S., and Fuhlbrigge, R.C. "Immune Surveillance in the Skin: Mechanisms and Clinical Consequences," *Nat Rev Immunol* 4:211-22, 2004.

23. Wolpowitz, D., and Gilchrest, B.A. "The Vitamin D Questions: How Much Do You Need and How Should You Get It?" *J Am Acad Dermatol* 54:301-17, 2006.

24. Fisher, G.J. "The Pathophysiology of Photoaging of the Skin," *Cutis* 75:5-8; discussion 8-9, 2005.

25. Venna, S.S.G., B.A. "Skin Aging and Photoaging," *Skin and Aging* 12:56-69, 2004.

26. Gilhar, A., et al. "Ageing of Human Epidermis: The Role of Apoptosis, Fas and Telomerase," *Br J Dermatol* 150:56-63, 2004.

27. Geriatric Nursing Resources for Care of Older Adults. *Normal Aging Changes.* Available at: GeronurseOnline.org. Accessed June 6, 2006.

28. Selden, S.T., et al. "Skin Tears: Recognizing and Treating This Growing Problem," *Extended Care Product News* 113(3):14-15, May-June, 2003.

29. Lee, B., and Tomic-Canic, M. "Tissue Specificity of Steroid Action: Glucocorticoids in Epidermis," in *Molecular Mechanisms of Action of Steroid Hormone Receptors.* Edited by Krstic-Demonacos, M., and Demonacos, C. Kerala, India: Research Signpost, 2002.

30. Wysocki, A.B. "Skin Anatomy, Physiology, and Pathophysiology," *Nurs Clin North Am* 34 (5):777-97, 1999.

31. Holloway, S., and Jones, V. "The Importance of Skin Care and Assessment," *Br J Nurs* 14:1172-176, 2005.

32. Baranoski, S. "Skin Tears: Staying on Guard Against the Enemy of Frail Skin," *Nursing* 33:(Suppl):14-20, 2003.

33. Centers for Medicare and Medicaid Services (CMS). "Guidance to Surveyors for Long Term Care Facilities," *Pressure Sores* Revised Tag F 314:144, November 2004.

34. Baranoski, S. "Meeting the Challenge of Skin Tears," *Advances in Skin & Wound Care* 18:74-75, 2005.

35. Payne, R.L., and Martin, M.L. "Defining and Classifying Skin Tears: Need for a Common Language," *Ostomy/Wound Management* 39(5):16-20, 22-24, 26, 1993.

36. Hanson, D.H., et al. "Skin Tears in Long-Term Care: Effectiveness of Skin Care Protocols on Prevalence," *Advances in Skin & Wound Care* 18:74, 2005.

37. Bank, D. "Decreasing the Incidence of Skin Tears in a Nursing and Rehabilitation Center," *Advances in Skin & Wound Care* 18:74-75, 2005.

38. Malone, M.L., et al. The Epidemiology of Skin Tears in the Institutionalized Elderly," *J Am Geriatr Soc* 39:591-95, 1991.

39. White, M.W., et al. "Skin Tears in Frail Elders: A Practical Approach to Prevention," *Geriatr Nurs* 15(2):95-99, 1994.

40. Birch, S., and Coggins, T. "No-Rinse, One-Step Bed Bath: The Effects on the Occurrence of Skin Tears in a Long-Term Care Setting," *Ostomy Wound Manage* 49:64-67, 2003.

41. Payne, R.L., and Martin, M.L. "The Epidemiology and Management of Skin Tears in Older Adults," *Ostomy Wound Manage* 26:26-37, 1990.

42. Baranoski, S. "Skin Tears: The Enemy of Frail Skin," *Advances in Skin & Wound Care* 13:123-26, 2000.

43. O'Regan, A. "Skin Tears: A Review of the Literature," *WCET Journal* 22:26-31, 2002.

44. Cuzzell, J. "Wound Assessment and Evaluation: Skin Tear Protocol," *Dermatology Nursing* 14:405-16, 2002.

45. Lukas, M. "Management of Multiple Skin Tears in a Patient with Chronic Liver and Renal Disease," *Advances in Skin & Wound Care* 18:75, 2005.

46. Lebwohl, M., et al. *Treatment of Skin Disease: Comprehensive Therapeutic Strategies.* London: Harcourt Publishers Limited (Mosby), 2002.

CHAPTER 5

Acute and chronic wound healing

Vanessa Jones, MSc, RN, NDN, RCNT, PGCE
Keith Harding, MB, ChB, MRCGP, FRCS
Joyce Stechmiller, ARNP, PhD, CS
Gregory Schultz, PhD

OBJECTIVES

After completing this chapter, you'll be able to:

• describe the physiology of wound healing

• discuss the cascade of wound healing events

• compare acute and chronic wound healing.

Wound healing events

When a patient experiences tissue injury it's essential that hemostasis is rapidly achieved and tissues are repaired to prevent invasion by pathogens and restore tissue function. The process of wound healing is a complex sequence of events that starts when the injury occurs and ends with complete wound closure and successful, functional scar tissue organization. Although tissue repair is commonly described as a series of stages, in reality, it's a continuous process during which cells undergo a number of complicated biological changes to facilitate hemostasis, combat infection, migrate into the wound space, deposit a matrix, form new blood vessels, and contract to close the defect.

However, wound closure isn't a marker of healing completion; the wound continues to change, in a process called remodeling, for up to 18 months postclosure. During this prolonged phase of remodeling and maturation, the closed wound is still quite vulnerable.

Wound healing cascade

The process of healing is usually divided into four phases—hemostasis, inflammation, proliferation, and maturation—each of which overlaps the others while remaining distinct in terms of time after injury. (See *Sequence of molecular and cellular events in skin wound healing.*)

Sequence of molecular and cellular events in skin wound healing

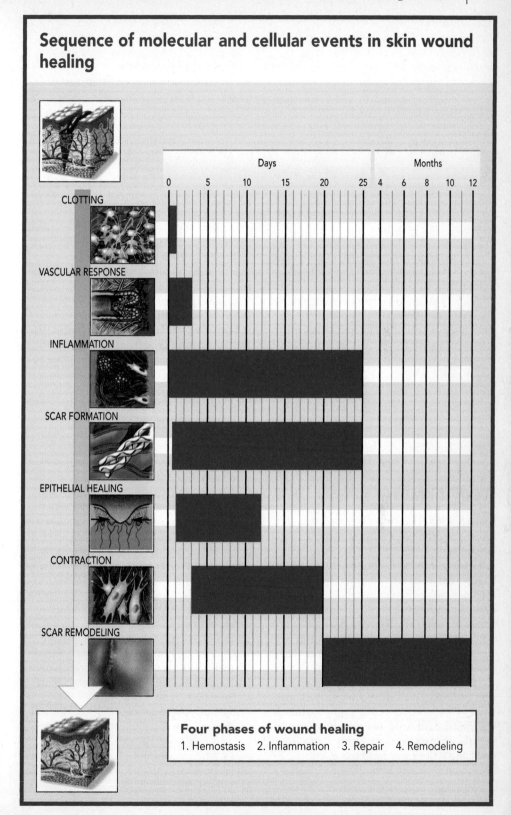

Four phases of wound healing
1. Hemostasis   2. Inflammation   3. Repair   4. Remodeling

Hemostasis

The disruption of tissues following injury causes hemorrhage, which initially fills the wound and exposes the blood to various components of the extracellular matrix (ECM).[1] Platelets aggregate and degranulate, which activates factor XII (Hageman factor), resulting in clot formation and hemostasis. Hemostasis stops hemorrhage at the site of blood vessel damage. This is essential as it preserves the integrity of the closed and high-pressure circulatory system to limit blood loss. A fibrinous clot forms during coagulation, acting as a preliminary matrix within the wound space into which cells can migrate.

After the fibrin clot forms, another mechanism is activated as part of the body's defense system—fibrinolysis—in which the fibrin clot starts to break down. This process prevents clot extension and dissolves the fibrin clot to allow ease of further cell migration into the wound space,[2] allowing the next stage of healing to proceed.

Inflammatory phase

As the fibrin clot is degraded, the capillaries dilate and become permeable, allowing fluid into the injury site and activating the complement system. The complement system is composed of a series of interacting, soluble proteins found in serum and extracellular fluid that induce lysis and the destruction of target cells. C3b, a complement molecule, helps bind (opsonize) neutrophils to bacteria, facilitating phagocytosis and subsequent bacterial destruction.

Cytokines and some proteolytic fragments that are hemoattractive are also found in the wound space.[2] Their abundance and accumulation at the site of injury initiate a massive influx of other cells. The two main inflammatory cells—neutrophils and macrophages—are attracted to the wound space to mount an acute inflammatory response.[3]

Neutrophils appear in a wound shortly after injury and reach their peak number within 24 to 48 hours and their main function is to destroy bacteria by the process of phagocytosis. Neutrophils have a very short life span and, after 3 days without infection, their numbers reduce rapidly.

Tissue macrophages are derived from blood monocytes and arrive approximately 2 to 3 days after injury, followed by lymphocytes. Like neutrophils, macrophages also destroy bacteria and debris through phagocytosis; however, macrophages are also a rich source of biological regulators, including cytokines and growth factors, bioactive lipid products, and proteolytic enzymes, which are also essential for the normal healing process.[2,4]

Cytokines, growth factors, and chemotaxis

Cytokine is a broad term that includes such molecules as growth factors, interleukins, tumor necrosis factors, and interferons. These molecules act on a variety of cells by exerting a wide range of biological functions by means of their specific receptors on target cells or proteins. Pathogens, endotoxins, tissue degradation products, and hypoxia are all factors that stimulate cells to produce cytokines following injury. The main cellular sources for these cytokines are platelets, fibroblasts, monocytes and macrophages, and endothelial cells. These cells are involved in physiological as well as pathological conditions (for example, tumors), though in wound healing they play an important role as mediators. Cytokines regulate cell proliferation, migration, matrix synthesis, deposition and degradation, and inflammatory responses in the repair process. (See *Major cytokines involved in wound healing*.)

Immediately after injury, platelet degranulation releases numerous cytokines, including platelet-derived growth factor (PDGF), transforming growth factor (TGF), and epidermal growth factor (EGF). These cytokines, together with other chemotactic agents, such as tissue debris and pathogenic materials, attract neutrophils and, later, macrophages. In time these cells contribute to a larger number and variety of cytokines, which participate in the healing process.[4]

Cytokines have diverse effects on the healing process, interacting in additive, synergistic, or inhibitory ways. (See *Major growth factor families,* page 68.) For example, keratinocyte growth factor enhances the stimulation of collagenase synthesis exerted by

Major cytokines involved in wound healing

Cytokine	Cell source	Biological activity
PRO-INFLAMMATORY CYTOKINES		
Tumor Necrosis Factor (TNF-α)	Macrophages	↑ PMN margination and cytotoxicity ↑ MMP synthesis
Interleukin-I (IL-1)	Macrophages, keratinocytes	↑ Fibroblast and keratinocyte chemotaxis ↑ MMP synthesis
Interleukin-6 (IL-6)	Macrophages, keratinocytes, PMNs	↑ Fibroblast proliferation
Interluekin-8 (IL-8)	Macrophages, fibroblasts	↑ Macrophage and PMN chemotaxis ↑ Collagen synthesis
Interluekin-γ	Macrophages, T-lymphocytes	↑ Macrophage and PMN activation ↓ Collagen synthesis ↑ MMP synthesis
ANTI-INFLAMMATORY CYTOKINES		
Interleukin-4 (IL-4)	T-lymphocytes, basophils, mast cells	↓ TNF-α IL-1, IL-6 synthesis ↑ Fibroblast proliferation, collagen synthesis
Interleukin-10 (IL-10)	T-lymphocytes, macrophages, keratinocytes	↓ TNF-α, IL-1, IL-6 synthesis ↓ Macrophage and PMN activation

insulin-like growth factor. TGF is inhibitory to fibroblast growth in the presence of EGF, but stimulates cell division when PDGF is present.

PRACTICE POINT

Keep in mind that the induration, heat, discomfort, redness, and swelling experienced during the inflammatory phase are part of the normal wound healing processes and aren't, at this stage, likely to be due to wound infection. Remember to share this information with your patients.

Proliferation phase

The proliferation phase usually begins 3 days after an injury and lasts for a few weeks. This phase is characterized by the formation of granulation tissue in the wound space. The new tissue consists of a matrix of fibrin, fibronectin, collagens, proteoglycans, glycosaminoglycans (GAGs), and other glycoproteins.[5] Fibroblasts move into the wound space and proliferate. Because the type III collagen in the wound has decreased tensile strength, the patient is at risk for such abnormalities as wound dehiscence or opening of wound edges in a previously closed wound that healed by primary intention. If organs are protruding from the now opened wound, it's called *evisceration*, which is a medical emergency, requiring immediate surgery.

PRACTICE POINT

The first 3 weeks after surgery, the patient is at high risk for wound dehiscence and evisceration.

Major growth factor families

Growth factor family	Cell source	Actions
Transforming growth factor (TGF) β TGF-β1 TGF-β2 TGF-β3	Platelets Fibroblasts Macrophages	Chemotatic for fibroblasts Promotes extracellular matrix formation ↑ Collagen and tissue inhibitors of metallproteinases (TIMP) synthesis ↓ matrix metaloproteinase (MMP) synthesis Reduces scarring ↓ Collagen ↓ Fibrinectin
Platelet-derived growth factor (PDGF) PDGF-AA; PDGF-BB; VEGF	Platelets Macrophages Keratinocytes Fibroblasts	Activates immune cells and fibroblasts Promotes ECM formation ↑ Collagen and TIMP synthesis ↓ MMP synthesis ↑ Angiogenesis ↑ Angiogenesis
Fibroblast growth factor (FGF) Acidic FGF, Basic FGF, KGF	Macrophages Endothelial cells Fibroblasts	↑ Angiogenesis ↑ Keratinocyte proliferation and migration ↑ ECM deposition
Insulin-like growth factor (IGF) IGF-I, IGF-II, Insulin	Liver Skeletal muscle Fibroblasts Macrophages Neutrophils	↑ Keratinocyte and fibroblast proliferation ↑ Angiogenesis ↑ Collagen synthesis ↑ ECM formation ↑ Cell metabolism
Epidermal growth factor (EFG) EGF, HB (Heparin-binding), TGF-α (alpha), Amphiregulin, Betacellulin	Keratinocytes Macrophages	↑ Keratinocyte proliferation and migration ↑ ECM formation
Connective tissue growth factor (CTGF) CTGF	Fibroblasts Endothelial cells Epithelial cells	↑ Collagen synthesis Mediates action of TGF-βs on collagen synthesis

Role of fibroblasts

Fibroblasts play a key role during the proliferation phase, appearing in large numbers within 3 days of injury and reaching peak levels on the 7th day. During this period they undergo intense proliferative and synthetic activity. Fibroblasts synthesize and deposit extracellular proteins during wound healing, producing growth factors and angiogenic factors that regulate cell proliferation and angiogenesis.[6]

Granulation tissue is comprised of many mesenchymal and non-mesenchymal cells with distinct phenotypes, inflammatory cells and new capillaries embedded in a loose ECM composed of collagens, fibronectin, and proteoglycans.

Role of ECM proteins

ECM consists of proteins and polysaccharides and their complexes produced by cells in the wound space. The two main classes of matrix proteins are fibrous (collagens and elastin) and adhesive proteins (laminin and fibronectin). In addition, the ECM contains polysaccharides called proteoglycans and GAGs.

Collagen is the most abundant protein in animal tissue and accounts for 70% to 80%

of the dry weight of the dermis.[7] The collagen molecule consists of three identical polypeptide chains bound together in a triple helix. Mainly made by fibroblasts, at least 19 genetically distinct collagens have been identified. Collagen synthesis and degradation is finely balanced.[4]

Elastin is a protein that provides elasticity and resilience[7] and is composed of fibrous coils that stretch and return to its former shape, much like metallic coils. Because of these properties, elastin helps maintain tissue shape. Elastin represents only 2% to 4% of the human skin's dry weight; it's also lungs and blood vessels. It's secreted into the extracellular space as a soluble precursor, tropoelastin, which binds with a microfibrillar protein to form an elastic fiber network.

Laminin and fibronectin are two fiber-forming molecules. Their function is to provide structural and metabolic support to other cells. Fibronectin is found in plasma and contains specific binding sites on its molecular wall for cells, collagens, fibrinogens, and proteoglycans. It plays a central role in tissue remodeling, acting as a mediator for physical interactions between cells and collagens involved in ECM deposition, thereby providing a preliminary matrix.

Proteoglycans consist of a central core protein combined with a number of GAG chains that may be one or several types. GAGs consist of long, unbranched chains of disaccharide units that can range in number from 10 to 20,000.[8] A highly complex group of molecules, proteoglycans are characterized by their many diverse structural and organizational functions in tissue. Forming a highly hydrated gel-like "ground substance," they can contain up to 95% (w/w) carbohydrates. Originally, however, they were thought to contribute to tissue resilience due to their capacity to fill much of the extracellular space.

Angiogenesis
Angiogenesis is the formation of new vessels in the wound space and is an integral and essential part of wound healing.[9] The vascular endothelial cell plays a key role in angiogenesis and arises from the damaged end of vessels and capillaries. New vessels originate as capillaries, which sprout from existing small

vessels at the wound edge. The endothelial cells from these vessels detach from the vascular wall, degrade and penetrate (invade) the provisional matrix in the wound, and form a knob-like or cone-shape vascular bud or sprout. These sprouts extend in length until they encounter another capillary, to which they connect to form vascular loops and networks, allowing blood to circulate. This pattern of vascular growth is similar in skin, muscle, and intestinal wounds.

Epithelialization
Epithelial healing, or epithelialization, which begins a few hours after injury, is another important feature of healing. Marginal basal cells, which are normally firmly attached to the underlying dermis, change their cell adhesion property and start to lose their firm adhesion, migrating in a leapfrog or train fashion across the provisional matrix. Horizontal movement is stopped when cells meet. This is known as contact inhibition.

Wound contraction
The final feature of the proliferation phase is wound contraction, which normally starts 5 days after injury. Wound contraction appears to be a dynamic process in which cells organize their surrounding connective tissue matrix, acting to reduce the healing time by reducing the amount of ECM that needs to be produced. The contractile activity of fibroblasts and myofibroblasts provides the force for this contraction. These cells may use integrins and other adhesion mechanisms to bind to the collagen network and alter its motility, bringing the fibrils and, subsequently, wound edges closer. Such contraction may not be important in a sharply incised, small, and noninfected wound; however, it's critical for wounds with large tissue loss.[10]

Although several theories exist to explain the wound contraction process, its exact mechanism remains unclear. In particular, the type and origin of fibroblasts that appear in the wound haven't yet been determined.[1,3,11-13]

The myofibroblast theory suggests that the contraction force occurs when the movement of microfilament (actin) bundles (also termed *stress fibers*) contracts the myofibroblast in a musclelike fashion. Because the myofibroblast displays many cell:cell and cell:matrix (fibronexus) contacts, the cellular contraction pulls collagen fibrils toward the body of the myofibroblast and holds them until they're stabilized into position. This gathering of collagen fibers toward the myofibroblast cell "body" leads to the shrinkage of granulation tissue. The ECM of the wound is continuous with the undamaged wound margin, enabling the granulation tissue shrinkage to pull on the wound margin, leading to wound contraction. The myofibroblast theory further proposes that the coordinated contraction (cellular shortening) of many myofibroblasts, synchronized with the help of gap junctions, generates the force necessary for wound contraction.[13]

The traction theory proposes that fibroblasts bring about a closer approximation of matrix fibrils by exerting "traction forces" (analogous to the traction of wheels on tarmac) on extracellular matrix fibers to which they're attached. This theory proposes that fibroblasts neither shorten in length nor do they act in a coordinated multicellular manner (as proposed by the myofibroblast theory); rather, a composite force, made up of traction forces of many individual fibroblasts, is responsible for matrix contraction. Such traction forces act as shearing forces tangential to the cell surface generated during cell elongation and spreading. According to the traction theory, the composite effect of many fibroblasts gathering collagen fibrils within the wound is thought to bring about wound contraction.[14]

Maturation phase

The maturation phase normally starts 7 days after injury and may last for 1 year or more. The initial component in the deposited ECM is fibronectin, which forms a provisional fiber network. Other components include hyaluronic acid and proteoglycans. The network has two main roles: as a substratum for the migration and growth of cells, and as a template for subsequent collagen deposition. Collagen deposition becomes the predominant constituent of the matrix and soon forms fibrillar bundles and provides stiffness and tensile strength to the wound.

Collagen deposition and remodeling contribute to the increased tensile strength of skin wounds. Within 3 weeks of injury, the tensile strength is restored to approximately 20% of normal, uninjured skin. As healing continues, the skin gradually reaches a maximum of 70% to 80% tensile strength. Different organs regain tensile strengths to differing degrees. The remodeling process involves the balance between the synthesis and degradation of collagen. A range of collagenases regulates the latter. This process is also characterized by a gradual reduction in cellularity and vascularity. Differentiation of fibroblasts into myofibroblasts with resultant apoptosis (programmed cell death) are also features of tissue remodeling.[13]

PRACTICE POINT

A patient history should always include information about prior wounds. Healed wounds never achieve the same tensile strength as uninjured skin, thereby increasing the potential for reinjury.

The scar is the final product of wound healing and is a relatively avascular and acellular mass of collagen, which serves to restore tissue continuity and some degree of tensile strength and function. However, the strength of the scar remains less than that of normal tissue, even many years following injury, and it's never fully restored. (See *Summary of wound healing*.)

PRACTICE POINT

The width of the resultant scar of a wound healing by secondary intention is about 10% of the original defect, primarily due to the process of wound contraction, working in conjunction with proliferation.

Role of matrix metalloproteases in wound healing

Proteases, especially the matrix metalloproteinases (MMPs), play essential roles in all phases of normal wound healing. (See *Role*

Summary of wound healing

The following is a summary of the events that occur during the phases of wound healing.

HEMOSTASIS

Platelets ⟶ Release cytokines (PDGF, TGFβ, EGF)

INFLAMMATORY PHASE

Tissue debris and pathogens ⟶ Attract macrophages and neutrophils, which are responsible for:
- phagocytosis
- producing biological regulators, bioactive lipids, and proteolytic enzymes.

PROLIFERATIVE PHASE

Fibroblasts ⟶ Responsible for:
- synthesizing and depositing extracellular proteins
- producing growth factors
- producing angiogenic factors.

Extracellular matrix (ECM) and granulation tissue ⟶ ECM comprised of:
- collagens and elastin
- adhesive proteins
- fibronectin and lamina
- polysaccharides
- proteoglycans
- glycosaminoglycans.

Angiogenesis ⟶ Capillary growth into ECM

ECM

Capillaries

Reepithelialization ⟶ Migration of marginal basal cells across the provisional matrix

Wound contraction ⟶ Contraction of fibroblasts and myofibroblasts to bring wound edges closer

(continued)

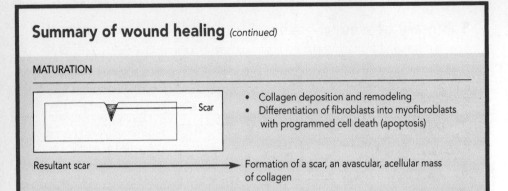

Summary of wound healing (continued)

MATURATION

Scar

Resultant scar

- Collagen deposition and remodeling
- Differentiation of fibroblasts into myofibroblasts with programmed cell death (apoptosis)

Formation of a scar, an avascular, acellular mass of collagen

Role of MMPs in wound healing

Proteases (especially matrix metaloproteinases [MMPs]) play important, beneficial roles in normal wound healing and perform the following:
- Contract wound matrix through use of myofibroblasts
- Implement angiogenesis (breakdown of capillary basement membrane)
- Migrate cells (epidermal cells, fibroblasts, vascular endothelial cells)
- Remodel scar ECM
- Remove damaged extracellular matrix (ECM) (especially during the inflammatory phase of healing)

of MMPs in wound healing.) For example, during the inflammatory phase, damaged extracellular matrix proteins (such as collagen) must be removed so that newly synthesized collagen molecules can correctly align with collagen molecules in the wound matrix, permitting migration of epidermal cells and fibroblasts into the wound bed. (See *Extracellular matrix proteins and MMPs: Critical factors for epithelial migration, angiogenesis, and contraction.*) To remove damaged collagen molecules, collagenases (see *Families of MMPs, TIMPs, and ADAMs*) make a single cut in collagen molecules, which permits the gelatinases to further de-

grade collagen molecules into small fragments that are then removed from the injury area by neutrophils and macrophages. MMPs also play key roles in angiogenesis, by first degrading the basement membrane that surrounds vascular endothelial cells (VECs). This causes new capillary buds to sprout and "channels" to erode through the ECM, through which the VECs migrate, eventually creating new capillary arcs. Furthermore, MMPs are required for myofibroblasts to contract ECM during the maturation and remodeling phase. The actions of MMPs are controlled by their natural inhibitors, the tissue inhibitors of metallproteinases (TIMPs).

Acute vs. chronic wound healing

Molecular and cellular abnormalities in chronic wounds

There would appear to be little consensus regarding the definition of acute and chronic wound etiologies. Chronicity implies a prolonged or lengthy healing process, whereas acute implies uncomplicated, orderly or organized, or rapid healing. Bates-Jensen and Wethe[15] define an acute wound as "a disruption in the integrity of the skin and underlying tissues that progress through the healing process in a timely and uncomplicated manner." Typically, surgical and traumatic wounds, which heal by primary intention, are classified as acute.

On the other hand, Sussman[16] defines a chronic wound as "one that deviates from ex-

Extracellular matrix proteins and MMPs: Critical factors for epithelial migration, angiogenesis, and contraction

Epithelial migration
Epidermal cells at the leading edge of migrating sheets secrete several types of matrix metaloproteases (MMPs); fibroblasts migrating through provisional wound matrix also secrete MMPs.

Angiogenesis
Endothelial cells secret MMPs that degrade the basement membrane surrounding capillaries, allowing endothelial cells to proliferate and migrate toward angiogenic factors produced by cells in ischemic areas.

Contraction
Fibroblasts transform into myofibroblasts, which express contractile fibers and MMPs, and as myofibroblasts contract, force is applied to collagen fibers which reduces the size of the wound.

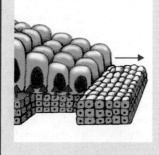
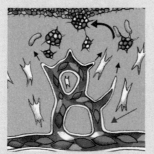
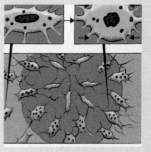

Families of MMPs, TIMPs, ADAMs

Collagenases
- Matrix metaloproteinase (MMP)-1, MMP-8, MMP-13, MMP-18
- Cut native type I collagen at one site

Gelatinases
- MMP-2, MMP-9
- Cut type collagen after collagenses make initial cut
- Cut native type IV collagen in basement membranes

Stromelysins
- MMP-3, MMP-10, MMP-11, MMP-19

- Cut core portein of prteoglycans

Metaloelastase/matrilysin
- MMP-7, MMP-12
- Cut multiple substrates including type IV collagen

Membrane-type (MT-MMPs)
- MT-MMP1 (MMP-14), MT-MMP2 (MMP-15), MT-MMP3 (MMP-16), MT-MMP4 (MMP-17)
- Attached to plasma membrane, active pro-MMPs

Tissue inhibitors of metaloproteinases (TIMPs)
- TIMP-1, TIMP-2, TIMP-3, TIMP-4
- Specific inhibitors for MMPs

A Disintegrin and metaloproteinase (ADAM)
- Aggrecanase 1 (ADAM-1)

TNFα converting enzyme (TACE)

TIME: Principles of wound bed preparation

Clinical observations	Molecular and cellular problems	Clinical actions
Tissue Nonviable or deficient	Defective matrix and cell debris impairing healing	Debridement (episodic or continuous) • Autolytic, sharp, surgical, mechanical, or biological • Biological agents
Infection or in-flammation	*High bacteria counts or prolonged inflammation* ↑ Inflammatory cytokines ↑ Proteases ↓ Growth factor activity	*Remove infected foci* *Topical/systemic* Antimicrobials Anti-inflammatories Protease inhibitors
Moisture imbalance	Dessication slowing epithelial cell migra-tion Excessive fluid causing maceration of wound	Apply moisture balancing dressings Compression, negative pressure and oth-er methods of removing fluid
Edge margin non-advancing or undermined	Epidermal margin not migrating Nonresponsive wound cells and abnor-malities in protease activities	Reassess cause, refer, or consider correc-tive advanced therapies: • Adjunctive therapies • Bioengineered skin • Debridement • Skin grafts

©Courtesy International WBP Panel.

Imbalanced molecular environments of healing and chronic wounds

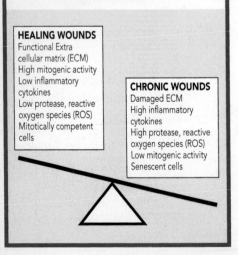

HEALING WOUNDS
Functional Extra cellular matrix (ECM)
High mitogenic activity
Low inflammatory cytokines
Low protease, reactive oxygen species (ROS)
Mitotically competent cells

CHRONIC WOUNDS
Damaged ECM
High inflammatory cytokines
High protease, reactive oxygen species (ROS)
Low mitogenic activity
Senescent cells

pected sequence of repair in terms of time, ap-pearance, and response to aggressive and ap-propriate treatment." The Wound Healing Society uses the definition of chronic wound as proposed in 1992 by Lazarus and colleagues: Chronic wounds "fail to progress through a normal, orderly, and timely sequence of repair or wounds that pass through the repair pro-cess without restoring anatomic and function-al results."[17] Such wounds usually heal by sec-ondary intention and are associated with path-ology; for example, diabetes, ischemic disease, pressure damage, and inflammatory diseases.

The physiological differences between wounds that heal slowly and those that heal rapidly have been studied in a variety of ways. (See *Imbalanced molecular environ-ments of healing and chronic wounds*.) One experiment explored the effect of chronic wound fluid on cell function.[18] Researchers cultured fibroblasts from human neonatal foreskin to use as a laboratory model of

Effects of clinical actions	Clinical Outcome
Restoration of wound base and functional extracellular matrix proteins	Viable wound base
Low bacteria counts or controlled inflammation ↓ Inflammatory cytokines ↓ Proteases ↑ Growth factor activity	Bacterial balance and reduced inflammation
Restore epithelial migration, desiccation avoided. Edema, excessive fluid controlled, maceration avoided	Moisture balance
Migrating keratinocytes and responsive wound cells. Restoration of appropriate protease profile in wound	Advancing epithelial margin

ma, ischemic reperfusion injury, subclinical bacterial contamination, and foreign bodies.

Because chronic wounds are typically characterized by full-thickness tissue loss, reepithelialization is prolonged due to the loss of appendages.[3] Normally, epithelial cells require the smooth, moist surface of the basement membrane to move across the wound. In chronic wounds, epithelial cells latch on to and pull themselves across the scaffolding of macromolecules of the provisional matrix, such as laminin and fibronectin.

Wound bed preparation

Wound bed preparation is a systematic approach to correcting the molecular and cellular abnormalities, which is critical to promoting healing of chronic wounds. Recently, the concept of wound bed preparation has emerged in a systematic, comprehensive approach to wound care management that addresses four key aspects of practice principles: tissue debridement, inflammation/infection, moisture balance, and edge of the wound (TIME).[20] (See *TIME: Principles of wound bed preparation.*)

Summary

acute wounds. They then exposed the model to either chronic wound fluid or a control and found that chronic wound fluid dramatically inhibited the growth of the fibroblasts. According to Phillips et al.,[18] these results indicate that the microenvironment of chronic wounds impairs wound healing.

Other researchers[5,19] theorize that prolonged inflammation is the most significant factor in delayed healing. Indeed, Hart[5] proposes that the prolonged inflammatory phase is due to the presence of inflammatory leukocytes, typically neutrophils and their production of proinflammatory cytokines that perpetuate inflammation. He also argues that the release of tissue-damaging proteinases, which degrade newly formed tissues, delay or prevent normal wound healing processes. In addition to prolonged inflammation, Hart[5] suggests several other factors that may induce chronicity, including recurrent physical trau-

In closing, the molecular and cellular environment of chronic wounds differs substantially from acute healing wounds. Specifically, nonhealing wounds have chronically elevated proinflammatory cytokines, which leads to chronically elevated levels of proteases (MMPs and neutrophil elastase) and reactive oxygen species (ROS) that degrade the components that are essential to healing, such as EMC components, growth factors, and receptors. Cells in the base of non-healing wounds often become insensitive to growth factors resulting in senesent cells. Clinical studies using topical application of protease or dressings that bind proteases or vacuum-assisted closure dressing have shown that reversing these molecular and cellular abnormalities promotes healing of chronic wounds.

Show what you know

1. Immediately following tissue injury, the priority is:

 A. to modify the immature scar tissue.
 B. to achieve rapid hemostasis.
 C. to rapidly fill the wounded area with granulation tissue.
 D. to destroy bacteria.

ANSWER: B. Rapid hemostasis is essential as it preserves the integrity of the closed and high-pressure circulatory system to limit blood loss.

2. The main mechanism by which chronic wounds fail to heal is believed to be:

 A. too rapid progress from hemostasis to maturation.
 B. a failure of fibroblasts and myofibroblasts to facilitate wound contraction.
 C. a dysfunction of collagen remodeling.
 D. a prolonged inflammatory phase.

ANSWER: D. Because chronic wounds contain abnormally high levels of proteinases and proinflammatory cytokines, prolonged inflammation is believed to be the most significant factor in delayed healing.

3. During the proliferative phase, the framework that new tissue grows into is commonly called:

 A. the extracellular matrix.
 B. the complement system.
 C. chemotaxis.
 D. apoptosis.

ANSWER: A. New tissue, or granulation tissue, grows into the extracellular matrix, which is composed of neovascular tissue, collagens, fibronectin, and proteoglycans.

References

1. Witte, M., and Barbul, A. "General Principles of Wound Healing," *Surgical Clinics of North America* 77:509, June 1997.
2. Steed, D. "The Role of Growth Factors in Wound Healing," *Surgical Clinics of North America* 77:575, June 1997.
3. Martin, P. "Wound Healing: Aiming for Perfect Skin Regeneration," *Science* 276:75, April 1997.
4. Slavin, J. "Wound Healing: Pathophysiology," *Surgery* 17(4):I-V, April 1999.
5. Hart, J. "Inflammation 2: Its Role in the Healing of Chronic Wounds," *Journal of Wound Care* 11:245-49, July 2002.
6. Stephens, P., and Thomas, D.W. "The Cellular Proliferative Phase of the Wound Repair Process," *Journal of Wound Care* 11:253-61, July 2002.
7. Wysocki, A.B. "Anatomy and Physiology of Skin and Soft Tissue," *Acute and Chronic Wounds: Nursing Management.* Edited by Bryant, R.A. St. Louis: Mosby–Year Book, Inc., 2000.
8. Clark, R.A.F. *The Molecular and Cellular Biology of Wound Repair,* 2nd ed. New York: Plenum Publishing Corp., 1996.
9. Neal, M. "Angiogenesis: Is It the Key to Controlling the Healing Process?" *Journal of Wound Care* 10(7):281-87, July 2001.
10. Calvin, M. "Cutaneous Wound Repair," *Wounds* 10(1):12, January 1998.
11. Rohovsky, S., and D'Amore, P. "Growth Factors and Angiogenesis in Wound Healing," in Ziegler, T., et al., eds. *Growth Factors and Wound Healing: Basic Science and Potential Clinical Applications.* New York: Springer-Verlag New York, Inc., 1997.
12. Berry, D.P., et al. "Human Wound Contraction: Collagen Organisation, Fibroblasts and Myofibroblasts," *Plastic and Reconstructive Surgery* 102(1):124-31, July 1998.
13. Tejero-Trujeque, R. "Understanding the Final Stages of Wound Contraction," *Journal of Wound Care* 10(7):259-63, July 2001.
14. Ehrlich, P. "The Physiology of Wound Healing: A Summary of the Normal and Abnormal Wound Healing Processes," *Advanced Wound Care* 11(7):326, November-December 1998.
15. Bates-Jensen, B.M., and Wethe, J. "Acute Surgical Wound Management," in Sussman, C., and Bates-Jensen, B.M., eds. *Wound Care: A Collaborative Practice Manual for Physical Therapists and Nurses.* Gaithersburg, Md.: Aspen Pubs., Inc, 2005.
16. Sussman, C. "Wound Healing Biology and Chronic Wound Healing," in Sussman, C., and Bates-Jensen, B.M., eds., *Wound Care: A Collaborative Practice Manual for Physical Therapists and Nurses.* Gaithersburg, Md.: Aspen Pubs., Inc, 2005.
17. Lazarus, G.S., et al. "Definitions and Guidelines for Assessment for Wounds and Evaluation of Healing," *Archives of Dermatology* 130(4):489-93, April 1994.
18. Phillips, T.J., et al. "Effect of Chronic Wound Fluid on Fibroblasts," *Journal of Wound Care* 7(10):527-32, November 1998.
19. Yager, D.R., and Nwomeh, B.C. "The Proteolytic Environment of Chronic Wounds," *Wound Repair and Regeneration* 7(6):433-41, November-December 1999.
20. Schultz, G.S. "Wound Bed Preparation, A Systemic Approach to Wound Bed Management," *Wound Rep Reg* 11 (supp1):S1-S28, 2003.

CHAPTER 6

Wound assessment

Sharon Baranoski, MSN, RN, CWOCN, APN, DAPWCA, FAAN
Elizabeth Ayello, PhD, RN, APRN, BC, CWOCN, FAPWCA, FAAN
Diane K. Langemo, PhD, RN, FAAN

OBJECTIVES

After completing this chapter, you'll be able to:

* state the reasons for performing a wound assessment

* differentiate between partial- and full-thickness injury

* list the parameters of a complete wound assessment.

The wound

The management of acute and chronic wounds has evolved into a highly specialized area of practice. An accurate and detailed wound assessment is vital in the care of patients with wounds and provides key elements about the current status of a wound. Care plans, treatment interventions, and ongoing management are all based on the initial and subsequent wound assessments. The total patient assessment, inclusive of any comorbid conditions and lifestyle, must also be a part of any comprehensive wound assessment. This chapter addresses the key assessment parameters of a patient with a wound admitted to any health care setting. The chapter content includes an explanation of the importance of a history and physical ex-amination, how to assess a wound, essential practice points, and documentation.

A wound is a disruption of normal anatomic structure and function.[1] Wounds are classified as acute or chronic. Acute wounds can be the result of trauma or surgery. According to Larazus,[1] acute wounds proceed through an orderly and timely healing process with the eventual return of anatomic and functional integrity. Chronic wounds, on the other hand, fail to proceed through this orderly and timely process and lose the cascade effect of wound healing and sustained anatomic and functional integrity. Simply stated, wounds may be classified as those that repair themselves or can be repaired in an orderly and timely process (acute wounds) and those that don't (chronic wounds).[1] In the United States, the Centers for Medicare and Medicaid Services

(CMS) is considering changing its current definition of a chronic wound. Their definition includes a time frame of greater than 30 days duration for complete healing.[2]

The pathology or cause of the wound must be determined before appropriate interventions can be implemented. States differ as to which clinicians can legally diagnose the wound, so check your specific practice act for your discipline. Wounds may have surgical-, traumatic-, neuropathic-, vascular-, or pressure-related etiology. For example, an acute wound caused by a bite (animal, insect, spider, or human) needs a different care plan than a wound caused by a burn. A patient who has an animal bite may require additional testing to rule out damage to nerves, tendons, ligaments, or bone, as well as determination of rabies or rabies vaccination status of the animal and the need for tetanus immunization.[3] The pathologic etiology will provide the basis for additional testing and evaluation to start the wound assessment process. (See *The nine Cs of wound assessment.*)

Initial assessment

Obtain a thorough history and a complete physical examination on every patient admitted into your care. Obtaining a patient history provides information on disease processes, medications the patient is taking, and a family history of conditions that can have an impact on the etiology of the wound. In addition, the patient history may reveal information that explains poor healing or warns of the likelihood of poor healing. A thorough patient history also helps focus your questioning on issues that could direct your initial interventions, such as vascular studies, glucose testing, and oxygen perfusion testing.[4] Therapies received as part of a prior health condition, such as radiation at the site of a wound, are also important factors that can contribute to impaired healing and delay appropriate management strategies.[1] (See "Radiation wounds" in chapter 21, Palliative wound care.)

Family support and functional abilities should be evaluated as well. Can the patient care for himself? Is there anyone at home, able and willing, to assist with care after discharge? Can the patient change his own dressings? Who will put on compression stockings? Can the patient afford to purchase the necessary items? These questions are an essential component of conducting a comprehensive assessment of the patient with a wound.

Physical examination

A head-to-toe physical examination should be performed to evaluate all skin areas, pressure points, old scars, indications of any prior surgeries, and the presence of vascular, neuropathic, or pressure ulcers. The appearance of the skin, nails, and hair on the extremities should be noted. Evaluation of skin color, temperature, capillary refill, pulses, and edema are also essential elements of a thorough physical examination.[4]

Different types of wounds require different considerations. Dehisced surgical wounds may have opened due to an infection, or may heal poorly due to underlying disease processes, current medications (such as steroids), or malnutrition. Hemosiderin staining due to the chronic leakage of red blood cells into the soft tissue of the lower leg is a classic sign of venous insufficiency. If not managed with compression, this leakage often leads to venous ulcers. Hemosiderin deposits (reddish-brown color) are often seen in patients with venous ulcers. Arterial ulcers often present with the classic signs of hair loss, weak or absent pulse, and very thin, shiny, taut skin. Neuropathic ulcers require intense evaluation of the extent of the neuropathy.[5,6] Patients with diabetes are prone to callus formations and off-loading tension pressure points, both of which are easily noted on an examination. Examination of the total patient will reveal areas of concern and areas that can relate to why the patient has a wound and, if it's not healing, why healing is not progressing. Developing a realistic goal and care plan, performing regular follow-up examinations, and ensuring patient compliance are all key markers for successful outcomes. (See chapters on specific wound types for more details.)

Wound assessment

Wound assessment—a written record and picture of the progress of the wound—is a cumulative process of observation, data collection, and evaluation. As such, it's an important component of patient care. A wound assessment includes a record of your initial assessment, ongoing changes, and treatment interventions. This initial assessment serves as the baseline for future comparisons, with ongoing assessments occurring throughout the healing process.

Frequency of wound assessment is often determined by the patient's health care setting but should occur at least weekly.[7] Acute-care patients often receive wound assessments daily or with each dressing change. Long-term care facilities must assess wounds on admission and with each dressing change.[8] Home-care assessments are usually based on the frequency of the home visits, but often occur weekly or with each licensed

nurse visit. Regardless of the setting, however, the frequency of assessments should be determined by the wound characteristics observed at the previous dressing change, as well as on the physician's or other practitioner's orders. The effectiveness of interventions can't be ascertained unless baseline assessment data are compared to follow-up data.[9] (See *When to reassess a wound,* page 80.)

No written standard exists outlining the type and amount of information to include in a wound assessment; likewise, no single documentation chart or tool has been designated as the most effective. Two studies found that wound assessments were documented significantly more frequently when an assessment chart is used and that using a chart improves the nurses' assessment skills.[10,11] Numerous documentation methods are available.[1,4,5,12] The assessment form that's used consistently by the facility's staff is the form that yields the most success. Also, forms that can be completed easily and quickly have a greater tendency of being used on a regular basis. If the staff finds a form too long or difficult, it won't be used.

A minimal wound assessment should include a thorough assessment of the whole patient, etiology or type of wound, and wound characteristics such as location, size, depth, exudate, and tissue type present.

PRACTICE POINT

CMS's suggestion for minimal pressure ulcer assessment includes[8]:
- Location and staging
- Size
- Exudate
- Pain
- Color and type of wound bed tissue
- Description of wound edges and surrounding tissue

Wounds can be classified using several different approaches. The partial- versus full-thickness model is used primarily by physicians and clinicians for wounds other than pressure ulcers. Damage to the epidermis and part of the dermis constitutes a partial-thickness wound. Abrasions, skin tears, blisters, and skin-graft donor sites are common examples of partial-thickness wounds. Full-

PRACTICE POINT ▬▬▬▬

When to reassess a wound

Assessment provides indicators of successful treatment interventions and attainment of achievable outcomes and guides decisions about product changes. Reassess the patient's wound:
• after the patient returns from surgery
• if the wound noticeably deteriorates
• if the wound becomes odorous or has new purulent exudate
• upon observing any other significant change in the condition of the wound
• after the patient has returned from another facility.

thickness wounds extend through the epidermis and dermis and may extend into the subcutaneous tissue, fascia, and muscle.[4] Partial-thickness wounds heal by resurfacing or reepithelialization. Full-thickness wounds heal by secondary intention through the formation of granulation tissue, contraction and, finally, reepithelialization, which of course requires a longer time period for healing.

Pressure ulcers and neuropathic ulcers have their own staging and classification systems to indicate the depth of injury and healing methods. (See chapter 13, Pressure ulcers, and chapter 16, Diabetic foot ulcers.)

Assessing the severity of a burn is a two-part process. Burn injuries are described by the extent of the body burned using one of several methods for estimating burn size, such as the Rule of Nines or Lund and Browder Chart. The depth of a burn injury is described by clinical observation of the anatomic layer of the skin involved (for example, superficial, partial-thickness, full-thickness, or subdermal burns).[6]

Obviously, there are many parameters to consider when performing a comprehensive wound assessment. Each clinical agency needs to develop a protocol that all clinicians should follow to ensure consistency. Whether using stage, grade, or partial- and full-thickness terminology, the one constant is clinical

assessment. Assessment data give the health care provider a mechanism to communicate, improve continuity among disciplines, and establish and modify appropriate treatment modalities.

Elements of a wound assessment

In 1992, Ayello developed a mnemonic for pressure ulcer and wound assessment and documentation.[12] (See *Pressure ulcer ASSESSMENT chart*. See also *Wound ASSESSMENTS chart*, page 82.) The mnemonic has been adapted for use with any type of wound to provide a thorough look at the parameters that complete and enhance an assessment. It provides a support structure for clinical decision-making regarding ongoing assessment and reassessment and may be used in any practice setting, according to the guidelines set up by your facility. This assessment chart may be used daily, weekly, or monthly. It's simple, fast, and can be further adapted to fit individual use.

Location and age of wound

Wound location should be documented using the correct anatomical terms—for example, right greater trochanter rather than right hip. Include a drawing of the human body, with the wound's location noted on the drawing, in your assessment record to provide complete admission documentation. If there are two or more wounds near one another, they should be labeled and numbered for clarity. How long has the patient had the wound? Are you dealing with a new, acute wound or a wound that has failed to heal for several weeks or months? Time alone isn't the sole determinant of acute versus chronic wound status. Although 30 days is often used for designation as chronic status, the more important criterion is whether or not the wound is making progress towards healing.[13,14]

In addition to wound duration, documentation of the cause of the wound, if known, is important. For example, if a patient reported that she spilled hot coffee on her amputated stump, which caused a blister that evolved into a full-thickness wound due to trauma and insufficient arterial supply, it would be

Pressure ulcer ASSESSMENT chart[12]

PATIENT'S NAME: AGE: _____ ❑ M   ❑ F

DATE: TIME: NUMBER OF PRESSURE ULCERS:

A ANATOMIC LOCATION OF WOUND
❑ Sacrum   ❑ Elbow ❑ R ❑ L
❑ Trochanter ❑ R ❑ L   ❑ Incisional
❑ Ischium ❑ R ❑ L   ❑ Other
❑ Heel ❑ R ❑ L
❑ Lateral malleolus ❑ R ❑ L

AGE OF WOUND
_____days or _____months patient has had the pressure ulcer

S SIZE
_____cm length _____cm width_____cm depth

SHAPE
❑ Oval ❑ Round
❑ Other _____

STAGE
Pressure ulcer stage:
❑ Stage I ❑ Stage II ❑ Stage III ❑ Stage IV
❑ Unable to determine stage; ulcer is necrotic
Wagner ulcer grade for neurotrophic ulcers:
❑ 0 ❑ 1 ❑ 2 ❑ 3 ❑ 4 ❑ 5

S SINUS TRACT, TUNNELING, UNDERMINING, FISTULAS
❑ Sinus tract, tunneling (narrow tracts under the skin) at ____ o'clock
❑ Undermining (bigger area [than tunneling] of tissue destruction — area is more like a cave than a tract)

E EXUDATE
Color
❑ Serous ❑ Serosanguineous ❑ Sanguineous
Amount
❑ Scant ❑ Moderate ❑ Large
Consistency
❑ Clear ❑ Purulent

S SEPSIS
❑ Local ❑ Systemic ❑ None

S SURROUNDING SKIN
❑ Dark ❑ Discolored ❑ Erythematous
❑ Intact ❑ Swollen
❑ Other _____

M MARGINS
❑ Attached (edges are connected to the sides of the wound)
❑ Not attached (edges aren't connected to the sides of the wound)
❑ Rolled (edges appear rounded or rolled over)

MACERATION
❑ Present ❑ Not present

E ERYTHEMA
❑ Present ❑ Not present

EPITHELIALIZATION
❑ Present ❑ Not present

ESCHAR (NECROTIC TISSUE)
❑ Yellow slough ❑ Black ❑ Soft ❑ Hard
❑ Stringy
Area around eschar is:
❑ Dry ❑ Moist ❑ Reddened

N NECROTIC TISSUE
❑ Present ❑ Not present

NOSE
❑ Odor present ❑ Odor not present

NEOVASCULARIZATION (BLOOD VESSELS ARE VISIBLE)
❑ Present ❑ Not present

T TISSUE BED
❑ Granulation tissue present ❑ Not present

TENDERNESS TO TOUCH
❑ No pain
❑ Pain present
❑ On touch
❑ Anytime
❑ Only when performing ulcer care
Patient getting pain medication:
❑ Yes ❑ No

TENSION
❑ Tautness, hardness present ❑ Not present

TEMPERATURE
❑ Skin warm to touch ❑ Skin cool to touch
❑ Normal

Wound ASSESSMENTS chart

PATIENT'S NAME:

AGE: _____

ASSESSMENT DATE: REASSESSMENT DUE DATE:

Wound etiology:
- ❏ Surgical ❏ Arterial ❏ Venous ❏ Pressure ulcer
- ❏ Diabetic or neurotrophic ulcer ❏ Other

A ANATOMIC LOCATION OF WOUND
- ❏ Upper/lower chest ❏ Abdomen ❏ Back
- ❏ Sacrum ❏ Foot ❏ R ❏ L ❏ Other ❏ R ❏ L
- ❏ Trochanter ❏ R ❏ L ❏ Ischium ❏ R ❏ L
- ❏ Elbow ❏ R ❏ L ❏ Arm ❏ R ❏ L
- ❏ Leg ❏ R ❏ L ❏ Heel ❏ R ❏ L
- ❏ Lateral malleolus ❏ R ❏ L
- ❏ Medial malleolus ❏ R ❏ L

AGE OF WOUND
- ❏ Acute: post op < 7 days ❏ Acute: post op > 7days
- ❏ Chronic: < 1 month
- ❏ Chronic: > 1 month _____ Days/months

S SIZE, SHAPE, STAGE
_____cm width_____cm length_____cm diameter

SHAPE
❏ Oval ❏ Round ❏ Irregular ❏ Other _____

STAGE
Stage of pressure ulcer
❏ I ❏ II ❏ III ❏ IV ❏ Unable to stage; ulcer necrotic
Wagner ulcer grade for neurotrophic ulcers
❏ 0 ❏ 1 ❏ 2 ❏ 3 ❏ 4 ❏ 5

S SINUS TRACT, TUNNELING, UNDERMINING, FISTULAS
❏ None ❏ Present: located _____ at
_____o'clock, _____cm depth

E EXUDATE
Amount
❏ None ❏ Scant ❏ Moderate ❏ Large
Color ❏ Serous ❏ Serosanguineous ❏ Sanguineous
Consistency: ❏ Thick ❏ Purulent ❏ Milky

S SEPSIS
❏ Systemic ❏ Local ❏ Both ❏ None
❏ Odor present

S SURROUNDING SKIN
- ❏ Intact ❏ Erythematous ❏ Edematous
- ❏ Induration ❏ Warm ❏ Cool
- ❏ Discolored ❏ Dry ❏ Other

M MACERATION
❏ Not present
❏ Present: _____cm, location_____

E EDGES, EPITHELIALIZATION
- ❏ Edge attached ❏ Edge not attached
- ❏ Edges rolled
- ❏ Surgical incision approximated
- ❏ Surgical incision open ❏ Sutures/staples intact
- ❏ Epithelialization present: _____ cm
- ❏ Epithelialization not present

N NECROTIC TISSUE
❏ Not Present ❏ Present
Type
❏ Yellow slough ❏ Black ❏ Soft ❏ Hard ❏ Stringy
Percentage of wound (check closest percentage):
- ❏ 100% of wound ❏ 75% of wound
- ❏ 50% of wound ❏ 25% of wound
- ❏ Other: _____ %

T TISSUE BED
- ❏ Granulation tissue not present
- ❏ Granulation tissue present _____ amount%
- ❏ Moist ❏ Dry
Tenderness or pain
(0 being no pain, 10 being intense pain)

Pain scale score

0	1	2	3	4	5	6	7	8	9	10

Circle appropriate number
Pain present:
- ❏ on touch ❏ anytime
- ❏ only when performing wound care
- ❏ other (specify) _____
Pain management: Specify method _____
❏ Not effective ❏ Effective

S STATUS
Wound status: Initial assessment date _____
- ❏ Improved: date _____ ❏ Unchanged: date _____
- ❏ Healing: date _____ ❏ Deteriorating:* date _____
*Notify physician
- ❏ Supportive therapy
  - ❏ compression ❏ off-loading
  - ❏ pressure relieving mattress ❏ other _____
- ❏ Patient's perception on quality of life _____
- ❏ Referrals Specify to whom _____
Initial assessment:
Signature _____Title _____ Date _____
Reassessment (per policy):
Signature _____Title _____ Date _____

© Baranoski, S., and Ayello, E.A.

incorrect to classify the wound as a pressure ulcer.

Wound size and stage

The National Pressure Ulcer Advisory Panel (NPUAP) staging system is only intended to be used for pressure ulcers and has been under review for how to incorporate deep-tissue injury into the definition. The staging system addresses the depth of insult in stages I through IV. Any pressure ulcer covered with eschar or necrotic tissue is unstageable except in long-term care where CMS recommends that it be documented on the Minimum Data Set (MDS) as a stage 4 ulcer.[8] (See chapter 13, Pressure ulcers.)

PRACTICE POINT

Even though the ulcer is necrotic and unstageable, you still need to document the outer visible wound size for length and width.

Partial-thickness wounds heal fairly quickly as they involve the epidermis and into, but not through, the dermis. Full-thickness wounds penetrate through the fat and involve muscle, tendon, or bone and take longer to heal. (See *Necrotic, unstageable pressure ulcer.*) Use the correct classification staging system for the specific wound type, for example, Meggit-Wagner for diabetic ulcers, CEAP for venous, or Payne-Martin for skin tears.

Wound measurement

Measurement of a wound is an important component of wound assessment and provides valuable information on wound progression or non-progression, as well as assessment of the effectiveness of clinical interventions. It's particularly important in determining clinical effectiveness for research purposes. Consistency and accuracy in how the wound is measured is important for determining change in the wound over time. Consistency is best assured when the agency develops and disseminates a protocol for wound measurement and staff follow the protocol.

The measurement method used can be either simple or sophisticated, and two-dimensional (wound surface area) or three-dimensional (wound volume). Change in wound measurement such as a decrease in size is used as an indicator of healing. Surgical incisions can be measured using length, for example, incision line is 8″ long. Wounds should not be measured using objects, for example, dime or half-dollar, but rather by centimeters (cm) or, if smaller, millimeters (mm).

Necrotic, unstageable pressure ulcer

Shown here is a pressure ulcer that's unstageable because its base is covered with eschar. Be sure to measure the pressure ulcer's length and width and document your findings.

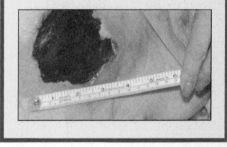

Area

The simplest and most common method of wound measurement is the linear method using a paper or plastic ruler marked in centimeters (cm) and millimeters (mm). One can measure the greatest head-to-toe length and greatest side-to-side width perpendicular to each other[15,16,17]; the greatest length and width, regardless of being perpendicular to one another; or the longest length head-to-toe and the longest width side-to-side. (See *Wound measurement,* page 84.) Linear measurement is inexpensive, readily available, causes little to no discomfort, and is frequently used by most clinicians.[15,18,19] However, use caution with this method, as it assumes that the wound area is a rectangle or square, which is rarely ever the case, and nearly always overestimates the size of the wound. Regardless of which method is used, what's most important is to have an agency

Wound measurement

Linear measurements of a wound should be taken at the greatest length and width perpendicular to each other, as shown below.

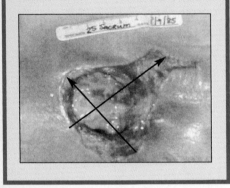

protocol and ensure that it's being implemented consistently. Another method to measuring area is by multiplying length by width for square centimeters (cm^2). This adds a third dimension of depth, which is then added to the linear measurement if desired.[15] If the wound is open, depth can be assessed, either by using a clean cotton-tipped applicator or a centimeter measuring device, placed into the deepest part of the wound, marking it, and then measuring it upon removal. (See *Determining wound depth.*)

Planimetry is a method where a wound tracing is made on metric graph paper with a 4-cm or 8-cm grid. The completed squares, within the traced wound edges, are then counted to yield an approximate area in square centimeters.[13] Minimal training is needed to use this method, the acetate tracing medium is inexpensive and disposable, and the wound area can be determined immediately.[15]

Wound area may also be measured by stereophotogrammetry (SPG), using a digital camera and computer software. A target plate is placed within the plane of the wound to be photographed. The photo is then downloaded to the computer screen where the wound edges are traced, along with the length and width, using a computer-pointing device or mouse. The computer automatically calculates the area as well as the length and width.[15] A color picture of the wound along with the measurements can be printed on a chart sheet for the patient record. This method allows for accurate, reproducible measurements of irregular wounds and is noninvasive.[15,20]

EVIDENCE-BASED PRACTICE

Using SPG to measure wounds is the most accurate and reliable method, with planimetry being the least trustworthy.[15]

Volume

As most wounds extend below the skin surface, they are three-dimensional, generally irregular, and, at times, more cone-shaped. To that end, volume becomes an important variable and needs to be measured and calculated. The most common wound volume measurement technique is measuring the three dimensions of length, width, and depth and multiplying those measurements by one another ($L \times W \times D$ = volume cm^3).[21] Caution should be used, however, as this equation assumes the base and surface area are the same size, which is generally not the case.

Other techniques include molds, fluid installations, the Kundin device, and SPG. However, molds and fluid installations are imprecise and time consuming, uncomfortable for the patient, and can potentially contaminate the wound.[13,22,23] The Kundin device is a plastic-coated, disposable, three-dimensional gauge with three arms for measuring length, width, and depth.[24] Wound volume is calculated via a mathematical formula, which assumes a shape somewhere between a cylinder and a sphere.[21,24] It's a convenient, relatively inexpensive, user-friendly technique.[21] As mentioned previously, SPG measures the depth and area of a wound and inputs that information into the software. The software calculates wound volume using the Kundin device formula. When the Kundin device and SPG were compared using wound models,

SPG was the more accurate method. However, more research is needed.

Wounds can also be photographed. Both the NPUAP and the Wound Ostomy and Continence Nurses Society (WOCN) have position statements about photographing wounds.[17,25] To that end, the NPUAP neither recommends nor discourages the use of photography. If it's used, however, it recommends that explicit protocols be established for each institution or agency and that the protocols be consistently followed.[17]

When using regular photography, it's necessary to permanently mark the date and time as well as to identify patient information on the photo. The photo should also include a sample measure in each frame (for example, a 10-cm strip of paper tape).[17] When digital photos are used, at least 1.5 megapixels are recommended to achieve the best clarity.[17] However, because digital photos can be altered, the identifying data must be encoded permanently. When regular photos are taken, distortion is a problem due to body contour, angle of the body in a bed, angle and distance of the camera from the patient, and lighting. Some photo software packages use a target plate in the photo and the software; once the photo is downloaded, it can automatically calculate wound area and volume as well as length and width.[14,17]

Sinus tracts, undermining, and fistulas

Sinus tracts, undermining, and fistula formation delay the healing cascade. Intervening early with the appropriate medical, surgical, and nursing actions is paramount to healing these complicated wounds.

Sinus tracts

A sinus tract (or tunnel) is a channel that extends from any part of the wound and may pass away from the wound through subcutaneous tissue and muscle. The channel or pathway, together with the wound itself, involves an area larger than the visible surface of the wound. The sinus or tunnel may result in dead space and abscess formation, further complicating the healing process. Sinus tracts are common in dehisced surgical wounds and may also be present in neuropathic and arter-

Determining wound depth

The depth of a wound can be measured by using a cotton swab applicator, as shown in the photographs below, or a centimeter measuring device.

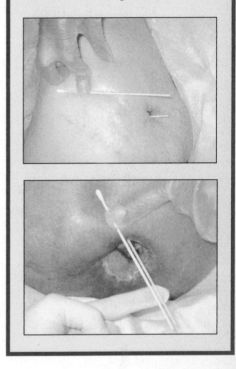

ial wounds. Documenting sinus tracts is an important element in assessment because it enables the clinician to evaluate potential treatment interventions. Treatment interventions involve loosely packing the dead space with an appropriate dressing to stimulate granulation and the contraction process. The goal is to close the sinus tract first, while allowing the outside of the wound to remain open and fully heal.

Measurement can be done using a clean cotton-tipped applicator or gloved finger, inserting it to the bottom or end, marking it, and measuring it upon removal. (See *Determining wound depth*.)

Undermining

Undermining, shown in the photographs below, is tissue destruction that occurs around the wound perimeter underlying intact skin.

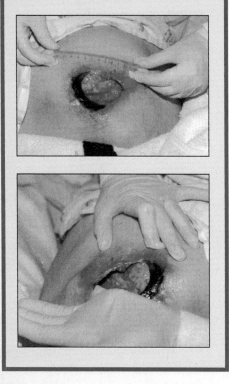

Undermining

Undermining is tissue destruction that occurs around the wound perimeter underlying intact skin; in these wounds, the edges have pulled away from the wound's base. (See *Undermining*.) Pressure ulcers that have been subjected to a shearing force often present with undermining in the area of the greatest shear. Undermining is also seen when the opening of the wound is smaller than the affected tissue below the dermis and in desiccated wound beds. Documentation of the location and amount of undermining is important. Clinicians can document using the clock figure, using the head as the 12 o'clock position (for example, "Undermining from 2 to 6 o' clock, measures 3 cm") or using percentages (for example, "75% of the wound has undermining measuring 2 cm from 12 to 9 o'clock"). Undermining may also be more extensive in one part of a wound than another. This, too, should be documented appropriately. Interventions include loosely packing or tucking all undermined areas to prevent buildup of debris and dead tissue, and applying an appropriate dressing, such as hydrogel, gauze, or alginate dressing.

The degree of undermining may be measured using the same method as for sinus tracts.

Fistulas

Fistulas can develop in surgical wounds and in deep, severe pressure ulcers. A fistula connects viscous organs together (for example, a rectovaginal fistula) or connect to the skin (for example, an enterocutaneous fistula).[4] Fistulas are named by using the point of origin, such as the rectum, and the point of exit, such as the vagina. Management of a patient with a fistula is complex and intense and demands critical thinking and technical skills.[13] Fistulas can take weeks or months to heal. In addition, the patient with a fistula is often malnourished and may require weeks of intense nutritional therapy to improve his condition.

Exudate and odor

Exudate is the accumulation of fluids in the wound, which may contain serum, cellular debris, bacteria, and leukocytes. Exudate may appear as dry, dehydrated, dead, or nonviable tissue (nondraining) or be moist and draining. Exudate assessment includes noting the amount (small, moderate, large), color, consistency, and odor.[26] For example, certain microorganisms have characteristic odors, such as *Pseudomonas aeruginosa*. (See *Classifying exudate*. See also *LOWE© skin barriers for wound margins: 20-second enablers for practice,* page 88.)

Exudate may be serous (clear or pale yellow), serosanguineous (serous or blood tinged), or sanguineous (bloody). The consistency may be thick, milky, or purulent.

Sepsis

Sepsis or bacteremia is caused by anaerobes and gram-negative bacteria and can occur in any susceptible wound. To determine the presence of sepsis, an assessment should include consideration of erythema, warmth, edema, purulent or increased drainage, induration, and increased tenderness or pain. If sepsis is present, it's important to determine whether the infection is local or systemic. Interventions are based on accurate assessment and laboratory support.

The best method to culture a wound to determine the presence of sepsis remains controversial. Typically, tissue biopsy followed by fluid aspiration is the gold standard.[7] These options, however, may not be available in all settings, and many clinicians lack the skill necessary to perform them. Many settings continue to use the swab method, in which the wound must be cleaned and thoroughly dried prior to swabbing for a culture. Culturing of wounds is important in determining sepsis. One must remember, however, that all pressure ulcers are considered colonized, as is any chronic wound.[13,14]

Malodorous wounds should also be documented. However, make sure the odor is from the wound—not the dressing change, which is a common mistake. Certain organisms—such as *Pseudomonas*—have a distinct odor that is easily recognized by the trained clinician. (See chapter 7, Wound bioburden, for more detailed information on infection and culturing.)

PRACTICE POINT

Remember that not all odor indicates infection; certain dressings develop a distinct odor when exudates interact with them (for example, hydrocolloids). Odor may also indicate the need to change the dressing more often.

Classifying exudate

Wound exudate can be classified in two ways—by type or amount.

Type (color and consistency)
These exudates may exist as a single form or in combinations (for example, serosanguineous):
- Serous or clear fluid
- Sanguineous for blood
- Purulent pus made up of inflammatory cells and tissue debris that can result from infection or an inflammatory process

Amount
The amount of exudate may indicate that the cause of the wound has not been treated (for example, edema due to venous insufficiency), that congestive heart failure is present (look for bilateral involvement and extension above the knee), that low albumen levels have occurred (malnutrition, kidney or liver disease), or that infection (check for signs or symptoms) is present. Amounts of exudate include:
- none
- small—there's just a detectable discharge when the dressing is removed, less than 33%
- moderate—discharge is covering less than 67% of dressing surface
- large—discharge is covering more than 67% of the dressing surface.

Surrounding skin
The skin surrounding a wound also provides valuable information to the assessing clinician. Erythema and warmth may indicate inflammation or infection. Interruptions in periwound skin integrity (denudation, erosion, papules, or pustules) may indicate allergic reactions to tape or dressing adhesive. Maceration or desiccation may be a sign that the dressing is too moist or too dry for the

amount or type of exudate. Palpation should be done with the fingertips around a wound surface. This may reveal induration or fluctuance, an abnormal fluid accumulation indicative of further tissue damage or abscess. Although new research provides us with a different understanding of where the wound ends[27] and the surrounding skin begins, assessment of surrounding tissue does provide useful information for the ongoing evaluation and future wound-care interventions.

LOWE© skin barriers for wound margins: 20-second enablers for practice

Exudate may indicate that the cause of the wound has not been treated (eg, edema due to venous insufficiency); congestive heart failure is present (look for bilateral involvement and extension above the knee); low albumen (malnutrition, or kidney or liver disease); or infection (check for symptoms or signs).

Periwound skin needs protection from exudate by using absorbent dressings over the wound and protecting the periwound skin. You can choose from 4 ways to protect the external skin of a wound. Try using this memory jogger to remember them: LOWE© (from Old English, meaning to approve of, prompt, or to humble oneself).

TYPE	ADVANTAGES	DISADVANTAGES
Liquid film Forming acrylate • No sting • Skin preparation etc.	• Transparent surface that resists removal • Low incidence of reactions	• Some skin sealants may evaporate and dry out • Lack of availability on some institutional formularies
Ointments • Petrolatum • Zinc oxide	• Relatively cheap and easy to apply	• Petrolatum liquefies with heat • Zinc oxide ointment does not allow visualization of underlying wound margin • Ointment vehicle may interfere with the action of ionized silver
Windowed dressing • Framing of wound margin with protective adhesive – Hydrocolloid – Film – Acrylate – Silicone etc.	• Provides a good seal around the wound edge • Some products facilitate visibility of the wound margins	• Reactions to the adhesive can occur • If seal is compromised, moisture may accumulate under the dressing
External collection devices	• External pouching may help in locations where an external seal is difficult (e.g., perirectal area)	• Devices need to monitored for external seal *Note: These devices do not replace a search for the cause of the excessive exudate and the need to correct the cause.*

Maceration

Maceration is a softening of the skin surrounding a wound due to excess drainage or pooling of fluid on intact skin and appears as a white, waterlogged area. It may be caused by inadequate management of exudate or an increase in exudate due to changes in the wound tissue. Maceration may be prevented by using an appropriate barrier cream around the wound, changing the dressing more often, or by selecting a more absorbent dressing. (See *color section, Wound assessment,* pages C3 to C5.)

Edges and epithelialization

Epithelialization is the regeneration of the epidermis across a wound surface.[13] The epithelial wound edge is continuous and often difficult to see. As wound migration occurs from the edges, the portion covered with epithelium is pearly or silver and shiny. It's also thin and fragile, and thereby easily insulted. The edge of a wound may be attached to the wound bed, unattached (undermining), or rolled inward. Wound edges should be assessed as part of a thorough evaluation of the wound.

Examining the wound edges may reveal whether the wound is acute or chronic and can often provide clues as to the wound's etiology. For example, a wound with inflamed edges or violaceous with undermined borders may indicate pyoderma gangrenosum. A wound with edges rolled inward may be too dry, causing the wound edges to seek more moisture from the wound bed. A wound covered in necrotic tissue, desiccated, or deprived of oxygenation will exhibit poorly defined wound margins.[13]

Epithelialization can also occur in the middle of a wound bed if hair follicles or new cell growth are present. The appearance of new tissue at the wound edge can be measured in centimeters or by the percentage of wound coverage (for example, "0.3 cm of epithelial tissue surrounds the wound," or "wound is 25% epithelialized"). The degree of epithelialization is often overlooked.

PRACTICE POINT

Be sure to assess and record the wound's epithelialization.

Necrotic tissue

Necrotic tissue is dead, devitalized, avascular tissue that provides an ideal medium for bacterial proliferation and may inhibit healing. It's a well-known theory that wound healing is optimized when all necrotic tissue is removed from the wound bed. Necrotic tissue may present as yellow, gray, brown, or black. As it becomes dry, it presents as thick, hard, leathery black eschar.[13,14] Yellow, stringy necrosed tissue is referred to as slough.[13]

Document necrotic tissue by quantifying the percentage of tissue in the wound bed. For example, the wound bed may be 100% necrotic or 25% granular with 75% necrotic tissue. (See color section, *Wound terminology*, page C5.)

Wound bed tissue

The wound bed tissue reveals the phase and progress of wound healing through observation of its tissue color, degree of moisture—a moist wound bed facilitates movement of fibroblasts and macrophages, as well as collagenase and other chemicals, resulting in healing—and amount of epithelialization. [13,14 28] The wound bed may be pale pink, pink, red, yellow, or black. Clean, granular wounds are typically described as red, and wounds with devitalized slough are described as yellow. Brown and black wounds are typically those with necrotic tissue or eschar or desiccated tissue, and need to be debrided because it slows the healing process.[13]

Is the wound bed moist or dry? The presence of moisture or dry tissue will guide you in selecting the right dressing to create an environment that supports healing. Do you see new tissue growth—epithelialization at the wound edges or within the wound bed? Is granulation tissue present—that is, beefy red tissue with a granular or gritty appearance?

Documentation should be based on your observations. Is the wound 100% granular tissue, or is it 25% filled with slough (yellow tissue) or necrotic (dead) tissue? All three tissue types can be found in the same wound, and assessing the amount of each type of tissue will help you document the outcome of care based on improvement or deterioration, as indicated by wound tissue characteristics. Outcomes can then be tracked by percentage of improvement toward a clean granular wound bed (for example, "the wound progressed from 75% necrotic tissue to 100% granular tissue").

Tenderness to touch or the amount of pain the patient reports—both in the wound itself and in the surrounding tissue—are also essential parts of your assessment. Wound pain is one of the secondary signs of infection. It's important to differentiate between constant and episodic pain (such as pain that occurs

Wound picture

When assessing wounds in your patient, use the mnemonic, **WOUND PICTURE,** for a fast and accurate assessment.

Wound or ulcer location

Odor? (In room or just when wound is uncovered?)

Ulcer category, stage (for pressure ulcer) or classification (for diabetic ulcer), and depth (partial-thickness or full-thickness)

Necrotic tissue?

Dimension of wound (shape, length, width, depth); drainage color, consistency, and amount (scant, moderate, large)

Pain? (When it occurs, what relieves it, patient's description, patient's rating on scale of 0 to 10)

Induration? (Surrounding tissue hard or soft?)

Color of wound bed (Red-yellow-black or combination)

Tunneling? (Record length and direction—toward patient's right, left, head, feet)

Undermining? (Record length and direction, using clock references to describe)

Redness or other discoloration in surrounding skin?

Edge of skin loose or tightly adhered? Edges flat or rolled under?

only with dressing changes). Use a pain assessment scale accepted by your facility. (See chapter 7, Wound bioburden, and chapter 12, Pain management and wounds.)

Measuring healing

Although assessing and measuring a wound are important, so is documenting wound healing. There is growing research on determining healing rates of different chronic wounds (pressure, venous, and diabetic neuropathic ulcers) as well as expected healing rates at 4 weeks.[29] In clinical practice, there are a variety of tools on the market to assess and document healing, including the Pressure Sore Status Tool (PSST),[5] the Pressure Ulcer

Scale for Healing (PUSH),[4,30] and the Sessing Scale.[31]

The PSST includes 11 wound factors to be tracked over time, and each are scored numerically. The total of the 11 factors reflects overall wound status. Although this tool provides a precise record, it's fairly time consuming; so, it's utilized more often in clinical research. The PUSH tool, developed and revised by the NPUAP, has been research-validated. It allows for quick and reliable assessments necessary to monitor healing over time. Three scores are developed: one is for surface area (L × W), one indicates drainage amount, and the third is for tissue type. The total score of these three factors is then plotted on a healing record (or graph) to depict healing over time. It's designed solely for pressure ulcers and should be used at least weekly.[4,30,32] The simple, easy-to-use, and reliable Sessing Scale measures granulation tissue, infection, drainage, necrosis, and eschar on a 7-point scale. Each characteristic is given a numeric value, and the positive or negative numeric changes from successive assessments over time yield a scale score.[31] Assessments should be done at least weekly by a qualified and trained health care professional.

Documentation essentials

Documentation is an essential component of wound assessment. Every wound assessment should be documented thoroughly, accurately, and legibly, with an accompanying signature as well as the date and time of the assessment. Wounds should be documented on the patient's admission, with each dressing change, upon any significant change in the wound, and upon discharge.

As mentioned previously in this chapter, the first assessment and documentation is a baseline comparison for all future assessments. It is recommended that each clinical agency have a consistent agency chart form and format for wound documentation. All facilities should follow the wound assessment policy as determined by their setting-specific regulations. These include the mandated Outcome and Assessment Information Set (OASIS) for home care, or the MDS for long-term care. Other assessment and documentation tools that might become part of the agency protocol include the aforementioned PSST, PUSH tool, or Sessing Scale.

PRACTICE POINT

It's important to remember that the OASIS and the MDS are regulatory documentation tools—neither tool is considered a comprehensive wound assessment.

Summary

Wound assessment—an appraisal of a patient's condition based on clinical signs and symptoms, laboratory data, and medical history—is an integral part of wound management. Assessment has become a highly specialized area of care, requiring well-developed observational skills and current knowledge. The use of current terminology is imperative to accurate assessment and communication. Use of the Wound ASSESSMENTS chart or the WOUND PICTURE mnemonic can provide a fast, ongoing, and accurate assessment for patients with wounds.[33] (See *Wound picture*.) Assessment of wound parameters provides clinicians with the information needed to make decisions affecting the outcome of care. These decisions will guide the wound care team to suitable interventions, management, and care strategies.

Show what you know

1. *Wound assessment involves all of the following* except:

   A. observation.
   B. data collection.
   C. evaluation.
   D. dressing change.

ANSWER: D. Wound assessment involves observation, data collection, and ongoing evaluation process. Dressing change is an intervention for the management of wound care.

2. *A wound that has tissue damage through the epidermis and partially into the dermis would be classified as:*

   A. superficial.
   B. partial-thickness.

   C. full-thickness.
   D. subdermal.

ANSWER: B. A superficial wound involves only the epidermis and the dermis is still intact. A full-thickness wound extends through the dermis. A subdermal wound extends into underlying structures below the skin such as bone, muscle, or tendon.

3. *In assessing a wound, you find an area of tissue destruction under the edge of the patient's wound. This is best described as:*

   A. a sinus tract.
   B. maceration.
   C. fistula.
   D. undermining.

ANSWER: D. A sinus tract is a channel that involves an area larger than the visible surface of the wound. Maceration is the softening of the surrounding skin usually from exposure to or excess wound drainage. A fistula is an opening between two organs or an organ and the skin.

References

1. Larazus, G.S., et al. "Definitions and Guidelines for Assessment of Wounds and Evaluation of Healing," *Archives of Dermatology* 130(4):489-93, April 1994.
2. Centers for Medicare and Medicaid Services (CMS). "Usual Care of Chronic Wounds Meeting, March 29, 2005." Available at: *www.cms.gov*. Accessed June 11, 2006.
3. Bower, M.G. "Evaluating and Managing Bite Wounds," *Advances in Skin & Wound Care* 15(2): 88-90, March-April 2002.
4. Stotts, N.A., and Cavanaugh, C.C. "Assessing the Patient with a Wound," in *Home Health Care Nurse*. Philadelphia: Lippincott Williams & Wilkins, 1999.
5. Bates-Jensen, B. "The Pressure Sore Status Tool a Few Thousand Assessments Later," *Advances in Wound Care* 10(5):65-73, 1997.
6. Richards, R. "Assessment and Diagnosis of Burn Wounds," *Advances in Skin & Wound Care* 12(9): 468-71, November-December 1999.
7. Wound, Ostomy, Continence Nurses Society. Guideline for Prevention and Management of Pressure Ulcers. WOCN Clinical Practice Guideline Series 2. Glenview, IL: WOCN Society, 2003.
8. Centers for Medicare and Medicaid Services (CMS) Tag F-314 Pressure Ulcers. Revised Guidance for Surveyors in Long Term Care. Issued November 12, 2004. Available at: *http://new.cms.hhs.gov/manuals/downloads/som107ap_pp_guidelines_ltcf.pdf.* Accessed June 11, 2006.
9. van Rijswijk, L. "The Fundamentals of Wound Assessment," *Ostomy/ Wound Management* 42(7):40-46, August 1996.
10. Banfield, K.R., and Shuttleworth, E. "A Systematic Approach with Lasting Benefits: Designing and Implementing a Wound Assessment Chart," *Professional Nurse* 8(4):234-38, January 1993.
11. Morison, M.J. "Wound Assessment," *Professional Nurse* 2(10):315-17, July 1987.
12. Ayello, E. "Teaching the Assessment of Patients with Pressure Ulcers," *Decubitus* 5(7):53-54, July 1992.

13. Bryant, R.A. *Acute and Chronic Wounds, Nursing Management,* 2nd ed. St. Louis: Mosby–Year Book, Inc., 2000.
14. Maklebust, J., and Sieggreen, M. *Pressure Ulcers: Guidelines for Prevention and Management,* 3rd ed. Springhouse, Pa.: Springhouse Corp., 2000.
15. Langemo, D.K., et al. Two-Dimensional Wound Measurement: Comparison of 4 Techniques. *Advances in Skin & Wound Care* 11(7):337-43, 1998.
16. Cutler, N.R., George, R., Seifert, R.D., et al. "Comparison of Quantitative Methodologies to Define Chronic Pressure Ulcer Measurements," *Decubitus* 6:22-30, 1993.
17. National Pressure Ulcer Advisory Panel. Documentation Photography. Available at: www.npuap.org. Accessed March 23, 2006.
18. Rodeheaver, G.T., and Stotts, N.A. "Methods for Assessing Change in Pressure Ulcer Status," *Advances in Skin & Wound Care* 8:28-34, 1995.
19. Thomas, A.C., and Wysocki, A.B. "The Healing Wound: A Comparison of Three Clinically Useful Methods of Measurement," *Decubitus* 3:18-25, 1990.
20. Frantz, R.A., and Johnson, D.A. "Stereophotogrammetry and Computerized Image Analysis: A Three-dimensional Method of Measuring Wound Healing," *Wounds* 4:58-64, 1992.
21. Langemo, D.K., et al. "Comparison of 2 Wound Volume Measurement Methods," *Advances in Skin & Wound Care* 2001,14(4):190-96.
22. Resch, C., et al. "Pressure Sore Volume Measurement: A Technique to Document and Record Wound Healing," *J Am Geriatr Soc* 36:444-46, 1988.
23. Berg, B., and Traneroth, C.A. "A Method for Measuring Pressure Sores," *Lancet* 1990,335:1445-446.
24. Kundin, J.I. "A New Way to Size Up a Wound," *Am J Nurs* 1:206-207, 1989.
25. Wound Ostomy and Continence Nurses Society (WOCN). *Photography in Wound.* Available at: *www.wocn.org.* Accessed March 23, 2006.
26. Ayello, E.A., and Sibbald, R.G. LOWE© "Skin Barrier for Wound Margins." E Alert April 2006.
27. Stojadinovic, O., et al. "Role of B-Catenin and C-myc in the Inhibition of Epithelialization and Wound Healing," *American Journal of Pathology* 167(1) 59-69, 2005.
28. *http://www.ruralfamilymedic*
29. Jessup, R.L. "What Is the Best Method for Assessing the Rate of Wound Healing? A Comparison of 3 Mathematical Formulas," *Advances in Skin & Wound Care* 19(3):138,140-42, 145-46, 2006.
30. National Pressure Ulcer Advisory Panel. PUSH Tool. Available at: http://www.npuap.org/PUSHinstr:html. Accessed March 18, 2006.
31. Ferrell, B.A., et al. "The Sessing Scale for Assessment of Pressure Ulcer Healing," *Journal of the American Geriatric Society* 43(1):37-40, 1995.
32. Stotts, N.A., et al. "Testing the Pressure Ulcer Scale for Healing (PUSH) and Variations of the PUSH," Paper presented at the 11th Annual Symposium on Advanced Wound Care, April 18-22, 1998, Miami Beach, Fla.
33. *Wound Care Made Incredibly Easy,* 2nd ed. Philadelphia: Lippincott, Williams, & Wilkins, 2006.

CHAPTER 7

Wound bioburden

Sue E. Gardner, PhD, RN, CWCN
Rita A. Frantz, PhD, RN, CWCN, FAAN

OBJECTIVES

After completing this chapter, you'll be able to:

- distinguish between colonization and infection in a chronic wound

- identify the most valid method of determining a wound infection

- explain the effects of antiseptics on chronic wound tissue

- identify conditions when antimicrobial therapy is indicated for treatment of a chronic wound.

Bioburden in wounds

The human body is in constant contact with multiple microorganisms originating from both endogenous and exogenous sources.[1] Usually, these microorganisms are present without any evidence of infection because a balance exists between host resistance and microbial growth. Infection occurs when this equilibrium is upset, either because of lowered host defenses or increased microorganism quantity or virulence. Infection is directly related to the number and virulence of the organisms, which overcome host resistance.[2]

The skin provides a physical and chemical barrier to microorganisms. Many microorganisms are able to survive on the skin and are known as skin colonizers, or normal flora. Normal flora may actually inhibit the growth of more virulent microorganisms

and, therefore, serve a protective function. This mutually beneficial relationship between host and microorganism is referred to as a *commensal relationship.* Some normal flora are transient colonizers; they merely survive, don't multiply, and can easily be removed. Resident flora, on the other hand, multiply and are permanent.

Breaks in the skin, including wounds, allow microorganisms to access deeper tissue and structures where they can more readily adhere and multiply.[2] Host response to microorganisms in the wound is multifaceted. Nonspecific host responses occur regardless of microbial species; whereas specific host responses are triggered by specific microorganisms and involve the immune system. Regardless, nonspecific and specific responses are essential for preventing invasion of wound microorganisms into vital tissues and organs.

Nonspecific responses include phagocytosis by polymorphonuclear leukocytes (PMNs) and macrophages and inflammation. Although the mechanism of inflammation evolved to protect humans from microorganisms in particular[3], the inflammatory response can be elicited from any type of tissue injury. Thus, the first phase of wound healing is referred to as the *inflammatory phase* (see chapter 5, Acute and chronic wound healing); the cascade of events that occur during this phase are essential to activating the healing process.

Inflammation

Inflammation is integral to microbial resistance. It's triggered by endogenous (host sources) and exogenous (microbial) mediators.

Endogenous mediators, such as cytokines and growth factors, arise from mast cells, PMNs, macrophages, the complement system, and immune cells. These cells release mediators in response to contact with microorganisms or microbial products. Endogenous mediators are also released in response to tissue injury unrelated to microorganisms, such as injury caused by surgical procedures or trauma.

Exogenous mediators are produced by microorganisms. Most notable is endotoxin, which is produced by gram-negative bacteria. If released into the blood, endotoxin activates all inflammatory mechanisms at once, resulting in septic shock. Exotoxins are inflammatory mediators released by bacteria. Many bacterial exotoxins are extremely chemotactic; that is, they attract leukocytes. However, many bacterial toxins don't elicit inflammation directly. They indirectly elicit inflammation by activating mast cells and macrophages or by evoking an adaptive immune response, which then produce inflammatory mediators.[3,4]

The release of inflammatory mediators results in localized vasodilation and increased blood flow to the area of injury. The accompanying increase in vascular permeability promotes a rapid influx of phagocytic cells, complement, and antibody to the wound site. Collectively, these events remove microorganisms and debris as well as bacterial toxins and enzymes. These physiological responses to injury are expressed by the signs of inflammation including erythema, heat, edema, and pain.[3,5,6]

Inflammation is characterized as being either acute or chronic.[3,7] Acute inflammation is the initial response to tissue invasion or injury and includes pronounced vascular changes and the predominance of PMNs at the site of injury.[7] Again, this type of inflammation can result from microorganisms or any type of tissue injury. Chronic inflammation occurs if the invasion or injury of tissue isn't resolved and persists over a long period of time. The vascular response becomes less pronounced during chronic inflammation and the predominant leukocyte at the site of injury shifts to macrophages.[3,7] Chronic inflammation is also characterized by the proliferation of fibroblasts and scar tissue.[6,7]

Infection

When host resistance fails to control the growth of microorganisms, localized wound infection results. Uncontrolled localized infection of a wound can lead to deep, more severe infections such as extensive cellulitis, osteomyelitis, bacteremia, and sepsis. More subtly, localized wound infection impairs healing and is thought to be an important cause of wound chronicity.[8]

The persistent presence of microorganisms leads to the influx of phagocytes, which release proteolytic enzymes, inflammatory mediators, and free radicals. The cumulative effect of these substances in the wound is additional tissue injury and wound deterioration.[9] Moreover, inflammatory mediators produce localized thrombosis and vasoconstriction resulting in a hypoxic wound environment, which, in turn, promotes further bacterial proliferation, thus establishing a destructive, prolonged inflammatory cycle.[10] The immune response (that is, specific host responses) may be down-regulated in an attempt to limit self-destruction.

The proliferative phase of wound healing is also affected by wound infection. Bacteria and bacterial toxins stimulate macrophages to produce an excessive angiogenic response. The resultant granulation tissue is edema-

tous, somewhat hemorrhagic, and more fragile.[11] Although the collagen content of infected wounds is higher than the collagen content of noninfected wounds, collagenolytic
activity is also higher, resulting in wound
breakdown.[12,13] Migration of epithelial tissue is inhibited by bacteria and bacterial toxins, and new epithelium is prone to lysis and
desiccation by neutrophil proteases.[14,15]
Finally, wound contraction is inhibited in the
presence of large numbers of bacteria.[16]

PRACTICE POINT

Wound infection prolongs the inflammatory phase and disrupts the proliferative
phase of wound healing.

> # Key elements of wound infection
>
> - Wound infection occurs in wound tis-
>   sue, not on the surface of the wound
>   bed.
> - Wound infection occurs in viable
>   wound tissue; it isn't a phenomenon
>   of necrotic tissue, eschar, or other
>   debris contained in the wound bed.
> - Wound infection is caused by inva-
>   sion and multiplication of microbes
>   in the wound.
> - Wound infection is manifested by a
>   host reaction or tissue injury.

Defining infection

Wound infection has been defined as the invasion and multiplication of microorganisms
in wound tissue resulting in pathophysiologic
effects or tissue injury.[22] Of particular importance in this definition is the fact that invasion and multiplication of microorganisms
occurs in the *wound tissue*. (See *Key elements
of wound infection*.) Thus, wound infection
can be differentiated from wound contamination and colonization.

Wound contamination is the presence of
bacteria on wound surfaces with no multiplication of bacteria.[23-25] Other organisms are
permanent colonizers and replicate, or multiply, on the wound surface. Wound colonization is characterized by the replication of microorganisms on the wound surface without
invasion of wound tissue and no host immune response.[2] Some of these colonizers
may be involved in a mutually beneficial relationship with the host preventing the adherence of more virulent organisms in the
wound bed. These organisms include
Corynebacteria species, coagulase negative
staphylococci, and viridans streptococci.[10]

The mere presence or multiplication of microorganisms on the wound surface doesn't
necessarily constitute wound infection.
Contamination and colonization with wound
microorganisms is a condition common to all
wounds healing by secondary intention and,
in fact, is a prerequisite to the formation of

granulation tissue.[1,26, 146.] In contrast,
wound infection is the invasion and multiplication of microorganisms in the wound tissue
beneath the wound surface. Thus, for an infection to be present, the microorganisms
must be present in viable tissue.

PRACTICE POINT

Contamination and colonization of
a wound with microorganisms doesn't constitute
infection.

The presence of microorganisms in wound
pus, necrotic tissue, or slough isn't evidence
of tissue invasion. These nonviable substances are known to support bacterial
growth[27], and debridement of this tissue is
essential to prevent infection. However, the
presence of microorganisms in necrotic tissue
that hasn't invaded viable tissue doesn't constitute wound infection.

Multiplication of microorganisms is another key element of the definition; that is, microorganisms must replicate and produce
large enough numbers to cause injury or impair healing.

Another key element in the definition is
that the invading organisms must produce
host responses or tissue injury. The concepts
of host response and pathophysiologic tissue
injury are interrelated; that is, they both pre-

sent clinical signs and symptoms. As previously described, host response produces the signs and symptoms associated with inflammation. Tissue injury produces other signs and symptoms.

Identifying infection

Despite the known deleterious effect of infection on healing[17,18], the identification and diagnosis of localized wound infection is fraught with ambiguity in clinical practice. This is especially true for chronic wounds, which heal by secondary intention. (See chapter 5, Acute and chronic wound healing.)

PRACTICE POINT

The first sign of critical colonization may be delayed wound healing as evidenced by no change in wound size (L × W) or increasing exudate. [146]

Conversely, the identification and diagnosis of localized infection of acute wounds—such as surgical incisions—is less equivocal because most of these wounds display a clinically apparent, robust inflammatory response. The normal time frame for inflammation associated with the wounding event (for example, a surgical procedure) is 3 to 5 days.[22] Inflammation that persists past 3 to 5 days is considered indicative of wound infection.[19]

Like acute wound infections, the identification of deep, more severe infections is often easier to identify due to the development of overt systemic signs and symptoms. For example, extensive erythema, elevated body temperature, elevated white blood cell count, and elevated blood sugar in people with diabetes are readily apparent. Similarly, osteomyelitis should always be considered if a wound can be probed to bone because exposed bone is usually indicative of osteomyelitis, especially in diabetic foot ulcers.[120]

EVIDENCE-BASED PRACTICE

A wound that has exposed bone or that can be probed to the bone with a sterile instrument should be evaluated for osteomyelitis.[20]

However, identifying milder, localized infection in chronic wounds is much more problematic for a variety of reasons. First, chronic wounds by definition are slow to heal or don't heal at all. Although many factors may account for impaired healing, wound bioburden has always been suspected as a major deterrent to healing and an important cause of wound chronicity. Second, the manifestation of inflammation may be altered in chronic wounds because of population-specific factors. For example, the inflammatory response to bacteria may be influenced by age[21], presence of diabetes, tissue perfusion and oxygenation, other aspects of immunocompetence, and anti-inflammatory drug use.

Finally, considerable disagreement exists regarding what constitutes wound infection in the chronic wound.[110] In addition to this lack of consensus, the value of wound cultures in identifying infection is a source of confusion for clinicians and a source of debate among experts. However, despite the confusion surrounding identification of localized chronic wound infection, an operative definition of wound infection can provide a foundation from which clinicians can approach identification and diagnosis in a rational, consistent manner.

Methods to identify wound infection

In practice, wound infection is identified and diagnosed based on clinical signs and symptoms of infection or on the findings from wound cultures. The advantages and disadvantages of using these methods can be evaluated in light of the key elements contained in the definition of wound infection. A practical clinical approach for clincans, using the mnemonic Nerds and Stones [146] can help identify superficial and deep infection. (See *Nerds© and Stones©*.)

Clinical signs and symptoms

The most common and clinically practical method for identifying wound infection is to monitor for clinical signs and symptoms of infection. Clinical signs and symptoms of wound infection reflect host response to inva-

Nerds© and Stones© [146]

Superficial infection
- **N**on-healing wounds
- **E**xudate wounds
- **R**ed and bleeding wound surface granulation tissue
- **D**ebris (yellow or black necrotic tissue) on the wound surface
- **S**mell or unpleasant odor from the wound

Deep infection
- **S**ize bigger
- **T**emperature increased
- **O**s (prone to or exposed bone)
- **N**ew or satellite areas of breakdown
- **E**xudate, erythema, edema
- **S**mell

sion or tissue injury. They can be detected by direct observation of the wound and periwound area or be reported by the patient. The clinical signs and symptoms of wound infection can be divided into those that comprise the classic signs of infection and those that are specific to secondary wounds (that is, tissue injury).

The classic signs and symptoms of infection are pain, erythema, edema, heat, and purulent exudate.[3,5,6] As indicators of infection, they're a reflection of the host's response to invading organisms. The first four of these signs are also known as the signs of inflammation, which can be elicited by tissue damage unrelated to infection.[3] Purulent exudate is the result of bacterial exotoxins recruiting white blood cells to the wound. However, it's the host reaction, expressed by the classic signs and symptoms of infection, that distinguishes an infected wound from one that's merely colonized or contaminated according to some authors.[26] For example, the American Diabetes Association (ADA) Consensus Conference on diabetic foot wound care (1999) defined localized infection in diabetic foot ulcers as purulence or two or more signs of inflammation.[118]

The enabler "NERDS"© can be used to diagnosis superficial bacteria burden. Look for two to three of the signs that spell out the term "NERDS." Once the bacteria sink to the deep layers of wound tissue or surrounding skin use the Enabler "STONES" to identify deep infection. Early recognition of infection is crucial so that appropriate systemic

treatment can be started and further damage can be prevented.[146]

PRACTICE POINT

The classic signs of infection are pain, erythema, edema, heat, and purulent exudate.

The classic signs and symptoms of infection are believed to be reliable indicators of infection in acute wounds such as surgical incisions. In surgical wounds, inflammation occurs after wounding, but should subside within 5 days.[28] The Centers for Disease Control and Prevention's (CDC) definition of a surgical site infection (SSI) reflects the confidence placed in clinical signs and symptoms to identify SSIs.[29] (See *CDC criteria for surgical site infection,* page 98.) SSIs are defined as infections occurring within 30 days of the operative procedure and are categorized as superficial incisional, deep incisional, or organ/space. The presence of purulent drainage is sufficient criteria as are signs of inflammation accompanied by a positive culture.

Unlike acute wounds, the classic signs and symptoms are not always present in chronic wounds[30] or diabetic foot ulcers[119] with high wound bioburden. This may be due to diminished systemic or local inflammatory responses among populations with high prevalence of chronic wounds, such as patients with diabetes and those with peripheral vascular disease or autoimmune disorders. Similarly, immunosuppressed patients with acute wounds may not express classic signs

CDC criteria for surgical site infection

The Centers for Disease Control and Prevention (CDC) has established the following criteria to define surgical site infection (SSI).

Superficial incisional SSI	Deep incisional SSI	Organ/space SSI
Involves only skin or subcutaneous tissue of the incision and at least one of the following: • purulent drainage from the superficial incision • organisms isolated from aseptically obtained culture of fluid or tissue from the incision • at least one of the following, unless negative culture: – pain or tenderness – localized swelling – redness or heat – incision opened by surgeon • diagnosis of SSI by the surgeon or attending physician.	Involves deep soft tissues (such as fascia and muscle layers) of the incision and at least one of the following: • purulent drainage from the deep incision but not organ/space • deep incision spontaneously dehisces or is deliberately opened by surgeon with one of the following symptoms, unless negative culture: – fever greater than 100.4° F (38° C) – localized pain • an abscess • diagnosis of deep SSI by surgeon or attending physician.	Involves any part of the anatomy (other than the incision) opened or manipulated during operation and at least one of the following: • purulent drainage from a drain placed in organ/space • organisms isolated from aseptically obtained culture of fluid or tissue in organ/space • an abscess or other evidence of infection • diagnosis of an organ/space SSI by a surgeon or attending physician.

of infection despite high wound bioburden. The only exception is the symptom of pain, which may occur in people with compromised immune function and be the only apparent symptom of infection.[32]

EVIDENCE-BASED PRACTICE

The classic signs and symptoms of infection may not be present in chronic wounds or in patients who are immunosuppressed.

EVIDENCE-BASED PRACTICE

Pain may be the only classic sign of wound infection present in immune compromised patients.

Additional signs and symptoms specific to secondary wounds have been proposed as in-dicators of infection.[33] These signs and symptoms include:
• serous drainage with concurrent inflammation
• delayed healing
• discoloration of granulation tissue
• friable granulation tissue
• pocketing at the base of the wound
• foul odor
• wound breakdown.

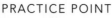

PRACTICE POINT

Granulation tissue bleeds easily due to bacteria stimulation of vascular endothelial growth factors (VEGF).[146]

All of these signs and symptoms, with the exception of pocketing, were found to be valid indicators of localized infection in a sample of chronic wounds.[30] Among a sample of diabetic foot ulcers, all were found to be valid with the exception of pocketing, friable granulation tissue, and wound breakdown.[119] Moreover, delayed healing may be the only sign apparent. According to the clinical practice guideline published by the Agency for Healthcare Research and Quality, "a clean pressure ulcer should show some evidence of healing within 2 to 4 weeks."[34] Although many factors have been associated with delayed healing, wound infection may be a primary contributor.[8] When it's the only sign readily apparent, delayed healing should stimulate further assessment of wound bioburden by clinicians.[34]

PRACTICE POINT

Delayed healing may be the only sign of infection in some wounds.

Although using clinical signs and symptoms of infection to monitor wounds for infection is congruent with the definition of infection, the assessment of these parameters is quite subjective.[35] Therefore, the clinical signs and symptoms checklist (CSSC) was developed to assess for the presence such signs and symptoms of infection in chronic wounds. (See *Clinical signs and symptoms checklist,* pages 100 and 101.) The CSSC provides a precise description for each of the clinical signs and symptoms. Although more research regarding the validity and reliability of this checklists needed, preliminary findings indicate that the reliability of the items on the CSSC are acceptable.[31, 121] Moreover, the CSSC provides clinicians with information on assessing the lesser-known signs and symptoms specific to secondary wounds.

Compounding the subjective limitations of using signs and symptoms to identify wound infection is the lack of clear guidelines regarding the number of signs and symptoms that need to be present to constitute infection. Increasing pain and wound breakdown were found to be sufficient signs of infection in a small study (n = 36) of chronic wounds, but none were necessary.[30] Further, it's unclear how assessment of clinical signs and symptoms leads to decisions regarding wound infection status.[35] As mentioned previously, the ADA suggests that purulent exudate or the presence of two signs of inflammation be used to define infection in diabetic foot ulcers.[118] In practice, the presence of frankly obvious signs and symptoms of infection often triggers treatment or wound cultures to guide selection of antimicrobials.

EVIDENCE-BASED PRACTICE

Increasing pain and wound breakdown are sufficient signs of wound infection.

PRACTICE POINTS

Wound cultures are used to diagnose wound infection when it isn't clinically obvious.

The ADA suggests that purulent exudate or the presence of two or more signs of inflammation are indicative of infection in diabetic foot ulcers.

Early idenitification of wound infection is crucial in wound management. Cutting and colleagues tried to determine which clinical signs and symptoms of infection are present in all wounds as well as any that are specific to a particular wound[147] by using a Delphi process of international interdisciplinary wound experts. They determined that cellulitis, malodor, pain, delayed healing, wound deterioration or breakdown, and an increased amount of exudate are common to all wounds (except for acute wounds healing by primary intention and full-thickness burns). Symptoms or criteria that had the highest score for infection in a particluar wound are as follows: crepitus for pressure ulcers, phlegmon for neuropathic/diabetic ulcers, increase in local skin temperature for venous ulcers, and dry necrosis, which may turn moist and boggy at the edges of the necrotic tissue, for arterial disease-associated tissue breakdown.[147] (See *Ranking of clinical infection indicators by wound type,* pages 102 and 103.)

Wound cultures and specimens

Like clinical signs and symptoms, the identification of wound infection based on culture findings may be inconclusive. Nonetheless, numerous methods are available for clinical and research purposes. The methods present-

Clinical signs and symptoms checklist

SIGNS AND SYMPTOMS   CHECK (+) IF PRESENT

Increasing pain in the ulcer area
The patient reports increased level of peri-ulcer pain since the ulcer developed. Ask him to select the most appropriate statement for current level of ulcer pain from the following choices:
1. I can't detect pain in ulcer area.
2. I have less ulcer pain now than I had in the past.
3. The intensity of the ulcer pain has remained the same since the ulcer developed.
4. I have more ulcer pain now than I had in the past.
If the patient selects number 4, his pain is increasing. Write n/a if the patient can't respond to
the question.

Erythema
The presence of bright or dark red skin or darkening of normal ethnic skin color immediately
adjacent to the ulcer opening indicates erythema.

Edema
The presence of shiny, taut skin or pitting impressions in the skin adjacent to the ulcer but within 4 cm from the ulcer margin indicates edema. Assess pitting edema by firmly pressing the
skin within 4 cm of ulcer margin with a finger, release and waiting 5 seconds to observe indentation.

Heat
A detectable increase in temperature of the skin adjacent to the ulcer but within 4 cm of the ulcer margin as compared to the skin 10 cm proximal to the wound indicates heat. Assess differences in skin temperature using the back of your hand or your wrist.

Purulent exudate
Tan, creamy, yellow, or green, thick fluid that's present on a dry gauze dressing removed from
the ulcer 1 hour after the wound was cleaned and dressed indicates purulent exudate.

Sanguinous exudate
Bloody fluid that's present on a dry gauze dressing removed from the ulcer 1 hour after the
wound was cleaned and dressed indicates sanguinous exudate.

Serous exudate
Thin, watery fluid that's present on a dry gauze dressing removed from the ulcer 1 hour after
the wound was cleaned and dressed indicates serous exudate.

Delayed healing of the ulcer
The patient reporting no change, or an increase in the volume or surface area of the ulcer, over
the preceding 4 weeks indicates delayed healing. Ask the patient if the ulcer has filled with tissue or is smaller around than it was 4 weeks ago.

Discoloration of granulation tissue
Granulation tissue that is pale, dusky, or dull in color compared to surrounding, healthy tissue.
Note variations of normal, beefy-red appearance of granulation tissue.

Friable granulation tissue
Bleeding of granulation tissue when gently manipulated with a sterile cotton-tipped applicator
indicates friable tissue.

Clinical signs and symptoms checklist *(continued)*

SIGNS AND SYMPTOMS	CHECK (+) IF PRESENT
Pocketing at base of wound The presence of smooth, nongranulating pockets of ulcer tissue surrounded by beefy red granulation tissue indicates pocketing.	☐
Foul odor The ulcer may have a putrid or distinctively unpleasant smell.	☐
Wound breakdown Small open areas in newly formed epithelial tissue not caused by reinjury or trauma indicate wound breakdown.	☐

Adapted with permission of HMP Communications from Gardner, S.E., et al. "A Tool to Assess Clinical Signs and Symptoms of Localized Chronic Wound Infection: Development and Reliability," *Ostomy/ Wound Management* 47(1):40-47, January 2001.

ed here are limited to those most commonly used in practice.

Wound cultures require two steps. The first step is the acquisition of a specimen from the wound. The second step includes the laboratory procedures used to grow, identify, and quantify the microorganisms. Clinicians are directly responsible for the first part and must be aware of laboratory processes included in the second to acquire an appropriate wound specimen and effectively transport the specimen to the laboratory.

The three most common types of wound specimens are:
- wound tissue
- needle-aspirated wound fluid
- swabs.

The tissue biopsy method consists of aseptically removing a piece of viable wound tissue with a scalpel or punch biopsy instrument. Wound tissue specimens are the most congruent with the first two elements that define wound infection if the specimens are samples from viable tissue rather than necrotic tissue. Among a sample of 41 wounds of mixed etiology, the quantitative tissue biopsy method had a sensitivity of 100%, a specificity of 93.5%, and an accuracy of 95.1% in predicting the success of delayed closure.[36] Based on this and other data, the tissue biopsy became the gold standard specimen for wound cultures.[37] Unfortunately, tissue biop-

sy cultures are invasive, skill-intensive (both from clinician and laboratory perspectives), and unavailable in many settings. Therefore, they aren't commonly used in practice, but are often used in research of wound microbiology.

 PRACTICE POINT

Wound tissue is considered the best specimen for culture from which to identify wound infection.

Needle-aspiration technique obtains fluid through multiple insertions of a 22G needle into the tissue surrounding the wound. The needle is attached to a 10-cc syringe.[38] Although studies have compared needle aspiration technique with both quantitative tissue biopsy and swab cultures, the sensitivity, specificity, and accuracy of quantitative needle-aspiration remains unclear due to methodological limitations.[37-39] However, this may be the best technique for specimen collection when focal collections of tissue fluid or abscess formations exist close to the wound.[40]

The most practical and widely available method for obtaining wound specimens is the swab culture. However, the usefulness of this method is extremely contentious. Since this method samples only wound surface organisms (as opposed to organisms within the tis-

Ranking of clinical infection indicators by wound type

Acute wounds: Primary

Cellulitis
Pus/abscess
Delayed healing
Erythema ± induration
Haemopurulent exudate
Malodor
Seropurulent exudate
Wound breakdown/enlargement
Increase in local skin temperature
Edema
Serous exudates with erythema
Swelling with increase in exudate volume
Unexpected pain/tenderness

Acute wounds: Secondary

Cellulitis
Pus/abscess
Delayed healing
Erythema ± induration
Haemopurulent exudate
Increase in exudate volume
Malodor
Pocketing
Seropurulent exudates
Wound breakdown/enlargement
Discoloration
Friable granulation tissue that bleeds easily
Increase in local skin temperature
Edema
Unexpected pain/tenderness

Diabetic foot ulcers

Cellulitis
Lymphangitis
Phlegmon
Purulent exudate
Pus/abscess
Crepitus in the joint
Erythema
Fluctuation
Increase in exudate volume

Induration
Localized pain in a normally asensate foot
Malodor
Probes to bone
Unexpected pain/tenderness
Blue-black discoloration and hemorrhage (halo)
Bone or tendon becomes exposed at base of ulcer
Delayed/arrested wound healing despite offloading and debridement
Deterioration of the wound
Friable granulation tissue that bleeds easily
Local edema
Sinuses develop in an ulcer
Spreading necrosis/gangrene
Ulcer base changes from healthy ink to yellow or grey

Arterial leg ulcers

Cellulitis
Pus/abscess
Change in color/viscosity of exudates
Change in wound bed color*
Crepitus
Deterioration of wound
Dry necrosis turning wet
Increase in local skin temperature
Lymphangitis
Malodor
Necrosis—new or spreading
Erythema
Erythema in peri-ulcer tissue — persists with leg elevation
Fluctuation
Increase in exudate volume
Increase in size in a previously healing ulcer
Increased pain
Ulcer breakdown

Venous leg ulcers

Cellulitis
Delayed healing despite appropriate compression therapy

Increase in local skin temperature
Increase in ulcer pain/change in nature of pain
Newly formed ulcers within inflamed margins of pre-existing ulcers
Wound bed extension within inflamed margins
Discoloration, e.g., dull, dark brick red
Friable granulation tissue that bleeds easily
Increase in exudate viscosity
Increase in exudate volume
Malodor
New onset dusky wound hue
Sudden appearance/increase in amount of slough
Sudden appearance of necrotic black spots
Ulcer enlargement

Pressure ulcer

Cellulitis
Change in nature of pain
Crepitus
Increase in exudate volume
Pus
Serous exudate with inflammation
Spreading erythema
Viable tissues become sloughy
Warmth in surrounding tissues
Wound stops healing despite relevant measures
Enlarging wound despite pressure relief
Erythema
Friable granulation tissue that bleeds easily
Malodor
Edema

Burns: Partial-thickness

Cellulitis
Ecthyma gangrenosum
Black/dark brown focal areas of discoloration in burn
Erythema

Ranking of clinical infection indicators by wound type (continued)

Hemorrhagic lesions in subcutaneous tissue of burn wound or surrounding skin	Opaque exudates	Sub-eschar pus/abscess formation
Malodor	Rejection/loosening of temporary skin substitutes	Unexpected increase in wound breadth
Spreading peri-burn erythema (purplish discoloration or edema)	Secondary loss of keratinized areas	Discoloration
Unexpected increase in wound breadth		Friable granulation tissue that bleeds easily
Unexpected increase in wound depth	**Burns: Full-thickness**	Malodor
Discoloration		Edema
Friable granulation tissue that bleeds easily	Black/dark brown focal areas of discoloration in burn	Opaque exudate
Sub-eschar pus/abscess formation	Cellulitis	Rapid eschar separation
Increased fragility of skin graft	Ecthyma gangrenosum	Rejection/loosening of temporary skin substitutes
Increase in exudate volume	Erythema	Secondary loss of keratinized areas
Increase in local skin temperature	Hemorrhagic lesions in subcutaneous tissue of burn wound or surrounding skin	
Loss of graft	Increased fragility of skin graft	**Key:**
Edema	Loss of graft	
Onset of pain in previously pain-free burn	Onset of pain in previously pain-free burn	
	Spreading peri-burn erythema (purplish discoloration or edema)	

Key:

HIGH	Mean score 8 or 9
MEDIUM	Mean score 6 or 7
LOW	Mean score 4 or 5

*black for aerobes, bright red for *Streptococcus*, green for *Pseudomonas*

Results of the Delphi process identifying criteria in six different wound types
Used with permission: Medical Education Partnership LTD, 2005.

---

sue), many believe it's ineffectual as a measure of infection.[34] In addition, it may be difficult to recover anaerobic organisms from swab specimens.[19] However, others defend the role of swab cultures in monitoring infection, emphasizing its entrenchment in clinical practice.[41]

The swab techniques most commonly used or advocated in the literature are swabs of wound exudate, swabs taken using a broad Z-stroke over the entire wound bed, and swabs using the technique described by Levine and colleagues.[19,40,43,47-51] Specimens obtained in this manner sample microorganisms on the surface and aren't congruent with the first or second key elements of infection.

Wound cleaning is advocated prior to obtaining swabs using either Z-stroke or Levine's technique in order for the culture to isolate wound tissue microorganisms as opposed to microorganisms associated with wound exudate, topical therapies, or nonviable tissue.[19,50] Moistening the swab with normal saline or transport medium is also recommended prior to specimen collection.[39,50] Moistening the swab is believed to provide more precise data than a dry swab.[52] Swabs using the broad Z-stroke entail rotating the swab between the fingers as the wound is swabbed from margin to margin in a 10-point zigzag fashion.[40] Because a large portion of the wound surface is sampled, the specimen collected may reflect surface contamination rather than tissue bioburden.[19]

The Levine technique consists of rotating a swab over a 1-cm square area with sufficient pressure to express fluid from within the wound tissue, as shown top of next page.[43]

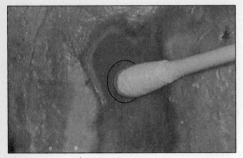

Photo courtesy of Dr. Rita Frantz

This technique is believed to be more reflective of "tissue" bioburden than swabs of exudate or swabs taken with a Z-stroke.[19] Theoretically, the Levine technique is the best technique of wound swabbing provided the wound is cleaned first and the area sampled is over viable tissue, not necrotic tissue or eschar.[19]

Although the accuracy of swab cultures as compared to biopsy cultures had been studied, the findings from these studies provided little information from which to base clinical practice.[39,41-46] The most serious methodological problem presented by these studies is that the specific swabbing techniques employed were not described. Swabbing techniques vary greatly according to wound preparation, area of the wound sampled, duration of sampling, and even the type of swab employed (for example, alginate).[37] To address this problem, we compared culture findings from swab specimens obtained using wound exudate, the Z-stroke technique, and Levine's technique with culture findings from viable wound specimens.[122] The findings from this study indicated that culture findings based on swab specimens obtained using Levine's technique were more accurate and concordant with culture findings based on tissue specimens than both wound exudate and Z-stroke technique.

PRACTICE POINT

Levine's technique provides culture findings most comparable to tissue specimens because this technique attempts to sample microorganisms from within the wound tissue, not just from the wound surface.

Analyzing cultures and specimens

Laboratory procedures for the microbiological analysis of wound specimens include isolation and identification of the microorganisms alone or in combination with quantification of the microorganisms isolated. When done alone, isolation and identification is referred to as qualitative culture, and when done in conjunction with quantification, it's referred to as quantitative culture. Quantitative cultures provide information regarding the type of organisms present in addition to the number of organisms present, which is usually expressed as number per gram of tissue, milliliter of fluid, or swab. The number of organisms present provides information regarding the rate of microorganism multiplication; therefore, quantitative cultures reflect the third key element of wound infection more completely than qualitative cultures.

Qualitative cultures

The recovery, isolation, and identification of microorganisms gained importance in identifying wound infection following the post-World War I (WWI) development of organism-specific antimicrobials.[53] According to the CDC, one sufficient criteria of surgical site infection is an "organism isolated from an aseptically obtained culture of fluid or tissue."[29] By this definition, an organism present in the tissues of the wound indicates infection. It's important to note that this CDC criterion implies that isolation of organisms must be from within the tissue or tissue fluid, not isolation of organisms from the wound surface. The CDC defines pressure ulcer infection as the presence of two of the following clinical findings: redness, tenderness, or swelling of wound edges and organisms are isolated from a needle aspiration, tissue biopsy, or blood culture.[54] Clinical signs and symptoms of infection must be present along with isolation of an organism known to cause disease.

Acute wounds often contain skin flora, such as staphylococci and diphtheroids.[2] Chronic wounds, with their distinctive environment, often contain larger numbers and types of microorganisms than acute wounds. These wounds have large amounts of exudate, necrotic tissue and eschar, large surface areas, and deep cracks and crevices suitable for a variety of microbial species. Chronic wounds have been associated with anaerobes and multiple types of organisms.[55-57] Common organisms isolated from chronic wounds are *Proteus mirabilis, Escherichia coli,* and *Streptococcus, Staphylococcus, Pseudomonas, Corynebacteria,* and *Bacteroides* species.[55,56,58-60]

Limited data indicate that the presence of *P. mirabilis, P. aeruginosa,* and *Bacteroides,* an anaerobe, deter chronic wound healing.[61,62] Nonhealing chronic wounds were also associated with the presence of *E. coli,* group D *Streptococci,* and other anaerobic cocci.[44]

Although the presence of methicillin-resistant *S. aureus* (MRSA) in chronic wounds presents a problem for infection control in health care settings, the association between colonization with MRSA and subsequent infection or bacteremia is unclear.[63] Only the presence of b-hemolytic *Streptococcus* is considered to be a notable threat in the chronic wound at levels less than 105 organisms per gram of tissue.[40,53,64] Nonetheless, qualitative cultures have a role in the monitoring of wounds and in guiding antibiotic selection for infected wounds. Qualitative cultures are accomplished by plating wound specimens on solid media, identifying isolates using standard microbiological procedures, and testing for antibiotic sensitivity. Qualitative cultures from swab specimens obtained using Levine's technique were found to be highly concordant to qualitative cultures from tissue specimens.[122] In terms of recovering any and all organisms, swab specimens obtained using Levine's technique were 78% concordant with tissue specimens. Concordance with respect to recovering the specific organisms *S. aureus, P. aeruginosa,* and b-hemolytic *Streptococcus* was 96%, 96%, and 99%, respectively.

PRACTICE POINT

Beta-hemolytic *Streptococcus* is considered a notable threat in wounds regardless of the number of these microorganisms present.

PRACTICE POINT

Gram+ organisms are first to invade wounds with decreased host resistance followed by Gram-, then anaerobic.[146]

Quantitative cultures

Although Pasteur suggested that the invasion of microorganisms in the body was related to quantity of inoculation, French WWI surgeons were the first to base wound management on the number of organisms present.[65-67] The relationship between bacterial quantity, wound infection, and sepsis was given attention in the 1960s. Krizek and Davis[68] found that fatal sepsis was associated with visceral or blood cultures greater than 106 or 107 organisms per gram of tissue or milliliter of blood. These researchers also demonstrated that fatal wound sepsis was related to the number of bacteria in the wound.[69] In addition, Noyes and colleagues[70] found that wound exudates with greater than 106 bacteria per milliliter were associated with invasive infection. The U.S. Army Surgical Research Unit provided a series of studies that found burn wound sepsis was associated with bacterial levels exceeding 105 organisms per gram of tissue.[71-73] Quantity of bacteria was also inversely linked to chronic wound healing.[17,36,61,62] These studies, along with earlier findings that clean wounds harbor microorganisms, provided the foundation from which quantitative culturing was added as a method of diagnosing infection.[36] The Agency for Healthcare Research and Quality (AHRQ) clinical practice guideline, Treatment of Pressure Ulcers, embraced quantitative cultures as the gold standard method to diagnose pressure ulcer infection.[34,74] Greater than 105 organisms per gram of tissue, milliliter of fluid, or swab has been adopted by many as the critical value for diagnosing wound infection.[17,21,26,34,53,75] Although references to greater than 105 have been interpreted as 100,000[1] or 1,000,000[76] organisms per gram of tissue, greater than 1,000,000 organisms per gram of tissue is the preferred critical value.[77]

Swab specimens can be quantitatively or semi-quantitatively processed. Wound tissue specimens must be of sufficient weight to ensure validity of findings—around 0.25 g of tissue.[76] Quantitative swab cultures are placed in 1 ml of dilutant and vortexed to release microorganisms from the swab. This fluid is then serially diluted, plated, and incubated, usually in aerobic conditions only. However, the recovery of anaerobes from swab specimens has been described through the use of an anaerobic transport container.[123] Plates are read for type and quantity of organisms and quantification is expressed as number or organisms per swab or gram of tissue. Similarly, wound aspirate is diluted, plated, and incubated. Quantification is expressed as the number of organisms per ml of fluid.[38]

We compared the quantitative culture findings from swab specimens obtained using Levine's technique to quantiative culture findings from tissue specimens in a sample of chronic wounds.[122] A critical threshold of 37,000 organisms per swab had a sensitivity of 90% and specificity of 57% when the true infection status of the wound was defined as 1,000,000 or more organisms per gram of tissue. Although this is the first study to examine different critical thresholds for swab specimens, further study is needed to identify the optimal critical threshold for practice.

Semi-quantitative swabs are inoculated onto solid media and streaked on four quadrants. The number of colony-forming units is counted in each quadrant and results are reported from 1 to 4+. Dow and colleagues[40] suggest 4+ should be used as the cut-off for diagnosing infection.

PRACTICE POINT

Wounds with greater than 1,000,000 organisms per gram of tissue are considered to be infected. The optimal critical threshold for swab specimens obtained using Levine's technique has yet to be established.

In summary, the identification of wound infection remains ambiguous and uncertain. Monitoring wounds for the clinical signs and symptoms of infection is an important component of wound assessment. Indicators of inflammation are especially important markers in acute wounds, such as SSIs. However, the signs and symptoms associated with inflammation may not be present in some patients with acute wounds or in patients with chronic wounds. The signs specific to secondary wounds may be useful in these cases and should be incorporated into clinical assessment. Wounds suspected of infection, especially those with delayed healing, are often

cultured to confirm the diagnosis. While qualitative cultures provide useful information in wounds that are demonstrating obvious clinical signs of infection, they may not be as useful in diagnosing infection in the absence of signs and symptoms unless certain pathogens are isolated. In the absence of clinical signs and symptoms, quantitative cultures are the gold standard method for diagnosing localized wound infection.

Managing wound bioburden

Controlling wound bioburden requires a multifaceted approach consisting of one or more of the following:
• correction of the host factors that contributed to the infection
• removal of devitalized tissue and foreign debris
• initiation of antimicrobial therapy.

Although not all of these interventions will be indicated in every case of wound infection, they each have a role to play in either reducing the number of microorganisms or enhancing host resistance.

The presence of host factors that reduce resistance to infection are often overlooked in management of wound bioburden. Judicious attention to restoration of adequate blood supply and tissue oxygen, provision of nutritional support, maintenance of glycemic control, reduction of edema, and protection from mechanical forces on the wounded tissue will aid in restoring the balance between host resistance and microorganisms. Failure to address these host factors may contribute to continued proliferation of microorganisms despite initiation of other treatment modalities.

PRACTICE POINT

In managing wound bioburden, attention should be given to supporting or restoring host defenses to microorganism invasion, such as adequate blood supply and tissue oxygen, nutrition, management of blood sugar, and control of edema.

Because necrotic tissue provides an excellent medium for growth of microorganisms, removal of devitalized tissue and debris is an essential step in treating wound infection,. When devitalized tissue is adherent to the wound bed, wound debridement is indicated. Methods of wound debridement are addressed in chapter 8, Wound debridement.

Wound cleaning

Host factors such as foreign debris and contaminants on the surface of the wound can harbor microorganisms or provide nutrients for their growth. Wound cleaning is a process that removes these less adherent inflammatory contaminants from the wound surface and renders the wound less conducive to microbial growth. However, the process of wound cleaning can also create tissue trauma. Effective wound cleaning requires selection of methods that minimize chemical and mechanical trauma to wound tissue while removing surface debris and contaminants. Although definitive research is lacking to guide selection of wound cleaning methods, the available practice evidence suggests using a nontoxic cleaning solution in combination with a delivery device that will create sufficient mechanical forces to remove the surface debris while limiting tissue injury.

Cleaning agents

The usefulness of specific agents to correct host factors depends on a balance between their antibacterial properties and their cytotoxicity to wound healing cells, such as white blood cells (WBCs) and fibroblasts.[78] For the majority of wounds, isotonic saline is adequate to clean the wound surface. A recent review by the Cochrane Collaboration concluded that water, although not isotonic, is a suitable alternative, as long as it's free of any potential contaminants.[124] Because the fluid has only brief contact with the wound surface, it isn't crucial that the solution be isotonic (0.9% sodium chloride). Although, if you choose to use an isotonic solution, an inexpensive saline solution can be prepared by combining two teaspoons of noniodized salt in one liter of boiling water. (See *Preparing saline solution at home,* page 108.)

If the wound surface is heavily laden with surface debris, a commercial wound cleaner may be used. These agents contain surface-active agents or surfactants that by the nature of their chemical polarity break the bonds that attach wound contaminants. The intensity of their chemical reactivity is directly related to their cleaning capacity and cytotoxicity. Thus, selection of a wound cleaner needs to weigh cleaning capacity against potential toxicity to cells in the wound.

Evidence regarding the safety of wound cleaners is difficult to interpret due to the lack of standardized methods for testing these agents. At present, the majority of available evidence comes from in vitro studies comparing wound cleaners under experimentally controlled conditions. The earliest such study evaluated the relative toxicity of various commercial wound and skin cleaners according to their effect on the viability of PMNs.[79] PMNs were exposed to increasing 1:10 dilutions of test cleaners for 30 minutes and analyzed for viability and phagocytic function. The toxicity index was defined as the amount of dilution required to achieve PMN viability and phagocytic function compared to that obtained by cells exposed to a balanced salt solution. Generally, toxicity levels of wound cleaners ranged from 10 to 1,000 while skin cleaners were 10,000. A second study of wound cleaner cytotoxicity evaluated the effects of five wound cleaning products on the viability of human fibroblasts, red blood cells, and white blood cells in culture.[80] Although the results were similar, the findings related to specific agents varied somewhat from those reported by Foresman et al.[79] One cleaner was found to be considerably more toxic in this study, a result of the sample tested failing to meet the manufacturer's specification for pH.

Collectively, these studies confirm that skin cleaners, which are formulated to break the

PATIENT TEACHING

Preparing saline solution at home

To prepare saline solution at home, tell the patient to bring 1 quart of water to a boil and allow it to boil for 5 minutes. He should then add 2 teaspoons of noniodized salt and stir until the salt is completely dissolved. Warn him to allow the solution to cool completely before using. The solution can be stored for up to 1 week, at room temperature, in a tightly covered glass or plastic container.

chemical bonds that bind fecal matter to the skin, are stronger and more toxic than wound cleaners.

EVIDENCE-BASED PRACTICE

Skin cleaners should never be used for wound cleaning due to their toxicity.

Antiseptic agents have historically been used to control bacterial levels in chronic wounds. This practice was based on the well-documented finding that bacteria suspended in a test tube of fluid medium are rapidly killed when exposed to an antiseptic. However, in order for an agent to be effective in the environment of a chronic wound, an agent must be able to penetrate into contaminated tissue in an active form and in sufficient concentration to achieve bactericidal activity. Because antiseptics bind chemically to multiple organic substrates that are normally present in chronic wounds, they may fail to reach bacteria in the wound tissue when used in standard clinical concentrations.[81-83] Thus, they're unable to create an effective antibacterial effect. Furthermore, antiseptics are toxic to all cells with which they come into contact, including white blood cells and fibroblasts.

The cytotoxic properties of antiseptics have been well documented in vitro and in vivo.[78,84-91] Furthermore, the addition of an antiseptic to wound cleaners has been shown to increase the toxicity index of the agent to 10,000 on average.[92] Although multiple clinical studies are cited to support the benefits of using antiseptic agents in healing chronic wounds, they fail to distinguish the antimicrobial effect of the antiseptic from other bacteria-reducing treatments that are being simultaneously administered, such as debridement or absorption of wound exudate, including bacteria and their toxins.[93-96] Although some clinicians have reported using antiseptics for specific clinical indications, such as to demarcate a gangrenous wound and limit bacterial invasion of surrounding tissue, to date, no scientifically valid clinical studies have documented the antibacterial benefits of using antiseptic agents in chronic wounds.[125-127]

PRACTICE POINT

Antiseptics shouldn't be used as a cleaning agent for wounds.

Cleaning devices

The effectiveness of wound cleaning is influenced by the type of cleaning device used to deliver the solution to the wound surface. It's essential that the method used provide sufficient force to remove surface contaminants and debris while minimizing trauma to the wound. A variety of scrubbing cloths, sponges, and brushes are available for wound cleaning. Although evidence related to their efficacy is limited, it has been demonstrated that wounds cleaned with coarse sponges were significantly more susceptible to infection than those scrubbed with a smoother sponge.[97] Furthermore, when compared to saline, wound cleaners containing surfactant were found to decrease the coefficient of friction between the scrubbing device and wound tissue.

Wound irrigation, as opposed to a cleaning device, promotes wound cleaning by creating hydraulic forces generated by the fluid stream. In order for the irrigation to be effective in cleaning the wound, the force of the irrigation stream must be greater than the adhesion forces that hold the debris to the surface of the wound. Multiple studies have substantiated that increasing pressure of a fluid stream improves removal of bacteria and debris from the wound.[98,99] Wound irrigation pressures of 10 lb per square inch (psi) and 15 psi are more effective than 1 psi and 5 psi in removing debris and bacteria from the wound surface; however, increasing the irrigation pressure to 20 psi or greater doesn't significantly improve the efficacy of cleaning.

When irrigation is delivered with a mechanical irrigation device, such as those used for dental hygiene, greater pressures are attainable than with other methods. Although clinical studies of mechanical irrigation devices used on crushing trauma wounds have confirmed that cleaning with 70 psi produces significantly more effective removal of bacteria and debris than 25 psi or 50 psi,[100-102] lower pressures are generally desirable in chronic wounds. However, even with pressures as low as 10 psi, bacteria and debris removal with mechanical irrigation devices was significantly more effective than results obtained from irrigation with a bulb syringe.

Although high pressure optimizes wound cleaning, the risk of dispersing fluid into adjacent wound tissue or along tissue planes is increased when higher pressures are used for irrigation.[103-105] The magnitude of this dispersion is related to the amount of fluid stream pressure. Research on the animal model established that irrigation at 70 psi produced greater dispersion of fluid into the tissues than irrigation with a 35-ml syringe and a 19G needle (8 psi).[105] Moreover, when a single orifice tip was used to irrigate experimental wounds, extensive fluid penetration occurred at pressures greater than 30 psi.[104] This dispersion of fluid did not occur when a multi-jet tip was used to deliver the irrigation stream. Collectively, this evidence supports avoiding irrigation pressures of greater than 15 psi for wound cleaning.

While high pressures should be avoided in performing wound irrigation, it's also necessary to create sufficient hydraulic forces with the fluid stream to overcome the adhesion forces holding debris to the wound surface. Research on experimental wounds in the animal model found that irrigation pressures of 1 psi and 5 psi produced significantly less removal of wound debris than results achieved with 10 psi and 15 psi.[99] The use of a needle and syringe to deliver fluid to wound tissue is generally regarded as a convenient method of providing effective irrigation pressure. A 35-cc syringe and a 19G needle or angiocatheter has been shown to deliver an irrigation stream at 8 psi.[106] This study also demonstrated that irrigation with a 19G needle and a 35-cc syringe was significantly more effective than a bulb syringe in removing wound bacteria and preventing the development of infection in experimental wounds.[106] Additional evidence of the effectiveness of a needle and syringe method of irrigation over the bulb syringe was established in a clinical experimental study of trauma wounds treated within 24 hours of injury with either a standard bulb syringe (0.05 psi) or a 12-cc syringe and 22G needle (13 psi).[107] A significant decrease was observed in both wound inflammation and wound infection in those wounds cleaned with the syringe and needle compared with the bulb syringe. The collective evidence regarding the effect of fluid stream pressure on removal of wound debris and bacteria supports using an irrigation pressure of 5 psi to 15 psi for wound cleaning.

A variety of needle and syringe combinations can be used to achieve the desired range of irrigation pressure. The size of the syringe and the needle gauge determine the amount of pressure of the fluid stream. Since the force depressing the plunger is distributed over a larger surface area, the larger the syringe, the less the force. With a 19G needle, 6-cc, 12-cc, and 35-cc syringes will produce pressures of 30, 20, and 8 psi, respectively. The opposite effect occurs by increasing the size of the needle. Since the larger the lumen of the needle, the greater will be the flow of fluid, needles of 25-, 21-, and 19G will create pressures of

4, 6, and 8 psi, respectively, when used with a 35-cc syringe.

A number of pressurized canisters capable of delivering saline under pressure are now available commercially. Although the claim is made that these devices produce a 19G stream at 8 psi, no evidence exists to support this assertion. In a preliminary report of the pressure dynamics of one of these devices, measurement of pressure was limited to the pressure within the pressurized canister system, not the actual force of the fluid stream against the wound surface.[108]

PRACTICE POINT

Wound irrigation can be accomplished with a variety of medical tools and specially made devices.

EVIDENCE-BASED PRACTICE

Research indicates that the optimum pressure for wound cleaning is between 5 and 15 psi.

In addition to varying the amount of pressure used for wound irrigation, the fluid stream can be delivered in either a pulsatile or continuous flow pattern. The benefit of delivering wound irrigation with a pulsatile as compared to a continuous fluid stream hasn't been substantiated in experimental studies.[98,101,102] Although several commercially available battery-powered, disposable irrigation systems (Davol, Inc., Cranston, Rhode Island; Stryker Instruments, Kalamazo, Michigan; Zimmer, Inc., Dover, Ohio) deliver pulsatile fluid streams with different spray patterns and remove the fluid and wound debris with suction, their efficacy in comparison to other irrigation methods remains to be established.[109-112] At the present time, their primary benefit appears to be their portability and capability to serve as an alternative to whirlpool therapy for patients with chronic wounds, which aren't amenable to whirlpool, or for patients when whirlpool therapy isn't accessible.

PRACTICE POINT

Pulsatile irrigation devices don't appear to be better than nonpulsatile devices, but they may be useful for patients who don't have access to a whirlpool.

An alternate approach to wound irrigation is the whirlpool bath. It cleans the wound by exposing the entire wound bed and surrounding skin to agitating water generated by jets in the sides of the whirlpool tub. Only two studies have investigated the cleaning effectiveness of whirlpool and these are methodologically confounded with wound irrigation, which was provided at the end of the whirlpool therapy.[113,114] The benefit of the whirlpool bath is thought to be derived from the prolonged exposure of the wound to water, which softens wound debris and makes it more amendable to removal. For this reason, the whirlpool is best suited for use with chronic wounds containing thick slough or necrotic tissue. Since it isn't possible to control the amount of pressure being exerted on the wound surface in a whirlpool bath, once the devitalized tissue has been cleared from the wound, the whirlpool should be discontinued to avoid disrupting new granulation tissue forming in the wound. Extreme caution must also be taken to ensure that the wound doesn't come in close contact with the water jets, since the high pressure they generate could cause further tissue injury.

A more recently developed technology that assists with removing fluids from a wound is negative-pressure wound therapy (NPWT). Fluid removal is accomplished by placing an open-cell reticulated foam dressing into the wound, sealing it with a semiocclusive covering and applying subatmospheric pressure through an evacuation tube coupled to a computer modulated pump. The suction action created by the subatmospheric pressure facilitates removal of stagnant fluid from a wound. Although removal of stagnant wound fluid with NPWT is thought to decrease wound bioburden, research findings have been mixed. In a randomized trial comparing NPWT and conventional moist gauze therapy, quantitative bacterial load, as measured by tissue biopsy, did not change significantly in either treatment group.[128] However, the NPWT wounds showed a significant decrease in nonfermentative gram negative bacilli and an increase in *staphylococcus aureus*. Similarly, in a study of 65 patients with acute or chronic wounds that were randomized to initial treatment with vacuum-assisted closure or a "modern" dressing, there was no significant reduction in bacterial clearance.[129] In contrast, others have reported a trend toward reduction in bacterial load using semiquantitative superficial swabs.[130-131] Additionally, Morykwas and colleagues found a 1000-fold decrease in the number of bacteria in experimentally innoculated wounds of pigs that had been treated with NPWT for four days. [132] Variation in sampling techniques and methods of analyses of wound specimens have contributed to these discrepant findings. The inconsistency of these findings dictate that further research be conducted to clarify the potential beneficial effects of NPWT in reducing wound bioburden.

Antimicrobial therapy

When removal of necrotic tissue doesn't reduce bacterial burden to a level compatible with healing, additional interventions to reduce the number of organisms on the wound surface are indicated. These antimicrobial therapies consist of elemental topical antimicrobials and antibiotics, both topical and systemic. These agents act directly on the microorganisms destroying the bacteria and preventing development of new colonies.

The clinical use of antimicrobials to control bacterial burden in chronic wounds has been characterized by misconceptions and controversy. As a result, they have frequently been used too extensively or for too long a time. The lack of valid indicators of chronic wound infection has further complicated the selection and use of antimicrobial therapy. Research evidence has documented that systemic antibiotics are of no value in reducing bacterial counts in chronic, granulating wounds.[115] Furthermore, the presence of purulent exudate, a recognized sign of infection in an acute wound, isn't a sufficient indicator of the need to initiate anitmicrobial therapy to treat a chronic wound. Given the current state of ambiguity regarding valid clinical signs and symptoms of chronic wound infection, the decision to initiate antimicrobial therapy is best guided by the failure of a wound to make progress toward healing despite the absence of devitalized tissue.

Topical elemental antimicrobials are formulated from elements such as silver, copper, gold or zinc. The specific formulation of the antimicrobial agent is crucial to its effectiveness in reducing bacterial burden without destroying cells essential to healing. Iodine is an example of an agent that, in its elemental form, is toxic to cells that promote healing. However, when formulated as *cadexomer iodine* gel, it slowly releases iodine from its microspheres while absorbing bacteria. [133-134] In vitro study of varying concentrations of cadexomer iodine demonstrated that it is nontoxic to human fibroblasts in culture in concentrations of up to 0.45% and chronic wounds treated with cadexomer iodine revealed reepithelialization on biopsy.

Topical agents formulated with silver have long been a part of the armamentarium of antibacterials. Using the ionized form of silver (Ag+), these agents exert bacteriostatic properties through the action of the silver cation on proteins. The Ag+ binds to proteins in the bacterial cell wall distrupting its integrity resulting in death of the cell. Silver containing wound care products include pure silver, creams, and sustained release dressings. Research evidence regarding the efficacy of these agents is most substantial for the cream formulations (silver sulfadiazine 2% or 7%). Topical cream formulations has been shown to reduce bacterial density, vascular margination and migration of inflammatory cells in chronic leg ulcers.[135] The efficacy of silver sulfadiazine cream in reducing bacterial burden in chronic wounds was substantiated in a randomized trial of 45 patients with a single infected pressure ulcer that were randomly assigned to receive silver sulfadiazine cream, povidone-iodine solution, or saline gauze dressings.[93] Standard care consisting of debridement, pressure reduction, and nutritional support was provided to all subjects. In 100% of the ulcers treated with silver sulfadiazine cream, the bacterial levels were reduced to 105 or less per gram of tissue during the 3-week protocol, while only 78.6%

of the povidone-iodine solution-treated ulcers and 63.6% of the saline gauze-treated ulcers achieved these reductions in bacterial levels. Overall, ulcers treated with silver sulfadiazine responded more rapidly, with one-third achieving bacterial levels of less than 105 within 3 days and half the ulcers reaching this level within 1 week. These data support limiting treatment with silver-based creams to no more than 2 weeks. If clinical evidence of improvement has not occurred in this time, other host factors that may be contributing to decreased bacterial resistance should be explored.

 EVIDENCE-BASED PRACTICE

Research suggests that topical elemental antimicrobial therapy with silver-based creams be limited to 2 weeks.

A more recently developed topical delivery system, the silver impregnated dressing, has been shown to have antimicrobial effects on a broad spectrum of organisms.[136] However, many questions remain regarding the dosage of silver released into the wound and the potential for delays in healing if the silver cation binds to fibroblasts and epithelial cells. Reports of industry conducted in vitro studies demonstrate that different silver-containing dressings release different amounts of silver over time.[137] There are preliminary indications that the toxic dosage of silver differs depending on whether the fibroblasts and epithelial cells are in a monolayer or in a three-dimensional matrix.[138] The potential adverse consequences in epithelializing wounds was demonstrated in a controlled study of matched pair skin graft donor sites treated with a non-antimicrobial foam dressing or a nanocrystalline silver dressing. Although there were no differences in bacterial counts between the two treatment groups, reepithelialization was significantly slower in the wounds treated with the silver dressing.[139] At the present, in vivo evidence to establish the safety and efficacy of silver containing dressings is lacking. Therefore, given the ambiguity in the evidence surrounding silver-containing dressings, discretion should be exercised in using them as a method of reducing

microorganisms on wound surfaces, and treatment periods should be limited to four weeks duration. Their use should be discontinued when reepithelialization is observed in the wound.

Topical antibiotics exert their antimicrobial effects through selective binding to chemical targets on the bacterial cell wall. Since human cell membranes lack these chemical targets, topical antibiotics have negligible effect on cells that promote wound healing. Although numerous antibiotics are available for topical application, research confirming the potential utility of topical antibiotics in reducing bacterial burden in chronic wounds is limited to one randomized controlled trial. In this study the 31 pressure ulcers comprising the experimental group were treated with topical gentamicin cream and standard treatment consisting of debridement, cleaning, pressure reduction and nutritional support. They demonstrated significant improvement, while only three of the nine given standard treatment alone improved.[61] Serial bacteriological and pathological observations made over a 1- to 4-week treatment period showed a rapid reduction in bacterial counts to levels less than 106 per ml in all ulcers treated with gentamicin. Furthermore, analysis of quantitative bacterial counts in relation to clinical outcome revealed an absolute correlation between significant clinical improvement and a fall in the bacterial count to less than 106 per ml and between no clinical improvement and the persistence of counts greater than 106 per ml.

Although clinical studies provide evidence supporting the utility of topical antibiotics in reducing bacterial burden in chronic wounds, these agents can cause adverse reactions in some patients. Reports of permanent hearing loss with topical 1% neomycin solution and acute anaphylactic reactions with topically applied Bacitracin suggest that careful monitoring is indicated when using these agents.[116,117] Additionally, since there's a risk of selecting out resistant strains of bacteria, antibiotics that are used to treat infections systemically shouldn't be used in a topical form on chronic wounds. For this reason, despite the reported effectiveness of gentamicin in reducing bacterial levels in pressure ulcers, alternative topical antibiotics are indicated that won't produce resistant bacterial strains to systemic forms of the antimicrobial agent. Furthermore, since topical antibiotics are limited in the range of species that they are effective against, it is important to judiciously select the specific antibiotic based on the organism present in the wound.

While topical antibiotics have demonstrated effectiveness in reducing bacterial burden when the area of involvement is localized, they're generally regarded as inadequate to control more extensive tissue involvement, such as advancing cellulitis. In these instances, systemic antibiotic therapy is indicated. Since the type of organisms and degree of invasiveness will vary, the choice of antimicrobial therapy will need to be individualized. Unfortunately, little research evidence exists to guide selection of antibiotics to treat chronic wound infections. Generally, chronic wound infections are treated empirically with antibiotics that have narrow, but sufficient spectrum of coverage. Care should be taken to avoid routine or extended periods of treatment. Less acute forms of chronic wound infection are treated with oral antibiotics. However, parenteral therapy may be indicated when the infection involves deeper tissue and is accompanied by systemic signs, such as fever, chills, and elevated WBC count. Regardless of the route, the effectiveness of any systemic antibiotic in reducing bacterial burden will be dependent on the adequacy of the patient's peripheral circulation. In those instances where peripheral vascular disease compromises the blood flow to the infected tissue, systemic antimicrobial therapy may produce no clinical improvement in the wound.

PRACTICE POINT

The effectiveness of systemic antibiotics is dependent on an adequate blood supply to the wound.

Several adjuvant therapies have shown potential as interventions for reducing bacterial burden in chronic wounds. Hyperbaric oxygen therapy, administered by intermittent inhalation of pure oxygen at a pressure greater than 1 atmosphere, has been shown to promote PMN microbicidal efficacy in diabetic foot ulcers.[140] Ultraviolet light (UV) has long been recognized for its bacteriocidal effects derived from in vitro studies. Recently, the effect of UV has been demonstrated in a clinical study of 22 patients with chronic wounds containing high bacterial levels as determined by quantitative swab culture.[141] Following one 180-second UV-C treatment session, cultures showed a statistically significant reduction of predominant bacteria ($P = 0.001$), and significant reductions of *MRSA* ($p<0.05$) and *S. aureus* ($p<0.01$).[142]

Additionally, exposure of wound tissue to electrical current using an electrical stimulation device has been shown in animal studies to exert bacteriostatic and bactericidal effects on microorganisms known to infect chronic wounds. In a study of 20 patients with burn wounds that had been unresponsive to conventinal therapy for 3 months to two years, application of direct current (DC) stimulation for 10 minutes twice weekly produced a quantitatively lower level of microorganisms.[142] However, the antibacterial effect of pulsed current (PC), the more commonly used electrical stimulation modality in current practice, remains unclear. There is evidence that the voltage that would be required to produce an antibacterial effect would create profound muscle contractions, making it not applicable in clinial practice.[143-145]

Summary

Most of our understanding of wound infection has been derived from the study of acute wounds. As wound healing science has evolved, it has become clear that chronic wounds are distinctly different environments where host resistance has been overwhelmed by bacterial burden. The classic signs and symptoms of infection are well recognized. However, they're based on assessments made of acute wounds and aren't valid in the chronic wound. While indicators of chronic wound infection remain ambiguous, substantial evidence exists showing that necrotic tissue harbors microorganisms. Therefore, debridement of necrotic tissue in the wound bed is an essential first step to reducing bacterial burden. Regular wound cleaning with a noncytotoxic solution, using sufficient force to remove surface contaminants and debris while minimizing trauma, is an important adjunct to reduce surface contaminants. In those instances where these measures aren't sufficient to restore a balance between host resistance and bacterial burden, antimicrobials that act directly on the bacteria are indicated.

Show what you know

1. Which of the following distinguishes a wound colonized with bacteria from one that's infected?

    A. An infected wound will have purulent exudate; a colonized wound won't.
    B. An infected wound will have organisms present in viable tissue; a colonized wound won't.
    C. An infected wound will always have necrotic tissue; a colonized wound won't.
    D. An infected wound will have a positive swab culture; a colonized wound won't.

ANSWER: B. For a wound to be infected, organisms must be present in viable tissue and not limited to the wound surface. Purulent exudate may be observed in a colonized wound as well as one that's infected. While necrotic tissue does contain organisms, a wound can be infected without the presence of necrotic tissue. Both an infected wound and a colonized wound will produce a positive swab culture. For the wound to be infected, the organisms must be present in the tissue and not limited to the surface of the wound that has contact with the culture swab.

2. Which of the following is the most valid indicator of a wound infection?

    A. A swab culture showing large amounts of *Staphylococcus*
    B. The presence of erythema in the periwound area
    C. Quantitative culture of tissue showing 1,000,000 organisms/g of tissue
    D. Large amounts of serosanguinous exudate on dressings

ANSWER: C. Quantitative cultures provide a count of the actual number of organisms present in a standard gram of tissue taken from beneath the wound surface in the wound tissue. Although quantitative swab cultures are fairly comparable to quantitative tissue cultures, tissue cultures remain the gold standard. Erythema is one of the classic signs of inflammation and may arise in response to any type of tissue injury, including, but not limited to, infection. Serosanguinous exudate contains serum and a small number of red blood cells, and may be indicative, but not conclusive, of infection.

3. Antiseptics are a deterrent to healing of clean, granulating wounds because they:

    A. interfere with absorption of nutrients.
    B. discolor the wound tissue.
    C. irritate surrounding skin.
    D. are harmful to fibroblasts and other cells.

ANSWER: D. Antiseptics have been documented as toxic to fibroblasts. Although some antiseptics can bleach out the color of wound tissue, this isn't what causes them to disrupt the repair process. While many antiseptics can cause skin irritation if allowed to come in contact with the periwound surface, this isn't the mechanism that interferes with wound repair.

4. The use of topical antibiotics for treatment of chronic wounds should be:

    A. used routinely to reduce high bacterial levels.
    B. used routinely to prevent infection.
    C. avoided unless necrotic tissue is present.
    D. avoided in absence of signs of infection.

ANSWER: D. Treatment with topical antibiotics is indicated only when signs of infection are present. However, it's important to recognize that a chronic wound may not present with the same signs of infection as an acute wound. Treatment with topical antibiotics isn't indicated unless the wound is infected. Routine use of topical antibiotics for prevention of infection is unnecessary and can lead to development of resistant organisms. Using topical antibiotics in the presence of necrotic tissue isn't effective.

5. Which of the following correctly describes the Levine Technique for wound culturing?

    A. Obtain a tissue specimen using a sterile scalpel.
    B. Aspirate wound fluid using a 21G needle and 10 cc syringe.
    C. Swap necrotic tissue prior to cleaning the wound.
    D. Rotate swab over a 1-cm square area with sufficient pressure to express fluid from within the wound tissue.

ANSWER: D. Rotating a swab over a 1-cm square area to express fluid from within the wound describes the Levine Technique. Using a sterile scalpel and aspirating wound tissue with a needle and syringe are alternate methods of obtaining a wound specimen for culture. C is incorrect. You should never culture necrotic tissue.

References

1. Robson, M.C. "Wound Infection: A Failure of Wound Healing Caused by an Imbalance of Bacteria," *Surgical Clinics of North America* 77(3):637-50, June 1997.
2. Bowler, P.G. "Wound Pathophysiology, Infection, and Therapeutic Options," *Annals of Medicine* 34:419-27, September 2002.

3 Majno, G. *Cells, Tissues, and Disease: Principles of General Pathology.* New York: Oxford University Press, 2004.

4. Abraham, S.N. "Discovering the Benign Traits of the Mast Cell," *Science and Medicine* 3(5):46-55, September-October 1997.

5. McGeer, A., et al. "Definitions of Infection for Surveillance in Long-term-care Facilities," *American Journal of Infection Control* 19(1):1-7, February 1991.

6. Thomson, P.D., and Taddonio, T.E. "Wound Infection," in Krasner, D., and Kane, D., eds., *Chronic Wound Care,* 2nd ed. Wayne, Pa.: HMP Communications, 1997.

7. Larocco, M. "Inflammation and Immunity," in Porth, C.M., ed., *Pathophysiology: Concepts of Altered Health States,* 4th ed. Philadelphia: Lippincott Williams & Wilkins, 1994.

8. Tarnuzzer, R.W., and Schultz, G.S. "Biochemical Analysis of Acute and Chronic Wound Environments," *Wound Repair and Regeneration* 4(3):321-26, July-September 1996.

9. Heggers, J.P., and Robson, M.C. "Prostaglandins and Thromboxanes," in Ninneman, J., ed., *Traumatic Injury-infection and Other Immunological Sequelae.* Baltimore: University Park Press, 1983.

10. Dow, G. "Infection in Chronic Wounds," in *Chronic Wound Care: A Clinical Source Book for Healthcare Professionals,* 3rd ed. Wayne, Pa.: HMP Communications, 2001.

11. Hunt, T.K., et al. "A New Model for the Study of Wound Infection," *Journal of Trauma* 7(2):298-306, March 1967.

12. Bucknall, T.E. "The Effect of Local Infection upon Wound Healing: An Experimental Study," *British Journal of Surgery* 67(12):851-55, December 1980.

13. Dunphy, J.E. "The Cut Gut," *American Journal of Surgery* 119(1):1-8, January 1970.

14. Lawrence, J.C. "Bacteriology and Wound Healing," in Fox, J.A., and Fischer, J., eds., *Cadexomer Iodine.* Stuttgart: Schattauer Verlag, 1983.

15. Orgill, D., and Demling, R.H. "Current Concepts and Approaches to Wound Healing," *Critical Care Medicine* 16(9):899-908, September 1988.

16. Stenberg, B.D., et al. "Effect of bFGF on the Inhibition of Contraction Caused by Bacteria," *Journal of Surgical Research* 50(1):47-50, January 1991.

17. Lookingbill, D.P., et al. "Bacteriology of Chronic Leg Ulcers," *Archives of Dermatology* 114(12):1765-68, December 1978.

18. Robson, M.C., et al. "Wound Healing Alterations Caused by Infection," *Clinics in Plastic Surgery* 17(3):485-92, July 1990.

19. Stotts, N.A., and Whitney, J.D. "Identifying and Evaluating Wound Infection," *Home Healthcare Nurse* 17(3):159-65, March 1999.

20 Grayson, M.L., et al. "Probing to Bone in Infected Pedal Ulcers: A Clinical Sign of Underlying Osteomyelitis in Diabetic Patients," *JAMA* 273(9):721-23, March 1995.

21. Gilchrist, B. "Infection and Culturing," in Krasner, D., and Kane, D., eds., *Chronic Wound Care,* 2nd ed. Wayne, Pa.: HMP Communications, 1997.

22. American College of Surgeons: Committee on the Control of Surgical Infections. *Manual on Control of Infection in Surgical Patients.* Philadelphia: Lippincott Williams & Wilkins, 1976.

23. Baxter, C., and Mertz, P.M. "Local Factors that Affect Wound Healing," *Nursing RSA Verpleging* 7(2):16-23, February 1992.

24. Gilchrist, B. "Treating Bacterial Wound Infection," *Nursing Times* 90(50):55-58, December 1994.

25. Hutchinson, J.J., and McGuckin, M. "Occlusive Dressings: A Microbiologic and Clinical Review," *American Journal of Infection Control* 18(4):256-68, August 1990.

26. Stotts, N.A., and Hunt, T.K. "Pressure Ulcers: Managing Bacterial Colonization and Infection," *Clinics in Geriatric Medicine* 13(3):565-73, August 1997.

27. Barnett, A., et al. "A Concentration Gradient of Bacteria within Wound Tissue and Scab," *Journal of Surgical Research* 41(3):326-32, September 1986.

28. Stotts, N.A. "Promoting Wound Healing," in Kinney, M.R., et al., eds., *AACN's Clinical Reference for Critical Care Nursing,* 4th ed. St. Louis: Mosby–Year Book, Inc., 1998.

29. Horan, T.C., et al. "CDC Definitions of Nosocomial Surgical Site Infections, 1992: A Modification of CDC Definitions of Surgical Wound Infections," *American Journal of Infection Control* 20(5):271-74, October 1992.

30. Gardner, S.E., et al. "The Validity of the Clinical Signs and Symptoms Used to Identify Localized Chronic Wound Infection," *Wound Repair and Regeneration* 9(3):178-86, May-June 2001.

31. Gardner, S.E., et al. "A Tool to Assess Clinical Signs and Symptoms of Localized Chronic Wound Infection: Development and Reliability," *Ostomy/Wound Management* 47(1):40-47, January 2001.

32. Steed, D.L. "Diabetic Wounds: Assessment, Classification, and Management," in Krasner, D., and Kane, D., eds., *Chronic Wound Care,* 2nd ed. Wayne, Pa.: HMP Communications, 1997.

33. Cutting, K.F., and Harding, K.G. "Criteria for Identifying Wound Infection," *Journal of Wound Care* 3(4):198-201, June 1994.

34. Bergstrom, N., et al. *Treatment of Pressure Ulcers. Clinical Practice Guideline, Number 15. AHCPR Publication No. 95-0652.* Rockville, Md.: Agency for Health Care Policy and Research, Public Health Service, U.S. Department of Health and Human Services, December 1994.

35. Cutting, K.F. "Identification of Infection in Granulating Wounds by Registered Nurses," *Journal of Clinical Nursing* 7(6):539-46, November 1998.

36. Robson, M.C., and Heggers, J.P. "Bacterial Quantification of Open Wounds," *Military Medicine* 134(1):19-24, January 1969.

37. Stotts, N.A. "Determination of Bacterial Burden in Wounds," *Advances in Wound Care* 8(4):46-52, July-August 1995.

38. Lee, P., et al. "Fine-needle Aspiration Biopsy in Diagnosis of Soft Tissue Infections," *Journal of Clinical Microbiology* 22(1):80-83, July 1985.

39. Rudensky, B., et al. "Infected Pressure Sores: Comparison of Methods for Bacterial Identification," *Southern Medical Journal* 85(9):901-903, September 1992.

40. Dow, G., et al. "Infection in Chronic Wounds: Controversies and Treatment," *Ostomy/Wound Management* 45(8):23-40, August 1999.

41. Donovan, S. "Wound Infection and Wound Swabbing," *Professional Nurse* 13(11): 757-59, August 1998.

42. Bill, T.J., et al. "Quantitative Swab Culture versus Tissue Biopsy: A Comparison in Chronic Wounds," *Ostomy/Wound Management* 47(1):34-37, January 2001.

43. Levine, N.S., et al. "The Quantitative Swab Culture and Smear: A Quick, Simple Method for Determining the Number of Viable Aerobic

Bacteria on Open Wounds," *Journal of Trauma* 16(2):89-94, February 1976.

44. Sapico, F.L., et al. "Quantitative Microbiology of Pressure Sores in Different Stages of Healing," *Diagnostic Microbiology of Infectious Diseases* 5(1):31-38, May 1986.

45. Basak, S., et al. "Bacteriology of Wound Infection: Evaluation by Surface Swab and Quantitative Full Thickness Wound Biopsy Culture," *Journal of the Indian Medical Association* 90(2):33-34, February 1992.

46. Herruzo-Cabrera, R., et al. "Diagnosis of Local Infection of a Burn by Semiquantitative Culture of the Eschar Surface," *Journal of Burn Care & Rehabilitation* 13(6):639-41, November-December 1992.

47. Morison, M.J. *A Colour Guide to the Nursing Management of Wounds.* Oxford: Blackwell Scientific, November-December 1992.

48. Pagana, K., and Pagana, T.J. *Mosby's Diagnostic and Laboratory Test Reference.* St. Louis: Mosby–Year Book, Inc., 1992.

49. Alvarez, O., et al. "Moist Environment for Healing: Matching the Dressing to the Wound," *Ostomy/Wound Management* 21:64-83, Winter 1988.

50. Cooper, R., and Lawrence, J.C. "The Isolation and Identification of Bacteria from Wounds," *Journal of Wound Care* 5(7):335-40, July 1996.

51. Cuzzell, J.Z. "The Right Way to Culture a Wound," *AJN* 93(5):48-50, May 1993.

52. Georgiade, N.G., et al. "A Comparison of Methods for the Quantitation of Bacteria in Burn Wounds I: Experimental Evaluation," *American Journal of Clinical Pathology* 53(1):35-39, January 1970.

53. Robson, M.C., and Heggers, J.P. "Quantitative Bacteriology and Inflammatory Mediators in Soft Tissue," in *Biological and Clinical Aspects of Soft and Hard Tissue Repair.* Edited by Hunt, T.K., et al. New York: Praeger Pubs., 1984.

54. Garner, J.S., et al. "CDC Definitions for Nosocomial Infections, 1988," *American Journal of Infection Control* 16(3):128-40, June 1988.

55. Peromet, M., et al. "Anaerobic Bacteria Isolated from Decubitus Ulcers," *Infection* 1(4):205-207, December 1973.

56. Chow, A.W., et al. "Clindamycin for Treatment of Sepsis by Decubitus Ulcers," *Journal of Infectious Disease* 135(suppl):S65-S68, March 1977.

57. Vaziri, N.D., et al. "Bacterial Infections in Patients with Chronic Renal Failure: Occurrence with Spinal Cord Injury," *Archives of Internal Medicine* 142(7):1273-76, July 1982.

58. Bryan, C.S., et al. "Bacteremia Associated with Decubitus Ulcers," *Archives of Internal Medicine* 143(11):2093-95, November 1983.

59. Gilchrist, B., and Reed, C. "The Bacteriology of Chronic Venous Ulcers Treated with Occlusive Hydrocolloid Dressings," *British Journal of Dermatology* 121(3):337-44, September 1989.

60. Trengove, N.J., et al. "Qualitative Bacteriology and Leg Ulcer Healing," *Journal of Wound Care* 5(6):277-80, June 1996.

61. Bendy, R.H., et al. "Relationship of Quantitative Wound Bacterial Counts to Healing of Decubiti: Effect of Topical Gentamicin," *Antimicrobial Agents and Chemotherapy* 4:147-55, 1964.

62. Daltrey, D.C., et al. "Investigation into the Microbial Flora of Healing and Non-healing Decubitus Ulcers," *Journal of Clinical Pathology* 34(7):701-705, July 1981.

63. Roghmann, M.C., et al. "MRSA Colonization and the Risk of MRSA Bacteraemia in Hospitalized Patients with Chronic Ulcers," *Journal of Hospital Infection* 47(2):98-103, February 2001.

64. Leaper, D.J. "Defining Infection," *Journal of Wound Care* 7(8):373, September 1998.

65. Absolon, K.B., et al. "From Antisepsis to Asepsis: Louis Pasteur's Publication on 'The Germ Theory and its Application to Medicine and Surgery'," *Review of Surgery* 27(4):245-58, July-August 1970.

66. Elek, S.D. "Experimental Staphylococcal Infections in the Skin of Man," *Annals of the New York Academy of Science* 65:85, 1956.

67. Hepburn, H.H. "Delayed Primary Suture of Wounds," *British Medical Journal* 1:181-83, 1919.

68. Krizek, T.J., and Davis, J.H. "Endogenous Wound Infection," *Journal of Trauma* 6(2):239-48, March 1966.

69. Krizek, T.J., and Davis, J.H. "Experimental Pseudomonas Burn Sepsis: Evaluation of Topical Therapy," *Journal of Trauma* 7(3):433-42, May 1967.

70. Noyes, H.E., et al. "Delayed Topical Antimicrobials as Adjuncts to Systemic Antibiotic Therapy of War Wounds: Bacteriologic Studies," *Military Medicine* 132(6):461-68, June 1967.

71. Lindberg, R.B., et al. "The Successful Control of Burn Wound Sepsis," *Journal of Trauma* 5(5):601-16, September 1965.

72. Shuck, J.M., and Moncrief, J.A. "The Management of Burns: Part I. General Considerations and the Sulfamylon Method," *Current Problems in Surgery* 352, February 1969.

73. Teplitz, C., et al. "Pseudomonas Burn Wound Sepsis. I. Pathogens of Experimental Burn Wound Sepsis," *Journal of Surgical Research* 4:200-16, May 1964.

74. Rodeheaver, G.T., and Frantz, R.A. "14. Guideline: Bacterial Control," in *Treating Pressure Ulcers. Guideline Technical Report, Number 15, Volume 1.* Edited by Bergstrom, N., and Cuddigan, J. Rockville, Md.: U. S. Department of Health and Human Services, Public Health Service, Agency for Health Care Policy and Research, AHCPR Publication No. 96-N014, 1994.

75. Krizek, T.J., and Robson, M.C. "Evolution of Quantitative Bacteriology in Wound Management," *American Journal of Surgery* 130(5):579-84, November 1975.

76. Heggers, J.P. "Variations on a Theme," in *Quantitative Bacteriology: Its Role in the Armamentarium of the Surgeon.* Edited by Heggers, J.P., and Robson, M.C. Boca Raton: CRC Press, 1991.

77. Robson, M.C. Personal communication, May 29, 2002.

78. Lineaweaver, W., et al. "Topical Antimicrobial Toxicity," *Archives of Surgery* 120(3):267-70, March 1985.

79. Foresman, P.A., et al. "A Relative Toxicity Index for Wound Cleansers," *Wounds* 5(5):226-31, September-October 1993.

80. Wright, R.W., and Orr, R. "Fibroblast Cytotoxicity and Blood Cell Integrity Following Exposure to Dermal Wound Cleansers," *Ostomy/Wound Management* 39(7):33-36, 38, 40, September 1993.

81. Zamora, J.L., et al. "Inhibition of Povidone-iodine's Bactericidal Activity by Common Organic Substances: An Experimental Study," *Surgery* 98(1):25-29, July 1985.

82. Fleming, A. "The Action of Chemical and Physiological Antiseptics in a Septic Wound," *British Journal of Surgery* 7:99-129, February 1919.

83. Lacey, R.W. "Antibacterial Activity of Povidone Towards Non-sporing Bacteria," *The Journal of Applied Bacteriology* 46(3):443-49, June 1979.

84. Cooper, M.L., et al. "The Cytotoxic Effects of Commonly Used Topical Antimicrobial Agents on Human Fibroblasts and Keratinocytes," *Journal of Trauma* 31(6):775-84, June 1991.

85. Teepe, R.G., et al. "Cytotoxic Effects of Topical Antimicrobial and Antiseptic Agents on Human Keratinocytes In Vitro," *Journal of Trauma* 35(1):8-19, July1993.

86. Branemark, P.I., and Ekholm, R. "Tissue Injury Caused by Wound Disinfectants," *Journal of Bone and Joint Surgery American* 49(1):48-62, January 1967.

87. Brennan, S.S., et al. "The Effect of Antiseptics on the Healing Wound: A Study Using the Ear Chamber," *British Journal of Surgery* 72(10):780-82, October 1985.

88. Cotter, J.L., et al. "Chemical Parameters, Antimicrobial Activities, and Tissue Toxicity of 0.1% and 0.5% Sodium Hypochlorite Solutions," *Antimicrobial Agents Chemotherapeutics* 9(1):118-22, July 1985.

89. Brennan, S.S., et al. "Antiseptic Toxicity in Wounds Healing by Secondary Intention," *Journal of Hospital Infection* 8(3):263-67, November1986.

90. Becker, G.D. "Identification and Management of the Patient at High Risk for Wound Infection," *Head and Neck Surgery* 8:205-10, January-February 1986.

91. Viljanto, J. "Disinfection of Surgical Wounds without Inhibition of Normal Wound Healing," *Archives of Surgery* 115:253-56, March 1980.

92. Hellewell, T.B., et al. "A Cytotoxicity Evaluation of Antimicrobial and Non-antimicrobial Wound Cleansers," *Wounds* 9(1):15-20, Janaury 1997.

93. Kucan, J.O., et al. "Comparison of Silver Sulfadiazine, Povidone-iodine and Physiologic Saline in the Treatment of Chronic Pressure Ulcers," *Journal of the American Geriatric Society* 29(5):232-35, May 1981.

94. Carrel, A., and Dehelly, G. *The Treatment of Infected Wounds.* New York: Hoeber, 1917.

95. American Medical Association. *AMA Drug Evaluation,* 10th ed. Chicago: American Medical Association, 1994.

96. Sundberg, J., and Meller, R. "A Retrospective Review of the Use of Cadexomer Iodine in the Treatment of Chronic Wounds," *Wounds* 9(3):68-86, May-June 1997.

97. Rodeheaver, G.T., et al. "Mechanical Cleaning of Contaminated Wounds with a Surfactant," *American Journal of Surgery* 129(3):241-45, March 1975.

98. Madden, J., et al. "Application of Principles of Fluid Dynamics to Surgical Wound Irrigation," *Current Topics in Surgical Research* 3:85-93, 1971.

99. Rodeheaver, G.T., et al. "Wound Cleaning by High Pressure Irrigation," *Surgical Gynecology and Obstetrics* 141(3):357-62, September 1975.

100. Grower, M.F., et al. "Effect of Water Lavage on Removal of Tissue Fragments from Crush Wounds," *Oral Surgery Oral Medicine Oral Pathology* 33(6):1031-36, June 1972.

101. Green, V.A., et al. "A Comparison of the Efficacy of Pulsed Mechanical Lavage with That of Rubber-bulb Syringe Irrigation in Removal of Debris from Avulsive Wounds," *Oral Surgery Oral Medicine Oral Pathology* 32(1):158-64, July 1971.

102. Stewart, J.L., et al. "The Bacteria-removal Efficiency of Mechanical Lavage and Rubber-bulb Syringe Irrigation in Contaminated Avulsive Wounds," *Oral Surgery Oral Medicine Oral Pathology* 31(6):842-48, June 1971.

103. Bhaskar, S.N., et al. "Effect of Water Lavage on Infected Wounds in the Rat," *Journal of Periodontology* 40(11):671-72, November 1969.

104. Carlson, H.C., et al. "Effect of Pressure and Tip Modification on the Dispersion of Fluid Throughout Cells and Tissues During the Irrigation of Experimental Wounds," *Oral Surgery Oral Medicine Oral Pathology* 32(2):347-55, August 1971.

105. Wheeler, C.B., et al. "Side Effects of High Pressure Irrigation," *Surgical Gynecology and Obstetrics* 143(5):775-78, November 1976.

106. Stevenson, T.R., et al. "Cleansing the Traumatic Wound by High Pressure Syringe Irrigation," *Journal of the American College of Emergency Physicians* 5(1):1721, January 1976.

107. Longmire, A.W., et al. "Wound Infection Following High-pressure Syringe and Needle Irrigation" [Letter to the editor], *American Journal of Emergency Medicine* 5(2):179-818, March 1987.

108. Singer, A.J., et al. "Pressure Dynamics of Various Irrigation Techniques Commonly Used in the Emergency Department," *Annals of Emergency Medicine* 24(1):36-40, July 1994.

109. Loehne, H. "Pulsatile Lavage with Concurrent Suction," In *Wound Care: A Collaborative Practice Manual for Physical Therapists and Nurses,* 1st ed. Edited by C. Sussman, C., and Bates-Jensen, B.M. Gaithersburg, Md.: Aspen Pubs., 1998.

110. Cicione, J. "Making Waves," *Case Review* 26-29, July-August 1998.

111. Ho, C., et al. "Healing with Hydrotherapy," *Advances for Directors in Rehabilitation* 7(5):45-49, 1998.

112. Morgan, D., and Hoelscher, J. "Pulsed Lavage: Promoting Comfort and Healing in Home Care," *Ostomy/Wound Management* 46(4):44-49, April 2000.

113. Bohannon, R.W. "Whirlpool Versus Whirlpool Rinse for Removal of Bacteria from a Venous Stasis Ulcer," *Physical Therapy* 62(3):304-308, March 1982.

114. Neiderhuber, S., et al. "Reduction of Skin Bacterial Load with Use of Therapeutic Whirlpool," *Physical Therapy* 55(5):482-86, May 1975.

115. Robson, M.C., et al. "The Efficacy of Systemic Antibiotics in the Treatment of Granulating Wounds," *Journal of Surgical Research* 16(4):299-306, April 1974.

116. Johnson, C.A. "Hearing Loss Following the Application of Topical Neomycin," *Journal of Burn Care and Rehabilitation* 9(2):162-64, March-April 1988.

117. Schechter, J.F., et al. "Anaphylaxis Following the Use of Bacitracin Ointment. Report of a Case and Review of the Literature," *Archives of Dermatology* 120(7):909-11, July 1984.

118. American Diabetes Association (1999). Concensus conference on diabetic foot management.

119. Gardner, S.E. et al. "Clinical Signs of Infection in Diabetic Foot Ulcers with High Microbial Loads." (submitted for publication).

120. Kravitz, S. "Infection: Are we defining it accurately?" *Advances in Skin and Wound Care* 19(4):176, May 2006.

121. Gardner, S.E. et al. "The Reliability of the Clinical Signs and Symptoms Checklist in diabetic Foot Ulcers" *Ostomy Wound Management* (in press).

122. Gardner, S.E. et al. "Diagnostic Validity of Three Swab Techniques for Identifying Chronic Wound

Infections," *Wound Repair and Regeneration* (in press)

123. Johnson, S. et al. "Use of an Anaerobic Collection and Transport Swab Device to Recover Anaerobic Bacteria From Infected Foot Ulcers in Diabetics," *Clinical Infectious Diseases* 20(Suppl 2):S289-S290, June 1995.

124. Fernandez R., et al. "Water for Wound Cleansing (Review)," *The Cochrane Database of Systemic Reviews Issue 4*, Hoboken, NJ: John Wiley & Sons, Ltd., 2006.

125. Sibbald, R.G. "Topical Antimicrobials," *Ostomy Wound Management* 49(5A Suppl):14-18, May 2003

126. Edwards, R. & Harding, K.G. "Bacteria and Wound Healing," *Current Opinions in Infectious Disease* 17(2):91-96, April 2004.

127. Falanga, V. "The Chronic wound: Impaired Healing and Solutions in the Contest of Wound Bed Preparation," *Blood Cells and Molecular Disease* 31(1):88-94, January-February 2004.

128. Moues, C.M., et al. "Bacterial Load in Relation to Vacuum-assisted Closure Wound Therapy: A Prospective Randomized Trial," *Wound Repair and Regeneration* 12(1):11-17, January-February 2004.

129. Braakenburg, A. et al.: "The Clinical Efficacy and Cost Effectiveness of the Vacuum-assisted Closure Technique in the Management of Acute and Chronic Wounds: A Randomized Controlled Trial," *Plastic and Reconstructive Surgery* 118(2):3907, August, 2006.

130. Deva, A.K., et al. "Topical Negative Pressure in Wound Management," *Medical Journal of Australia* 173(3):128-31, August 2000.

131. Pinocy, J., et al. "Treatment of Periprosthetic Soft Tissue Infection of the Groin Following Vascular Surgical Procedures by Means of a Polyvinyl Alcohol-vacuum Sponge System," *Wound Repair Regeneration* 11(2):104-9, March-April 2003.

132. Morykwas, M.J., et al. "Vacuum-assisted Closure: A New Method for Wound Control and Treatment: Animal Studies and Basic Foundation," *Annals of Plastic Surgery* 38(6):553-62, June 1997.

133. Stadelmann, W.K., et al. "Impediments to Wound Healing," *American Journal of Surgery,* 176(Suppl 2A):39S-47S, August 1998.

134. Zhou, L.H., et al. "Slow Release Iodine Preparation and Wound Healing: *In Vitro* Effects Consistent with Lack of *In Vivo* Toxicity in Human Chronic Wounds," *British Journal of Dermatology,* 146(3):365-74, March 2002.

135. Fumal, I., et al. "The Beneficial Toxicity Paradox of Antimicrobials in Leg Ulcer Healing Impaired by a Polymicrobial Flora: A Proof-of-Concept Study," *Der-matology* 70(Suppl 1):70-74, 2002.

136. Bowler, P.G., et al. "Microbicidal Properties of a Silver-containing Hydrofiber Dressing Against a Variety of Burn Wound Pathogens," *Journal of Burn Care Rehabilitation*, 25(2):192-96, March-April 2004.

137. Ovington, L.G. "The Truth About Silver," *Ostomy Wound Management,* 50(9A Suppl):1S-10S, September, 2004.

138. Poon, V.K.M., et al. "*In vitro* Cytotoxicity of Sliver: Implications for Clinical Wound Care," *Burns* 30(2):140-47, March 2004.

139. Innes, M.E., et al. "The Use of Silver Coated Dressings on Donor Site Wounds: a Prospective, Controlled Matched Pair Study," *Burns* 27(6):621-27, September 2001.

140. Zamboni, W.A., et al. "Evaluation of Hyperbaric Oxygen for Diabetic Wounds: A Prospective Study," *Undersea Hyperbaric Medicine* 24(3):175-79, September 1997.

141. Thai, T.P., et al. "Effect of Ultraviolet Light C on Bacterial Colonization in Chronic Wounds," *Ostomy Wound Management* 51(10):32-45, October 2005.

142. Fakhri, O., et al. "The Effect of Low-Voltage Electric Therapy on the Healing of Resistant Skin Burns," *Journal of Burn Care Research* 8(1):15-18, January-February 1987.

143. Guffey, J.S., et al. "*In Vitro* Bactericidal Effects of High Voltage Pulsed Current Versus Direct Current Against *Staphylococcus aureus*," *Journal of Clinical Electrophysiology* 1(1):5-9, January 1989.

144. Kincaid, C., et al. "Inhibition of Bacterial Growth *In Vitro* Following Stimulation with High Voltage, Monophasic, Pulsed Current," *Physical Therapy* 69(8):651-55, August 1989.

145. Szuminsky, N.J., et al. "Effect of Narrow, Pulsed High Voltages on Bacterial Viability," *Phyical Therapy* 74(7):660-67, July 1994.

146. Sibbald R.G., et al. "Increased Bacterial Burden and Infection The Story of Nerds and Stones," *Advances in Skin & Wound Care* 19 (8) 447-61, October 2006.

147. Cutting KF, et al. "Clinical identification of wound infection:a Delphi approach," In: *EWMA Position Document—Identifying Criteria for Wound Infection*, London: MEP Ltd, 6-9, 2005.

CHAPTER 8

Wound debridement

Elizabeth A. Ayello, PhD, RN, APRN,BC, CWOCN, FAPWCA, FAAN
Sharon Baranoski, MSN, RN, CWOCN, APN, DAPWCA, FAAN
Janet Cuddigan, PhD, RN, CWCN, CCCN
R. Gary Sibbald, MD, FRCPC (Med)(Derm), MEd, FAPWCA
The contributions of Morris D. Kerstein, MD, to the first edition of this chapter
are greatly acknowledged.

OBJECTIVES

After completing this chapter, you'll be able to:

• state the purpose of debriding a wound

• list criteria for *not* debriding a necrotic wound

• describe types of debridement that include sharp/surgical, mechanical, maggot, enzymatic, and autolytic

• compare advantages and disadvantages of each type of debridement

• select the most appropriate method of debridement depending on patient preference, clinician expertise, and health care system resources.

Speeding the healing process

Debridement is the removal of necrotic tissue, exudate, bacteria, and metabolic waste from a wound in order to improve or facilitate the healing process. Accumulation of necrotic tissue usually results from poor blood supply, a prolonged inflammatory process, bacterial damage, or an untreated cause of the wound (for example, increased interstitial pressure, or other mechanical, chemical, or traumatic injury). In otherwise healthy people, natural debridement keeps pace with the accumulation of dying tissue in a wound. If the host resistance is impaired by poor nutrition, continued pressure damage, or other comorbidities such as diabetes, medical intervention is required to facilitate wound healing.

The primary purpose of debridement is to reduce or remove dead and necrotic tissue that serves as a proinflammatory stimulus and a culture medium for bacterial growth. The removal of this tissue is necessary to reduce the biological burden of the wound in order to control and prevent wound infection, especially in deteriorating wounds.[1] Debridement allows the practitioner to visualize the walls and base of a wound more accurately to determine the presence of viable tissue. (Keep in mind that a pressure ulcer that has not been debrided cannot be staged). If necrotic tissue isn't removed, it not only impedes wound healing but also results in protein loss, spread of bacterial damage to deeper tissue causing surrounding cellulitis and osteomyelitis, and the possibility of septicemia, limb amputation, or death. By removing necrotic tissue, debridement creates an acute wound within a chronic wound, restoring circulation and allowing adequate oxygen delivery to the wound site.[2]

For a wound to heal, it must have a microenvironment free from the nonviable tissue that serves as a bacterial culture medium to increase organism proliferation.[3] Oxygen is a primary requirement for this energy-dependent metabolic process to occur. The production of free radicals kills bacteria, facilitating the proliferation of fibroblasts and epithelial cells, which are crucial for wound healing. However, when bacteria is present in hypoxic conditions, it competes with healing tissue for nutrients and produces exotoxins and endotoxins that damage newly generated, mature cells. This setting of hypoxia and bacteria interrupts the fundamental wound healing process of fibroblast migration into the extracellular matrix. Fibroblasts, which produce the fibrils of collagen, help lay the foundation for new cell growth. This process allows a chronic wound stuck in the inflammatory stage to move to the proliferative stage promoting new tissue formation and laying the foundation for healing with the necessary recruitment of fibroblasts to deposit collagen.[3]

Leukocytes—primarily polymorphonuclear leukocytes—are the primary cells of the inflammatory process of wound healing. They enter the wound and remove devitalized tissue and foreign material. Collaboration of local enzymes (proteolytic, fibrinolytic, or collagenolytic) also helps to dissolve and remove devitalized tissue. Because collagen comprises approximately 75% of the skin's dry weight, the overall endogenous collagenase is considered to be one of the main regulators of tissue remodeling in the process of wound healing. Remodeling is part of the healing process in which the wound restructures into its final functional image.

After a wound is cleaned, macrophages are recruited; they, in turn, recruit fibroblasts, which deposit collagen and fill the wound with scar tissue. An acute wound with a good blood supply and essential nutrients generally "heals" within 14 days—but this doesn't represent the total healing process. Remodeling typically takes another 4 weeks, making the total healing process about 6 weeks. Other factors may be involved in the healing process. For example, a wound that appears in an area of rich blood supply such as the scalp will heal faster than a wound in an area with a lesser blood supply. Collagen breakdown and collagen buildup occur in equal degrees, resulting in an appropriate-appearing scar. However, excess collagen can form a keloid or hypertrophic scar. A hypertrophic scar represents disordered collagen within the scar tissue of a healed wound. A keloid extends beyond the wound margin with a greater disorganization of collagen fibers.

Identifying necrotic tissue

Dead or necrotic tissue may be loose and moist, or dry and firm. This tissue is identified by its moist, yellow, green, or gray appearance, and may become thick and leathery with a dry black eschar due to dehydration. Oxygen and nutrients can't penetrate a wound impaired by necrotic tissue. Dead tissue is the breeding ground for bacteria, and the eschar may mask an underlying abscess.[4] Necrotic tissue that's moist, stringy, and yellow is referred to as slough (devitalized connective tissue).

In general, removing necrotic tissue restores the local vascular supply to the wound and improves healing. However, debriding too much tissue can destroy the collagen structural framework for healing. Some wounds shouldn't be debrided at all. Exercise caution, for example, in dealing with necrotic ulcers on the heels or toes, which may have poor perfusion. Debriding heel ulcers remains a controversial issue due to problems with perfusion and the small amount of tissue that covers the calcuteanous bone. Conversely, some wounds can become larger with debridement. Pyoderma gangrenosum is one example of a wound that should not be debrided when there is a raised active border. The raised active border indicates acute inflammatory reaction and debridement would stimulate the infiltrate even more through a process called *pathergy*.

PRACTICE POINT

Monitor stable necrotic heels for odor and signs of edema, erythema, fluid wave, or drainage, which signal the need for debridement.[5]

PRACTICE POINT

It's often important to watch the interphase between viable and necrotic tissue for further tissue breakdown or softening eschar that could signal proximal bacterial spread.

Guidelines from the Agency for Health Care Policy and Research (AHCPR), now called the Agency for Health Care Research and Quality (AHCRQ),[5] and the Wound, Ostomy and Continence Nurses Society (WOCN)[6] recommend against disturbing a dry, stable eschar ulcer of the heel without signs of edema, erythema, fluctuance (fluid wave), or drainage. In these wounds, eschar acts as a natural barrier to infection. Some clinicians have questioned this recommendation and are actively debriding heel wounds.[7] In clinical practice, others leave the eschar intact and focus on preventing trauma to the wound. Wrap the foot in a soft dressing material and monitor it for signs of infection and changes in eschar.

Chronic wound care begins with treating the cause and patient-centered concerns including pain and activities of daily living. Assess individual patients to determine if the wound is healable, maintenance, or nonhealable. To assess healability, adequate blood supply needs to be present.[8] A palpable pulse in the foot indicates a pressure in excess of 80 mm Hg and enough blood supply for healing to occur. This finding could equate to an Ankle Brachial Pressure Index of 0.6 or higher. If there is enough blood supply and the cause has been corrected (compression for venous ulcers and pressure offloading for diabetic neurotrophic foot ulcers), the ulcer is healable. For pressure ulcers, the source of

tissue damage needs to be corrected including high blood pressure, poor nutrition, friction and shear, decreased mobility, or excess local moisture. Active debridement can be coupled with moisture and bacterial balance.

A maintenance wound occurs when a wound has enough blood supply to heal but due to patient or health delivery system factors, the wound does not have the ability to heal. Debridement and local wound care should then be conservative for maintenance wounds. A nonhealable or palliative wound, does not have enough blood supply to heal and debridement should be conservative and limited to soft slough with a local antimicrobial (such as povidone iodine or chlorhexidine) and moisture reduction to reduce local bacteria.

Debridement is a critical first step in preparing the wound bed for healing. Wound bed preparation (WBP) is the management of a wound to accelerate endogenous healing or to facilitate the effectiveness of other therapeutic measures.[9] The original TIME model—**T**issue nonviable or deficient, **I**nfection or inflammation, **M**oisture imbalance, **E**pidermal margin non-advancing or undermining[9]—has recently been reconceptualized to the DIME model.[8,10,11] (See *New wound bed preparation (DIME) model,* page 122.)[11] As mentioned, you should first examine patient-centered concerns and wound cause prior to beginning local wound healing. (See *Best practices for preparing the wound bed,* page 123.)[8]

PRACTICE POINT

Save time and use the DIME acronym in preparing the wound bed for healing.
- Debridement
- Infection or inflammation
- Moisture imbalance
- Epidermal margin nonadvancing or undermining[8,10]

Predebridement teaching

Patient-centered care should include teaching about the purpose and usual expectations of the debriding process. This process needs to be explained and understood by the patient

New wound bed preparation (DIME) model

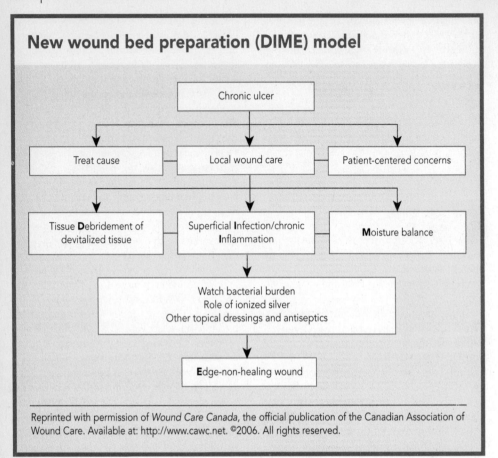

Chronic ulcer

Treat cause — Local wound care — Patient-centered concerns

Tissue **D**ebridement of devitalized tissue — Superficial **I**nfection/chronic Inflammation — **M**oisture balance

Watch bacterial burden
Role of ionized silver
Other topical dressings and antiseptics

Edge-non-healing wound

and family *prior* to initiating treatment. Include in your teaching the debridement method that will be used and the desired outcome. It is vital that the patient and family understand why the necrotic tissue is being removed. Some laypersons mistakenly believe that necrotic tissue is a "scab" (eschar) and is a sign of healing. They need to know that epithelium needs a firm granulation base to migrate optimally towards the center of a wound. Delayed healing will result if epithelial margins need to migrate down valleys under eschar or over hypertrophic or unhealthy granulation tissue. Similarly, patients and families need to know that the wound will change during the debridement process because an acute wound is created within a chronic wound to stimulate the healing process. For example, tell them to expect a wound to become larger in size.

Debridement methods

Mechanical, sharp/surgical, enzymatic, and autolytic are the common methods of debridement.[10,12,13,14] However, a resurgence in the use of older methods, such as maggots (biological or larval therapy), has become accepted practice in some wound care centers.[10,12] (See *Overview of debridement methods,* pages 124 to 126.)[10]

Mechanical debridement

Methods of mechanical debridement include wet-to-dry dressings, hydrotherapy (whirlpool), and wound irrigation (pulsed lavage).[10,12,13,14] Mechanical debridement may be more painful than other debridement methods and the health care provider should consider premedicating the patient for pain. Both whirlpool and pulsed lavage (see chap-

Best practices for preparing the wound bed[8]

Identify and treat the cause
- Diagnose and correct or modify treatable causes of tissue damage
- Differentiate the wound's ability to heal: healable, maintenance, or nonhealable wound

Address patient-centered concerns
- Assess and support the management of patient-centered concerns to enable healing
- Provide patient education and support to increase adherence to the treatment plan

Provide local wound care
- Assess and monitor the wound history and physical characteristics (location and measurements)
- Debride healable wounds, removing non-viable, contaminated, or infected tissue (surgical, autolytic, enzymatic, mechanical, or maggot)

- Clean wounds with low-toxicity solutions (such as normal saline or water); reserve topical antiseptic solutions for wounds that are non-healable or those in which the bacterial burden is of greater concern than the stimulation of healing
- Assess and treat the wound for increased bacterial burden or infection; distinguish from persistent inflammation of nonbacterial origin
- Select a dressing that is appropriate for the needs of the wound, the patient, and the caregiver or clinical setting
- Monitor the quantity and quality of wound exudate to prevent periwound maceration
- Evaluate expected rate of wound healing; if suboptimal, reassess patient according to recommendations 1 to 9

Provide organizational support
- For improved outcomes, education and evidence base must be tied to interprofessional teams with cooperation of health care systems

Reprinted with permission of *Wound Care Canada*, the official publication of the Canadian Association of Wound Care. Available at: http://www.cawc.net. ©2006. All rights reserved.

---

ter 9, Wound treatment options) require special equipment and skill. All of the mechanical methods are nonselective; that is, they don't always discriminate between viable and nonviable tissue. Mechanical methods may be harmful to healthy granulation tissue on the surface of the wound and lead to bleeding, trauma, and disruption of the collagen matrix along with the necrotic tissue.

PRACTICE POINT

Mechanical debridement may be painful; consider premedicating the patient for pain.

Wet-to-dry dressings

Despite the drawbacks, such as pain and the necessary application of up to 3 times per day, the use of wet-to-dry dressings to debride a wound unfortunately remains a common treatment in all health care settings. This method involves placing a moist saline gauze dressing on the wound surface and removing it when it's dry. The removal of the dried gauze dressing facilitates removal of devitalized tissue and debris from the wound bed. However, newly formed granulation tissue and new cell growth are also removed. To prevent pain and to help remove the dry gauze, clinicians often wet the dressing before removal. However, this defeats the purpose

(Text continues on page 126.)

Overview of debridement methods[10]

Method	Considerations	Contraindications
SURGICAL/SHARP		
Necrotic tissue is removed using a scalpel, scissors, forceps, or curette	• Urgent need for debridement • Highly selective • Rapid results • Pain unless the patient has neuropathy; analgesia often needed • Risk of hemorrhage/complications • Cost; use of special equipment • Requires patient consent • Requires special training and expert comfort level (including anatomic knowledge) • Must distinguish between necrotic and healthy tissues • Can be done at bedside • May require the need for operating room and systemic anesthetics for extensive procedures • Anticoagulant therapy	• Malignant wounds • Patients with clotting/bleeding abnormalities • Ischemic tissue • Unstable • Underlying dialysis fistula, prosthesis, or arterial bypass graft • Caution with wounds involving hands and face • Caution with immunocompromised patients
AUTOLYIC		
Endogenous enzymes present in wound fluid interact with moist dressing to soften and remove necrotic tissue	• Need for minor or moderate debridement • Patient has a decreased or minimal risk of wound infection • Performed in any setting • Can be used with other methods • Selective • Safe, easy to use • Painless and soothing when dressing in place • Slow • Risk of maceration to surrounding skin • Removal of some dressings may be painful • Odor • Secondary dressing needed for some types of primary dressings • Absorptive dressing can dehydrate the wound bed	• Some dressings cannot be used with infected wounds • Exposed tendon/bone • Friable skin • Deep extensive wounds • Severe neutropenia • Immunocompromised patients
MECHANICAL		
Wet-to-dry: moist dressing is applied to wound, allowed to dry, and removed with force	• Larger wounds • Nonsurgical candidates • Nonselective • Painful	• Clean wounds

Overview of debridement methods *(continued)*

Method	Considerations	Contraindications
MECHANICAL *(continued)*		
	• Frequent dressing changes required, can be done up to 3 times a day; not cost-effective • May macerate surrounding skin • Bleeding • Dressing fibers stick to wound and can cause a foreign body reaction • May disperse bacteria when removed • Traditional more than a modern accepted practice	
Hydrotherapy: moving water dislodges loose debris	• Increases circulation to wound bed • May macerate periwound skin • Time consuming • May cause trauma to wound bed and lead to bacterial contamination of wound and environment • Labor-intensive • Theoretical risk of fluid embolism or promotion of infection with irrigation • Health care professional needs personal protective equipment due to aerolization • Can impede venous blood flow in legs	• Clean wounds • Presence of diabetic neuropathy
Pulsed lavage: irrigation combined with suction	• Bed-bound patients	• Clean wounds
MAGGOT LARVAE (*LUCILLIA SERICATA* GREEN BOTTLE FLY)		
Consume necrotic tissue and bacteria	• Psychological distress • Allergic reaction • Potential for increased pain in ischemic wounds • Time consuming • Selective • Rapid • Costly • May be painless • Decrease bacterial load • Bedside use • Can be used for various wound types, including infected wounds	• Allergies to adhesives, fly larvae, eggs, soybeans • Patients with bleeding abnormalities • Deep, tunneled wounds

(continued)

Overview of debridement methods (continued)

Method	Considerations	Contraindications
ENZYMATIC		
Enzymes degrade and remove necrotic tissue	• Patient on anticoagulants • Can be used on infected wounds • Cost effective • Bedside use • Can be selective • Decreased wound trauma • Cost varies • Daily or twice-a-day application depending on type of enzyme • Sting/inflammation around wound with some enzymes • Not used with heavy metal salts (silver and mercury) • May need cross-hatching of eschar • Clinicians need to document in patient's medication record because enzymes are prescribed drugs • Match type of enzyme used to type of nonviable tissue in the wound	• Clean wound • Allergy to component of the enzyme preparation

of aggressively removing dead tissue. This type of debridement requires significant nursing time and although the materials may be relatively inexpensive, the overall cost can often be greater than other techniques.

A wet-to-dry dressing can be used when a moderate to large amount of necrotic tissue is present and surgical intervention is not an immediate option. Because of pain and the removal of viable tissue, the Centers for Medicare and Medicaid Services (CMS) has stated in its revised surveyors guidance on pressure ulcers that use of wet-to-dry dressings should be limited.[15] CMS also states that wet-to-dry dressings should not be used in a clean, granulating wound. Instead, they recommend use of moist wound therapy dressings, which are discussed in chapter 9, Wound treatment options.

Hydrotherapy

Hydrotherapy (or whirlpool) debridement may be indicated for patients with large wounds that need aggressive cleaning or softening of necrotic tissue. It is contraindicated in granulating wounds because it can macerate and injure the wound bed. Hydrotherapy should be discontinued after necrotic tissue has been removed from the wound bed.

Hydrotherapy is performed by putting the patient's wound in a whirlpool bath and letting the swirling waters soften and loosen dead tissue. This procedure is usually performed in the physical therapy department, with an average treatment duration of 10 to 20 minutes up to twice per day. Operators should carefully monitor the water temperature to prevent burns. The water should be tepid (80° to 92° F [26.7° to 33.3° C]) or close to body temperature (92° to 96° F [33.3° to 35.5° C]).

This type of debridement may cause periwound maceration, traumatize the wound bed, and put the patient at risk for waterborne infections such as *Pseudomonas aeruginosa*. The potential for cross-contamination between patients is also a concern. Both patient and health care workers may be exposed to health risks associated with aerosolization. To minimize infection risks, the whirlpool tank must be thoroughly cleaned with an appropriate disinfectant after each use.

Pulsed lavage

Pulsed lavage debridement is often indicated for patients with large amounts of necrotic tissue and for those whom other debridement methods are not an option. It is accomplished by using specialized equipment that combines a pulsating irrigation fluid with suction.[16] With pulsed lavage, you can clean and debride a wound at variable irrigation pressures (measured in pounds per square inch [psi]). The pulsatile action and effective wound bed debridement may improve granulation tissue growth. This treatment takes 15 to 30 minutes and should be done twice daily if more than half of the wound contains necrotic tissue.

Patients may need to be premedicated for comfort before beginning the procedure. Safe and effective ulcer irrigation pressures ranges from 4 to 15 psi.[5] Controlling the amount of water pressure is critical during this procedure. Because fluid is being forced at the wound directly, the risk of driving organisms deep into the wound tissue is a concern. In addition, inhalation of contaminated water droplets or mist is possible for the clinician and the patient.

 PRACTICE POINT

Always use appropriate equipment to prevent excess lavage pressure. Wear personal protective equipment to prevent splash injury, including eye and face protectors as well as an impervious gown. Remember to administer pain medication to the patient before the procedure.

Sharp/surgical debridement

Sharp/surgical debridement includes the use of a scalpel, forceps, scissors, hydrosurgery devices, or lasers to remove dead tissue.[13,14,17,18] Sharp debridement is considered the 'gold standard' of debridement by many clinicians.[18] It can cause pain so a topical anesthetic, such as lidocaine cream or gels, may be required.[19] Patients may also need follow-up appointments for serial debridement.

Because viable tissue may also be inadvertently removed with this method, excellent judgment must be used when performing sharp debridement.[13,14,18-20] The clinician must be able to differentiate where and what to cut; for example, being able to identify a tendon versus slough because both are yellow in color.[13,14,18-20] Clinicians need guidance as to where the line of demarcation between viable and non-viable keratinocytes are at the wound edge. Recent research by Tomic-Canic and colleagues focuses on an easy way for clinicians to identify how far from the wound edge to perform debridement, based on the pathology of the abnormal keratinocytes at the wound edge.[21]

Nonviable surgical debridement must be distinguished from sharp/surgical debridement that may remove viable tissue on the wound surface to a bleeding base creating an acute wound within a chronic wound.[8-10,18] This procedure is usually done by experienced physicians or surgeons. In the United States, only physicians can perform surgical debridement in the operating room with hydrosurgery devices. Individual states may allow nurses, physical therapists, and physician assistants with appropriate licensing and training to perform some sharp debridement procedures with a scalpel, forceps, or scissors.

The use of sharp debridement is based on expert opinion and clinical data. Steed[22] reanalyzed data from multisite clinical trials that tested the use of growth factor rhPDGF in neuropathic diabetic foot ulcers. The study found significantly higher healing rates in treatment facilities performing more frequent and complete surgical debridement to bleeding tissue and not just the removal of the pericallus. The removal of loose bright friable granulation tissue from the surface of an ulcer removes senescent fibroblasts as well as bacteria that may be arranged in biofilms leading to damage to the underlying tissue. Surgical debridement is used for adherent eschar and devitalized or dead slough on the wound surface. This method can be used in infected wounds and should be the first choice for wounds demonstrating signs of advancing cellulitis or sepsis. Small wounds may be debrided at the bedside, but extensive

Versajet

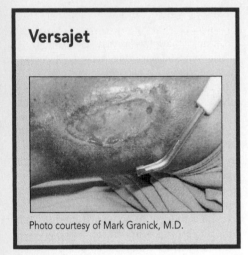

Photo courtesy of Mark Granick, M.D.

wounds—for example, a stage IV pressure ulcer—may require debridement in the operating room. Physicians have reported that use of hydrosurgery devices has decreased the number of times that debridement was needed.[17] (See *Versajet*.) Surgical/sharp debridement must be performed with extreme caution in patients taking anticoagulant medications. The medication may need to be held for a short period of time prior to the procedure. Patients with prolonged bleeding may be best treated with other methods of debridement.

PRACTICE POINT

Exercise caution when performing surgical/sharp debridement on any patient who has been on a prolonged course of anticoagulant therapy.

Enzymatic debridement

Enzymatic debridement is considered safe, effective, and easy to use. Enzymes are effective wound surface cleaning agents that accelerate eschar degradation and debridement. The removal of debris helps a chronic wound move from the inflammatory stage to the proliferative stage resulting in enhanced wound healing.[23] Enzymatic agents are an ideal option for patients who are not candidates for surgery, and for patients receiving care in a long-term care facility or at home where other debridement methods may not be available. Enzymatic debridement is accomplished by applying topical enzymatic agents to devitalized tissue. These agents will digest and dissolve necrotic tissue in the wound bed through breaking down collagen, elastin, and other parts of the abnormal devitalized wound matrix.[2,8,10] Before applying the topical enzymatic agent, crosshatching or scoring can be performed to enhance the local penetration of the agent.

If infection has spread beyond the ulcer (as in advancing cellulitis), immediate removal of necrotic tissue is usually recommended. Surgical debridement and then nonenzymatic debridement should be considered. Enzymes often can be used alone to break down the eschar before sharp debridement, or in conjunction with mechanical debridement. Some topical antibiotics are compatible with enzymatic debriding agents and may be used in conjunction with the treatment.[13,14]

Enzymes that act on necrotic tissue are categorized as proteolytics, fibrinolytics, and collagenases, depending on the tissue component they target. Because papain urea enzymatic debriding agents target eschar, they are often used on wounds with necrosis. Collagenases target nonviable collagen tissue while sparing viable tissue thereby making them useful in necrotic wounds with slough tissue at the wound base.[13,14]

You should be aware of the specific advantages and disadvantages to derive maximum benefit from each particular type and brand of enzyme in the wound. Enzymes with chlorophyllin may stain the wound bed green making assessment and differentiation from infection more challenging. Some enzymes are selective and can be used throughout the treatment phase. Others are nonselective and can harm healthy surrounding tissue; these enzymes should be applied only to the area of eschar or slough. Avoid the use of nonselective enzymes on healthy tissue, such as granulation tissue adjacent to exposed tendons. The surrounding wound margin can be protected by applying a protective barrier ointment or film-forming liquid acrylate around the wound.[13,14] Zinc oxide ointment may interfere with the therapeutic activity of some enzymes.

Silver and other metals including zinc oxide can inactivate enzymes; be careful when selecting cleaning agents and dressings that contain any ingredients that can interfere with enzyme action.

Enzymes are a prescription drug and require a physician or prescriber's order. Some are applied once per day, while others require twice-per-day application. Before reapplying the enzymatic agent, thoroughly clean the wound to remove any residual enzymatic ointment and loose wound debris. To use an enzymatic debriding agent, thoroughly clean the wound with normal saline solution to remove debris on the wound bed. Avoid solutions with metal ions, such as mercury or silver for collagenase and papain-urea agents. Hydrogen peroxide may inactivate papain urea agents.[14]

If within your state's scope of practice and permitted by your facility, crosshatching or scoring the eschar with a scalpel (#11 or #15 blade), without cutting deep enough to cause bleeding, is recommended prior to applying the enzyme to let the debriding agent penetrate into the eschar. After scoring is complete, apply a thin layer (about the thickness of a nickel) of enzymatic ointment onto the necrotic tissue. Cover the wound with an appropriate dressing to keep it moist and let the debriding agent work. Various types of dressings can be used with enzymatic debriders. Avoid covering the wound with a dressing that contains any component that could interfere with the effectiveness of the enzyme. For example, because heavy metals are known to interfere with papain-urea and collagenase enzymatic debriders, do not use them in combination with a silver antimicrobial dressing. (For more information on dressing types, see chapter 9, Wound treatment options.) Follow the specific manufacturer's directions for the particular enzyme you're using. Because these are prescribed drugs, also be sure to record the application of the enzyme in the patient's medication record.

Papain, which comes from the Carica papaya, is a cysteine protease. In the United States, it is usually combined with urea. This combination alters the structures of protein substrates thus enhancing the action of the papain.[23] The papain-urea combination may be more effective in degrading fibrin within the wound bed and is thought to work from the top of the wound down.[24] Most papain-urea preparations are applied once or twice per day. Healthy skin surrounding the wound may be irritated from this enzyme combination due to the production of exudate and its nonselective enzymatic actions.[25] Pain may also be associated with its use. Papain-urea has been shown to interfere with the action of platelet derived growth factor while collagenase is selective and has a similar harmful effect.[26] Because of the nonelective action, the papain-urea combination should be discontinued as soon as the majority of wound debridement has been completed and replaced with agents that will stimulate moist interactive healing.

Another type of enzymatic debriding agent, collagenase, is derived from *Clostridium histolyticum*. It may be more effective at degrading collagen and elastin and is thought to work from the bottom of the wound up.[25] Research supports collagenase as a more selective enzyme and when compared to debridement it controls and may reduce pain caused by debridement.[27] Collagenase upregulates the migration of keratinocytes over the wound bed and stimulates granulation.[28,29] Muller and colleagues found collagenase to be quicker and more cost-effective than autolytic debridement with a hydrocolloid dressing in 24 patients with pressure ulcers.[30] Research by Riley and Herman[31] has shed new light on the role keratinocytes play in wound healing and how it is influenced by different substances including enzymes. This research found that collagenase doubled keratinocyte growth and migration; the increase was fivefold when heparin-binding epidermal-like growth factor was added.[31] An in vitro study by Mekkes and colleagues found increased healing rates with collagenase and ineffective debridement with firbrinolysin (desoxyribonuclease).[32] Collagenase has also been shown to reduce scarring in partial-thickness burn wounds, which has crucial implications for a patient's quality of life.[33]

The optimal method for enzymatic debriding agents has been the subject of much controversy. Research has also shown some differences between papain-urea and collagenase use. While overall healing rates for papain-urea and collagenase were not significantly different in one study, papain-urea did debride eschar at a faster rate.[34] However another study found that papain-urea decreased keratinocyte migration by 50%.[31]

The search for new enzymes continues. Mekkes et al have reported on Antarctic krill as an effective debriding agent.[35] While a systematic review by Bradley and colleagues failed to provide evidence to support the use of enzymatic agents over other methods.[36]

Autolytic debridement

Autolytic debridement uses the body's endogenous enzymes to slowly remove necrotic tissue from the wound bed. In a moist wound, phagocytic cells and proteolytic enzymatic enzymes can soften and liquefy the necrotic tissue that is then digested by macrophages. Autolytic debridement can be facilitated with appropriate dressings in the superficial wound that contains little necrotic tissue, or a larger, deeper pressure ulcer.[13,14] Underlying these concepts is a requirement of adequate circulation and nutrition.[10] Autolytic debridement may take longer than other methods; however, it represents a less stressful method to the patient and wound than mechanical debridement. This method of debridement is contraindicated in infected wounds.

Autolytic debridement is easy to perform and involves applying a moisture-retentive topical dressing, such as a semiocclusive or occlusive dressings; types include transparent films, hydrocolloids, hydrogels, and calcium alginate dressings.[10] (See chapter 9, Wound treatment options.) Wound fluid accumulates under the dressing, aiding in the lysis of necrotic tissue. This method is pain-free in patients with adequate tissue perfusion.

Studies have compared the efficacy of hydrogel dressings and mechanical debridement with wet-to-dry dressings.[37,38,39] Several researchers[37,38,39] have concluded that autolytic debridement with a hydrogel is more time- and cost-effective, resulting in faster healing

when compared with wet-to-dry dressings. One case report found that use of a clear acrylic dressing promoted autolytic debridement and had the added advantage of being able to view the wound without removing the dressing.[40] Schimmelpfenning & Mollenhauer[40] and Konig et al[41] found that autolytic debridement with moist interactive dressings was equal in efficacy to enzymatic methods using collagenase. The Cochrane review on debridement in diabetic ulcers concluded that hydrogels were more effective than gauze.[42]

PRACTICE POINT

Be sure to tell the patient and his family that fluid accumulating under the dressing is a normal part of the debridement process. Discolored wound fluid may not signal a wound infection.

Monitor the wound for signs of infection, such as odor, increasing exudate or wound size, periwound erythema, edema, warmth, or increased pain, and discontinue autolytic debridement if these symptoms occur. Immunocompromised patients should be assessed frequently for any indication of infection. Autolytic debridement isn't the treatment of choice in severely infected wounds; in fact, it may lead to more severe infection and is therefore contraindicated in these situations. Surgical consult is warranted with appropriate medical management of the infection.

Maggot therapy (biological or larval therapy)

Maggot therapy was widely used in the early part of the 20th century. It fell out of favor due in part to the "disgust factor" and the use of newer modalities such as antimicrobial agents in wound treatments. With Europe leading the way, a resurgence in larval therapy use has occurred in the United States.[43,44] In this type of debridement, several applications of sterilized medicinal *Lucilia sericata* (greenbottle fly) maggots are placed in the wound bed every 2 to 3 days.[45] (See *Maggots in heel wound.*) The specific application technique for how the maggots are actually put in the wound varies. Some place the maggots directly into the wound so they can roam around (free-range) and others place the maggots contained in a device such as a pouch or tea bag-like sack. Early evidence supports that free-range maggot therapy maximizes debridement benefits compared to maggots that are contained in pouches or sacks and then placed in the wound.[46]

Just how do these larvae accomplish debridement? The mechanism by which maggot therapy works is believed to be by the enzymes the maggots secrete. These substances are proteinases that degrade the necrotic tissue.[47] The maggots also digest bacteria making them effective in wounds with resistant bacterial strains.[48,49] Maggots also encourage healing by stimulating granulation tissue.

Prospective trials on the efficacy of maggot therapy have reported debridement and evidence of decrease in wound size.[50,51] Some case studies have reported the efficacy and selectivity of maggot debridement therapy.[52,53] Mumcuologlu[54] has reported significant debridement (80% to 85%) with clinical application of maggots as well as the prevention of amputation and bacterial spread.

Maggots can be used in almost all wounds. Richardson[55] and Thomas[56] reviewed current best practices. However, some contraindications for their use include a life- or limb-threatening wound, psychological distress or the "ick factor," bleeding abnormalities, and deep-tracking wounds.[43] The literature is unclear about some aspects of maggot use. Sherman[57] says that maggots should not be used in the presence of osteomyelitis or critical ischemia associated with arterial insufficiency while Claxton et al disagrees.[43] Maggots are cost-effective when used properly and have the potential to help in situations where other resources are not available.[58] Despite the potential for psychological distress, most patients, as well as health care professionals, were satisfied with the treatment in one study.[52]

Something else to consider with maggot therapy is the level of pain it causes. Currently, there are conflicting reports about the level of expected pain with maggot debridement therapy. Sometimes, pain is minimal or absent.[59] In another report, 25% of patients with superficial painful wounds complained of increased pain during treatment with maggots.[47] These patients need analgesics for

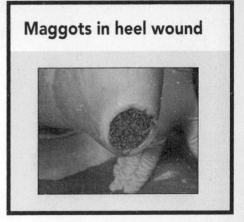

Maggots in heel wound

pain management. The type of wound might make a difference as to whether the patient has pain during therapy. A retrospective study by Steenvorde et al.[60] found that diabetic patients, the majority who had neuropathy (n = 21), did not experience increased pain, while 40% (n = 8) of nondiabetic patients experienced pain when being treated with maggots.

Choosing a debridement method

Does it matter which type of debridement you use on a wound? "No one method of debridement has been proven optimal for pressure ulcers", according to the Wound Ostomy and Continence Society (WOCN).[6]

Given the various and conflicting evidence about the different debridement options, choosing the right way to debride wounds can be challenging. Answering the following questions can help guide you in choosing the best debridement method for your patient.[8,10,13,14,61] (See *Debridement decision-making algorithm,* page 132.) Remember, your choice may be limited by the availability of the various debridement methods in your facility or health care system.

How much time do you have to debride?

Infected wounds require immediate attention and may require surgical debridement after systemic antimicrobial therapy has been initiated. The patient's clinical condition and the

Debridement decision-making algorithm

The following patient factors drive the debridement decision-making process:

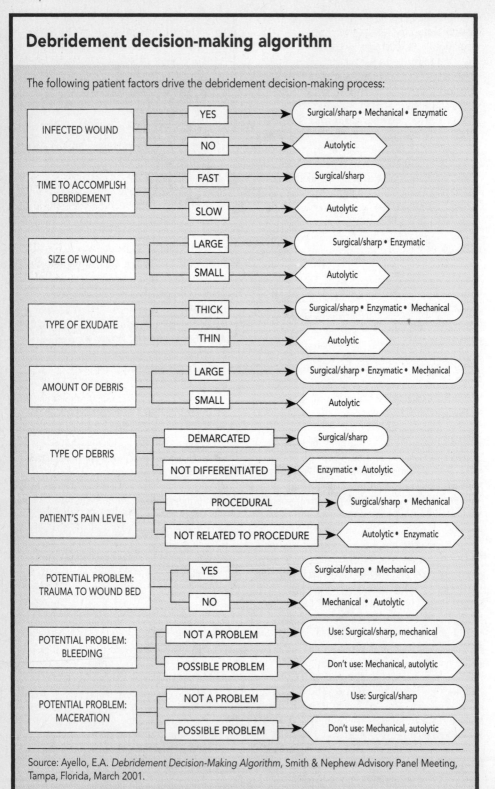

Source: Ayello, E.A. *Debridement Decision-Making Algorithm*, Smith & Nephew Advisory Panel Meeting, Tampa, Florida, March 2001.

Library & Student Services

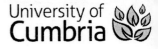

University of Cumbria

Dear student,
The enclosed item(s) are due for return or renewal on or before the date(s) stamped in each item. You can return them in person to any University of Cumbria library or you can post them back. If you are returning by post please send them to the address at the bottom of this letter and ensure that you obtain a certificate of posting from the Post Office. The certificate is free and will provide up to £30 of compensation should the item be lost by Royal Mail.

You are responsible for the item until it is received at the library. You will also be liable for fines if the items are received after the return due date.

To conserve resources please post the item(s) back to us in this envelope.

Contact details for off campus support:

Fusehill Street, Carlisle
Tel: 01228-616218   email LiSSfusehill@cumbria.ac.uk
Lancaster
Tel: 01524-590871   email LiSSlancaster@cumbria.ac.uk

Further information about the Certificate of Posting can be found at
www.royalmail.com

If you live near one of our libraries or gateway campuses you may find it quicker to have books sent there for collection. Details of the locations and opening hours can be found at:
http://www.cumbria.ac.uk/StudentLife/Learning/Resources/Libraries/Home.aspx

Fusehill Library
University of Cumbria
Fusehill Street
Carlisle
Cumbria
CA1 2HH

amount of time that you can devote to a treatment may influence your choice.

What are the wound characteristics?

Consider the size, depth, location, amount of drainage (and if it is increasing), presence (and extent) or absence of infection, and etiology of the wound.

How selective a method is needed?

Determine the risk for damage to healthy tissue when necrotic tissue is removed.

What methods are permitted?

Check that the intended debridement method is allowed by your state's practice act and by your facility. For example, using a scalpel to crosshatch eschar requires specialized training and licensure.

What's the care setting?

Some resources available in a hospital aren't practical in the home and may not even be available in a long-term care facility.

How much debridement is enough?

How do you know when you've debrided enough? Assess the tissue in the wound bed: When most of the wound surface is covered with granulation tissue and the necrotic tissue is gone, you've debrided enough.

Saap and Falanga[62] developed a method to assess adequacy of wound debridement. Their Debridement Performance Index may make more effective comparisons between different debridement methods and facilitate more predictive prognostic information.[62]

Falanga[63] has proposed that chronic wounds need constant debridement because maintenance debridement is an important part of the wound-bed preparation in these wounds. In the past, debridement was regarded as a singular event based on the visible assessment of the wound. Now, however, it's thought that frequent, limited, maintenance debridement will keep the biological burden low and stimulate growth factors.[9,64-66] Maintenance debridement may prove challenging in the future due to proposed reimbursement changes in the United States based on the place in which debridement can be done as well as the frequency of the procedure.

Summary

Debridement is an essential step in the wound bed preparation management process. Although surgical debridement is the fastest way of removing necrotic tissue from a wound, it may not be appropriate for all patients in all health care settings. The selection of the correct method of debridement should be based on the individual patient and the degree of necrosis present. By knowing the options for debridement, you can help prepare the wound bed and assist your patient on the road to healing.

Show what you know

1. *Which statement about the purpose of debridement is correct? Debridement:*

    A. is nonessential for wound healing.
    B. removes debris so cell movement is enhanced.
    C. removes necrotic tissue in order to enhance the wound's biologic burden.
    D. reduces the need for moist wound healing.

ANSWER: B. Debridement is the removal of debris so that cell movement can be enhanced. A is incorrect; most wounds need debridement to heal; C is incorrect because necrotic tissue increases the wound's biologic burden; and D is incorrect because wounds need moist healing.

2. *Which sign in a stable necrotic heel would signal a need for debridement?*

    A. Edema
    B. Presence of thick, leathery eschar
    C. An impending inspection by a regulator
    D. Yellow slough

ANSWER: A. Edema is a sign of infection, which signals the need for debridement. Other signs are erythema, fluid wave, and drainage. The other options are incorrect.

3. *Which method is an example of mechanical debridement?*

    A. Collagenases
    B. Maggots
    C. Film dressings
    D. Pulsed lavage

ANSWER: D. Pulsed lavage is a method of mechanical debridement. Collagenases are enzymes, maggots secrete natural collagenase, and film dressings are a method of autolytic debridement.

4. A resident in a long-term care facility is on Coumadin and needs debridement for a necrotic ulcer on his forearm. Which of the following methods of debridement would be least indicated?

A. Surgical
B. Enzymatic
C. Mechanical
D. Autolytic

ANSWER: A. Because the resident is on Coumadin and bleeding can occur, surgical debridement would be least indicated. Also, the appropriate personnel and equipment may not be available in the patient's long-term care facility. The other options are incorrect.

5. Which method of debridement would be best to use initially for a hospitalized client with an infected large sacral pressure ulcer?

A. Surgical
B. Enzymatic
C. Mechanical
D. Autolytic

ANSWER: A. Time is of the essence and surgical debridement is the quickest method that can be used with infected wounds. Because the client is hospitalized, the appropriate personnel and equipment to perform this method of debridement are available. The other options are incorrect.

References

1. Ramasastry, S.S. "Chronic Problem Wounds," *Clinical Plastic Surgery* 25(3):367-96, July 1998.
2. Ayello, E.A., et al. "Skip the Knife: Debriding Wounds Without Surgery," *Nursing 2002* 32(9):58-63, September 2002.
3. Wysocki, B. "Wound Fluids and the Patho-genesis of Chronic Wounds," *Journal of Wound, Ostomy, and Continence Nursing* 23(6):283-90, November 1996.
4. Edlich, R.F., et al. "The Biology of Infections: Sutures, Tapes, and Bacteria," in *Wound Healing and Wound Infection: Theory and Surgical Practice.* Edited by Hunt, T.K. New York, NY: Appleton-Century-Crofts, 1980.
5. Bergstrom, N., Bennett, M.A., Carlson, C.E., et al. *Treatment of Pressure Ulcers. Clinical Practice Guideline, No. 15,* AHCPR Publication No. 95-0652. Rockville, MD: Agency for Health Care Policy and Research, December 1994.
6. Wound Ostomy and Continence Nurses Society. *Guideline for Prevention and Management of Pressure Ulcers # 2 WOCN Clinical Practice Guideline Series,* Glenview, Ill.: WOCN, 2003.
7. Brem, H., et al. "Protocol for Treatment of Diabetic Foot Ulcers," *Am J Surg* 187(suppl 1):1S-10S, 2004.
8. Sibbald, R.G., et al. "Best Practice Recommendations for Preparing the Wound Bed: Update 2006," *Wound Care Canada* 4(1):15-29, 2006.
9. Schultz, G.S., et al. "Wound Bed Preparation: A Systematic Approach to Wound Management," *Wound Repair and Regeneration* 11(suppl 1):S1-S28, March 2003.
10. Kirshen, C., et al. "Debridement: A vital Component of Wound Bed Preparation," *Advances in Skin and Wound Care* 19(9):506-17, quiz 518-519, November-December, 2006.
11. Canadian Association of Wound Care. Available at: http://www.cawc.net. 2006.
12. Beitz, J.M. "Wound Debridement: Therapeutic Options and Care Considerations," *Nursing Clinics of North America* 40(2):233-49, 2005.
13. Ayello, E.A, Cuddigan, J.E. "Debridement: Controlling the Necrotic/Cellular Burden," *Adv Skin Wound Care* 17(2):66-75; quiz 76-78, March 2004.
14. Ayello, E.A., Cuddigan, J.E. "Conquer Chronic Wounds with Wound Bed Preparation," *Nurse Pract* 29(3):8-25; quiz 26-27, 2004.
15. Centers for Medicare and Medicaid Services (CMS) Tag F-314 *Pressure Ulcers. Revised Guidance for Surveyors in Long Term Care.* Issued Nov 12, 2004. Available at: http//new.cms.hhs.gov/manuals/download/som107ap_pp_guidelines_ltcf.pdf. Accessed on December 1, 2006.
16. Scott, R., and Loehne, H. "Five Questions and Answers About Pulsed Lavage," *Advances in Skin & Wound Care* 13(3, part I):133-34, May-June 2000.
17. Mosti, G., and Mattaliano, V. "The Debridement of Chronic Leg Ulcers by Means of a New, Fluidjet-based Device," *Wounds* 18(8):227-37, August 2006.
18. Leaper, D. Sharp techniques for wound debridement. World Wide Wounds. Available at : http://www.worldwidewounds.com/2002/december/Leaper/Sharp-Debridement. Html. Accessed on July 17, 2006.
19. Williams, D., Enoch, S., Miller, D., et al. "Effect of Sharp Debridement Using Curette on Recalcitrant Nonhealing Venous Leg Ulcers: A Concurrently Controlled, Prospective Cohort Study," *Wound Repair Regen* 13:131-37, March-April 2005.
20. Ashworth, J., and Chivers, M. "Conservative Sharp Debridement: The Professional and Legal Issues," *Professional Nurse* 17(10):585-88, June 2002.
21. Brem, H., et al. "Molecular Markers in Patients with Chronic Wounds to Guide Surgical Debridement," *Molecular Medicine* 13(1-2):30-39, 2007.
22. Steed, D.L., et al. "Effect of Extensive Debridement and Treatment on the Healing of Diabetic Foot Ulcers. Diabetic Ulcer Study Group," *Journal of the American College of Surgeons* 183(1):61-64, July 1996.
23. Wright, J.B., and Shi, L. "Accuzyme Papain-Urea Debriding Ointment: A Historical Review," *Wounds* 15(4):2S-12S, April 2003.
24. Hebda, P.A., and Lo, C. "Biochemistry of Wound Healing: The Effects of Active Ingredients of Standard Debriding Agents–Papain and Collagenase–on Digestion of Native and Denatured Collagenous Substrates, Fibrin and Elastin," *Wounds* 13(5):190-94, 2001.
25. Hebda, P.A., et al. "Evaluation of Efficacy of Enzymatic Debriding Agents for Removal of Necrotic Tissue and Promotion of Healing in Porcine Skin Wounds," *Wounds* 10(3):83-96, 1998.
26. Falanga, V. "Wound Bed Preparation and the Role of Enzymes: A Case for Multiple Actions of Therapeutic Agents," *Wounds* 14(2):47-57, February 2002.

27. Hansbrough, J.F., et al. "Wound Healing in Partial-Thickness Burn Wounds Treated with Collagenase Ointment versus Silver Sulfadiazine Cream," *J Burn Care Rehabil* 16(Pt 1):241-47, 1995.

28. Pilcher, B.K., Dumin, J.A., Sudbeck, B.D., et al. « The Activity of Collagenase-1 is Required for Keratinocyte Migration on a Type I Collagen Matrix," *J Cell Biol* 137:1445-57, 1997.

29. Burgos, A., Gimenez, J., Moreno, E., et al. "Collagenase Ointment Application at 24- versus 48-hour Intervals in the Treatment of Pressure Ulcers. A Randomized Multicentre Study," *Clin Drug Invest* 19:399-407, 2000.

30. Muller, E., van Leen, M.W., Bergmann, R. "Economic Evaluation of Collagenase-containing Ointment and Hydrocolloid Dressings in the Treatment of Pressure Ulcers," *Pharmacoeconomics* 19:1209-1216, 2001.

31. Riley, K.N., and Herman, I.M. "Collagenase Promotes the Cellular Responses to Injury and Wound Healing In Vivo," *J Burns Wounds* 4:112-24, July 2005.

32. Mekkes, J.R., et al. "Quantitative and Objective Evaluation of Wound Debriding Properties of Collagenase and Fibrinolysin/Desoxyribonuclease in a Necrotic Ulcer Animal Model," *Arch Dermatol Res* 290:152-57, 1998.

33. Frye, K.E., Luterman, A. "Decreased Incidence of Hypertrophic Burn Scar Formation with the Use of Collagenase, An Enzymatic Debriding Agent," *Wounds* 17(12):32-36, December 2005.

34. Alvarez, O.M., et al. "A Prospective, Randomized, Comparative Study of Collagenase and Papain-urea for Pressure Ulcer Debridement," *Wounds* 14:293-301, 2002.

35. Mekkes, J.R., et al. "Efficient Debridement of Necrotic Wounds Using Proteolytic Enzymes Derived from Antarctic Krill: A Double-blind, Placebo-controlled Study in a Standardized Animal Wound Model," *Wound Repair Regen* 6(1):50-57, January 1998.

36. Bradley, M., et al. "The Debridement of Chronic Wounds: A Systematic Review," *Health Technol Assessment* 3(17 Pt 1):iii-iv, 1-78, 1999.

37. Mulder, G.D. "Cost-effective Managed Care: Gel versus Wet-to-dry for Debridement," *Ostomy Wound Management* 41(2):68-70, 72, 74 passim, March 1995.

38. Thomas, S., et al. "Clinical Experience with a New Hydrogel Dressing," *J Wound Care* 5:132-33, 1996.

39. Trudgian, J. "Investigating the Use of Aquaform Hydrogel in Wound Management," *Br J Nurs* 9:943-48, 2000.

40. Schimmelpfenning, D., and Mollenhauer, S. "Use of a Clear Absorbent Acrylic Dressing for Debridement," *JWOCN* 33(6):639-42, November/December 2006.

41. Konig, M., Vanscheidt, W., Augustin, M., Kapp, H. "Enzymatic versus Autolytic Debridement of Chronic Leg Ulcers: A Prospective Randomised Trial," *J Wound Care* 14:320-23, July 2005.

42. Smith, J. "Debridement of Diabetic Foot Ulcers," *Cochrane Database Syst Rev* (4):CD003556, 2002.

43. Claxton, M.J., et al. "5 Questions—and Answers—About Maggot Debridement Therapy," *Adv Skin Wound Care* 16:99-102, 2003.

44. Bolton, L.L. "Evidence Corner, Maggot Therapy," *Wounds* 18(9):A19-A22, September 2006.

45. Courtenay, M., et al. "Larva Therapy in Wound Management," *J R Soc Med* 93(2):72-74, 2000.

46. Steenvorde, P., et al. "Maggot Debridement Therapy: Free-range or Contained? An In Vivo Study," *Adv Skin Wound Care* 18:430-35, October 2005.

47. Chambers, L., et al. "Degradation of Extracellular Matrix Components by Defined Proteinases from the Greenbottle larva *Lucilia sericata* Used for the Clinical Debridement of Non-healing Wounds," *Br J Dermatol* 148:14-23, 2003.

48. Wollina, U., et al. "Biosurgery in Wound Healing: The Renaissance of Maggot Therapy," *J Eur Acad Dermatol Venereol* 14:285-89, 2000.

49. Rayner, K. "Larval Therapy in Wound Debridement," *Prof Nurse* 14:329-33, February 1999.

50. Sherman, R.A. "Maggot versus Conservative Debridement Therapy for the Treatment of Pressure Ulcers," *Wound Rep Regen* 10:208-14, 2002.

51. Sherman, R.A. "Maggot Debridement Therapy for Treating Non-healing Wounds," *Wound Rep Regen* 8:327, 2000.

52. Sherman, R.A.,et al. "Maggot Debridement Therapy in Outpatients," *Arch Phys Med Rehabil* 82:1226-29, 2001.

53. Tanyuksel, M., et al. "Maggot Debridement Therapy in the Treatment of Chronic Wounds in a Military Hospital Setup in Turkey," *Dermatology* 10:115-18, 2005.

54. Mumcuoglu, K.Y. "Clinical Applications for Maggots in Wound Care," *Am J Clin Dermatol* 2:219-27, 2001.

55. Richardson, M. "The Benefits of Larval Therapy in Wound Care," *Nurs Stand* 19(7):70, 72, 74 passim, 2004.

56. Thomas, S., Andrews, A., Jones, M. "The Use of Larval Therapy in Wound Management," *J Wound Care* 7:521-24, 1998.

57. Sherman, R.A. "Maggot Therapy for Foot and Leg Wounds," *Int J Low Extrem Wounds* 1:135-142, June 2002.

58. Wayman, J., et al. "The Cost Effectiveness of Larval Therapy in Venous Ulcers," *J Tissue Viability* 10(3):91-94, 2000.

59. Kitching, M. "Patients' Perceptions and Experiences of Larval Therapy," *J Wound Care* 13(1):25-29, 2004.

60. Steenvoorde, P., et al. "Determining Pain Levels in Patients Treated with Maggot Debridement Therapy," *J Wound Care* 14:485-88, November 2005.

61. Mosher, B.A., et al. "Outcomes of Four Methods of Debridement Using a Decision Analysis Methodology," *Advances in Wound Care* 12(2):81-88, March 1999.

62. Saap, L.J., and Falanga, V. "Debridement Performance Index and Its Correlation with Complete Closure of Diabetic Foot Ulcers," *Wound Repair Regen* 10:354-59, 2002.

63. Falanga, V. "Wound Bed Preparation and the Role of Enzymes: A Case for Multiple Actions of Therapeutic Agents," *Wounds* 14(2):47-57, March 2002.

64. Steed, D.L. "Debridement," *Am J Surg* 187(5A):71S-74S Review, May 2004.

65. Vowden, K.R., and Vowden, P. "Wound Debridement, Part 1: Non-sharp Techniques," *J Wound Care* 8:237-40,1999.

66. Vowden, K.R., and Vowden, P. "Wound Debridement, Part 2: Sharp Techniques," *J Wound Care* 8:291-94, June 1999.

CHAPTER 9

Wound treatment options

Sharon Baranoski, MSN, RN, CWOCN, APN, DAPWCA, FAAN
Elizabeth A. Ayello, PhD, RN, APRN,BC, CWOCN, FAPWCA, FAAN
Andrea McIntosh, RN, BSN, CWOCN, APN
Linda Galvan, RN, BSN, CWOCN, APN
Pamela Scarborough, PT, MS, CDE, CWS, FACCWS

OBJECTIVES

After completing this chapter, you'll be able to:

* explain moist wound therapy

* select dressings based on assessment of wound characteristics

* list indications for use of dressings by categories

* state the advantages and disadvantages for each dressing category

* use the principles of care in dressing selection

* discuss the use of advanced therapies.

A challenge for clinicians

Wound healing in the 21st century is a different and complex process. Although we are gaining new knowledge as to the biology of wound healing, "we can no longer care only for the wound itself; we must step back and look at the entire human being who happens to have a wound that needs healing."[1] This is an exciting, but challenging time for wound care clinicians as new understanding of the biology of healing wounds has given rise to many new wound care treatments. Being able to differentiate among the various treatment options, when and how to apply them, in what combinations, and when to change them has indeed become an art and science. "With the emergence of more complex products, we will be increasingly required to use

these products appropriately to maximize their impact. As a better understanding of the wound environment becomes available, our ability to tailor our approach and better treat the patient as a whole increases."[2]

Providing quality care for your wound care patients should start with understanding wound products, cost-effective treatment modalities, and the principles of optimal wound interventions. Wound dressings can present a challenging decision for clinicians. As clinicians try to heal wounds faster, the marketplace continues to provide many more treatment choices. Keeping abreast of wound dressing choices and various application techniques, as well as which product to use and when, is an ambitious task for all clinicians. Essential dressing competency recommendations have been suggested. (See *Clinician com-*

petencies for dressing selection.) Clinicians can benefit from a working knowledge of wound management including dressing options, cost, frequency of product changes, and how they correlate with successful outcomes.

Moist wound healing

Health and wound care have certainly changed! During the past 3 decades, wound care has made more advances than over the past 2,000 years. The wound care revolution has occurred due in part to Dr. Winter's discovery (in the 1960s) of the importance of moist wound healing in experimental animals.[3] Hinman and Maibach[4] paralleled these findings of faster resurfacing in partial thickness wounds in humans. This new concept of moist wound healing, coupled with advancement in wound dressing materials, has changed the practice of wound management.

EVIDENCE-BASED PRACTICE

Partial-thickness wounds in pigs covered with a plastic material had two times faster epithelialization than identical wounds left open to air.[3]

We now understand that wound healing must take place in a moist environment. Epithelial cells require moisture to migrate from the wound edges to reepithelialize or close the wound. This process is likened to "leap-frogging" of the cells. In a dry wound, these cells have to burrow down underneath the wound bed to find a moist area upon which to "march" or move forward. (See *Epithelial cell migration in an open wound,* page 138.)

The importance of moist wound healing based on wound physiology requires that new dressing materials be developed. Rather than the passive coverings used in the past, which have evolved from "natural" coverings such as feathers and leafs, to gauze, to more sophisticated dressings based on current research, today's wound dressings actively change, enhance, remove detrimental substances in wound fluid, and some even accelerate the rate of wound closure.[5]

Formerly, wound dressings were primarily used to protect the wound from secondary

Clinician competencies for dressing selection

- Conduct a thorough wound assessment to identify wound characteristics and treatment options.
- Know the principles of wound care.
- Be able to differentiate among the different types of dressings.
- Know the characteristics of an ideal dressing.
- Consider the patient's health care coverage, financial abilities, and access to appropriate products, and factor in cost as well as clinical benefit when selecting products.
- Take advantage of conferences, seminars, and self-study opportunities to keep abreast of the latest treatment techniques and products.

Adapted with permission from Baranoski, S. "Wound Dressings: A Myriad of Challenging Decisions," *Home Healthcare Nurse* 23(5): 307-317, May 2005.

infection by forming a barrier against bacteria and absorbing wound fluid. The greatest advantage of contemporary dressings is the maintenance of moist wound conditions in contrast to the "classical gauze techniques" that lead to the formation of a dry, firmly adhering scab.[6] Today's dressings promote rapid healing, act as a barrier, decrease or eliminate pain, require fewer changes, provide autolytic debridement, and can be cost-effective, if used appropriately.[7]

Ovington[8] states "despite the benefits of newer dressing products, gauze is still the most widely used dressing and may be erroneously considered a standard of care." This is based on a study by Pieper and colleagues[9] of 1,638 wounds in the home care setting. The most commonly used dressing for all types of wounds (n = 406) was dry gauze. No dressing (that is, an uncovered wound) was the second most common (n = 252), and saline-moistened gauze (n = 145) was third.[9]

Epithelial cell migration in an open wound

In a moist environment, epithelial cells can migrate on the wound bed surface to close the wound, as shown below.

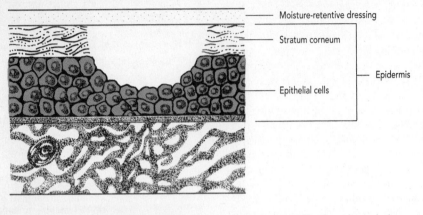

- Moisture-retentive dressing
- Stratum corneum
- Epithelial cells
- Epidermis

In a dry wound bed, epithelial cells burrow underneath the wound bed, as shown below.

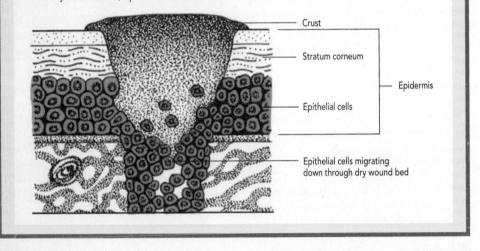

- Crust
- Stratum corneum
- Epithelial cells
- Epidermis
- Epithelial cells migrating down through dry wound bed

Advanced moisture-retentive dressings comprised less than 25% of all dressings used.

Ovington[8] cautions clinicians about using gauze dressings. (See *The case against gauze dressings*.) Although intended for wet-to-moist use, gauze dressings are often allowed to dry out before removal. Research by Kim[10] suggests that a saline gauze dressing acts as an osmotic dressing. As water evaporates from the saline dressing, it becomes hypertonic. Because the body wants to maintain homeostasis by reestablishing isotonicity, wound fluid is drawn into the gauge dressing.

In addition to water, wound fluid includes blood and proteins. These substances form an impermeable layer on the dressing that prevents wound fluid from "wetting" the dressing; the net result is the dressing dries out. Ovington[8] states that "removal of a wet-to-moist dressing that has dried may then cause reinjury of the wound, resulting in pain and delayed wound healing." Decreased pain, including at time of dressing change, has been found when semiocclusive dressings rather than gauze dressings are used.[11,12] The mechanism for this reduction in pain is that nerve endings in the wound aren't exposed and don't become dehydrated.

Local tissue cools as a gauze dressing becomes dry. As water evaporates from the wound surface, wound temperature decreases. Reduced tissue temperatures (up to 10° below normal) have been found in wounds left open and uncovered (69.8° F [21° C]) as well as those where gauze dressings are used (77° to 80.6° F [25° to 27° C]).[13] Reduced wound temperature results in physiologic effects (effects of local vasoconstriction, hypoxia, impaired leukocyte mobility, phagocytic efficiency, and increased affinity of hemoglobin for oxygen), all which contribute to impaired wound healing.[8] Higher temperatures of 91.4° to 95° F (33° to 35° C) are found in wounds covered with transparent films or foam dressings. Semiocclusive dressings impede moisture loss from the wound, thus preventing local cooling and its associated negative healing effects.[8]

Gauze dressings don't present a barrier to bacteria. An in vitro study by Lawrence[14] demonstrated that bacteria can pass through up to 64 layers of dry gauze. Once the gauze is moistened, it's even less effective as a barrier to bacteria.[8] Infection rates are higher in wounds where gauze is used as compared to wounds covered with transparent films or hydrocolloids.[15,16] Gauze dressings are also labor intensive as they require several changes per day.[8] (See *Why are gauze dressings still used?* page 140.)

Film dressings and hydrocolloid dressings were among the first of the dressing materials that could maintain a moist wound-healing environment. New application techniques had to be learned and, more importantly, the clinical significance of wound fluid findings understood. The accumulation of light greenish-yellow fluid seen collecting under film dressings has caused us to relearn what is a normal expectation in a healing wound. Even the different nuance of wound odors has been cause for new learning. For example, different odors occur as wound fluid interacts with different dressing materials. A wound being treated with alginate dressings, which are made from seaweed, may smell like "low tide."

The case against gauze dressings

- A gauze dressing can impair wound healing because it lowers the wound temperature and impedes fluid evaporation.
- Wet-to-dry gauze dressings are a nonselective mechanical debridement method. Removal of healthy tissue causes injury to the wound and pain.
- Clinical studies have shown higher infection rates in wounds for which gauze dressings were used compared to wounds dressed with transparent films or hydrocolloids.
- Changing a dressing more than once per day isn't always effective for patient outcomes and may not be reimbursable.
- Research has shown that bacteria are released into the air when gauze dressings (wet or dry) are removed from the wound.
- Semiocclusive dressings are more financially feasible from a total cost perspective.

Adapted with permission from Ovington, L.G. "Hanging Wet-to-Dry Dressings Out to Dry," *Advances in Skin & Wound Care* 15(2):79-84, March-April 2002.

Treatment decisions

The myriad of products available for wound care have enhanced the overall management of patients, but have also created confusion about selecting the appropriate product. Optimal wound interventions should be dependent on the basic principles of wound care, attentive wound assessment, and expected outcomes. A complete wound assessment should be the driving element in all treatment decisions. (See chapter 6, Wound assessment.) Wound assessment should be based on the principles of wound care. (See *Principles of care: MEASURES acronym,* page 140.)

Why are gauze dressings still used?

Ovington[8] suggests reasons for the continued use of gauze dressings.

- Gauze dressings have a long tradition in wound care—gauze and saline are familiar and readily available.
- Gauze is perceived as being inexpensive; advanced dressings may be incorrectly perceived as being expensive. Frequency of dressing change and caregiver costs must be considered in addition to the cost of the dressing itself when calculating the total cost of dressing changes.
- Most advanced dressings are of discrete dimensions and can't always be adjusted

for wounds of different sizes, requiring health care facilities to stock multiple sizes. Gauze, on the other hand, is easily tailored to fit the wound.

- Many practitioners are unaware of the broad array of alternative dressing products available and the way they work. The variations in appearance and performance of new types of dressings may initially confuse the health care provider.
- Advanced dressings may be perceived as more expensive than gauze due to individual rather than bulk purchase pricing.

Adapted with permission from Ovington, L.G. "Hanging Wet-to-Dry Dressings Out to Dry," *Advances in Skin & Wound Care* 15(2):79-84, March-April 2002.

Principles of care: The MEASURES acronym

Minimize trauma to wound bed

Eliminate dead space (tunnels, tracts, undermining)

Assess and manage the amount of exudate

Support the body's tissue defense system

Use non-toxic wound cleansers

Remove infection, debris, and necrotic tissue

Environment maintenance, including thermal insulation and a moist wound bed

Surrounding tissue, protect from injury and bacterial invasion

Adapted with permission from Baranoski, S. "Wound Dressings: Challenging Decisions," *Home Healthcare Nurse* 17(1):19-25, January 1999.

Wound treatment decisions must be patient centered. What are the patient's goals and preferences? Local wound care starts with a thorough assessment of the wound and a comprehensive collection of data about the patient's overall status. Wound assessment parameters can assist with treatment choices and decisions for appropriate dressing selection. (See *Wound care decision algorithm.*)

Once a thorough wound assessment is complete, choosing dressings and treatments

becomes a clinical decision, that is mutually arrived at with the patient, based on data collected during the assessment and the overall expected outcome.

PRACTICE POINT

Dressing choices = Wound assessment + Principles of wound care

Wound care decision algorithm

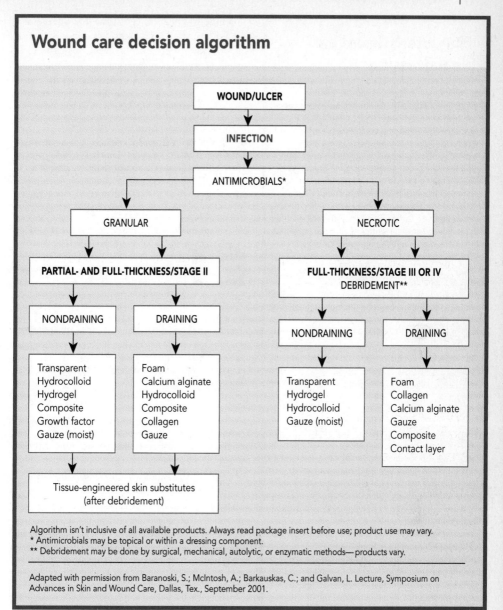

```
                    ┌─────────────────┐
                    │   WOUND/ULCER   │
                    └─────────────────┘
                             │
                    ┌─────────────────┐
                    │    INFECTION    │
                    └─────────────────┘
                             │
                    ┌─────────────────┐
                    │ ANTIMICROBIALS* │
                    └─────────────────┘
```

GRANULAR	NECROTIC
PARTIAL- AND FULL-THICKNESS/STAGE II	**FULL-THICKNESS/STAGE III OR IV** DEBRIDEMENT**

GRANULAR → PARTIAL- AND FULL-THICKNESS/STAGE II

NONDRAINING	DRAINING
Transparent Hydrocolloid Hydrogel Composite Growth factor Gauze (moist)	Foam Calcium alginate Hydrocolloid Composite Collagen Gauze

Tissue-engineered skin substitutes
(after debridement)

NECROTIC → FULL-THICKNESS/STAGE III OR IV DEBRIDEMENT**

NONDRAINING	DRAINING
Transparent Hydrogel Hydrocolloid Gauze (moist)	Foam Collagen Calcium alginate Gauze Composite Contact layer

Algorithm isn't inclusive of all available products. Always read package insert before use; product use may vary.
* Antimicrobials may be topical or within a dressing component.
** Debridement may be done by surgical, mechanical, autolytic, or enzymatic methods—products vary.

Adapted with permission from Baranoski, S.; McIntosh, A.; Barkauskas, C.; and Galvan, L. Lecture, Symposium on Advances in Skin and Wound Care, Dallas, Tex., September 2001.

Treatment goals may aim to achieve a clean wound, heal the wound, maintain a clean wound bed, or place the patient in another setting to continue care.[17] Clinicians need to match the wound assessment characteristics with the dressing characteristics. The goal of care then becomes *using the right product on the right wound at the right time*. For example, a granular, nondraining moist or wet wound needs to maintain a moisture balance conducive to healing. The primary dressing choice would be a product that maintains a moist environment but doesn't cause maceration or desiccation of the wound bed. In another example, the goal of dressing selection for a necrotic draining wound is to loosen the eschar for surgical debridement or to autolytically debride the wound (see chapter 8, Wound debridement),

Characteristics of an ideal dressing

Use the following characteristics to determine the ideal dressing for your patient. The ideal dressing should:

- maintain a moist environment
- facilitate autolytic debridement
- be comfortable for the range of use needed (such as to fill tunneling, undermining, or sinus tracts to eliminate dead space)
- come in numerous shapes and sizes
- be absorbent
- provide thermal insulation
- act as a bacterial barrier
- reduce or eliminate pain at the wound site and not cause pain on dressing removal.

The following considerations can be used to evaluate the dressing:

- number of days the dressing can remain in place
- reason for change or removal
- appearance of dressing (soiled or intact)
- ease of dressing application
- ease of dressing removal
- ease of dressing maintenance
- ease of teaching about dressing to caregiver.

Adapted with permission from Seaman, S. "Dressing Selection in Chronic Wound Management," *Journal of the American Podiatric Medical Association* 92(1):24-33, January 2002.

absorb the excess exudate, and prevent trauma to surrounding tissue.

 PRACTICE POINT

If the wound is dry, add moisture. If the wound has drainage, absorb it. If the wound has necrotic tissue, debride it.

Clinicians need to reassess the wound status when completing dressing changes so that appropriate treatment interventions can be implemented. It's important to also understand that once the characteristics of the wound assessment change, so may the dressing choice. All wound products come with product information and instructions to guide the user in appropriate use of that product. The most appropriate dressing should be selected, considering the patient, the wound, and the site. (See *Characteristics of an ideal dressing* and *NICE© for dressing decision making*. See also *Wound dressings categories*, pages 160 to 169.)

 PRACTICE POINT

Wound dressings should be changed to meet the characteristics of the wound bed.

 PRACTICE POINT

Read and understand the information in the package insert before using a wound care product.

Dressings that come in contact with the wound bed are considered primary dressings. Secondary dressings are those dressings that cover a primary dressing or secure a dressing in place. Clinicians should know which dressings are safe to be put into the actual wound and those that are used as securement products. Several dressings on the market act as primary and secondary dressings. Again, what are the wound characteristics that you are addressing?

Dressing selections should also include an assessment of the patient outcome for treatment. High-priced, inappropriate dressings are often used when a more cost-effective product would apply. Outcome is commonly driven by institutional setting. Acute care patients with length of stays of 4 to 5 days usually won't achieve healing as their outcome, but will achieve a moist, clean wound bed that supports the healing environment. Home care and long-term care settings may have a goal of healing or maintaining the current

NICE© for dressing decision making

There are thousands of dressings available and the clinician needs to decide which dressing to select for a particular wound. Ask yourself the following questions about the wound to help determine the dressing that is NICE© to use:

- Is there any **N**ecrotic tissue that needs to be debrided? (Make sure the wound has the ability to heal; if not, however, moist interactive dressings and active surgical debridement to bleeding tissue are contraindicated.)
- Is the wound **I**nfected or inflamed? (Clinicians often look for more than one sign or symptom before diagnosing infection.)
- Do the specific wound **C**haracteristics, such as location, need to be considered? (If the wound is around the anus, a waterproof adhesive dressing may be preferred.) Is pain an issue?
- Is there any **E**xudate; if so, why, how much, and what is the color and consistency?

Exudate may indicate that the cause of the wound has not been treated (for example, edema due to venous insufficiency); that congestive heart failure is present (look for bilateral involvement and extension above the knee); that albumin levels are low (malnutrition, kidney, or liver disease); or that infection is present. Periwound skin needs protection from exudate by using absorbent dressings and protecting the periwound skin. Select a dressing by answering the four questions. Remember, it's NICE© to pick the right dressing.

Letter	Key information to know	Caution
Necrotic tissue Slough, eschar	• Wet to dry dressings are a non-selective method of mechanical debridement. • Autolytic debridement of tissue is best accomplished with hydrogels, hydrocolloids, and alginate dressings. • With dressing-stimulated autolytic debridement, watch for secondary infection and remove unwanted slough with dressing change.	• Dressings are a slower method of debridement compared to sharp/ surgical methods. • There is limited use of wet-to-dry dressings as a debridement method • Some dressings cannot be used or caution is urged in necrotic wounds; check with the manufacturer for any contraindications for use. Removal of non-viable tissue is a critical step in preparing the wound bed for healing.
Infection/ inflammation	• Consider using antimicrobial dressings (for example, silver or iodine). • Infected wounds may require more frequent dressing changes.	• Not all dressings can be used in infected wounds; check with the manufacturer for the specific brand indicated for use.
Characteristics	• Select and reassess a dressing based on location of the wound, such as the use of conformable dressings for hard-to -fit areas. • Waterproof dressings may be used if incontinence is an issue. • Consider the patient's pain and select dressings that may promote comfort and pain reduction.	• Change dressings when they become soiled from feces or urine. • Different dressings can remain in place for different lengths of time; check with the manufacturer for recommended frequency for dressing changes. • Avoid dressings that may increase or contribute to wound pain and consider systemic pain management strategies.

(continued)

NICE© for dressing decision making *(continued)*

Letter	Key information to know	Caution
Exudate	• Match the absorbency of the dressing (none, low, moderate, heavy) to the amount of exudate from the wound. • Assess surrounding skin to evaluate for macerations.	• Surrounding skin needs to be protected from wound drainage; refer to the enabler LOWE©. Search for the cause of the excessive exudate and the need to correct the cause. Exudate may be an indicator of infection.

© E.A. Ayello and R.G. Sibbald.

Economic considerations for nurses

- Clean rather than sterile dressings can usually be used in the home with chronic wounds (refer to your facility's policy).
- Saline solution can be made at home by adding 8 teaspoons of salt to 1 gallon of boiling water.[18]
- Dressings shouldn't be left at the patient's bedside.
- Cost of product selected and resources available for financial assistance should be considered.
- Frequency of dressing changes and cost-effective use of materials affect economy.
- Fistula management may use pouching versus dressing.
- Hydrogen peroxide, povidone-iodine, hypochlorite solution, and acetic acid should be avoided as wound cleansers. All contribute to delayed healing of wounds.[18]

Adapted with permission from Baranoski, S. "Wound Dressings: Challenging Decisions," *Home Healthcare Nurse* 17(1):19-25, January 1999.

The practice of using the same wound dressing during the entire healing time is no longer valid. *All* wounds under the care of clinicians should be assessed at a minimum of once a week and more often if notable changes occur. The type of wound, status of the wound, clinical setting, and regulatory compliance may dictate a different interval of assessment, however. (See chapter 6, Wound assessment.)

Wound assessment is the cumulative process of observation of the actual wound as well as observing the patient, data collection, and evaluation. For many patients, weekly reassessment will provide the indices of a successful treatment and guide decisions that suggest product changes. As the wound characteristics change, so too should the choice of the wound dressings. Indeed, several different types of products may be needed as the wound progresses through the stages of healing.

Dressings should be carefully matched to the wound, the patient, and the setting. For example, a deep wound with a large amount of drainage will require a highly absorbent dressing such as an alginate or foam. As the depth and amount of drainage decreases, a dressing such as a hydrogel, hydrocolloid, or film might be used.

 PRACTICE POINT

Don't use film dressings with higher moisture vapor rates developed for use over I.V. line sites on open wounds.

status of the wound based on the overall health status of the patient. Wound outcomes need to be patient-focused and realistic to the length of time a patient is cared for.

Over the course of healing, the treatment plan will change as the wound is filled with granulation tissue and epithelialization occurs. Economic factors should also be considered when selecting dressings. (See *Economic considerations for nurses.*)

The notion that all wounds are alike has also changed. Understanding of the etiology of the wound is essential for appropriate care.[18] Local wound care products as well as supportive care must be individualized for the particular wound. For example, a venous stasis ulcer might require a highly absorptive dressing as well as the necessary compression therapy. A variety of layered bandages beyond the classic "Unna boot" are now used. Further, checking for ankle-brachial index and pulses using a Doppler is part of the total care of a patient with a peripheral vascular ulcer.

Using wound healing biology to select treatment

An example of increased understanding of the "biology" of wound healing and technology is the use of growth factors. Growth factors are now available either derived from a patient's own platelets or in a drug form dispensed in a tube to apply to diabetic wounds. Research continues as to what combination, what quantity, and when growth factors will best enhance wound healing. Yet another way technology is providing new options for wound management is in the use of tissue-engineered skin equivalents for healing chronic wounds.

Moist wound therapy and dressing options

The essential role and function of a wound dressing is to provide the right environment to enhance and promote wound healing. Research over the last 40 years has lead to the generally accepted phenomena that moist wound dressings create an optimal environment for wounds to heal faster and with less scar formation. The work of Orland[19] and Winter[3] led to the development of moist wound dressings as a clinical intervention to treat wounds.

George Winter is often cited as the father of moist wound healing. His laboratory work comparing air drying to occlusive dressings and effect on epithelialization in the animal model is generally considered to be a landmark study.[3,20] Fear of increasing infection with occlusive therapy slowed the development of the first moist wound therapy dressing. Sixteen years passed before the development of what is considered the first moist wound therapy dressing, Opsite. Continued research, clinician experiments, and interest in wounds in general has led many companies to develop a potpourri of moist wound treatment dressings. However, this has created a challenge for health care providers, who struggle to keep up with the ever-increasing number of new products.

The following synopsis will review the major dressing categories and assist with helpful practice points on what, when, and how to use these dressings.

Transparent film dressings
Transparent film dressings, so named for their "see-through" properties, are thin polyurethane membranes. They are coated with an adhesive that allows them to adhere to the wound margins without sticking to the actual wound, as shown below.

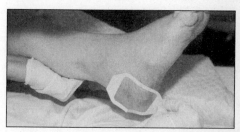

Transparent films have no absorptive capacity but do transmit moisture vapor and are semipermeable to gases. These dressings imitate the outer skin layer to provide a moist environment, similar to a blister. This covering allows epithelial cells to migrate over the surface of the wound. Fluid may accumulate under these dressings. This fluid is sometimes mistaken for pus, a sign of infection. The fluid is a useful adjunct to create an autolytic environment, thereby inducing a cleaner wound surface. When excess fluid accumulates or leaks out from the sides of the dressing, it needs to be changed. Maceration of periwound skin can occur if not changed in a timely manner.

The dressings provide a valuable protective barrier against outside contaminates, fluid, and bacteria. Transparent films also provide protection from friction and aid in autolytic debridement and pain control. Film makes an excellent secondary dressing as well. Most films can be left on for up to 7 days. Transparent films can be used on a variety of wound types, such as stages I and II pressure ulcers, superficial wounds, minor burns, or lacerations; over sutures, catheter sites, donor sites, and superficial dermal ulcers; and for protection of the skin against friction. Transparent dressings can be used on central lines, peripheral inserted central catheter (PICC) lines, and infected wounds.

In addition, some of the newer transparent films currently on the market also contain ionic silver.

Practice essentials
• Apply transparent film dressings to healthy skin; use with caution on aging and fragile skin. These dressings aren't recommended for infants and small children.
• These dressings may be used on dry to minimally moist wounds.
• Don't use transparent film dressings on exudating wounds.
• Transparent film dressings make excellent secondary dressings.
• Not all film dressings can be used on infected wounds.
• Change the dressing when fluid reaches the edge of the dressing, when the seal is broken, or as needed.
• When removing the dressing, lift the corner and pull the film toward the outside of the wound to break the adhesive barrier.
• Avoid roughness when pulling the film off; gently stretch the dressing and support the skin as you're removing the dressing.
• Skin protective wipes and sprays can be used on the periwound area before applying the dressing. Skin wipes also provide an additional seal to prevent the dressing edges from rolling. (See *LOWE© skin barriers for wound margins: 20-second enablers for practice*, page 88.)
• Always read the package insert before applying the dressing because product usage may vary.
• Numerous sizes and shapes are available.

Hydrocolloid dressings

Hydrocolloid dressings were introduced in the 1980s. These new wafer-shaped dressings, as shown below, became the mainstay

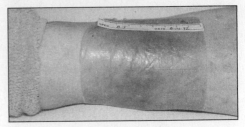

for wound management for many years. Hydrocolloids are impermeable to gases and water vapor.[21] They are composed of opaque mixtures of adhesive, absorbent polymers, pectin gelling agents, and sodium carboxymethylcellulose. Hydrophilic particles within the dressing react with the wound fluid to form a soft gel over the wound bed. According to Choucair,[21] some hydrocolloid dressings provide an acidic environment and some act as a bacterial or viral barrier. Their translucent appearance allows for viewing of the amount of exudate absorbed and fluid accumulation under the dressing.

Hydrocolloid dressings may have a noticeable odor during dressing changes. This is normal in the absence of clinical signs of infection. Some hydrocolloids may also leave residue in the wound bed.

Hydrocolloid dressings have evolved into a shape to fit most wounds and locations. They're available in wafers, sheets, pastes, powders, and in numerous sizes. Adhesive properties and ability to absorb exudate vary by product. Because most of these dressings are adhesive, care must be taken when using on fragile skin. Correct application requires the dressing to be bigger then the actual wound size. For optimal dressing adherence, the dressing must extend at least 1″ (2.5 cm) onto the healthy skin surrounding the wound. The dressing should be changed as recommended by the manufacturer. This could be from 3 to 7 days and often depends on the amount of exudate. Many of the newer hydrocolloids have other absorptive ingredients added, such as alginate, collagen, and sustained-released silver ions.

Hydrocolloids are indicated for minimally to moderately heavy exudating wounds, abrasions, skin tears, lacerations, pressure ulcers, dermal wounds, granular, or necrotic wounds and under compression wraps. Some of the second generation hydrocolloids are more absorptive and can be used in heavily exudating wounds. They also provide a moist environment conducive to autolytic debridement. Excessive granulation (hyper-granulation tissue) and maceration can occur if the dressing isn't changed appropriately. Hydrocolloids are often used as a preventive dressing on high-risk areas and around surgical wounds to protect the skin from frequent tape removal.

Practice essentials
• Change the dressing every 3 to 7 days, or before it reaches its maximal absorption or when fluid reaches within 1″ of the edge.
• Not all hydrocolloid dressings can be used on infected wounds.
• These dressings aren't recommended for undermining, tunnels, or sinus tracts.
• Hydrocolloid dressings may be cut to fit the wound area, such as on an elbow or heel.
• These dressings may be used as primary or secondary dressings or over other wound filler products.
• Remove the dressing by starting at a corner and gently rolling it off the wound; don't pull to remove.
• Flush out any residue with saline.
• Skin protective wipes or sprays may be used on the periwound area to enhance adherence.
• Picture-framing with tape may prevent the dressing edges from rolling.

Hydrogel dressings
Hydrogel dressings, as shown below, have provided clinicians with a viable means to hydrate dry wound beds.

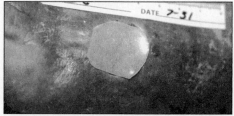

Amorphous hydrogel dressings, as shown at top of next column, are water in a gel

form or matrix. Their unique cross-linked polymer structure entraps water and reduces the temperature of the wound bed by up to 5° C.[21,22] This moist environment facilitates autolysis and removal of devitalized tissue.

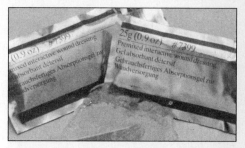

The main application for hydrogels is hydrating dry wound beds and softening and loosening slough and necrotic wound debris. Hydrogels have a limited absorptive capacity due to their high water concentration. Some hydrogels have other ingredients, such as alginates, collagen, or starch, to enhance their absorptive capacity and will absorb low to moderate amounts of exudate. Absorptive capability varies by product and type of gel. They can be used for many types of wounds, including pressure ulcers, partial- and full-thickness wounds, and vascular ulcers. The soothing and cooling properties also make them excellent choices for use in skin tears, dermabrasion, dermal wounds, donor sites, and radiation burns.

Maceration can be a concern for clinicians. Periwound skin areas need to be protected from excess hydration; therefore, protective barriers are often recommended. One of the benefits of a hydrogel is the ability to be used with topical medications or antibacterial agents. Hydrogels are packaged as sheets, tube gels, sprays, and impregnated gauze pads or strips for packing tunneling and undermined areas within the wound bed. Some require a secondary dressing to secure the hydrogel; new versions have adhesive borders. Some newer versions also contain ionic silver.

Practice essentials
• Don't use hydrogels with heavily draining wounds or on intact skin.
• Daily dressing changes may be necessary due to evaporation of the hydrogel. Some sheet hydrogels may last for several days.

Check daily to maintain a moist environment.
• Protect the surrounding skin with a skin barrier ointment, wipe, or spray.

Foam dressings

Foam dressings, as shown below, are highly absorbent and are usually made from a

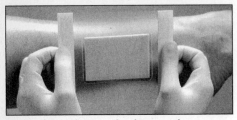

polyurethane base with a heat- and pressure-modified wound contact layer.[23] Foam dressings are permeable to both gases and water vapor, and their hydrophilic properties allow for absorption of exudate into the layers of the foam.

Foam dressings are some of the most adaptable dressings for wound care. They are indicated for wounds with moderate to heavy exudate, prophylactic protection over bony prominences or friction areas, partial- and full-thickness wounds, granular or necrotic wound beds, skin tears, donor sites, under compression wraps, surgical or dermal wounds, in combination with other primary dressings, and wounds of any etiology. They can also be used on infected wounds, if changed daily.[24] The second generation of foams are also available with ionic silver.

Foams shouldn't be used on dry eschar wound beds because they could cause further desiccation of the wound site. Foams may be used in combination with topical treatments and or enzymatic debriders. Foams are available in many sizes and shapes, and as cavity (pillow type) dressings. Many foams don't have an adhesive border, so they'll need to be secured with tape. However, new foam products have emerged with adhesive borders. Caution with fragile skin may be warranted.

Practice essentials
• Not all foams have FDA approval for use on infected wounds—be sure to check the package insert.

• Foam dressings can be left in place for up to 7 days, depending on the amount of exudate absorption.
• Removal of these dressings is trauma-free.
• Foam dressings can be cut to fit the size of the wound.
• Skin wipes or sprays can be used to protect the periwound area from maceration.
• Nonadhesive border dressings will require taping or wraps to secure.
• Make sure you put the *correct* side of the foam dressing in contact with the wound bed.

Calcium alginate dressings

Calcium alginate dressings, as shown below, provide yet another choice for clinicians to

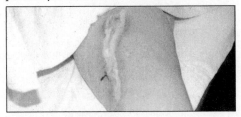

use in managing highly exudative wounds. Alginate dressings are absorbent, nonadherent, biodegradable, nonwoven fibers derived from brown seaweed, composed of calcium salts of alginic acid and mannuronic and guluronic acids.[21-23]

When alginate dressings come in contact with sodium-rich solutions such as wound drainage, the calcium ions undergo an exchange for the sodium ions, forming a soluble sodium alginate gel. This gel maintains a moist wound bed and supports a therapeutic healing environment. Alginates can absorb 20 times their weight; this may vary based on the particular product. They are extremely beneficial in managing large draining cavity wounds, pressure ulcers, vascular ulcers, surgical incisions, wound dehiscence, tunnels, sinus tracts, skin graft donor sites, exposed tendons, and infected wounds. Additionally, their hemostatic and absorptive properties make them useful on bleeding wounds. Alginates are contraindicated for dry wounds, eschar covered wounds, surgical implantation, or on third-degree burns.

Alginates are available in sheet, pad, and rope formats and in numerous sizes; some newer versions of calcium alginate dressings also contain controlled-release ionic silver. They are usually changed daily or as indicated by the amount of drainage. Early wound care interventions may warrant more frequent dressing changes due to high volume of drainage. As fluid management is attained, the frequency of dressing changes can be decreased.

Practice essentials
• Calcium alginate dressings provide easy application and trauma-free removal.
• These dressings are a good choice for undermined or tunneled, draining wounds.
• These dressings require a secondary dressing.
• These dressings may leave fiber residue, which may be flushed with saline to remove.
• Calcium alginate dressings facilitate autolytic debridement.
• These dressings are cost-effective if used appropriately.

Hydrofiber

A hydrofiber dressing is made from sodium carboxymethylcellulose, which interacts with wound fluid or exudate to form a gel. These dressings may also contain controlled-released ionic silver. They are comfortable, easy to remove, and and are very absorptive products.

Practice essentials
• Hydrofiber dressings may require a secondary dressing to secure to the wound.
• These dressings are used to maintain a moist environment.
• These dressings should not be used on a dry wound bed, on third-degree burns, or for heavy bleeding.

Composite dressings

A combination of materials makes up a single layered composite dressing. These dressings provide multiple functions, such as a bacterial barrier, an absorptive layer, foam, hydrocolloid, or hydrogel.[23] Additionally, they must have an adhesive border and semiadherent or nonadherent properties. These dressings are conformable and are available in numerous sizes and shapes.

However, not all composite dressings provide a moist environment; many are used or created with a secondary dressings. They are also referred to as *island dressings*.

Practice essentials
• Use composite dressings with caution when treating a patient with fragile skin.
• Composite dressings are easy to apply.
• These dressings may be used on infected wounds and with topical products.
• They may facilitate autolytic or mechanical debridement.
• Frequency of dressing change depends on the wound type and manufacturers' recommendations.
• These dressings may adhere to wound bed; use caution when removing.

Collagen dressings

Collagen is a major protein of the body and is necessary for wound healing and repair. Collagen dressings are derived from bovine hide (cowhide). Collagen dressings are either 100% collagen or may be combined with alginates or other products. They are a highly absorptive hydrophilic moist wound dressing.

Seaman[24] suggests that collagen powders, particles, and pads are useful in treating highly exudating wounds. If the wound has low to moderate exudate, sheets should be used. If the wound is dry, gels should be used. Collagen dressings can be used on granulating or necrotic wounds and on partial- or full-thickness wounds.[24]

A collagen dressing should be changed a minimum of every 7 days. If wound infection is present, then daily dressing change is recommended. Collagen dressings require a secondary dressing for securement.

Practice essentials
• Use collagen dressings with caution when treating patients with fragile skin if adhesive secondary dressings are also being used.
• These dressings are contraindicated for patients sensitive to bovine products.
• Don't use these dressings on dry wounds or third-degree burns.
• Collagen dressings are easy to remove.
• Their gel properties prevent these dressings from adhering to the wound bed.

• These dressings facilitate a moist wound environment and may be used with other topical products.
• Change collagen dressings daily if used on infected wounds.

Contact layer dressings

Contact layer dressings are a single layer of a woven net that acts as a low adherence material when applied to wound surfaces.[23] A contact layer dressing is applied directly to the wound and acts as a protective interface between the wound and the secondary dressings. Their main purpose is to allow exudate to pass through the contact layer and into the secondary dressing. They are often used with ointments, creams, or other topical products such as growth factors or tissue-engineered skin substitutes. Contact layer dressings aren't recommended for dry wounds or third-degree burns. Check the package insert for clarification as to which wounds the product can be used on. Various sizes and shapes are available. Frequency of dressing changes is dependent on the etiology of the wound and the amount of exudate.

Practice essentials
• Contact layer dressings aren't recommended for dry wounds or third-degree burns.
• Contact layer dressings are easy to apply and are secured with a secondary dressing.
• They protect the wound bed during dressing changes.

Gauze dressings

Gauze dressings have been used in wound care for many years and were once considered a standard of care. Today, gauze still remains one of the most widely used dressings. Numerous variations of woven and nonwoven gauze products are available. Many are used as packing agents, primary and secondary dressings, for infected wounds, and for mechanical debridement. Woven gauze may leave lint fibers in the wound bed, contributing to inflammation and possible infection. Nonwoven gauze is absorbent and doesn't leave fibers in the wound. Should gauze be included in the wound dressing list

of products? Yes, but not as a moist wound therapy intervention but as a secondary dressing when used with other moist wound products. Even if moistened with saline, gauze doesn't create an optimal moist healing environment. Gauze impedes healing, increases the risk of infection, requires numerous dressing changes, and is a substandard of care in today health care environment.[8] Clearly, the benefits of gauze dressings are over-shadowed by the disadvantages.

Practice essentials
• Gauze dressings are easy to apply.
• They don't provide an adequate moist wound environment.
• Gauze dressings require frequent changes; check your facility's policy for guidelines.
• These dressings may traumatize the wound bed when being removed.
• Woven gauze may leave lint fibers in the wound bed.
• Gauze dressings are labor-intensive.

Antimicrobial dressings

Antimicrobial dressings have added a new dimension to the wound dressing arena. Clinicians now have several choices of dressings when dealing with wound infections. These new dressings are different than topical antibiotic therapy. They provide the benefit of an antimicrobial effect against bacteria and a moist environment for healing. The active ingredient may be silver ions, cadexomer iodine, or polyhexamethylene biguanide. Antimicrobial dressings do not replace the need for systemic antibiotic therapy; rather, they serve as an adjunct in treating wound infections As research continues and new products become available, this classification of wound dressing will expand. Antimicrobial dressings are available in a variety of forms: transparent dressings, gauze, island dressings, foams, and absorptive fillers to name a few. Some of these dressings can remain in place for 7 days.

Practice essentials
• Antimicrobial dressings are an adjunct in treating wound infections.
• Frequency of dressing change varies among antimicrobials.

• Antimicrobial dressings are used in wounds with high bacterial bioburden or in wounds that are critically colonized to prevent wound infection.

• Antimicrobial dressings may be used under compression wraps to prevent infection in wounds with high bacterial bioburden.

Advanced therapies

Tissue-engineered skin substitutes

New technology has spawned a new generation of materials to advance wound healing and provide all of the characteristics of natural skin. Tissue engineering involves the development of materials that combine novel materials with living cells to yield functional tissue equivalents, such as skin substitutes.[24] Two tissue-engineered products containing living cells are approved for use in the United States. Apligraf and Dermagraft both contain living cells derived from neonatal foreskin. A single foreskin can produce over 200,000 units of the product.[20] Apligraf is a bilayered skin product consisting of a dermal equivalent composed of type I bovine collagen that contains living human dermal fibroblasts as an overlying cornified epidermal layer of living human keratinocytes. Apligraf doesn't contain Langerhans' cells, melanocytes, or endothelial cells, perhaps explaining why it isn't clinically rejected. It contains only human fibroblasts and is extensively tested for infectious agents. Dermagraft is a cryopreserved human fibroblast-derived dermal substitute indicated for use in the treatment of full-thickness diabetic foot ulcers.[25]

Different tissue-engineered skin products are approved for various applications such as use on venous ulcers, diabetic ulcers, and burns . Additional applications will most likely be available in the future. Skin substitutes are surgically applied by a physician; however, several applications may be needed before healing is attained. Prior to application, the wound bed preparation process needs to be strictly followed. Wounds are debrided, moisture balance maintained, and infection monitored.

The wound may be cultured prior to the procedure and appropriate oral antibiotic therapy used, as well as an antimicrobial wound dressing, to prevent "losing" the graft. If infection does occur, it can be successfully handled with various topical medications. The graft site must be protected from injury; the secondary dressing is changed without disturbing the graft site. Tissue-engineered skin holds a promising future for wound care patients.

Practice essentials

• Skin substitutes will only adhere to a clean wound bed.

• Watch for signs and symptoms of infection.

• *Don't* debride the yellow caramelized crust at the edges or in the wound; this is the growth factor and you are removing the tissue-engineered skin substitute. This is important to teach physicians and staff who are changing the wound dressings.

• Don't allow graft site to adhere to secondary dressing.

Negative pressure wound therapy

Negative pressure wound therapy (NPWT) was developed in the early 1990s. NPWT applies subatmospheric pressure, or suction, to the wound bed via a unit attached to a dressing. Application and type of the dressing varies by the specific manufacturer. The VAC (KCI) uses an open-celled foam sponge that's placed in the wound and secured with an adhesive drape. The adhesive drape provides a semiocclusive environment that supports moist wound healing. The drape is vapor permeable to facilitate gas exchange, an important consideration when treating wounds infected with anaerobic organisms.[26] The suction effect removes excess fluid from the wound bed via a tubing system attached to a canister. Removal of interstitial fluid allows for enhanced circulation and disposal of cellular waste from the lymphatic system (see photo below). Stagnant wound fluid has been shown to contain elements that delay wound healing by suppressing proliferation.[27]

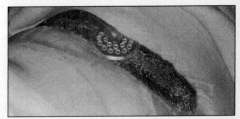

With another similar system, The Versatile One™ (Blue Sky), any type of dressing can be used including gauze.

Use of the system varies by manufacturer as to the frequency of dressing changes, amount of pressure and length of time the NPWT is turned on. The NPWT guidelines for appropriate wounds are acute and traumatic wounds; surgical dehiscence; pressure ulcers; diabetic, arterial and venous ulcers; fresh flaps; and any compromised flap. With the VAC , dressing changes vary between 48 hours and 72 hours. Untreated infected wounds should have the dressing changed every 12 hours. Two types of foam densities are utilized for different types of wounds. The black, sterile, polyurethane foam has large pores and is more effective for stimulating granulation tissue and wound contraction. The white, sterile, polyvinyl alcohol soft foam is denser with smaller pores and is recommended when growth of granulation tissue is less needed or when patient can't tolerate the polyurethane foam due to pain. For the Versatile One™, the dressing change depends on frequency of system use as per physician orders. Impregnated, non-adherent gauze is recommended to minimize pain and maximize safety. Because the specifics of each of the NPWT systems are different, clinicians need to be familiar with the correct dressing for the wound bed and drape and how to use the tubing and power unit. Lastly, NPWT has greatly enhanced the ability of clinicians to deal with many complex, heavily draining, and difficult to management wounds.

Practice essentials
• Dressing changes should be performed as per specific manufacturer's directions.
• Be sure to apply skin sealant to the entire periwound area under the drape to assist in preventing blistering and excoriation when removing the adhesive drape (VAC).
• Check with manufacturer directions to see how long the suction unit can be off until the dressing must be changed.

Electrical stimulation
Electrical stimulation (ES) has been used for more than three decades to accelerate the rate of chronic wound healing. It is one of the most cost effective, therapeutically efficacious modalities in today's arsenal of wound healing interventions.[28] Based on the research in this area of study, the strength-of-evidence rating for this modality was increased from Level B to Level A in 1999.[29] The Paralyzed Veterans of America published a Clinical Practice Guideline titled: *Pressure Ulcer Prevention and Treatment Following Spinal cord Injury,* which stated that ES qualified as a stand-alone intervention and no longer classified it as an adjunctive therapy.[30] The therapeutic effects of ES include increased blood flow [31], increased tissue oxygenation,[32, 33] increased angiogenesis,[34] decreased wound pain,[35] increased wound tensile strength[36,37] and decreased diabetic peripheral neuropathic pain.[38] Application for wound healing includes therapeutic exogenous (externally applied) electric currents that are delivered to the wound tissues via at least two electrodes (as shown below), which

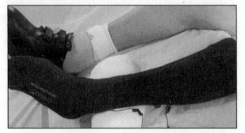

are placed directly into the wound or around the wound (periwound tissue), or by using a stocking or glove electrode garment to the affected limb (as shown top of next column).

ES uses an electrical current to transfer energy to the tissue producing a number of cellular processes and physiological responses that are important to wound healing. This includes the following:
• stimulation of fibroblasts to enhance collagen and DNA synthesis
• increased number of receptor sites for growth factors
• alteration in the direction of fibroblast migration, activation of cells in the wound site, improved tissue perfusion, and decreased edema.[39]

The electrical current may be delivered as low-intensity direct current , high-voltage pulsed current (HVPC), transcutaneous electrical nerve stimulation , or pulsed electromagnetic energy. However, high voltage

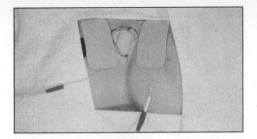

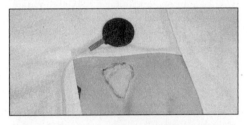

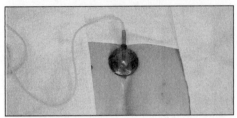

when using the VitalStim™ stimulator for treating dysphagia patients.
• ES can be a first line of treatment and should be used in combination with other moist wound therapy interventions.
• When using silver products ensure that the residue has been well irrigated from the wound prior to using electrical stimulation.

Low-level laser therapy in wound healing

Used in Europe and Russia for over thirty years as an adjunctive modality for wound healing, laser therapy for wound healing is still in its infancy in the United States. Laser is an acronym for light amplification by stimulating emissions of radiation. Low-level laser therapy or low-intensity laser therapy (LLLT or LILT), is also known as *cold laser therapy, photobiomodulation,* and *monochromatic infrared light therapy.* Laser light is always one single color (therefore monochromatic) and is in the infrared (nonvisible) area of the light spectrum. Several studies regarding the use of LLLT (or LILT) have indicated a positive effect on the three overlapping phases of wound healing: inflammation, proliferation, and remodeling. The proposed outcome of LLLT is more rapid wound healing. Dyson and colleagues [41-48] have suggested that this modality can reduce the inflammatory phase, cause earlier initiation of the proliferative phase and augment the rate of contraction as angiogenesis increases.

There are more than 2,000 scientific, peer-reviewed studies world-wide that have been published on the uses of LLLT. Specific topics have included chronic wound healing, acute soft tissue injuries, shingles, regeneration for both nerve injuries and diabetic peripheral neuropathy, and reduction of postoperative pain. There is also a significant number of research articles describing the effects of LLLT on keratinocytes, mast cells, and macrophages and fibroblasts, all of which are critical to the wound healing processes.

Light is applied by a multicluster diode probe (as shown top of next page), a single diode probe, or a multicluster diode pad. The literature and anecdotal reports indicate that most chronic wounds, including diabetic neuropathic foot ulcers, venous insufficiency, arterial insufficiency, and pressure ulcers, re-

pulsed current (HVPC) has become the current used most often for wound treatments in the last decade.

ES is performed by physical therapists or other clinicians trained and educated in identifying how and when to apply and change the ES treatment parameters (for example, ES dosage, polarity, electrode placement) according to the wound characteristics. According to Myer,[40] HVPC has a waveform of paired short-duration pulses with a long interpulse interval. It's a pulsed or interrupted monophasic waveform. The duration of treatment is usually 45 to 60 minutes, 5 to 7 times per week. ES is contraindicated for basal or squamous cell carcinoma in the wound or periwound tissue, for osteomyelitis (if not responding to systemic treatment with antibiotics), for ion residues of iodine or silver in the wound, or over electronic implants or over the heart.[28]

Practice essentials
• Don't place ES electrodes over the carotid sinus, close to the heart, or near the laryngeal musculature. The exception to this rule is

spond well to this treatment intervention.[49-59]

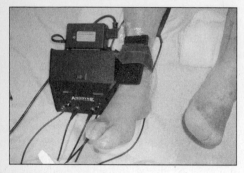

Practice essentials
• When treating directly over or in an open wound, apply a thin plastic transparent barrier, such as Saran Wrap™, over the wound or place the pad(s) or probe in a plastic bag to keep them clean from contaminates.

Ultraviolet light
Ultraviolet light (UV) has been used for centuries to treat a myriad of health and skin problems in the form of natural sunlight and more recently by artificial UV generated sources. Ultraviolet light A (UVA) and ultraviolet light B (UVB) are responsible for the pigmentation and erythema (and sometimes blistering) often seen in light-skinned individuals after significant sun exposure. UVB light assists in wound healing by inducing an inflammatory reaction, stimulating the growth of granulation tissue, and promoting breakdown and elimination of dead tissue from the wound.[60]

Ultraviolet light C (UVC) (light wavelength 200 nm to 290 nm) is the form of UV 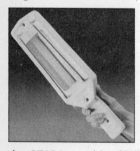 light most often used in the treatment of chronic wounds specifically for its bactericidal effects (see Dermawand, at left). Recent research demonstrated that UVC is capable of killing strains of bacteria in laboratory cultures, animal tissue, and in patients with chronic ulcers infected with methicillin-resistant *Staphylococcus au-*

reus.[61-62] In patients with chronic wounds, UVC treatment also reduced the wound bioburden and facilitated wound healing.[63] In addition, in vitro studies have shown that UVC therapy destroyed 100% of antibiotic-resistant bacteria.[64]

Suggested application of UVC is as follows: remove dressing, debride if not contraindicated, protect periwound area with petroleum jelly, hold light perpendicular to wound bed at a distance of 1″, and apply UV light.

PRACTICE POINT

Contemporary UV light equipment is usually equipped with distance guards, which ensures correct distance and reproducibility of UV treatments.

Practice essentials
• Provide appropriate eye protection for both clinician and patient to prevent retinal damage with use of UV light therapy.
• Other precautions include care when patient is taking photosensitizing medications such as psoralens (treats psoriasis), phenothiazines (treats anxiety), amiodarone hydrochloride and quinidines (treats cardiac arrhythmias), gold-based medications (treats rheumatoid arthritis), and tetracyclines, sulfonamides, and quinolones (treats infection).
• In addition, added caution should be used with the patient who's recently undergone x-ray therapy and in individuals with known photosensitivity, such as blondes or redheads.[65]

Compression therapy
Compression therapy dressings
Compression therapy is the foundation for successful vascular management in patients with venous ulcers. Compression therapy wraps are used to manage edema and promote sufficient return of venous blood to the heart. Several types of compression wraps are available and instructions on their application technique vary. Some are applied in a spiral fashion while others are wrapped in a figure eight configuration. The degree of compression ranges from high to low and short stretch to long stretch. Clinicians need

to be proficient at applying the correct techniques based on the product they select. Detailed package inserts describe how to apply these products. Compression therapy dressings aren't recommended for arterial ulcer patients. If the patient presents with a mixed etiology, he should be aggressively monitored to be sure vascular compromise isn't occurring. (See chapter 14, Venous ulcers, lymphedema, and compression therapy.)

Practice essentials
• Vascular assessment and an ankle-brachial index Doppler study are recommended prior to the use of compression therapy dressings.
• Application techniques vary according to product; read package insert before applying.

Compression modalities

External pneumatic compression therapy or intermittent compression therapy (ICT) contributes to the healing of venous insufficiency ulcers by collapsing the superficial venous system and forcing blood into the deep system, thus increasing subcutaneous pressure. ICT prevents the leakage of blood, fibrin, and protein from the skin capillaries. In addition to the hemodynamic effect of ICT, enhancement of fibrinolysis has been proposed to be important outcome of this intervention.[66-67] ICT results in improved circulation with an increase in oxygenated blood flow and the removal of potentially harmful toxic waste from the wound and periwound area.[68]

Application of ICT (when compression sleeve is applied to affected limb) is best accomplished with the patient positioned supine and the lower extremities elevated above the heart. Treatment time varies but usually lasts from 45 to 60 minutes.

Practice essentials
• ICT is contraindicated for patients with acute deep vein thrombosis or severe peripheral vascular disease.
• Vascular studies should be done prior to compression to rule out peripheral vascular disease.
• Although not an absolute contraindication, precaution and vigilant observation and communication with the patient with a history of congestive heart failure must be practiced when using any type of compression system. This is important in order to ensure that the heart is not overloaded with the increase in fluids.

Growth factors

Growth factors are proteins (polypeptides) that naturally occur in the body. Growth factors are primarily found in platelets and macrophages. Various types of growth factors are being researched: epidermal growth factors, platelet-derived growth factor (PDGF), transforming growth factors, and fibroblast growth factors, to list a few. The types of growth factors used in research can be categorized into two major groups: single growth factors manufactured through recombinant DNA technology and multiple growth factors secured from human platelet releasate.[69]

PDGF is the most widely recognized growth factor today. It has been found to be efficacious in the management of diabetic ulcers and in granulating wounds. Becaplermin gel is a PDGF that is available by prescription for use in diabetic wounds.

 PRACTICE POINT

Becaplermin gel (Regranex) *must* be kept refrigerated.

Another approach to healing chronic wounds, especially diabetic ulcers, is the use of the exogenous application of autologous platelet-derived concentrate, such as platelet-rich plasma (PRP). PRP contains multiple growth factors. Unlike becaplermin, which is produced by the manufacturer and comes ready to use, PRP is prepared at the point of care for the patient. Blood taken from the patient is mixed with a small amount of anticoagulant citrate dextrose and the solution is then centrifuged to separate the platelets and serum.[70] The concentrated platelets are then placed into the specially provided syringe that mixes the concentrate as it is applied to the prepared wound bed as a gel.[70]

Although growth factor research is still in its infancy, it holds a promising future for wound care patients.

Hyperbaric oxygen therapy

Most chronic wounds are hypoxic, requiring an increase in oxygen for adequate wound healing to take place. Hyperbaric oxygen therapy (HBOT) is the delivery of oxygen at pressures greater than one atmosphere; this requires that the entire body be placed in a pressure vessel and the patient be allowed to breathe oxygen at this increased pressure. Systemic oxygen's physiological effects on the human body are more similar to a drug than a physical modality and, like any drug, there is the chance of an overdose (oxygen toxicity) and side effects.[71]

The Undersea and Hyperbaric Medical Society endorses HBOT for the following conditions and type of wounds: air or gas embolism, carbon monoxide poisoning, clostridial myositis and myonecrosis (gas gangrene), crush injury, compartment syndrome and other acute traumatic ischemias, decompression sickness, enhancement of healing in selected problem wounds; exceptional blood loss (anemia), intracranial abscess, necrotizing soft-tissue infections, refractory osteomyelitis, delayed radiation injury (soft tissue and bony necrosis), compromised skin grafts and flaps. [72] The treatment is delivered (as shown below) by the patient breathing 100% oxygen either in a

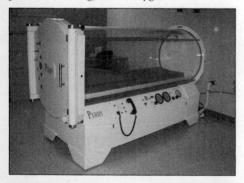

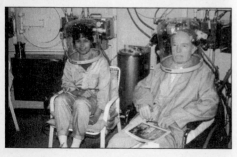

monoplace chamber where the entire chamber is usually pressurized with 100% oxygen or in a multiplace chamber which accommodates two or more people which are usually pressurized with air and in which the patients breathe oxygen via a mask or hood.

Studies have demonstrated that the oxygenation of hypoxic tissue is one of the key mechanisms by which HBOT accelerates wound healing.[73] When patients breathe oxygen at 2 to 3 times atmospheric pressure the amount of dissolved oxygen in the blood significantly increases. The subsequent effect is that more oxygen is delivered to the afflicted area by the circulating blood *plasma,* thereby alleviating the wound hypoxia. Although the actual HBOT treatment is only one to two hours in length, the systemic and local effects are prolonged. The following is a partial list of the principal methods by which HBOT is capable of affecting wound healing.

• *Vasoconstrictive effects of oxygen:* Vasoconstriction takes place in both arterial and venous vessels, which reduces edema and congestion while the amount of oxygen supplied by the plasma is increased.[74]

• *Hyperoxygenation of ischemic tissue:* Chronic wounds are frequently hypoxic. HBOT increases tissue pO_2 correcting wound hypoxia intermittently. It then allows for acceleration of the wound healing process through a series of actions which continue long after the HBOT session has ended and tissue oxygen levels have returned to pretreatment values.[75-76]

• *Improved wound metabolism:* PO_2 elevation promotes wound healing by increasing fibroblast replication, collagen synthesis, and the processes of neovascularization and epithelialization.[77]

• *Up-regulation of growth factors:* HBOT causes the up-regulation of cytokines including PDGF, which may be one of the mechanisms by which HBOT enhances angiogenesis.[78-79]

• *Antibacterial effects:* The increase in available O_2 enhances the leukocyte bactericidal effect including the killing of aerobic gram-positive (*Staphylococcus aureus*) and gram-negative organisms in addition to being cytotoxic to anaerobes. Neutrophils or polymorphonuclear cells (PMNs) require oxygen for phagocytosis and killing of bacteria to take place. Should the oxygen tension fall below 30 mm Hg, the efficiency of bacteriocidal action of PMNs decreases dramatically, leaving the patient at higher risk for infections.[80]

HBOT must be supervised by a hyperbaric-certified physician with expertise and training in this highly specialized treatment modality. HBOT has been shown to improve and accelerate wound healing in all types of chronic wounds including pressure ulcers, venous, and arterial insufficiency ulcers, burns (thermal), crush injuries, refractory osteomyelitis, costridial and myonecrosis (gas gangrene), delayed radiation injury (soft tissue and bony necrosis, and compromised skin grafts and flaps.[41] Transcutaneous oximetry can be used to predict the effectiveness of hyperbaric therapy. Levels greater than 200 mm Hg measured in a hyperbaric chamber correlate with a high likelihood of benefit from HBOT.

Practice essentials
• Patients should undergo revascularization when possible. HBOT is used when tissue hypoxia persists after adequate revascularization or if revascularization is not possible, but some flow remains.
• HBOT is an adjunctive therapy accompanying good wound care practices.

Ultrasound energy in wound care and healing

Therapeutic ultrasound delivers energy through mechanical vibrations in the form of sound waves at frequencies above detection by the human ear (>20 kHz). High-frequency ultrasound in the range of 1 to 10 MHz is currently used for fetal imaging and duplex scanning and has been used in the 1 to 3 MHz range for over six decades to promote soft tissue injury healing. In addition, high-frequency ultrasound has been implemented to facilitate wound healing. The high frequency ultrasound devices create their effect by running electricity through a crystal in the sound head, causing the crystal to "vibrate." The vibrations are then passed through the sound head via an ultrasound coupling medium into the tissues, causing them to vibrate and creating a local thermal effect.

Ultrasound effects tissue through thermal and nonthermal mechanisms. The thermal effects with greater tissue absorption increases with higher frequencies, whereas nonthermal effects are predominant with lower frequencies and when ultrasound is pulsed.[81]

Recently, low-frequency ultrasound has been added to the arsenal of tools available for wound care. Delivery of low-frequency ultrasound to wounds has been shown to effectively debride the wound of necrotic tissue, eradicate some strains of bacteria from the wound, and facilitate the wound healing process.[82]

This therapy is believed to promote wound healing through the processes of cavitation (production and vibration of micron-sized bubbles within the coupling medium and fluids within the tissues) and microstreaming (movement of fluids along acoustical boundaries).

The combination of cavitation and microstreaming, both of which occur more frequently with kilohertz than megahertz ultrasound, provides a mechanical energy capable of altering cell membrane activity and, therefore, cellular activity.

The mechanical energy from an ultrasound wave is absorbed by an individual protein molecule, theoretically inducing a conformational change. Signal transduction pathways can also be stimulated from ultrasound-generated mechanical energy. This may result in a broad range of cellular effects that impact wound healing including leukocyte adhesion, growth factor and collagen production, increased angiogenesis, increased macrophage responsiveness, increased fibrinolysis, and increased nitric oxide levels.

There are currently two delivery mechanisms for low-frequency ultrasound energy to wounds; contact and non-contact.

The SonicOne™ (Misonix UWD™ (Misonix, Inc.) (22.5MHz) and the Sonoca 180™ (Soring, Inc.) (25 MHz) both deliver their ultrasound energy in a "contact" mode. Meaning the ultrasound probe is in direct contact with the wound surface.

The non-contact ultrasound modality, MIST Therapy® System (Celleration®) (40 kHz) promotes wound healing through cleansing and maintenance debridement. Its effects are by the continuous ultrasonic energy being delivered via an atomized saline solution to the wound bed without direct con-

Low-frequency comparison chart

Features	SonicOne Misonix™	Sonoca 180™	MIST® Therapy
Frequency	22.5 kHz	20-80 kHz	40 kHz
Intensity	Variable (auto gain control)	Variable 40-100%	Preset—based on wound size
Mode	Continuous or pulsed	Continuous	Continuous
Fluid delivery	Sterile saline vapor	Sterile saline vapor	Sterile saline mist
Controls	Foot pedal	Foot pedal	Button on hand piece
Treatment time	Usually 2-5 min	Usually 2-5 min	Wound size dependent 3-20m
Wound bed contact	Yes; autoclavable metal probes	Yes - autoclavable metal probes	No; 0.5-1.5 cm Disposable applic.
Aerosolization	Yes	Yes	No
Selective debridement	Yes, immediate	Yes, immediate	Yes, ongoing

Low-frequency comparison chart. Adapted and used with permission Luther Kloth PT, MS, FAPTA, CWS, FCCWS

tact of the device to the body or the wound. The mist acts as a conduit for transmitting ultrasonic energy to the treatment site. (See *Low-frequency comparison chart*.)

Various clinical studies have evaluated the safety and efficacy of low-frequency therapeutic ultrasound in patients with a variety of wounds, including recalcitrant pressure ulcers, chronic lower extremity leg and foot ulcers, and diabetic foot ulcers. Among these, a randomized, controlled, double-blind trial, demonstrated improved healing of recalcitrant diabetic foot ulcers compared with a sham procedure in patients receiving standard wound care therapy.

PRACTICE POINT

Ultrasound cannot be used near parts of the body containing electronic implants/prosthesis or on areas of malignancy or over the lower back or abdomen during pregnancy.

Summary

Selection of appropriate wound treatment options must be patient centered and are driven by the specific goals of care. A succinct overview of the important characteristics and use of wound dressing products has been provided. (See *Wound dressing categories*, pages 160 to 169.)

Selecting from the abundant number of wound dressings that are now available can pose a challenge. Use of tools, such as the wound product chart and enablers, such as NICE© give clinicians a model to enhance their clinical decision making.

The concepts of moist wound healing and the significance of clinical treatment decisions regarding wound care dressing options described herein are essential elements of your wound care arsenal. Other therapies such as ES, HBOT, ultrasound, and growth factors, to name a few, are also important parts of the wound healing options available for consideration. By using the helpful practice points, tables, figures, and product algorithms, the clinician is guided through the milieu of product alternatives. Improving technology and evolving research into wound care dressings and modalities will continue to create new and challenging opportunities for all of us.

Show what you know

1. Wound dressings have evolved into a new concept of:

   A. dry gauze.
   B. moist wound therapy.
   C. open to air.
   D. wet to dry.

ANSWER: B. A, C, and D are all old concepts of wound management.

2. The following are categories of moist wound care dressings, except:

   A. hydrogel dressing.
   B. calcium alginate dressing.
   C. roller gauze dressing.
   D. foam dressing.

ANSWER: C. Gauze is a form of dry dressing therapy. A, B, and D are moist wound therapy dressings.

3. Wound dressing selection should be based on the characteristics of the wound. All of the following should be considered when selecting dressings except:

   A. size of dressing.
   B. nurse preference.
   C. moist or dry wound bed.
   D. drainage.

ANSWER: B. Nurse preference shouldn't be a parameter of dressing selection. A, C, and D are appropriate dressing parameters.

4. A disadvantage of transparent film is that it:

   A. is nonabsorptive.
   B. is conformable.
   C. allows wound inspection.
   D. is impermeable to bacteria.

ANSWER: A. Transparent film doesn't absorb fluid. B, C, and D are all advantages of transparent film use.

5. The acronym "MEASURES" is a useful tool for remembering the principles of wound care.

   A. True
   B. False

ANSWER: A

6. Which one of the following is a dermal skin substitute:

   A. Accuzyme
   B. Tegaderm
   C. Allevyn
   D. Apligraf

ANSWER: D. Apligraf is a bilayered skin substitute. A, B, and C are all moist wound therapy choices.

7. Which one of the following treatment options would not be an appropriate treatment option for a heavily draining wound?

   A. Negative pressure therapy
   B. Foam dressing
   C. Calcium alginate dressing
   D. Hydrogel amorphorus gel

ANSWER: D. Hydrogel amorphorus gel has minimal ability to absorb drainage so it is not indicated for use in heavily draining wounds. A , B, and C are all specifically used for heavily draining wounds.

8. Prior to the application of tissue-engineered skin substitute, the clinician needs to evaluate:

   A. that the wound bed is free of necrotic tissue.
   B. the patient's immune system status.
   C. that anti-rejection drugs have been administered.
   D. the patient's weight.

ANSWER: A. Tissue-engineered skin substitutes must be applied to a wound bed that is free of necrotic tissue and infection. B and C are incorrect as rejection of these products is not an issue. Although the patient's weight may be part of the total care plan, it is not essential to evaluate for use of this product.

9. All of the following are therapeutic effects of electrical stimulation except:

   A. increase blood flow.
   B. decreased tissue oxygenation.
   C. increased angiogenesis.
   D. decreased wound pain.

ANSWER: B. Tissue oxygenation is *increased* with the use of electrical stimulation. A, C, and D are all correct.

10. Which one of the following is not a method by which hyperbaric oxygen therapy affects wound healing:

   A. Increased fibroblast replication
   B. Up-regulation of growth factors
   C. Vasodilation effects of oxygen on the blood vessels
   D. Enhanced leukocyte bactericidal effects

ANSWER: C. Hyperbaric oxygen therapy causes *vasocontriction* in both arterial and venous vessels. A, B, and D are all ways in which hyperbaric oxygen therapy enhances wound healing.

Wound dressing categories

Andrea McIntosh RN, BSN, CWOCN, APN and Linda Galvan RN, BSN, CWOCN, APN

Generic category	Description/composition	Trade name	
Transparent film	Polyurethane or co-polymer with porous adhesive layer that varies in thickness and allows oxygen to pass through the membrane and moisture vapor to escape	3M Tegaderm 3M Tegaderm HP Bioclusive Blisterfilm CarraSmartFilm ClearSite Comfeel Film Dermatell	DermaView DermaViewII Mefilm Opsite Polyskin II ProCyte Suresite Transeal
Transparent film with silver	Ionic silver from a controlled-release barrier film	Arglaes	
Hydrocolloid	Hydrophilic colloid particles bound to polyurethane foam; some composed of gelatin, pectin, and carboxymethylcellulose Impermeable to bacteria and other contaminants	3M Tegasorb 3M Tegasorb Thin Comfeel Plus Cutinova Hydro DermaFilm Duoderm CGF Duoderm Extra Thin & Paste Duoderm Signal Exuderm LP Exuderm OdorShield Exuderm Satin	Hydrocol MPM Excel Nu-DERM Procol RepliCare RepliCare Thin Restore Restore CX Restore Plus SignaDres Sorbex Ultec Ultec Pro
Hydrocolloid with silver	Sustained-release of silver ions	Contreet	
Hydrogel	Water or glycerin based, non-adherent, crossed-linked polymer. Variable absorptive properties; contains 80 to 99% water; numerous sizes and forms (gels, sheets, strips, and gauze available)	3M Tegaderm Hydrogel Wound Filler Amerigel Aqua Flo AquaSite Aquasorb Biolex CarraDres	CarraSmart Carrasyn Gel Curafil Gel Curagel Curasol Gel DermaGauze Elastro-Gel, Plus Elta FlexiGel

Indications	Advantages and benefits	Disadvantages
Donor sites Primary and secondary dressings Partial-thickness wounds Pressure ulcers, Stages I and II Superficial burns Secondary dressing Peripheral I.V.s Abrasions	Wound inspection Impermeable to external fluids and bacteria Conformable Promote autolytic debridement Prevention/reduces friction Change every 5 to 7 days or prn if leakage noted Numerous sizes available Waterproof	Nonabsorptive May adhere to some wounds and fragile skin Not for draining wounds Fluid retention may lead to maceration of periwound area Third-degree burns
Post-op incisions Central lines, CVPs, and PICC lines Infected wounds Highly colonized wounds	Antimicrobial Same advantages as transparent films	Sensitivity to silver Can't use silver with enzymatic debriding agents Same disadvantages as transparent films
Pressure ulcers, Stages I to IV Partial- and full-thickness wounds Dermal ulcers Under compression wraps/stockings Necrotic wounds Preventive dressing for high-risk friction areas Secondary dressing or under taping procedures	Facilitates autolytic debridement Self-adherent Impermeable to fluids/bacteria Conformable Reduces wound pain Thermal insulation Absorptive, minimal to moderate drainage Long wear time—3 to 7 days, depending on exudate	Some dressings are opaque Not recommended for heavily draining wounds, sinus tracts, or fragile skin Some contraindicated for full-thickness wounds and/or with infection (check package inserts) Some may be difficult to remove Leakage can be a problem; edges roll up Some may leave a residue in wound bed
Infected wounds Highly colonized wounds	Antimicrobial Can be left on up to 7 days Same advantages as hydrocolloid dressing	Sensitivity to silver Must have exudate for ionic silver to be released Can't use silver with enzymatic debriding agents Same disadvantages as hydrocolloid
Pressure ulcers, Stages II to IV Partial- and full-thickness wounds Dermabrasion Painful wounds Dermal ulcers Radiation tissue damage	Nonadherent Trauma-free removal/soothing to patient Rehydrates the wound bed Reduces wound pain Can be used with topical medications	Some require secondary dressing to secure May macerate periwound skin Not recommended for heavily draining wounds

(continued)

Wound dressing categories (continued)

Generic category	Description/composition	Trade name	
Hydrogel (continued)		Hypergel	Skintegrity
		Iamin Hydrating Gel	SoloSite
			TenderWet
		IntraSite Gel	Transigel
		Normlgel	Vigilon
		Purilon Gel	Woun'Dres
		Restore Gel	Hydrogel
		SAF-Gel	Xcell
Hydrogel with silver	Controlled-release ionic silver	SilvaSorb Gel3	
Foam	Hydrophilic polyurethane or gel film coated foam, nonocclusive, nonadherent layer absorptive wound dressing	3M Foam	Lyofoam
		Allevyn	Mepilex
		Allevyn Cavity	Mitraflex
		Biatain	Optifoam
		CarraSmart	Polyderm
		COPA	Polymem
		COPA Island	PolyWic
		COPA Plus	Quadrifoam
		DermaFoam	Sof-Foam
		DermaLevin	Tielle
		Flexzan	Tielle Plus
		Gentleheal	VigiFoam
		LoProfile Foam	
Foam with silver	Controlled-release ionic silver	Contreet Foam	
		Polymem Silver	
		Optifoam AG	
Calcium alginate	Nonwoven composite of fibers from calcium-sodium alginate, a cellulose-like polysaccharide, highly absorptive dressing manufactured from brown seaweed; forms a soft get when mixed with wound fluid	3M Tegagen HI & HG Alginate	Maxorb Extra
		Algicell	CMC/Alginate
		Algiderm	Melgisobr
		AlgiSite	NU-DERM
		CarraGinate	Alginate
		Carrasorb H	Polymem
		Curasorb	Alginate
		Dermaginate	Restore
		Kalginate	CalciCare
		Kaltostat	SeaSorb
		Kaltostat Fortex	Sorbsan

Indications for use	Advantages and benefits	Disadvantages
Minor burns Donor sites Necrotic wounds	Can be used in infected wounds and in cavities or tunnels Softens and loosens necrosis, slough, to aid debridement Water-soluble 24- to 72-hour dressing change, depending on the form of gel	
Infected wounds Highly colonized wounds	Antimicrobial Can be left on up to 3 days Nonadherent Rehydrates the wound bed	Sensitivity to silver Not recommended for use in conjunction with topical medications Can't use silver with enzymatic debriding agents Same disadvantages as hydrogel
Partial- and full-thickness wounds with minimal to heavy drainage Pressure ulcers, Stages II to IV Surgical wounds Dermal ulcers Under compression wraps/stocking Infected and noninfected wounds (varies; check package insert) Tunneling and cavity wounds (varies; check package insert)	Nonadherent Trauma-free removal Absorptive, minimal to heavy drainage Conformable, easy to apply and remove Frequency of dressing change depends on amount of drainage 3- to 5-day dressing change Available with adhesive and nonadhesive border in various shapes and forms	Not recommended for nondraining wounds Not recommended for dry eschar Not all foams recommended for infected wounds and for use in tunnels and tracts (check package insert) May require secondary dressing or tape to secure May macerate periwound area if not changed appropriately
Infected wounds Highly colonized wounds	Antimicrobial Some can be left on up to 7 days Same advantages as foam dressing	Sensitivity to silver Must have exudate for silver to be released Can't use silver with enzymatic debriding agents Same disadvantages as foam
Partial- and full-thickness wounds Moderate- to heavy-draining wounds Pressure ulcers, Stage III and IV Dermal wounds Surgical incision/Dehisced wounds Post-op wounds for hemostasis Sinus tracts, tunnels, or cavities Infected wounds Donor sites	Highly absorbent and nonocclusive Trauma-free removal Can be used on infected wounds with tunneling and undermining Hemostatic properties for minor bleeding Reduced frequency of dressing changes, every day to every other day Available in sheets, ropes, and within other composite type dressings	Contraindicated for dry eschar, third-degree burns, surgical implantation, and heavy bleeding May require secondary dressing to secure Gel may have odor during dressing change Can desiccate the wound bed if wound has small amount of exudate or dressing not changed appropriately

(continued)

Wound dressing categories *(continued)*

Generic category	Description/composition	Trade name	
Calcium alginate with silver	Controlled-release ionic silver	Algidex Ag Alginate	Maxorb Ag (Alginate & Hydrofiber) Silvercel
Hydrofiber	Made from sodium carboxymethyl-cellulose that interacts with wound exudate and forms a gel	Aquacel	
Hydrofiber with silver	Controlled-release ionic silver	Aquacel Ag Maxorb Extra Ag (Hydrofiber and Alginate)	
Composites	Combination of two or more physically distinct products manufactured as a single dressing that provides multiple functions; may include a bacterial barrier, absorptive layer, foam, hydrocolloid, or hydrogel; semi-adherent or nonadherent	3M Tegaderm Absorbent Pad Alldress CombiDERM CombiDERM ACD Comfortell CompDress Island	Covaderm Plus Covrsite DermaDress Epigard Stratasorb Telfa Island Viasorb
Composites with silver	Transparent film with an alginate pad	Arglaes Island	
Enzymatic debriders	Proteolytic, chemical agent that breaks down devitalized tissue; requires a prescription	Accuzyme Ethezyme Gladase Panafil Santyl collagenase	

Indications	Advantages and benefits	Disadvantages
Infected wounds Highly colonized wounds	Antimicrobial Change every 3 days or prn if leakage noted Same advantages and benefits as calcium alginate dressing	Sensitivity to silver Must have exudate for silver to be released Can't use silver with enzymatic debriding agents Same disadvantages as calcium alginate
Partial- and full-thickness wounds Moderate- to heavy-draining wounds Donor sites Surgical wounds Pressure ulcers, Stages III and IV Sinus tracts, tunnels, or cavities Surgical incision/Dehisced wounds	Highly absorptive Trauma-free removal Reduced frequency of dressing changes Available in sheets and ribbons	Contraindicated for dry eschar, nonexudating wounds, third-degree burns, and heavy bleeding Requires secondary dressing to secure
Infected wounds Highly colonized wounds	Antimicrobial Antimicrobial action effective up to 7 days Same advantages and benefits as Hydrofiber dressing	Sensitivity to silver Must have exudate for silver to be released Can't use silver with enzymatic debriding agents Same disadvantages as hydrofiber
Primary and secondary dressings for partial- and full-thickness wounds Pressure ulcers, Stages I to IV (varies with each product) Minimal- to heavy-draining wounds Dermal ulcers Surgical incisions	Facilitates autolytic debridement Conformable Multiple sizes and shapes available Easy to apply and remove Most include adhesive border Frequency of dressing change dependent on wound type (check package insert)	Adhesive borders may limit use on fragile skin Some contraindicated for Stage IV ulcers (check package insert) Not all dressings provide moist wound therapy; may dessicate the wound bed (check package insert)
Infected wounds Highly colonized wounds	Antimicrobial Can be left in place up to 5 days Advantages and benefits same as composite dressing	Sensitivity to silver Must have exudate for silver to be released Can't use silver with enzymatic debriding agents Same disadvantages as composites
To debride full-thickness necrotic wounds, pressure ulcers, dermal ulcers, post-op wounds, infected wounds	Nonsurgical method of debridement Requires daily and/or twice-daily dressing changes (check package insert)	Inactivated by soaps, detergents, acidic solutions, and metallic ions (silver) Must be covered by secondary dressing Some enzymatics may damage healthy tissue

(continued)

Wound dressing categories (continued)

Generic category	Description/composition	Trade name
Collagen	Major protein of the body; dressing stimulates cellular migration and contributes to new tissue development and wound debridement; derived from bovine, porcine, or avian sources	Cellerate Rx Gel Cellerate Rx Powder ColActive Fibracol Kollagen-Medifil Particles/Gel/Pads Kollagen-SkinTemp Promogran Matrix Stimulen
Collagen with silver	Releases silver ions that are antimicrobial while collagen binds with MMP (matrix metalloproteases) in chronic wound exudate	ColActive Ag Prisma Matrix
Drugs	Prescription drugs	Cloderm Cream Triamcinolone Granulex ointment or Prudoxin Cream cream
Antimicrobial dressings	Nonadherent antimicrobial dressings that protect against bacteria and/or decrease bacterial load Cardexomer iodine-impregnated: Immediate and controlled-release of Cadexomer Iodine	Cadexomer Iodine-impregnated: Iodoflex Pad Iodosorb Gel
Silver dressings	Immediate and sustained release of ionic silver; effective barrier to bacterial penetration	Acticoat Silverseal Actisorb 3M Tegaderm SilvaSorb Ag Mesh SilverDerm7 Dressing with Silverlon Silver

ADVANCED WOUND CARE THERAPIES

Negative pressure therapy	Noninvasive active therapy using localized negative pressure to promote healing	Wound V.A.C.—Vacuum-Assisted Closure (KCI) The Versatile One (Blue Sky Medical)

Indications	Advantages and benefits	Disadvantages
Partial- and full-thickness wounds Pressure ulcers, Stage III and some Stage IVs (check package insert) Dermal ulcers Donor sites Surgical wounds	Absorbent, nonadherent Biodegradable gel Conforms well May be used in combination with topical agents 1- to 3-day dressing change, daily if infection present	Contraindicated for third-degree burns and sensitivities to collagen or bovine products Not recommended for necrotic wounds Requires secondary dressing May require rehydration
Infected wounds Highly colonized wounds	Antimicrobial Can be left on up to 7 days Same advantages as collagen dressing	Sensitive to collagen and silver Can't use silver with enzymatic debriding agents Same disadvantages as collagens
Varies by product	See package insert for use	Prescription needed
Infected wounds—any type (pressure ulcers, venous, arterial, diabetic, or surgical wounds) Partial- or full-thickness wounds Colonized, chronic nonhealing wounds	Decreases bacterial load in wound Reduces risk of infection	Cadexomer Iodine contraindicated in patients sensitive to iodine Secondary dressing required
Infected wounds Highly colonized wounds All wounds except: Stage I pressure ulcers, third-degree burns, and nonexuding wounds Under compression wraps/stockings Over grafts or skin substitutes	Inhibits growth of pathogens, especially antibiotic-resistant strains Reduces cost due to antimicrobial action effective up to 7 days	Sensitivity to silver Secondary dressing required Must be removed and wound cleansed prior to MRI Not recommended for use in conjunction with topical medications Incompatible with oil based products, including petroleum jelly May stain or discolor surrounding tissue due to silver turning black when it oxidizes Can't use silver with enzymatic debriding agents
Granular draining wounds Partial- and full-thickness wounds with moderate to heavy exudate Venous, arterial, and diabetic ulcers	Decreases edema Decreases bacterial colonization Increases blood supply and granular tissue formation Ability to individually adjust settings based on patient and wound type	Healthcare worker needs training to apply and operate equipment Not reimbursed in acute and long term care facilities Can increase pain in some wounds May adhere to some wounds

(continued)

Wound dressing categories (continued)

Generic category	Description/composition	Trade name	
Negative pressure therapy (continued)			
Skin substitutes	Skin substitutes developed in the laboratory from human fibroblasts	Apligraf DermaGraft GammaGraft	GraftJacket Orcel TransCyte
Extracellular matrix	Extracellular matrix material derived from the submucosal layer of porcine small intestines	Oasis Wound Matrix	
Becaplermin gel	Genetically engineered platelet-derived growth factors produced in yeast and then formulated into a gel	Regranex	

The products listed are representative of type and are not meant to be an all-inclusive listing; indication, advantages and disadvantages are some examples, more suggestions may apply. Numerous references were utilized in compiling this chart, refer to references.

References

1. Ayello, E.A. "20 Years of Wound Care: Where we have been, where We Are Going," *Advances in Skin & Wound Care* 19(1):28-33, January-February 2006.
2. Queen, D. "A Personal Perspective," *International Wound Journal* (1):1, March 2006.
3. Winter, G.D. "Formation of the Scab and the Rate of Epithelialization of Superficial Wounds in the Skin of Young Domestic Pigs," *Nature* 193:293-94, 1962.
4. Hinman, C.D., and Maibach, H.I. "Effect of Air Exposure and Occlusion on Experimental Human Skin Wounds," *Nature* 200:377, 1963.
5. Baranoski, S. "Wound Dressings: A Myraid of Challenging Decisions," *Home Healthcare Nurse* 23(5) 307-17, May 2005.
6. Hatz, R.A., et al. *Wound Dressings, Wound Healing and Wound Management: A Guide for Private Practice.* New York: Springer-Verlag, 1994.
7. Field, C., and Kerstein, M. "Overview of Wound Healing in a Moist Environment," *American Journal of Surgery* 167(suppl 1A):2S-5S, January 1994.
8. Ovington, L.G. "Hanging Wet-to-dry Dressings Out to Dry," *Advances in Skin & Wound Care* 15(2):79-86, March-April 2002.
9. Pieper, B., et al. "Wound Prevalence, Types, and Treatments in Home Care," *Advances in Skin & Wound Care* 12(3):117-26, May-June 1999.
10. Kim, J.K., et al. "Normal Saline Wound Dressing—Is It Really Normal?" *British Journal of Plastic Surgery* 53(1):42-45, January 2000.
11. Hedman, L.A. "Effect of a Hydrocolloid Dressing on the Pain Level from Abrasions on the Feet during Intensive Marching," *Military Medicine* 153(4):188-90, April 1988.
12. Nemeth, A.J., et al. "Faster Healing and Less Pain in Skin Biopsy Sites Treated with an Occlusive Dressing," *Archives of Dermatology* 11:1679-683, November 1991.
13. Thomas, S. *Wound Management and Dressing.* London: The Pharmaceutical Press, 1990.
14. Lawrence, J.C. "Dressings and Wound Infection," *American Journal of Surgery* 167(suppl 1A):1S-24S, January 1994.
15. Hutchinson, J.J. "Prevalence of Wound Infection under Occlusive Dressings: A Collective Survey of Reported Research," *Wounds* (1):123-33, 1989.
16. Hutchinson, J.J. "A Prospective Clinical Trial of Wound Dressings to Investigate the Rate of

Indications	Advantages and benefits	Disadvantages
Pressure ulcers, Stages II to IV Surgical wounds Flaps and grafts Acute traumatic wounds	Generally, dressing changed every 48 to 72 hours (specifics for dressing and equipment vary by manufacturer)	Not recommended for nondraining wounds and wounds with eschar Contraindicated for wounds with malignancy and untreated osteomyelitis
Partial- and full-thickness wounds Venous and diabetic ulcers Granular wounds Burns	Growth factors present in skin equivalent Decrease wound healing time No donor site Decrease in pain for many patients	Cost Wound has to be granular Check manufacturer's directions for storage and shelf life
Partial- and full-thickness wounds Diabetic ulcers Second-degree burns Graft sites	Biological dressing Strength and flexibility	Sensitivity to porcine- or bovine-derived products
Neuropathic wounds Diabetic ulcers Granular wounds	Decreases healing time Increases growth of new tissue, cell division and movement, protein	Can't be used on infected wounds or wounds with necrotic tissue Cost Must be refrigerated

*Antimicrobials: may be topical or within a dressing component
**Surgical, Mechanical, Autolytic or Enzymatic debridement methods
© A. McIntosh, L. Galvan, C. Barkauskas, S. Baranoski, October 2003.
© A. McIntosh and L. Galvan revised April 2006.

Infection under Occlusion," *in* Harding, K (ed.) *Proceedings of the First European Conference on Advances in Wound Management*. London: Macmillan, 1993.

17. Baranoski, S. "Wound Assessment and Dressing Selection," *Ostomy & Wound Management* 41(suppl 7A):7S-14S, August 1995.

18. Rodeheaver, G. "Wound Cleansing, Wound Irrigation, Wound Disinfection," in *Chronic Wound Care*, 2nd ed. Edited by Krasner, D., and Kane, D. Wayne, Pa.: Health Management Publications, Inc., 1997.

19. Orland, G. "The Fine Structure of the Interrelationship of Cells in the Human Epidermis," *Journal of Biophysical and Biochemical Cytology* 4:529-35, 1958.

20. Eaglstein, W.H. "From Occlusive to Living Membranes," *Journal of Dermatology* 25(12):766-74, December 1998.

21. Choucair, M., and Phillips. "Wound Dressings," *in* Fitzpatrick (ed.) *Dermatology in General Medicine*. New York: McGraw-Hill Book Co., pp 2954-2958, 2000.

22. Ovington, L.G. "The Well-dressed Wound: An Overview of Dressing Types," *Wounds* 10:1A-11A, 1998.

23. Hess, C.T. *Clinical Guide: Wound Care*, 5th ed. Philadelphia: Lippincott Williams & Wilkins, 2006.

24. Seaman, S. "Dressing Selection in Chronic Wound Management," *Journal of the American Podiatric Medical Association* 92(1):24-33, January 2002.

25. InfoLink, Hess, C.T. editor Advanced BioHealing Will Offer Dermagraft, TransCyte Vol *Advances in Skin and Wound Care* 19(7):348 Sept 2006.

26. Mendez-Eastman, S. "Guidelines for Using Negative Pressure Wound Therapy," *Advances in Skin & Wound Care* 14(6):314-22, November-December 2001.

27. Falanga, V. "Growth Factors and Chronic Wounds: The Need to Understand the Microenvironment," *Journal of Dermatology* 19(11):667-72, November 1992.

28. Kloth, LC. "5 Questions and Answers about Electrical Stimulation," *Advances in Skin & Wound Care* 14(3):156-58, May-June, 2001.

29. Ovington, LG. "Dressing and Adjunctive Therapies: AHCPR Guidelines Revisited," *Ostomy/Wound Management* 45(suppl 1a):94S-106S, 1999.

30. Garber, S.L., et al. "Pressure Ulcer Prevention and Treatment Following Spinal Cord Injury: A Clinical Practice Guideline for Health Care Professionals," *Consortium for Spinal Cord*

Medicine Clinical Practice Guidelines. Washington D.C.: Paralyzed Veterans of America, 2000.

31. Junger, M., et al. "Treatment of Venous Ulcers with Low Frequency Pulsed Current (Dermapulse): Effects on Cutaneous Microcirculation," *Der Hautartz* 18:879-903, 1997.

32. Gagnier, K.A., et al "The Effects of Electrical Stimulation on Cutaneous Oxygen Supply in Paraplegics," *Physical Therapy* 68:835, 1988,

33. Dodgen, P.W., et al "The Effects of Electrical Stimulation on Cutaneous Oxygen Supply in Paraplegics," *Physical Therapy* 67:793, 1987.

34. Greenberg, J., et al. "The Effect of Electrical Stimulation (RPES) on Wound Healing and Angiogenesis in Second-degree Burns," Abstract # 44 in *Program and Abstracts of the 13th Annual Symposium on Advanced Wound Care,* Dallas, Tx., April 1–4, 2000.

35. Kloth, L.C., McCulloch, J.M. *Wound Healing Alternatives in Management,* 3rd ed. Philadelphia: F.A. Davis, pp 271-315, 2002.

36. Brown, M., et al. "Electrical Stimulation Effects on Cutaneous Wound Healing in Rabbits," *Physical Therapy* 68:955, 1988,

37. Demir, H., et al. "A Comparative Study of the Effects of Electrical Stimulation and Laser Treatment on Experimental Wound Healing in Rats," *Journal of Rehabilitation Research & Development* 41(2):147-54, March 2004.

38. Kumar, D., and Marshall, H.J. "Diabetic Peripheral Neuropathy: Amelioration of Pain with Transcutaneous Electrostimulation," *Diabetes Care* 20:1702, 1997.

39. Houghton, P.E., and Campbell, K.E. "Therapeutic Modalities in the Treatment of Chronic Recalcitrant Wounds," *In* Krasner, D., et al., (eds.) *Chronic Wound Care: A Clinical Source Book for Healthcare Professionals,* 3rd ed. Wayne, Pa.: Health Management Publications, Inc., pp 455-468, 2001.

40. Myer, A. "The Role of Physical Therapy in Chronic Wound Care," *In* Krasner, D., et al., (eds.) *Chronic Wound Care: A Clinical Source Book for Healthcare Professionals,* 3rd ed. Wayne, Pa.: Health Management Publications, Inc., 2001.

41. Steinlechner, C., Dyson, M. "The Effect of Low Level Laser Therapy on the Proliferation of Keratinocytes," *Laser Therapy* 5(2):65, 1993.

42. Dyson, M., and Young, S. "Effect of Laser Therapy on Wound Contraction and Cellularity in Mice," *Lasers in Medical Science* 1:125, 1986.

43. Dyson, M. "Cellular and Subcellular Aspects of Low Level Laser Therapy," *In* Ohshiro, T., and Calderhead, R.G. (eds.) *Progress in Laser Therapy* London: John Wiley & Sons, p. 221, 1991

44. Bolton, P.A., et al. "Macrophage Responsiveness to Light Therapy.A Dose Response Study," *Laser Therapy* 2:101-106, 1990.

45. Bolton, P.A., et al. "The effect of polarised light on the release of growth factors from the U-937 macrophage-like cell line. Laser Therapy. 1992; 4: 33-42.

46. Cheetham, M.J., et al. "Histological Effects of 820 nm Laser Irradiation on the Healthy Growth Plate of the Rat," *Laser Therapy* 2:59, 1992.

47. Bolton, P.A., et al. "The Direct Effect of 860 nm Light on Cell Proliferation and on Succinic Dehydrogenase Activity of Human Fibroblasts In Vitro," *Laser Therapy* 7:55-60, 1995.

48. el Sayed, S.O., Dyson, M. "Effect of Laser Pulse Repetition Rate and Pulse Duration on Mast Cell Number and Degranulation," *Laser in Surgery and Medicine* 19(4):433-3, 1997.

49. Nicolopoulos, N., et al. "The Use of Laser Surgery in the Subtotal Meniscectomy and the Effect of Low-level Laser Therapy on the Healing Potential of Rabbit Meniscus: An Experimental Study," *Lasers in Medical Science* 1(2):109-15, 1996.

50. Crous, L.C., and Malherbe, C.P. "Laser and Ultraviolet Light Irradiation in the Treatment of Chronic Ulcers," South African Journal of Physiotherapy 44(3):73-77, 1988.

51. Franek, A., et al. "Does Low Output Laser Stimulation Enhance the Healing of Crural Ulceration? Some Critical Remarks," Medical Engineering and Physics 24(9):607-15, 2002.

52. Iusim, M., et al. "Evaluation of the Degree of Effectiveness of Biobeam Low Level Narrow Band Light on the Treatment of Skin Ulcers and Delayed Postoperative Wound Healing," *Orthopedics* 15(9):1023-1026, 1992.

53. Lagan, K.M., et al. "Low-intensity Laser Therapy/Combined Phototherapy in the Management of Chronic Venous Ulceration: A Placebo-controlled Study," *Journal of Clinical Laser Medicine and Surgery* 20(3):109-16, 2002.

54. Lucas, C., et al. "The Effect of Low Level Laser Therapy (LLLT) on Stage III Decubitus Ulcers (pressure sores); A Prospective Randomised Single Blind, Multicentre Pilot Study," *Lasers in Medical Science* 15(2):94-100, 2000.

55. Lucas, C., et al. "Efficacy of Low-level Laser Therapy in the Management of Stage III Decubitus Ulcers: A Prospective, Observer-blinded Multicentre Randomised Clinical Trial," *Lasers in Medical Science* 18(2):72-77, 2003.

56. Lundeberg, T., and Malm, M. "Low-power HeNe Laser Treatment of Venous Leg Ulcers," *Annals of Plastic Surgery* 27(6):537-39, 1991.

57. Malm, M., and Lundeberg, T. "Effect of Low Power Gallium Arsenide Laser on Healing of Venous Ulcers," *Scandinavian Journal of Plastic Reconstructive Surgery and Hand Surgery* 25(3):249-51, 1991.

58. Nussbaum, E.L., et al. "Comparison of Ultrasound/Ultraviolet-C and Laser for Treatment of Pressure Ulcers in Patients with Spinal Cord Injury," Physical Therapy 74(9):812-23, 1994.

59. Kloth, L.C., and McCulloch, J.M. Wound Healing Alternatives in Management, 3rd ed. Philadelphia: F.A. Davis, pp. 326-339, 2002.

60. Conner-Kerr, T. et al: UVC reduces antibiotic-resistant bacteria in vitro. Ostomy/Wound Management 45:84, 1999.

61. Thai, T., et al. "Effect of Ultraviolet Light C on Bacterial Colonization in Chronic Wounds," Ostomy/Wound Management 51(10):32-45, 2005.

62. Thai, T., et al. "Ultraviolet Light C in the Treatment of Chronic Wounds with MRSA: A Case Study," Ostomy/Wound Management 48(11):52-60, 2002.

63. Conner-Kerr, T., et al. "The Effects of Ultraviolet Irradiation on Antibiotic-resistant Bacteria In Vitro," Ostomy/Wound Management 44:508-11, 1998.

64. Kloth, L.C., and McCulloch, J.M. *Wound Healing Alternatives in Management,* 3rd ed. Philadelphia: F.A. Davis, p 335, 2002.

65. Dai, G.M.S., et al "An In Vitro Cell Culture System to Study the Influence of External Pneumatic Compression on Endothelial Function," *Journal of Vascular Surgery* 32:977-87, 2000.

66. Kessler, C.M., et al. "Intermittent Pneumatic Compression in Chronic Venous Insufficiency Favorably Affects Fibrinolytic Potential and Platelet Activation," *Blood Coagulation and Fibrinolysis* 7:437, 1996.

67. Alpagut, U., Dayioglu, E. "Importance and Advantages of Intermittent External Pneumatic Compression Therapy in Venous Stasis Ulceration," *Angiology* 56(1), 2005.

68. Fylling, C.P. "Growth Factors: A New Era in Wound Healing," *In* Krasner, D., and Kane, D., *Chronic Wound Care,* 2nd ed. Wayne, Pa.: Health Management Publications, Inc., 344-47, 1997.

69. McAleer, J.P., et al. "Use of Autologous Platelet Concentrate in a Nonhealing Lower Extremity Wound," *Advances in Skin & Wound Care* 19(7):354-62, September 2006.

70. Dyson, M. *In* Morrison M., et al. (eds.) *Chronic Wound Care: A Problem-Based Learning Approach.* London: Mosby, 2004.

71. http://www.uhms.org/Indications/indications.htm

72. Gottrup, F., et al. "The Dynamic Properties of Tissue Oxygen in Healing Flaps," *Surgery* 95(5):527-36, 1984.

73. Fife, C. "Hyperbaric Oxygen Therapy Applications in Wound Care," *In* Sheffield, P., et al., (eds.) *Wound Care Practice.* Flagstaff, Az: Best Publishing, p 664, 2004.

74. Wright, J. "Hyperbaric Oxygen Therapy for Wound Healing," *World Wide Wounds,* May 2001.

75. http://www.worldwidewounds.com/2001/april/Wright/HyperbaricOxygen.html.

76. Knighton, D., et al. "Regulation of Wound Healing Angiogenesis-effect of Oxygen Gradients and Inspired Oxygen Concentration," *Surgery* 90:262-70, 1981.

77. Bonomo, S.R., et al. "Hyperbaric Oxygen as a Signal Transducer: Upregulation of Platelet Derived Growth Factor-beta Receptor in the Presence of HBO2 and PDGF," *Undersea Hyperbaric Medicine* 25(4):211-16, 1998.

78. Wu, L., et al. "Effects of Oxygen on Wound Responses to Growth Factors: Kaposi's FGF, But not Basic FGF Stimulates Repair in Ischemic Wounds," *Growth Factors* 12(1):29-35, 1995.

79. Knighton, D.R., et al. "Oxygen as an Antibiotic. The Effect of Inspired Oxygen on Infection," *Archives in Surgery* 119(2):199-204, 1984.

80. Stanisic, M.M., et al. "Wound Debridement with 25 kHz Ultrasound," Advances in Skin and Wound Care 18(9):484-90, November-December 2005.

81. Ennis, W.J., et al. "Ultrasound Therapy for Recalcitrant Diabetic Foot Ulcers: Results of a Randomized, Double-blind, Controlled, Multicenter Study," Ostomy/Wound Management 51(8): 24-26, 28-29, 32-39, August 2005

82. Ennis, W.J., et al. "Evaluation of Clinical Effectiveness of MIST Ultrasound Therapy for the Healing of Chronic Wounds," *Advances in Skin & Wound Care* 19(8):437-46, October 2006.

CHAPTER 10

Nutrition and wound care

Mary Ellen Posthauer, RD, CD, LD
David R. Thomas, MD, FACP, AGSF, GSAF

OBJECTIVES

After completing this chapter, you'll be able to:

- describe the process of screening to identify nutritional problems/concerns
- identify the parameters involved in completing a nutritional assessment
- describe the role of nutrients in wound prevention and healing
- define the role of nutrition management for malnutrition.

Nutritional concerns

Nutrition plays a key role in both the prevention and treatment of wounds. The goal in preventing pressure ulcers is to screen and identify individuals at risk for ulcer development. A nutritional assessment should be completed both for individuals at high risk for pressure ulcers and those currently with wounds. Data derived from the assessment are then used to develop a nutritional care plan.

Based on the assessment, nutrition interventions are selected that are most appropriate to manage the current condition. These interventions are based on standard protocols that should be reviewed as new research data becomes available.

Daily caloric requirements

Daily caloric requirements range from 25 kcal/kg/day for sedentary adults to 40 kcal/kg/day for elderly patients under moderate stress. Various formulas, including the Harris-Benedict equation, can be used to calculate caloric requirements, but controversy exists over accuracy in obese or severely undernourished individuals.[23] Other formulas have been adjusted for severely stressed hospitalized subjects.[24]

Nutritional screening

As defined by the American Dietetic Association (ADA), a nutritional screening is the process of identifying characteristics known to be associated with nutritional problems. It's purpose is to pinpoint individuals who are malnourished or at nutritional risk and then determining appropriate intervention. There are a number of nutrition screening tools available including the Mini-Nutritional Assessment (MNA) from Nestle Nutrition, which is validated in the United States and abroad. It includes 15 questions and four anthropometric measures to assess nutrition and may be found at www.nestle-nutrition.com/tools/mna.aspx.[60] The Council for Nutrition Appetite Questionnaire (CNAQ) is a screening tool for predicting anorexia-related weight loss in long- term care residents, but may also be used in a variety of clinical settings. This tool has been revised and is now called the Simple Nutrition Appetite Questionnaire (SNAQ).[26]

Screening may be completed by any member of the health care team, including the dietitian, dietetic technician nurse, physician, or other qualified health professional.[25]

The screening process should identify risk factors for the development of pressure ulcers as well as identify those individuals who are malnourished or at risk for malnutrition:
• Significant weight loss: 5 lb or more in 1 month; 5% in 30 days; 10% in 180 days
• Disease states and conditions: diabetes, dementia, malnutrition, chronic obstructive pulmonary disease (COPD), cancer, renal disease, obesity
• Immobility and inactivity: hip fracture, spinal cord injury (SCI), stroke
• Chewing and swallowing problems: dysphagia, stroke, Parkinson's disease, cerebral palsy
• Poor food and fluid intake
• Medication adverse effects.

Significant weight loss without any known medical condition places a patient at risk for malnutrition.

Disease states and conditions can increase the risk of pressure ulcer development.

Diabetes with chronic hyperglycemia may both cause and affect poor wound healing. High levels of glucose compete with transport of ascorbic acid into the cells, which is necessary for deposition of collagen. Delivery of leukocytes and antibiotics to the wound is impaired due to the lack of blood flow and oxygen to the tissues. For such patients, glycosylated hemoglobin (HgbA1C) is the best indicator of glucose status as it indicates blood glucose control over 2 to 4 months. In a small study of diabetic foot ulcers, successful control of diabetes was associated with improved healing rates.[28] However, in a larger trial, there were no differences in short-term metabolic control, as assessed by HgbA1C, levels between patients who healed primarily and those who healed after amputation.[29] Additional information can be found at www.diabetes.org.[61]

The primary nutritional goal for patients with diabetes is to improve metabolic control of glucose and lipids and provide the appropriate calories. The term *ADA diet* is no longer used as the American Diabetes Association does not recommend or endorse a single meal plan. The Consistent Carbohydrate Diabetes meal plan is now recommended by the ADA and incorporates carbohydrates daily at each meal and at snack time. In general, 50% of the calories are from carbohydrates, 20% from protein, and 30% from fat with an emphasis on mono and polyunsaturated fats. The consistent carbohydrate approach has been successful in the management of type 2 diabetes in the nursing home.[27]

Patients with renal disease often have multiple medical conditions, such as diabetes or heart disease, which complicates the nutrient parameters of their diet. For example, a renal diet limited in calories, protein, potassium, phosphorus, sodium, and fluid often results in poor dietary intake that doesn't meet the patient's needs.

Obese patients—those whose body weight is greater than 130% of the ideal body weight—usually have excessive weight placed on bony prominences, which can lead to skin impairment. A diet lacking in adequate calories and protein wouldn't be appropriate for obese patients as it wouldn't promote healing.

Altered mental status often limits patients' abilities to feed themselves or to comprehend the importance of consuming a balanced diet. Advanced dementia often results in weight loss, dysphagia, malnutrition, and pressure ulcers. When patients become incapable of responding to caregivers' assistance to nourish them, the probability of developing pressure ulcers increases.

Definition of high risk for pressure ulcer development

The Centers for Medicare and Medicaid Services has identified the following risk factors for the development of pressure ulcers:
- impaired mobility or transfer
- end-stage renal disease
- malnutrition
- coma.

Clinical conditions that are the primary risk factors for developing pressure sores include, but aren't limited to, resident immobility and:

1. The resident has two or more of the following diagnoses:
- Continuous urinary incontinence or chronic voiding dysfunction
- Severe peripheral vascular disease
- Diabetes
- Severe chronic obstructive pulmonary disease
- Chronic bowel incontinence

- Paraplegia
- Quadriplegia
- Sepsis
- Terminal cancer
- Chronic end-stage renal, liver, or heart disease
- Disease- or drug-related immunosuppression
- Full body cast

2. The resident receives two or more of the following treatments:
- Steroid therapy
- Radiation therapy
- Chemotherapy
- Renal dialysis
- Head of bed elevated most of the day due to medical necessity

Reprinted from F tag 314; Procedures: 483.25(c): Federal Register, Vol 56, No 187, Sept 1991.

Immobility affects a patient's ability to either prepare meals or travel to a restaurant for meals and perhaps not get the proper nutrients in his diet as a result. For example, hip fracture and SCI restrict mobility, often resulting in increased pain, thereby making it difficult for the patient to concentrate on or be able to prepare healthy meals. Functional limitation, such as difficulty chewing or swallowing, affects the ability of the patient to ingest adequate calories and fluids. Poor hearing and vision compromise the patient's communication skills, often resulting in poor intake at meals.

Drug therapy can often cause adverse effects, such as nausea and gastric disturbances, that curtail a patient's food and fluid intake. For instance, corticosteroids increase the risk of infection and inhibit protein synthesis. Corticosteroids also cause depletion of vitamin A from the liver, plasma, adrenals, and enzymes and interfere with collagen synthesis and resistance to infection.[30]

The Centers for Medicare and Medicaid Services (CMS), which regulates long-term-care facilities, has targeted pressure ulcers, inadequate nutrition, and inadequate hydration as key survey issues. The development of a pressure ulcer in a person who was at low risk is automatically considered a sentinel event. In 2004, the CMS[62] revised the F 314 tag, which is the guidance to surveyors as part of the State Operations Provider Certification manual that impacts 13,000 skilled nursing facilities in the United States. The revised guidance contains a section on undernutrition and hydration deficits. The document notes "continuing weight loss and failure of a pressure ulcer to heal, despite reasonable efforts to improve caloric and nutrient intake, may indicate that the resident is in multisystem failure or in an end-stage or end-of-life condition warranting an additional assessment of the resident's overall condition." The interdiscipinary team should assist in the development of nutritional goals considering the individual's prognosis and projected clinical course. (See *Definition of high risk for pressure ulcer development.*)

Nutritional assessment

Nutritional assessment is a systematic process of obtaining, verifying, and interpreting data in order to make decisions about the nature and cause of nutrition-related problems. It's an on-going process that also includes continued reassessment and analysis of the patient's needs. The assessment includes the patient's nutritional status using medical, nutritional, and medication histories; physical examination; anthropometric measurements; and laboratory data. The assessment also includes interpretation of data from the screening process as well as a review of data from other disciplines (such as speech, occupational, or physical therapy) that may affect the assessment process. Nutrition assessment precedes a care plan, intervention, monitoring, and evaluation.

As part of the nutritional assessment, observation during mealtime provides the health care professional the opportunity to determine if the patient has chewing or swallowing problems that may require the services of either a speech therapist or occupational therapist. Adequate intake of food and fluid is a concern for those with swallowing problems, and this, in turn, places them at risk for pressure ulcers. The speech therapist defines the diet texture and also assesses the patient's needs for special feeding techniques, which are implemented by the dietary department. For example, patients may require thickened liquids to prevent dehydration or aspiration. The occupational therapist often determines the need for self-feeding devices that promote eating independence. Physical therapy sessions often result in the need for both increased calories and fluid, which the dietitian will calculate and arrange provision at appropriate times.

Signs of malnutrition

Assess the patient's skin condition, checking for loss of subcutaneous fat as evidenced by loose skin in the extremities. Observe for listlessness, muscle wasting, and the presence of peripheral edema in the absence of cardiac disease or circulatory disorder. Dull, dry, sparse hair can be a possible protein energy deficiency. For further signs, see *Physical signs of malnutrition,* pages 176 to 178.

The older adult is particularly prone to pressure ulcers as a result of decreased mobility, multiple comorbid conditions, poor nutrition, and loss of muscle mass. Nutritional factors that contribute to skin breakdown include protein deficiency, which creates a negative nitrogen balance; anemia, which inhibits the formation of red blood cells; and dehydration, which causes dry, fragile skin.

In addition, immune function declines with age, increasing the risk of infection. With advancing age also comes decreased skin response to temperature, pain, and pressure. This affects the skin's elasticity and the healing process.

The CMS has distributed nutrition care alerts to long-term-care facilities, listing warning signs and recommending strategies for dehydration, weight loss, and pressure ulcers. (See *CMS nutrition care alerts,* pages 179 and 180.)

The prevention of pressure ulcers nutrition decision tree serves as a guide for the nutritional assessment and considerations for treatment. (See *Nutrition guideline policy for prevention of pressure ulcers,* page 181.)

Additionally, medications have an influence on a patient's nutritional status and have been identified as a cause of weight loss.[36] (See *Prescription drugs linked to anorexia,* page 182.) Drugs may either inhibit or induce metabolism of a nutrient or increase the excretion of a nutrient. Medications designed to calm and reduce agitation may in turn reduce mobility and activity levels and place patients at risk for pressure ulcer development. Drugs may increase or decrease appetite, alter sense of taste or smell, or cause gastric disturbances. Radiation therapy, chemotherapy, and renal dialysis can result in increased nausea and vomiting as well as decreased activity, placing the patient at risk.

(Text continues on page 178.)

Physical signs of malnutrition

Signs	Possible causes
HAIR	
Dull, dry, lack of natural shine	Protein-energy deficiency
	Essential fatty acid deficiency (EFA)
Thin, sparse, loss of curl, color changes, depigmentation, easily plucked	Zinc deficiency
	Other nutrient deficiencies: manganese, copper
EYES	
Small, yellowish lumps around eyes	Hyperlipidemia
White rings around both eyes	
Angular inflammation of eyelids, "grittiness" under eyelids	Riboflavin deficiency
Pale eye membranes	Vitamin B_{12}, folacin, and/or iron deficiency
Night blindness, dry membranes, dull or soft cornea	Vitamin A, zinc deficiency
Redness and fissures of eyelid corners	Niacin deficiency
Ring of fine blood vessels around cornea	General poor nutrition
LIPS	
Redness and swelling of mouth	Niacin, riboflavin, iron, and/or pyridoxine deficiency
Angular fissures, scars at corner of mouth	Niacin, riboflavin, iron, and/or pyridoxine deficiency
Soreness, burning lips, pallor	Pyridoxine deficiency
GUMS	
Spongy, swollen, bleeds easily, redness	Vitamin C deficiency
Gingivitis	Folic acid, vitamin B_{12} deficiency
MOUTH	
Cheilosis, angular scars	Riboflavin, folic acid deficiency, pyridoxine deficiency
Soreness, burning	Riboflavin deficiency
TONGUE	
Sores, swollen, scarlet, raw	Folacin, niacin deficiency
Soreness, burning tongue, purplish color	Riboflavin deficiency
Smooth with papillae (small projections)	Riboflavin, vitamin B_{12}, pyridoxine deficiency
Glossitis	Iron, zinc deficiency, pyridoxine deficiency
TASTE	
Sense of taste diminished	Zinc deficiency
TEETH	
Gray brown spots	Increased fluoride intake
Missing or erupting abnormally	Generally poor nutrition

Physical signs of malnutrition *(continued)*

Signs	Possible causes
FACE	
Skin color loss, dark cheeks and eyes, enlarged parotid glands, scaling of skin around nostrils	Protein-energy deficiency, specifically niacin, riboflavin, and pyridoxine deficiencies
Pallor	Iron, folacin, vitamin B_{12}, and vitamin C deficiencies
Hyperpigmentation	Niacin deficiency
NECK	
Thyroid enlargement	Iodine deficiency
Symptoms of hypothyroidism	Iodine deficiency
NAILS	
Fragility, banding	Protein deficiency
Spoon-shaped	Iron deficiency
SKIN	
Slow wound healing	Zinc deficiency
Psoriasis	Biotin deficiency
Eczema	Riboflavin deficiency
Scaliness	Biotin deficiency, pyridoxine deficiency
Black and blue marks due to skin bleeding	Vitamin C and/or K deficiency
Dryness, mosaic, sandpaper feel, flakiness	Increased or decreased vitamin A
Swollen and dark	Niacin deficiency
Lack of fat under skin or bilateral edema	Protein-energy deficiency
Yellow colored	Carotene deficiency or excess
Cutaneous flushing	Niacin
Pallor	Iron, folic acid deficiencies
GASTROINTESTINAL	
Anorexia, flatulence, diarrhea	Vitamin B_{12} deficiency
MUSCULAR SYSTEM	
Weakness	Phosphorus or potassium deficiency
Wasted appearance	Protein-energy deficiency
Calf tenderness, absent knee jerks	Thiamin deficiency
Peripheral neuropathy	Folacin, pyridoxine, pantothenic acid, phosphate, thiamine deficiencies
Muscle twitching	Magnesium or pyridoxine excess or deficiency
Muscle cramps	Chloride decreased, sodium deficiency
Muscle pain	Biotin deficiency
SKELETAL SYSTEM	
Demineralization of bone	Calcium, phosphorus, vitamin D deficiencies
Epiphyseal enlargement of leg and knee	Vitamin D deficiency
Bowed legs	Vitamin D deficiency

(continued)

Physical signs of malnutrition (continued)

Signs	Possible causes
NERVOUS SYSTEM	
Listlessness	Protein-energy deficiency
Loss of position and vibratory sense, decrease and loss of ankle and knee reflexes, depression, inability to concentrate, defective memory, delirium	Thiamin, vitamin V_{12} deficiencies
Seizures, memory impairment, and behavioral disturbances	Magnesium, zinc deficiencies
Peripheral neuropathy, dementia	Pyridoxine deficiency

Reprinted with permission from *Physical Signs of Malnutrition. Pocket Resource for Nutrition Assessment.* 2005 CD-HCF, pp 69-73.

Anthropometric factors

Anthropometry—the measurement of body size, weight, and proportions—is used to evaluate a patient's nutritional status. A change in anthropometric values can signal problems such as wasting or edema, reflecting nutritional excess or deficit. Accurate heights and weights are critical as they are the basis for determining caloric and nutrient requirements. Adjustment or notations should be made for casts and other appliances that alter true weight.

PRACTICE POINT

Weigh your patient each time on the same scale, at the same time of day, and with minimal clothing.

Body mass index (BMI) is a weight-to-height ratio composed of body weight in kilograms divided by the square of the height in meters:

$$\frac{\text{Weight (kg)}}{\text{Height (m}^2)}$$

OR

$$\text{BMI} = \frac{\text{Weight (lb)}}{\text{Height (in}^2)} \times 705$$

A normally hydrated person with a BMI greater than 30 is considered obese.[31] A BMI less than 19 places the patient at nutritional risk.[32]

Stress as a result of injury, surgery, burn, fracture, or wounds results in depletion of nutrient stores required for healing. Protein stores are used as energy sources if adequate carbohydrate and fat aren't provided.

Ideal body weight, sometimes called recommended body weight or desired body weight, can be approximated using specific calculations. However, any deviation from usual body weight is a more reliable measurement of the severity of malnutrition.

$$\% \text{ ideal weight} = \frac{\text{Actual weight} \times 100}{\text{Usual body weight}}$$

When evaluating the severity of weight variances, it's important to determine possible causes such as recent surgery, diuretic therapy, or other new treatments that may affect weight status. (See *Severity of weight loss*, page 183. See also *Estimating kilocalorie needs based on activity and injury factors*, pages 184 and 185.)

Biochemical and laboratory values

Biochemical tests are evaluated as part of the nutrition assessment process. (See *Useful lab values to screen for hydration status*, page 186.)

Protein status can be evaluated through a nitrogen-balance study, visceral protein blood levels, and tests of immune function such as total lymphocyte counts.

PRACTICE POINT

CMS nutrition care alerts

The chart below sets out the Centers for Medicare and Medicaid Services (CMS) warning signs and interventions for unintended weight loss, dehydration, and pressure ulcers.

Warning signs	Interventions
UNINTENDED WEIGHT LOSS	
The following are some signs that a patient may be at risk of or suffer from unintended weight loss: • Needs help to eat or drink • Eats less than half of meals and snacks served • Has mouth pain • Has dentures that don't fit • Has a hard time chewing or swallowing • Coughs or chokes while eating • Has sadness, crying spells, or withdrawal from others • Is confused, wanders, or paces • Has diabetes, COPD, cancer, HIV, or other chronic disease	Below are some action steps to increase food intake, create a positive dining environment, and help patients get enough calories: • Report observations and warning signs to nurse and dietitian! • Honor food likes and dislikes. • Offer many kinds of foods and beverages. • Provide oral care before meals. • Position the patient correctly for feeding. • Encourage the patient to eat. • Notify nursing staff if the patient has trouble using utensils. • Help the patient who has trouble feeding himself. • Allow enough time to finish eating. • Record meal and snack intake. • If the patient has had a loss of appetite or seems sad, ask what's wrong.
DEHYDRATION	

The following are some signs that a patient may be at risk of or suffer from dehydration:
• Drinks less than 6 cups of liquids daily
• Has one or more of the following:
  – Dry mouth
  – Cracked lips
  – Sunken eyes
  – Dark urine
• Needs help drinking from a cup or glass
• Has trouble swallowing liquids
• Has frequent vomiting, diarrhea, or fever
• Is easily confused or tired
	Most patients need at least 6 cups of liquids to maintain hydration. Below are some action steps to help patients get enough fluids:
	• Report observations and warning signs to nurse and dietitian!
	• Encourage the patient to drink every time you see him.
	• Make sure pitcher and cup are near enough and light enough for the patient to lift.
	• Offer the appropriate assistance as needed if the patient can't drink without help.
	• Offer 2 to 4 oz of water or liquids frequently.
	• Offer ice chips frequently (unless patient has a swallowing problem).
	• Check swallowing precautions, then, if appropriate, offer sips of liquid between bites of food at meals and snacks.
	• Drink fluids with the patient, if your facility permits you to do so.
	• Be sure to record fluid intake and output.

(continued)

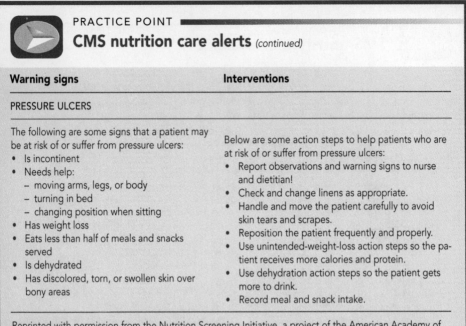

CMS nutrition care alerts (continued)

Warning signs	Interventions
PRESSURE ULCERS	

The following are some signs that a patient may be at risk of or suffer from pressure ulcers:
• Is incontinent
• Needs help:
  – moving arms, legs, or body
  – turning in bed
  – changing position when sitting
• Has weight loss
• Eats less than half of meals and snacks served
• Is dehydrated
• Has discolored, torn, or swollen skin over bony areas
	Below are some action steps to help patients who are at risk of or suffer from pressure ulcers:
	• Report observations and warning signs to nurse and dietitian!
	• Check and change linens as appropriate.
	• Handle and move the patient carefully to avoid skin tears and scrapes.
	• Reposition the patient frequently and properly.
	• Use unintended-weight-loss action steps so the patient receives more calories and protein.
	• Use dehydration action steps so the patient gets more to drink.
	• Record meal and snack intake.

Reprinted with permission from the Nutrition Screening Initiative, a project of the American Academy of Family Physicians and the American Dietetic Association, funded in part by a grant from Ross Products Division, Abbott Laboratories, Inc. HCFA Pub No. 10177.

The albumin level is dependent upon hepatocyte function. The half-life of albumin is 12 to 21 days; so, significant changes in liver function specific to albumin synthesis may go undetected. This long half-life also makes albumin a poor indicator of early malnutrition. Infection decreases the level of albumin. Acute stress, such as surgery or cortisone excess, reduces albumin even when protein intake is adequate. Edema and dehydration also affect levels. When albumin levels are low, serum calcium levels are low. Decreases in serum albumin may reflect the presence of inflammatory cytokine production or comorbidity rather than nutritional status.[33] (See *Nutrition markers linked to pressure ulcers*, pages 187 and 188.)

Pre-albumin (transthyretin and thyroxine-binding albumin) has a half-life of 2 to 3 days. Pre-albumin is a sensitive indicator of protein deficiency and of improvement in protein status with refeeding. Levels aren't greatly affected by mild liver or renal disease or fluid changes. (See *Laboratory values for nutritional assessment*, pages 189 to 191.)

Although some laboratory test may help clinicians evaluate nutritional issues in patients with pressure ulcers, no laboratory test is patient-specific or sensitive enough to warrant repeated testing. Serum albumin, pre-albumin, and cholesterol may be useful to help establish overall prognosis; however, they may not correlate well with clinical observation of nutritional status.[34,35]

Role of nutrients in healing

There are six major classes of nutrients: carbohydrates, proteins, fats, vitamins, minerals, and water. Through the process of metabolism, organic nutrients are broken down to yield energy, rearranged to build body structures, or used in chemical reactions for body processes.

The quick guide to nutrient needs for pressure ulcers provides a guide for practitioners to use when developing nutrition interventions for individual patients. (See *Quick*

Nutrition guideline policy for prevention of pressure ulcers

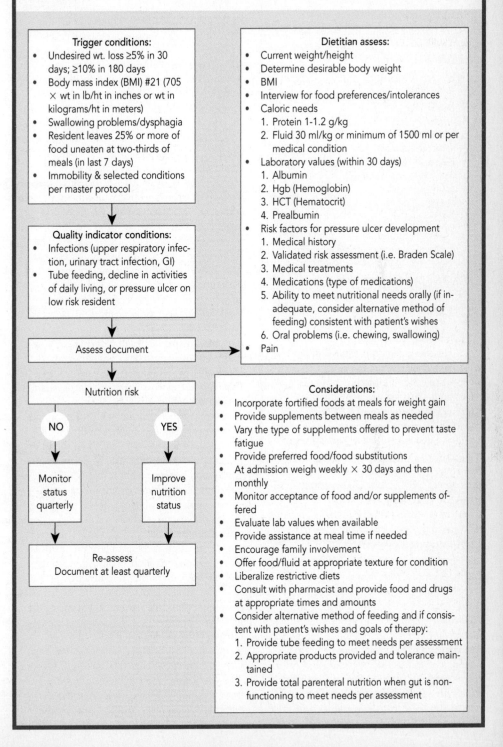

Trigger conditions:
- Undesired wt. loss ≥5% in 30 days; ≥10% in 180 days
- Body mass index (BMI) #21 (705 × wt in lb/ht in inches or wt in kilograms/ht in meters)
- Swallowing problems/dysphagia
- Resident leaves 25% or more of food uneaten at two-thirds of meals (in last 7 days)
- Immobility & selected conditions per master protocol

Quality indicator conditions:
- Infections (upper respiratory infection, urinary tract infection, GI)
- Tube feeding, decline in activities of daily living, or pressure ulcer on low risk resident

Assess document

Nutrition risk

NO / YES

Monitor status quarterly

Improve nutrition status

Re-assess
Document at least quarterly

Dietitian assess:
- Current weight/height
- Determine desirable body weight
- BMI
- Interview for food preferences/intolerances
- Caloric needs
  1. Protein 1-1.2 g/kg
  2. Fluid 30 ml/kg or minimum of 1500 ml or per medical condition
- Laboratory values (within 30 days)
  1. Albumin
  2. Hgb (Hemoglobin)
  3. HCT (Hematocrit)
  4. Prealbumin
- Risk factors for pressure ulcer development
  1. Medical history
  2. Validated risk assessment (i.e. Braden Scale)
  3. Medical treatments
  4. Medications (type of medications)
  5. Ability to meet nutritional needs orally (if inadequate, consider alternative method of feeding) consistent with patient's wishes
  6. Oral problems (i.e. chewing, swallowing)
- Pain

Considerations:
- Incorporate fortified foods at meals for weight gain
- Provide supplements between meals as needed
- Vary the type of supplements offered to prevent taste fatigue
- Provide preferred food/food substitutions
- At admission weigh weekly × 30 days and then monthly
- Monitor acceptance of food and/or supplements offered
- Evaluate lab values when available
- Provide assistance at meal time if needed
- Encourage family involvement
- Offer food/fluid at appropriate texture for condition
- Liberalize restrictive diets
- Consult with pharmacist and provide food and drugs at appropriate times and amounts
- Consider alternative method of feeding and if consistent with patient's wishes and goals of therapy:
  1. Provide tube feeding to meet needs per assessment
  2. Appropriate products provided and tolerance maintained
  3. Provide total parenteral nutrition when gut is non-functioning to meet needs per assessment

Prescription drugs linked to anorexia

This list of commonly prescribed medications have anorexia as a major adverse effect, which may lead to weight loss.

- Amlodipine (Norvasc)*
- Ciprofloxacin (Cipro)
- Cisapride (Propulsid)*
- Conjugated estrogens (Premarin)
- Digoxin (Lanoxin)
- Enalapril maleate (Vasotec)
- Famotidine (Pepcid)
- Fentanyl transdermal system (Duragesic)*
- Furosemide (Lasix)
- Ipratropium bromide (Atrovent)
- Levothyroxine sodium (Synthroid)
- Opioid analgesics (Propacet)
- Nifedipine (Procardia XL)
- Nizatidine (Axid)*
- Omeprazole (Prilosec)*
- Paroxetine hydrochloride (Paxil)*
- Phenytoin (Dilantin)
- Potassium replacement (K-Dur)
- Ranitidine (Zantac)
- Risperidone (Risperdal)*
- Sertraline (Zoloft)
- Warfarin (Coumadin)

* Indicates drugs with fastest growing usage.

guide to nutrient needs for pressure ulcers, pages 192 and 193.)

Carbohydrates

Carbohydrates provide energy and prevent gluconeogenesis from protein stores. Carbohydrate calories should comprise 50% to 60% of the patient's total caloric intake. An inadequate supply of carbohydrates results in muscle wasting (when the body is forced to convert protein stores for energy use), loss of subcutaneous tissue, and poor wound healing. Good sources of complex carbohydrates include whole grain breads, cereals, legumes, fruits, vegetables and milk.

Protein and amino acids

Protein is the only nutrient containing nitrogen in addition to carbon, hydrogen, and oxygen; some protein also contains sulfur and phosphorus. These elements combine to form amino acids, the smallest molecular units of protein. Protein is responsible for repair and synthesis of enzymes involved in wound healing, cell multiplication, and collagen and connective tissue synthesis. Protein is a component of antibodies needed for immune system function; 20% to 25% of calories should be obtained from protein sources.

The protein requirement for patients with pressure ulcers is arguable, but it's higher than the adult recommendation of 0.8 g/kg per day. Aging often leads to a decrease in skeletal muscle as well as a decline in protein turnover which decreases to 20% or less by age 70. Protein tissue accounts for 30% of whole body turnover prior to age 70. This decline may alter the ability of the body to fight infection and heal wounds. The recommendation for protein for older adults is 1.0 g/kg body weight.[1] Current recommendations for dietary intake of protein in stressed patients ranges between 1.2 and 1.5 g/kg per day. Many chronically ill elderly people can't maintain nitrogen balance at this level. Increasing protein intake beyond 1.5 g/kg per day may not increase protein synthesis and may cause dehydration.[2]

The association of dietary protein intake with wound healing has led to the investigation of specific amino acids. When the body is under stress, glutamine and arginine become conditionally essential amino acids. However, although glutamine is essential for immune system function, it hasn't shown noticeable effects on wound healing.[3]

L-Arginine is composed of 32% nitrogen, and its function is to stimulate the insulin-like growth factor that promotes healing. Arginine enhances immune function and wound collagen deposition in healthy elderly people.[4,5] One study tried to determine the level of oral arginine supplementation required, how it's metabolically tolerated, and its effectiveness in enhancing immune function in elderly patients with pressure ulcers. The study concluded that pharmacologic doses of arginine were well tolerated but didn't enhance lymphocyte proliferation or interleukin-2 production in nursing home residents with pressure ulcers.[6] Another study looked at the use of enteral formulas supplemented with arginine and concluded that elderly patients with normal renal function and appropriate fluids could tolerate the increased nitrogen loads. All of the systematic reviews have found no evidence to argue for the use of arginine alone or combined in the healing of pressure ulcers.[7]

One recent randomized, prospective, controlled, multicenter trial[8] at 23 long-term care facilities used a concentrated, fortified, collagen protein hydrolysate supplement. Ninety residents with stage II,III or IV pressure ulcers in four states participated in the study. Residents were randomized to receive standard care plus the protein hydrolysate supplement; or, standard care plus a placebo three times a day for eight weeks—standard care meant that residents in the study continued to receive any supplement or fortified foods they received prior to entering the study. The outcome was measured using the Pressure Ulcer Scale for Healing (PUSH). By week eight, there was a reduction of 50% in the PUSH scores in the treatment group compared with the control group, who received the placebo. Therefore, a concentrated, fortified, collagen protein hydroslysate supplement may be of benefit to residents with pressure ulcers residing in long-term care facilities. Additional research is needed to determine the effectiveness of high-protein supplements fortified with arginine and glutamine.[8]

Fats and fatty acids

Fat is the most concentrated source of energy and provides a reserve source of energy in the form of stored triglycerides in adipose tissue. Fat calories should comprise 20% to 25% of total caloric intake. Lean meats, poultry, fish, low-fat dairy products, and vegetable oils are appropriate sources of fat.

Vitamins

Vitamins are organic compounds that the body requires for proper functioning. Because the body doesn't produce vitamins, they must be obtained from food and beverages or synthetic supplements.

Severity of weight loss

Weight loss may be categorized as significant or severe. Significant weight loss consists of:
- 10% in 6 months
- 7.5% in 3 months
- 5% in 1 month
- 2% in 1 week.
  Severe weight loss consists of:
- >10% in 6 months
- >7.5% in 3 months
- >5% in 1 month
- >2% in 1 week.

© 1998, American Dietetic Association. *Nutrition Care of the Older Adult.* Used with permission.

Fat-soluble vitamins

Fat-soluble vitamins A, D, E, and K remain in the liver and fat tissue of the body until used. Because the body doesn't excrete excess fat-soluble vitamins, the risk of toxicity from overdose exists.

PRACTICE POINT

Look for signs and symptoms of overdose toxicity from fat-soluble vitamins A, D, E, and K if the patient is receiving supplements.

Vitamin A is responsible for epithelium maintenance. It also stimulates cellular differentiation in fibroblasts and collagen formation. Vitamin A deficiency, which is uncommon, results in delayed wound healing and increased susceptibility to infection.[9] Vitamin A supplementation has been shown to be effective in counteracting delayed healing in patients with non-pressure related wounds on corticosteroids.[10] Patients receiving high-dose steroids are often administered oral supplementation of 25,000 IU per day for 10 days.[11,12]

Vitamin E is an antioxidant and is responsible for normal fat metabolism and collagen synthesis. Vitamin E deficiency doesn't appear to play an active role in wound healing,[13] and it impedes the absorption of

Estimating kilocalorie needs based on activity and injury factors

Use the following formulas and charts to determine a patient's nutritional status and needs. Estimated daily calorie levels are determined by multiplying the patient's basal energy expenditure (BEE) and the appropriate injury and activity factors.

Total kilocalorie requirements = BEE × Activity factor × injury factor

ACTIVITY FACTOR (AF)

Confined to bed
Out of bed
Seated at work, little movement, little leisure activity
Seated at work with requirement to move, little leisure activity
Standing at work
Strenuous work or highly active leisure activity
30-60 minutes strenuous leisure activity 4-5 times per week

INJURY FACTORS

Blunt trauma
Burns (% total body surface):
0-20
20-40
40-100
Cancer
Closed head injury
Elective surgery
Fever
Post operative (no complication)
Multiple/long bone fracture
Multiple trauma with patient on ventilator
Multiple trauma
Peritonitis
Sepsis
Severe infection/multiple trauma
Trauma with steroids
Wound healing

Shortcut method for estimating adult energy needs per kilogram [8-10]	**KCals required**
Non obese population	
Obese, critically ill population	
Paraplegics*	
Quadriplegics*	

*Estimated energy needs for paraplegics and quadriplegics are adjusted by reducing calculated desirable body weight because immobilized patients lose muscle.

Estimating kilocalorie needs based on activity and injury factors *(continued)*

Protein needs for adults[3, 11]

	Albumin level	Protein requirement
CONDITION		
Normal nutrition (healthy adults)	3.5 g/dL	0.8 g/kg/day
Normal nutrition (elderly adults)	> 3.5 g/dL	0.8 to 1.0 g/kg/day
Mild depletion	2.8-3.5 g/dL	1.0-1.2 g/kg/day
Moderate depletion	2.1-2.7 g/dL	1.2-1.5 g/kg/day
Severe depletion	2.1 g/dL	1.5-2.0 g/kg/day
COPD	—	100-125 g protein/day total
EXCEPTION		
Renal failure		
Non-dialyzed		0.5-06 g/kg/day
Hemo-dialyzed		1.0-1.2 g/kg/day
Peritoneal-dialyzed		1.2-1.5 g/kg/day
Hepatic failure		0.25-0.5 g/kg/day

Another method of calculating protein needs: ratio of non-protein calories to grams of nitrogen (6.25 g protein = 1 g N).

Patient conditions	Ratio of nonprotein kcal: 1 g N
Adult medical	125-150 : 1
Minor catabolic	125-180 : 1
Severe catabolic	150-250 : 1
Hepatic or renal failure	250-400 : 1

vitamin A by reducing the rate of hepatic retinyl ester hydrolysis.[14]

Water-soluble vitamins

Water-soluble vitamins C and B play a role in wound healing. Vitamin C is essential for collagen synthesis. Collagen and fibroblasts compose the basis for the structure of a new wound bed. A deficiency of vitamin C prolongs the healing time and contributes to reduced resistance to infection. However, there's no clinical evidence that wound healing is improved by providing doses of vitamin C above the recommended daily allowance (RDI of 73-90 mg per day).[15] In a multicenter, blinded trial, 88 patients with pressure ulcers were randomized to either 10 mg or 500 mg twice daily of vitamin C. The trial failed to demonstrate any improved healing or closure rate between groups.[16] Even supertherapeutic doses of vitamin C haven't been shown to accelerate wound healing.[17]

Coenzymes (B vitamins) are necessary for the production of energy from glucose, amino acids, and fat. Pyridoxine (B_6) is important for maintaining cellular immunity and forming red blood cells. Thiamine and riboflavin are needed for adequate cross-linking and collagenation but their effect has not been demonstrated in pressure ulcers.

Useful lab values to screen for hydration status

Test	Normal values	Dehydration	Overhydration
Osmolality	280-303 mOsm/kg	> 303 mOsm/kg > 320 mOsm/kg (critical)	< 280 mOsm/kg
Serum sodium	135-145 mEq/L	> 145 mEq/L	< 130 mEq/L
Albumin	3.4-5.4 g/dL	Higher than normal	Lower than normal
Blood urine nitrogen (BUN)	7-20 mg/dL	> 35 mg/dL	< 7 mg/dL
BUN/creatine ratio	10:1	> 25:1	<10:1
Urine specific gravity	1.002-1.028 g/mL	> 1.028 g/mL	< 1.002 g/mL

Reproduced from Medline Plus Medial Encyclopedia, Healing Solutions, Hydration Care for Wound Prevention and Healing. Courtesy of Novartis Medical Nutrition. 2004, p. 25

Minerals

Minerals also contribute to a patient's well-being. zinc, a cofactor for collagen formation, also metabolizes protein, liberates vitamin A from storage in the liver, interacts with platelets in blood clotting, and assists in immune function. Deficiency can occur rapidly through wound drainage or excessive GI fluid loss or from long-term poor dietary intake. No clinical evidence exists to support supplementation (such as with zinc sulfate 200 to 300 mg daily). In a small study of patients with pressure ulcers, no effect on ulcer healing was seen at 12 weeks in zinc-supplemented versus non–zinc-supplemented patients.[18] Further, high serum zinc levels may inhibit healing, impair phagocytosis, and interfere with copper metabolism.[19-21] The U.S. Recommended Daily Intakes (USRDI) for zinc is 8 to 11 mg but most elderly people consume 7 to 11 mg of zinc per day,[22] chiefly from meats and cereals.

Copper is responsible for collagen cross-linking and erythropoiesis; the daily requirement for adult men and women is 900 mcg per day.

Iron is a constituent of hemoglobin, collagen transport, and oxygen transport; the daily requirement for adult men and women ages 50 to 70 is 8 mg per day. A multivitamin and mineral supplement with up to 100% of the USRDI's is the general recommendation if deficiencies are suspected or confirmed.

Water

Water, which constitutes about 60% of the adult body weight, may be the most important nutrient. It's distributed in the body in three fluid compartments (intracellular, interstitial, and intravascular). Water serves many vital functions in the body, including:
• aiding in hydration of wound sites and in oxygen perfusion
• acting as a solvent for minerals, vitamins, amino acids, glucose, and other small molecules and enabling them to diffuse into and out of cells
• transporting vital materials to cells as well as taking waste away from cells.

Patients with draining wounds, emesis, diarrhea, elevated temperature, or increased perspiration need additional fluids. Patients on air-fluidized beds require 500 ml of additional fluids daily. The dehydrated patient exhibits weight loss (2%, mild; 5%, moderate; and 8%, severe), dry skin and mucous membranes, rapid pulse, decreased venous pressure, subnormal body temperature, low blood pressure, and altered sensation.

(Text continues on page 191.)

Nutrition markers linked to pressure ulcers

This chart lists the nutritional markers that are—and aren't—associated with development of pressure ulcers.

First author	Clinical setting	Markers associated with presence of pressure ulcer	Markers not associated with presence of pressure ulcer
Allman [a]	Acute care	Albumin	Weight, hemoglobin, TLC, nutritional assessment
Gorse [b]	Acute care	Albumin	Nutritional assessment score
Inman [c]	Acute care, intensive care unit	Albumin (measured at 3 days)	Serum protein, hemoglobin, weight
Abbasi [d]	Acute care	Body mass index (BMI), total lymphocyte count (TLC)	Albumin, triceps skinfold thickness (TSF), arm circumference, weight loss, hemoglobin, nitrogen balance
Hartgrink [e]	Acute care, orthopedic	—	Nocturnal enteral feeding
Anthony [f]	Acute care	Albumin < 32 g/dL	—
Moolten [g]	Long-term care	Albumin < 3.5 g/dL	—
Pinchcofsky-Devin [h]	Long-term care	Severe malnutrition by biochemical markers	Mild-to-moderate malnutrition or normal nutrition
Berlowitz [i]	Long-term care	Impaired nutritional intake	Albumin, serum protein, hemoglobin, TLC, BMI/weight
Bennett [j]	Long-term care	—	Weight, BMI, weight gain
Brandeis [k]	Long-term care	Dependency in feeding	BMI/weight, TSF
Trumbore [l]	Long-term care	Albumin, cholesterol	—
Breslow [m]	Long-term care	Albumin, hemoglobin	Serum protein, cholesterol, zinc, copper, transferrin, weight, BMI, TLC
Bergstrom [n]	Long-term care	Dietary protein intake 93% of recommended daily allowance, dietary iron	Serum protein, cholesterol, zinc, copper, transferrin, weight, BMI, TLC
Ferrell [o]	Long-term care	—	Albumin, serum protein, BMI, hematocrit

(continued)

Nutrition markers linked to pressure ulcers (continued)

First author	Clinical setting	Markers associated with presence of pressure ulcer	Markers not associated with presence of pressure ulcer
Bourdel-Marchasson[p]	Long-term care	—	Oral nutritional supplement (26% vs. 20% incidence)
Guralnik[q]	Community	—	Albumin, BMI, impaired nutrition, hemoglobin

[a] Allman, R. "Pressure Sores: A Randomized Trial," *Annals of Internal Medicine* 107:641-48, 1987.

[b] Gorse, G.J., and Messner, R.L. "Improved Pressure Sore Healing with Hydrocolloid Dressings," *Archives of Dermatology* 123:766-71, 1987.

[c] Inman, K.J., et al. "Clinical Utility and Cost-effectiveness of an Air Suspension Bed in the Prevention of Pressure Ulcers," *JAMA* 269:1139-43, 1993.

[d] Abbasi, A.A., and Rudman, D. "Undernutrition in the Nursing Home: Prevalence, Consequences, Causes, and Prevention," *Nutrition Reviews* 52(4):113-22, April 1994.

[e] Hartgrink, H.H., et al. "Pressure Sores and Tube Feeding in Patients with a Fracture of the Hip: A Randomized Clinical Trial," *Clinical Nutrition* 17:287-92, 1998.

[f] Anthony, D., et al. "An Investigation into the Use of Serum Albumin in Pressure Sore Prediction," *Journal of Advanced Nursing* 32:359-65, 2000.

[g] Moolten, S.E. "Bedsores in the Chronically Ill Patient," *Archives of Physical Medicine & Rehabilitation* 53:430-38, 1972.

[h] Pinchcofsky-Devin, G., and Kaminski, M. "Correlation of Pressure Sores and Nutritional Status," *Journal of the American Geriatric Society* 34:435-40, 1986.

[i] Berlowitz, D.R., and Wilking, S.V. "Risk Factors for Pressure Sores: A Comparison of Cross-sectional and Cohort-derived Data," *Journal of the American Geriatric Society* 37:1043-50, 1989.

[j] Bennett, R.G., et al. "Air-fluidized Bed Treatment of Nursing Home Patients with Pressure Sores," *Journal of the American Geriatrics Society* 37:235-42, 1989.

[k] Brandeis, G.H., et al. "Epidemiology and Natural History of Pressure Ulcers in Elderly Nursing Home Residents," *JAMA* 264:2905-09, 1990.

[l] Trumbore, L.S., et al. "Hypocholesterolemia and Pressure Sore Risk with Chronic Tube Feeding," *Clinical Research* 38:760A, 1990.

[m] Breslow, R.A., et al. "Malnutrition in Tubefed Nursing Home Patients with Pressure Sores," *Journal of Parental and Enteral Nutrition* 15:663-68, 1991.

[n] Bergstrom, N., and Braden, B. "A Prospective Study of Pressure Sore Risk Among Institutionalized Elderly," *Journal of the American Geriatrics Society* 40:747-58, 1992.

[o] Ferrell, B.A., et al. "A Randomized Trial of Low-air-loss Beds for Treatment of Pressure Ulcers," *JAMA* 269:494-97, 1993.

[p] Bourdel-Marchasson, I., et al. "Prospective Audits of Quality of PEM Recognition and Nutritional Support in Critically Ill Elderly Patients," *Clinical Nutrition* 18:233-40, 1999.

[q] Guralnik, J.M., et al. "Occurrence and Predictors of Pressure Sores in the National Health and Nutrition Examination Survey Follow-up," *Journal of the American Geriatrics Society* 36:807-12, 1988.

Laboratory values for nutritional assessment

This chart contains additional laboratory value information to use in the nutritional assessment process.

Test	Normal values	Some implications
Albumin-Alb	3.5-5 g/dL (SI, 35-50 g/L)	**Function:** Maintain colloidal osmotic pressure, transport molecule for ions, hormones, some drugs, enzymes, fatty acids, amino acids, bilirubin, pigments **Site of synthesis:** Liver **Half Life:** 12-18 days **Increased:** Dehydration, diarrhea, Hodgkin's disease **Decreased:** Overhydration, liver disease, severe burns, malnutrition, pre-eclampsia, malabsorption, CHF, nephritic syndrome, infection, stress, advanced malignancies, protein losing enteropathies, thyroid disease, renal disorders, pregnancy, vasculitis, ulcerative bowel disease, individuals >70 yrs, trauma, sepsis, pernicious anemia, spinal cord injury, decubitus ulcer, cystic fibrosis, excessive administration of I.V. glucose in water, starvation, burns, surgery, MI, cirrhosis, leukemia, alcohol abuse, beri beri, cholecystitis, Crohn's disease, dementia, diabetes mellitus, meningitis, metastatic carcinomatosis, multiple myeloma, myasthenia, neoplasms, nephrosis, osteomyelitis, peptic ulcer, pneumonia, rheumatic fever, rheumatoid arthritis, scleroderma, sprue, systemic lupus erythematosus, ulcerative colitis, sarcoidosis, steatorrhea
Blood urea nitrogen-BUN	10-20 mg/dL (SI, 3.6-7.1 mmol/L)	**Function:** Detoxified product of protein metabolism, indicates recent protein intake **Site of synthesis:** Liver **Increased:** Dehydration, increased protein intake, urinary obstruction, renal failure/insufficiency, increased catabolism of protein due to infection, tumors, starvation, stress, trauma, myocardial infarction, diabetes mellitus, increased age, steroid therapy, bleeding ulcers, CHF, shock, GI hemorrhage, chronic gout, burns, sepsis, renal vein thrombosis, hypovolemia, Addison's disease, amyloidosis, analgesic abuse, Fanconi syndrome, glomerulonephritis, Goodpasture stain syndrome, heavy metal poisoning, intestinal obstruction, multiple myeloma, pancreatitis, peritonitis, pneumonia, polyarteritis nodosa **Decreased:** Overhydration, liver damage, advanced cirrhosis, liver failure, low protein diet, malnutrition, pregnancy, impaired absorption, acromegaly, celiac sprue, alcohol abuse, nephritic syndrome
Cholesterol (total)	<200 g/dL (SI< <5.20 mmol/L)	**Function:** Used to form bile salts, hormones, and cell membranes **Site of synthesis:** Liver **Increased:** CVC, atherosclerosis, myocardial infarction, hypothyroidism, uncontrolled DM, biliary cirrhosis, pregnancy, hyperlipoproteinemia, nephritic syndrome, biliary obstruction, high cholesterol and/or saturated fat diet, hypertension, obesity, smoking, xanthomatosis, stress, jaundice, leukemia

(continued)

Laboratory values for nutritional assessment (continued)

Test	Normal values	Some implications
Cholesterol (total)		**Decreased:** Hyperthyroidism, malnutrition, malabsorption, liver disease, anemia, stress, severe infection, cancer, pernicious anemia, hemolytic anemia, acute MI, cirrhosis, depression, epilepsy, gastric by-pass surgery, uremia
Cholesterol: high-density lipoprotein (HDLs)	>40 mg/dL (SI, 0.66 mmol/L) and < or = to 60 mg/dL (SI, 1.0 mmol/L)	**Function:** Carries cholesterol from tissues and transports it to the liver for catabolism and excretion, may inhibit cellular uptake of LDL **Site of synthesis:** Liver **Increased:** Chronic liver disorder, weight reduction, exercise, maintenance of weight loss, primary biliary cirrhosis, chronic hepatitis, alcoholism, hyperalphalipoproteinemia, hypobetalipoproteinemia **Decreased:** Genetics, lack of exercise, obesity, hypertriglycerides, hyperthyroidism, end stage liver disease, CRF, uncontrolled DM, nephritic syndrome, hypoproteinemia, metabolic syndrome, smoking, arteriosclerosis, bacterial infections, polycystic ovary syndrome, viral infections
Cholesterol: low-density lipoproteins (LDL)	<100 mg/dL (SI, 2.59/mmol/L) Desirable	**Function:** Carries cholesterol in plasma **Site of synthesis:** Liver **Increased:** MI, hypothyroidism, DM, nephritic syndrome, diet high in saturated fat and/or cholesterol, familial hypercholesterolemia, pregnancy, hepatic disease, Cushing's disease **Decreased:** Nephrotic syndrome, hypoproteinemia, hyperthyroidism, COPD, hypoalbuminemia, inflammatory joint disease
Creatinine	Male: 0.6-1.2 mg/dL (SI, 53-106 μmol/L) Female: 0.5-1.1 mg/dL (SI< 44-97 μmol/L)	**Function:** Nitrogenous by-product in the breakdown of muscle creatine phosphate due to energy metabolism. **Site of synthesis:** N/A **Increased:** Impaired renal function, shock, diabetic nephropathy, CHF, AMI, some cancers, dehydration, chronic nephritis, urinary tract obstruction, muscle disease, nephro-toxic drugs, gigantism, acromegaly, rhabdomyolysis, hyperthyroidism, multiple myeloma, surgery, rapid muscle loss, gout, azotemia, rheumatoid arthritis, systemic lupus erythematosus **Decreased:** Overhydration, muscular dystrophy, pregnancy, eclampsia, increased age, severe wasting
Prealbumin	15-36 mg/dL (SI< 150-360 mg/L)	**Function:** Transport thyroxine, complexes with retinol-binding protein for vitamin A transport **Site of synthesis:** Liver **Half Life:** 2-3 days **Increased:** Renal failure, dehydration, Hodgkin's, pregnancy, alcohol abuse, shigellosis **Decreased:** Liver disease, malnutrition, catabolic states, metabolic stress, inflammation, surgical trauma, hyperthyroidism, overhydration, protein losing enteropathy, infection, inflammation, cystic fibrosis, zinc deficiency

Laboratory values for nutritional assessment *(continued)*

Test	Normal values	Some implications
Total lymphocyte count (TLC)	3000-2500 cells/mm^3	**Increased:** Leukemia, infections bacterial disease, leukocytosis, thymoma viral infections, Addison's disease, parasites **Decreased:** Corticosteroid therapy, cancer, chemotherapy, radiotherapy, surgery, lymphopenia, malnutrition, AIDS, bone marrow failure, Cushing's syndrome, renal failure **Degrees of depletion:** mild = 1500-1800, moderate = 900-1500, severe <900

Signs of dehydration

Sufficient hydration is essential for all patients, and no less so for the patient with a wound. Use the following guidelines to prevent dehydration—and to recognize and treat it should it occur.
- If the patient can drink independently, keep water or other beverages at bedside so that they're easily accessible and in a container the patient can handle easily.
- If the patient doesn't consume fluids on his own, offer water at least every 2 hours.
  If you suspect dehydration, look for:
- dry skin
- cracked lips
- thirst (often diminished in elderly patients)
- poor skin turgor (The pinch test for skin turgor may be an unreliable indicator for dehydration in elderly patients. If you use this test, use only the skin on the forehead or sternum, and pinch gently. If well-hydrated, the skin goes back into place in 2 seconds.)
- fever
- appetite loss
- nausea
- dizziness
- increased confusion
- laboratory values (Serum creatinine, hematocrit, blood urea nitrogen, potassium, chloride, and osmolarity are increased. Sodium can be increased, normal, or low, depending on the underlying cause of dehydration.)
- decreased blood pressure
- increased pulse rate
- constipation (Recent diarrhea may explain the dehydrated state, and constipation is common when dehydration exists.)
- concentrated urine.

Patients who are at risk of dehydration require careful monitoring, such as weighing the patient daily. (See *Signs of dehydration.*) A weight loss of 2 kg in 48 hours indicates a corresponding loss of 2 L of fluid. Elderly patients, whose sense of thirst often declines, should be offered fluids more frequently.

Nutritional interventions

The management for malnutrition is extremely important for clients with wounds such as pressure ulcers. Areas such as nutritional status, undernutrition, nutritional support and, nutritional intake are all critical to this process.

Does nutritional status influence the incidence, progression, and severity of pressure

Quick guide to nutrient needs for pressure ulcers

Nutrient needs: Based on individual assessment	Prevention	Stage I	Stage II
Calories/kg body weight*	28-30 30-35 if additional calories needed	30-35	30-35
Protein, grams/kg body weight to promote a positive nitrogen balance††	1.0 1.2-1.5 if additional protein needed (Increase fluids/Monitor renal function)	1.2-1.5 if additional protein needed (Increase fluids/Monitor renal function)	1.2-1.5 if additional protein needed (Increase fluids/Monitor renal function)
Fluids, cc/kg body weight**	30	30-33	30-33
Vitamins/Minerals *if* deficiencies are confirmed or suspected: • Multivitamin & mineral supplement (up to 100% USRDI) • Elemental Zinc 25-50 mg daily	• Daily • NA	• Daily • NA	• Daily • NA

* Note: Alternate method of calculation: BEE X Activity Factor X Injury Factor of 1.2-1.6

**Note: Adjusted depending on condition, with less fluid possibly needed for residents with severe renal problems or CHF; and additional fluids needed for air fluidized beds, dehydration, draining wounds, ostomy losses, etc. Alternate calculation: 1 ml/calorie or 1500 ml minimum per day. Additional fluids needed for draining wounds, fever, other fluid losses; an extra 10-15 ml/kg body weight may be needed for air fluidized beds.

*** Unstageable may be defined as pressure ulcers with eschar and/or necrotic tissue covering wound; deep tissue injury (may appear as a stage I, but has underlying damage or necrotic underlying tissue, such as boggy or mushy heels, etc.) [1, 2, 3, 4, 5, 6, 7]

†† Use clinical judgment to determine amount of protein needed based on individualized nutrition assessment. Those who are nutritionally compromised (PEM, unintended weight loss, etc.) will need higher amounts of protein.

Note on weight: Dietetics professionals should use professional judgment in calculating weight (based on actual, ideal, adjusted, BMI) being careful to be consistent within their practice. At this time, there is no definitive evidence-based reference.

References

1. The Long Term Care Survey: Regulations, Forms, Procedures, Interpretive Guidelines. Washington, DC: American Health Care Association, 1999.
2. Department of Health & Human Services, Pub. 100-07 State Operations Provider Certification. CMS Transmittal 4, 11-12-04. Guidance to Surveyors for Long Term Care Facilities, Summary Of Changes: Appendix PP, Tag F314.
3. *Nutrition Care Manual Online*, American Dietetic Association, www.eatright.org, Chicago, IL, 2005.

sores? A review of several epidemiological studies supports this concept.[36,37] Research supports the finding that undernourishment on admission to a health care facility increas- es a person's likelihood of developing a pressure ulcer. In one prospective study, high-risk patients who were undernourished (17%) on admission to the hospital were twice as likely

Stage III	Stage IV (or Unstageable***)
35-40	35-40
1.2-1.5 if additional protein needed (Increase fluids/Monitor renal function)	1.2-1.5 if additional protein needed (Increase fluids/Monitor renal function)
30-33	30-33
• Daily	• Daily
• Reevaluate in 10 days to 2 weeks	• Reevaluate in 10 days to 2 weeks

4. The National Pressure Ulcer Advisory Panel, www.npuap.org, Frequently Asked Question: What is the role of nutritional support for patients in the prevention and treatment of pressure ulcers? 2003.
5. Bergstrom N, Bennett MA, Carlson CE, et. al. *Treatment of pressure ulcers. Clinical Practice Guideline, No. 15.* Rockville, MD: U.S. Department of Health and Human Services, Public Health Service, Agency for Health Care Policy and Research. Dec 1994: AHCPR Publication No. 95-0652.
6. Niedert K, et al. *Pocket Resource for Nutrition Assessment,* Consultant Dietitians in Health Care Facilities, a dietetic practice group of the American Dietetic Association, Chicago, IL, 2001.
7. Litchford M. *The Advanced Practitioners Guide to Nutrition & Wounds.* CASE Software, Greensboro NC, 2004.

to develop pressure ulcers as adequately nourished patients (9%).[38,39] Similarly, one study found that 59% of residents were undernourished and 7.3% were severely under-

nourished on admission to a long-term care facility. Pressure ulcers occurred in 65% of these severely undernourished residents, while no pressure ulcers developed in the mild-to-moderately undernourished or well-nourished residents.[40]

Epidemiological studies in the long-term care setting have correlated development of pressure ulcers with poor dietary intake. Studies revealed that residents with lower protein intake developed pressure ulcers. No other nutritional variable was significant for predicting ulcer development, including total intake of calories, vitamins A and C, iron, and zinc.[41] The use of pharmacologic agents to stimulate appetite, or orexigenic agents, has demonstrated weight gain, chiefly in patients with cancer or acquired autoimmune deficiency disease. Clinical studies using oxandrolone have shown weight gain in similar populations. Although it has been hypothesized that weight gain in undernourished patients with wounds would lead to better outcomes in terms of wound healing, there are currently no published studies that test the value of these agents in pressure ulcers or other chronic wounds.[42]

Effects of undernutrition

Undernutrition, or protein-energy malnutrition (PEM), is defined as "a wasting and excessive loss of lean body mass resulting from too little energy being supplied to body tissues that can be reversed solely by the administration of nutrients."[43] PEM is also characterized by starvation, not cachexia.[43] Functional deficits, such as impaired mobility, severe visual losses, poor dentition, and difficulty chewing, can predispose patients to PEM.[44] PEM has also been associated with changes in immune function, increasing susceptibility to infection, and delayed recovery from illness. (See *Consequences of protein-energy malnutrition,* page 194.)

The three types of PEM are marasmus, kwashiorkor, and marasmic kwashiorkor. Marasmus results from severe deprivation or impaired absorption of protein, energy, vitamins, and minerals. Typically, the person has weight loss, but the visceral protein stores (serum albumin, pre-albumin, and transfer-

Consequences of protein-energy malnutrition

Immunologic
- Impaired cell-mediated and humoral immunity
- Nosocomial infections (such as tuberculosis, *Helicobacter pylori*, or *Clostridium difficile*)

Integumentary
- Skin breakdown and development of pressure ulcers
- Delayed wound healing
- Sparse, dry, easily plucked hair
- Dermatitis

Musculoskeletal
- Decreased physical activity causing decreased muscle strength

- Recurrent falls
- Reduced ADLs

Cardiac
- Loss of cardiac muscle leading to decreased cardiac output

Pulmonary
- Impaired diaphragmatic movement
- Impaired clearance of secretions
- Increased susceptibility to aspiration

Gastrointestinal
- Atrophy of mucosal cells

Adapted with permission from *Nutrition Management and Restorative Dining for Older Adults*, Consultant Dietitians in Health Care Facilities, the American Dietetic Association, 2001.

Serving supplements

Remember that supplements should be offered between meals and not with a meal.

Photo courtesy of Aline Holmes, RN, APNC, MSN, APRN, BC, CNAA, BC

rin) remain normal. Cancer and COPD are also common causes of marasmus.

Kwashiorkor, or hypoalbuminemic malnutrition, is more difficult to detect because muscle mass is preserved. The patient may even appear well nourished, especially if edema is present. Serum albumin and cellular immunity are impaired, resulting in infection, poor wound healing, skin breakdown, and pressure ulcers.

Marasmic kwashiorkor, a combination of both types of malnutrition, is associated with the highest risk of morbidity and mortality.[45]

Increasing knowledge of the complexity of wound healing has led to the hypothesis that providing hypercaloric feeding in the form of nutritional supplements to patients at risk for undernutrition might reverse undernutrition and prevent the development of pressure ulcers. Indeed, one trial in France suggested that incidence of pressure ulcers may be decreased by nutritional supplements. Six-hundred seventy-two people older than age 65 and in an acute phase of a critical illness, were followed for 15 days or until discharge. At 15 days, the cumulative incidence of pressure ulcers was 40% (118/295) in the nutritional intervention group versus 48% (181/377) in the control group. This equates to a relative risk of developing a pressure ulcer (while taking a supplement) as 0.83 (95% CT 0.70 to 0.99). The proportion of erythema was 90% for both groups, thus no significant differences in the development of erythema was detected between the two groups.[46]

Providing nutritional support

Nutritional support is available for use when a person can't meet his nutritional needs by normal ingestion of food. Options include such strategies as providing additional liquid supplements or various snack foods to the person's oral diet; feeding through a tube placed into the GI tract; or, when the GI tract isn't functional, giving nutrients through the venous system as total parenteral nutrition. (See *Serving supplements.*)

Nutritional support is used to place the patient into positive nitrogen balance (the body maintains the same amount of protein in its tissues from day to day), according to the goals of care and whether it's compatible with the patient's and family's wishes. Enteral feeding (tube feeding) may be initiated when the ability to chew, swallow, and absorb nutrients through normal GI route is compromised. This occurs in conditions such as stroke, Parkinson's disease, cancer, and dysphagia, or when patients can't meet their nutritional needs orally. Most enteral tube feeding formulas are nutritionally complete and are designed for a specific purpose. Parenteral nutrition is the delivery of nutrient solutions directly into a vein, bypassing the intestine. It's necessary in patients when enteral tube feeding is contraindicated, is insufficient to maintain nutritional status, or has led to serious complications. (See *Nutritional assessment and support,* page 196.)

Does providing enteral feedings prevent pressure ulcers? The answer may lie in the limited number of studies that have been completed involving the use of tube feedings in patient with pressure ulcers. No difference in the number or healing of pressure ulcers was found in 49 long-term residents with pressure ulcers who received enteral feedings for 3 months.[47] Although pressure ulcers occur frequently in patients with hip fractures, randomized clinical trials of enteral nutrition in this population haven't been successful in preventing pressure ulcer development.[48] It's possible that poor tolerance of the feedings may have contributed to this result. In another study of 135 long-term-care residents with severe cognitive impairment, provision of tube feedings didn't increase survival or have an apparent effect on the prevalence of pressure ulcers.[49]

Ways to enhance nutritional intake

Many elderly people are chronically dehydrated, thus assuring adequate oral fluid intake can be challenging. (See *Beverage consumption,* page 197.) Use creative ways to encourage daily fluid intake. For example, in warm climates give frozen Popsicles, while in cooler climates, provide hot soup. Avoid beverages with caffeine, alcohol, or high glucose content, as they will act as diuretics, causing fluid loss.

Rather than just relying on supplemental shakes to increase calories and nutrients, consider adding powdered milk to foods the patient is already eating, such as pudding or yogurt. Offer small, frequent meals and snacks, such as high-calorie snacks, bars, and other forms of nutrient-rich products. You may also individualize feedings based on the person's preferences. To that end, make a contract with your patient to eat or drink some portion or percentage of his meals in return for something he loves that doesn't have as much nutritional value; this might enhance his overall food and nutrient intake.

Exploring why a patient isn't eating is the first step in helping him meet his nutritional needs.[63] (See *Unwanted foods,* page 197.) For example, is there an emotional or physical reason why eating is a problem? Find out if something is bothering the patient that's preventing him from eating. Provide an environment that reduces noxious smells, which may decrease appetite, while increasing pleasing aromas of food being prepared or other pleasant smells like cinnamon. A quiet, unhurried eating environment with frequent cueing is particularly helpful for cognitively impaired persons. Similarly, in evaluating physical ability to eat, consider the following questions:

• How much time does it take the patient to eat? Fatigue or fear of choking may cause him to eat slowly.

• Does the patient have the physical ability to bring the food to his mouth? Can he handle eating utensils? Neuromuscular impair-

Nutritional assessment and support

This algorithm can be used to determine when to consider enteral and parenteral feeding.

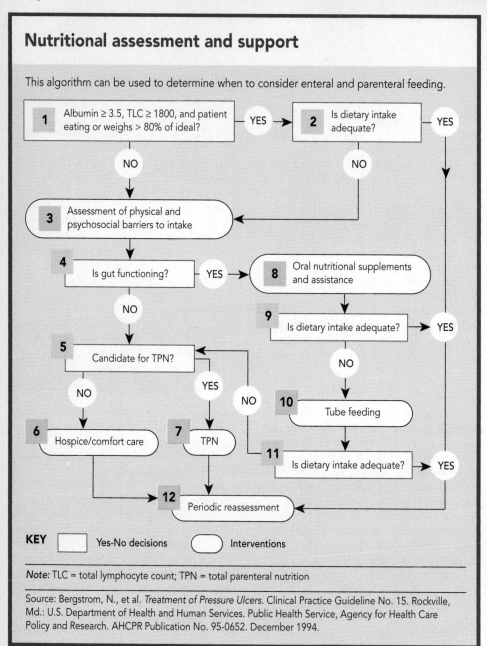

KEY

☐ Yes-No decisions   ◯ Interventions

Note: TLC = total lymphocyte count; TPN = total parenteral nutrition

Source: Bergstrom, N., et al. *Treatment of Pressure Ulcers.* Clinical Practice Guideline No. 15. Rockville, Md.: U.S. Department of Health and Human Services. Public Health Service, Agency for Health Care Policy and Research. AHCPR Publication No. 95-0652. December 1994.

ments, fatigue, or decreased endurance can interfere with the patient's ability to feed himself. Consider use of assistive devices and consultation from an occupational therapist. Some patients may prefer "finger" foods. Even with appropriate utensils, consider if the patient has the coordination to bring the food to his mouth.

• Can the patient see the food on his tray? Changes in visual fields from stroke, cataracts, glaucoma, or diabetes may alter his ability to see food on all or part of the tray. Arrange food so the patient can see and reach it.
• Can the patient chew? Check on the condition of his oral cavity. Provide appropriate mouth care to optimize taste buds and stimu-

Beverage consumption

The fluid on this tray is untouched; note the tops remain on the coffee, milk, and juice. Employees who deliver trays should open and uncover all liquids and encourage patients to drink beverages. A frail older adult, with arthritis for example, may not be able to open sealed containers.

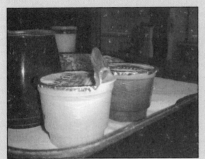

Photo courtesy of Aline Holmes, RN, APNC, MSN, APRN, BC, CNAA, BC

Unwanted foods

The patient ate the main entrée on this tray but left the pasta and broccoli. A survey of the patient's food preferences helps prevent the serving of unwanted foods.

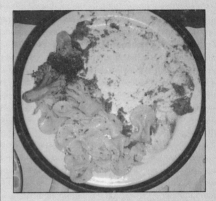

Photo courtesy of Aline Holmes, RN, APNC, MSN, APRN, BC, CNAA, BC

late appetite. Evaluate his oral hygiene and proper fitting or use of any dentures.
• Can the patient swallow? Cranial nerve and other neurologic conditions can cause swallowing difficulties. Evaluate the patient for any signs of abnormal swallowing. Teach the patient and family members to direct food to the unaffected side of the patient's mouth. Consultation from a speech therapist for management of swallowing difficulties and recommendations about food textures may be helpful.

 PRACTICE POINT

Evaluating if a person can swallow is critical for preventing aspiration. Signs of abnormal swallowing include drooling, collection of food in the cheeks, frequent coughing, gagging, or clearing the throat during the meal, and leakage of fluid from the nose after swallowing.

Involuntary weight loss, reduced appetite, and severe undernutrition are common in the geriatric population, and often go unexplained.[50] A common cause may be loss of

appetite due to a variety of psychological, GI, metabolic, and nutritional factors.[51] Loss of appetite may initiate a vicious cycle of weight loss and increasing undernutrition.

Cytokine-induced cachexia rather than simple starvation may be the reason that hypercaloric feedings in patients with pressure ulcers aren't effective. Hypercaloric feeding has positive results in all but the terminally undernourished patients. Cytokine-induced cachexia is remarkably resistant to hypercaloric feeding.[52,53]

Cytokine-mediated anorexia and weight loss are common in those who develop pressure ulcers. (See *Associations between cytokines, undernutrition, and chronic wounds,* page 199.) Serum interleukin (IL)-1 is elevated in patients with pressure ulcers.[54] Levels of IL-1 are elevated in pressure ulcers but low in acute wound fluid.[55] Circulating serum levels of IL-6, IL-2, and IL-2R are higher in patients with spinal cord injuries compared to normal controls, and highest in patients with pressure ulcers. The highest concentration of cytokines were found in patients with the slowest healing pressure ulcers.[56] In other

Monthly medical nutrition therapy pressure ulcer progress note

NAME: _____ GENDER: ☐ M   ☐ F
TARGET WEIGHT _____ lb. HEIGHT: _____ AGE: _____ years

DIET ORDER: FLUID INTAKE: _____ % intake _____ ml	DIET ORDER: FLUID INTAKE: _____ % intake _____ ml
SUPPLEMENT TYPE: TIME: _____ _____ % intake	SUPPLEMENT TYPE: TIME: _____ _____ % intake
FORTIFIED FOODS:	FORTIFIED FOODS:
TUBE FEEDING: FLUSH:	TUBE FEEDING: FLUSH:

FEEDING ABILITY   Dependent ☐   Independent ☐
             Limited assist ☐   Set-up only ☐
             Self-help devices ☐   Type _____
	FEEDING ABILITY Dependent ☐ Independent ☐
	             Limited assist ☐ Set-up only ☐
	             Self-help devices ☐ Type _____

NUTRIENT NEEDS: BEE _____ Activity factor _____ Injury factor _____ Total calories _____ Protein _____ gm/kg Total protein _____ Fluid _____ cc/kg Total fluids _____ ml	NUTRIENT NEEDS: BEE _____ Activity factor _____ Injury factor _____ Total calories _____ Protein _____ gm/kg Total protein _____ Fluid _____ cc/kg Total fluids _____ ml
CURRENT WEIGHT_____ (lb) ____ % change ☐ 30 days ☐ 90 days ☐ 180 days	CURRENT WEIGHT_____ (lb) ____ % change ☐ 30 days ☐ 90 days ☐ 180 days
PRESSURE ULCER(S) STAGE: 1 2 3 4 LOCATION: _____ SIZE: _____ Exudate: Light Moderate Heavy Pressure Ulcer Scale for Healing (PUSH) score:____	PRESSURE ULCER(S) STAGE: 1 2 3 4 LOCATION: _____ SIZE: _____ Exudate: Light Moderate Heavy Pressure Ulcer Scale for Healing (PUSH) score:____
PRESSURE ULCER(S) STAGE: 1 2 3 4 LOCATION: _____ SIZE: _____ Exudate: Light Moderate Heavy Pressure Ulcer Scale for Healing (PUSH) score:____	PRESSURE ULCER(S) STAGE: 1 2 3 4 LOCATION: _____ SIZE: _____ Exudate: Light Moderate Heavy Pressure Ulcer Scale for Healing (PUSH) score:____
RECOMMENDATIONS:	RECOMMENDATIONS:
RD SIGNATURE: _____	RD SIGNATURE: _____

studies, IL-6 serum levels were increased in patients with pressure ulcers but IL-1 and tumor necrosis factor were not elevated.[57]

Documentation in medical record

Medical nutrition therapy documentation in the medical record should include:
- amount of food consumed in both quantity and quality or type of food related to amount needed
- average fluid consumed daily (ml), related to amount required
- ability to eat—assisted, supervised, or independent
- acceptance or refusal of diet, meals, or supplements
- current weight and percentage gained or lost
- new conditions affecting nutritional status, such as introduction of thickened liquids or new diagnosis
- new medications affecting nutritional status
- current laboratory results (previous 3 months)
- wound condition and stage
- current calorie, protein, or fluid requirements
- recommendation for care plan.

(See *Monthly medical nutrition therapy pressure ulcer progress note.*)

Summary

Nutrition is an important consideration when treating the patient with pressure ulcers, chronic wounds, or diabetic ulcers because it not only facilitates healing, but also improves or stabilizes the patient's quality of life. The focus should be on optimal nutrition for each patient, which for some patients, may be achieved by a diet that includes supplements and allows the patient to enjoy his favorite foods. For others, enteral and parenteral nutritional support may be necessary. The amount and type of nutritional support provided to patients with pressure ulcers should be consistent with medical goals and the patient's wishes.[58,59]

Associations between cytokines, undernutrition, and chronic wounds

Proinflammatory cytokines
- Suppressed appetite
- Promotion of or interference with wound healing

Undernutrition
- Poor wound healing
- Increased risk of infection
- Increased incidence of pressure ulcers

Chronic wounds
- Source of cytokines
- Increased association with undernutrition
- Increased serum levels of cytokines

Show what you know

1. A patient who is 68″ tall and weighs 188 lb has a body mass index of:

   A. 20.5.
   B. 28.6.
   C. 27.1.
   D. 25.4

ANSWER: D. Weight (188 lb) ÷ height (68″) × 705 = 25.4.

2. A patient who weighs 125 lb with a stage IV pressure ulcer, poor appetite, and a pre-albumin level of 25 mg/dL has a recommended daily protein requirement of:

   A. 57 to 118 g.
   B. 68 to 107 g.
   C. 85 to 113 g.
   D. 68 to 86 g.

ANSWER: D. 125 ÷ 2.2 = 57 kg × 1.2 − 1.5 = 68.4 g to 85.5 g.

3. Clinical signs of kwashiorkor include:

   A. well-nourished appearance, edema.
   B. decreased energy intake, normal serum protein.
   C. decreased protein intake, infections.
   D. A and C.
   E. all of the above.

ANSWER: D. Clinical signs of kwashiorkor include a well-nourished appearance, edema, decreased protein intake and infections.

4. Recommendations for a severely stressed patient with a stage IV pressure ulcer whose nutritional status is compromised include:

A. calories of 30 to 35 g/kg of body weight; protein 1.5 g/kg per day; zinc sulfate 220 mg per day; 6 to 8 cups fluid per day.
B. calories of 20 to 30 g/kg of body weight; protein 1.5 g/kg per day; multivitamin; 6 to 8 cups fluid per day.
C. calories of 40 to 35 g/kg of body weight; protein 1.5 g/kg per day; ascorbic acid supplements 500 mg per day; 6 to 8 cups fluid per day.
D. calories of 30 to 35 g/kg of body weight; protein 1.5 g/kg per day; multivitamin; 6 to 8 cups fluid per day.

ANSWER: D. There's no evidence to prove supplementation of zinc or ascorbic acid benefits healing unless there's a deficiency. Calories, protein and fluid requirements are increased in stressed patients.

References

1. Chernoff, PhD., R.D., FADA. "Protein and Older Adults" *Journal of the American College of Nutrition*, Vol. 23, No.90006,601S, 2004
2. Long, C.L., et al. "A Physiologic Basis for the Provision of Fuel Mixtures in Normal and Stressed Patients," *Journal of Trauma* 30(9):1077-86, September 1990.
3. McCauley, R., et al. "Effects of Glutamine Infusion on Colonic Anastomotic Strength in the Rat," *Journal of Parenteral and Enteral Nutrition* 15(4):437-39, July-August 1991.
4. Barbul, A., et al. "Arginine Enhances Wound Healing and Lymphocyte Immune Response in Humans," *Surgery* 108(2):331-37, August 1990.
5. Kirk, S.J., et al. "Arginine Stimulates Wound Healing and Immune Function in Aged Humans," *Surgery* 114(2):155-60, August 1993.
6. Langkamp-Henken B., et al. "Arginine Supplementation is Well Tolerated but Doesn't Enhance Mitogen-induced Lymphocyte Proliferation in Elderly Nursing Home Residents with Pressure Ulcers," *Journal of Parenteral and Enteral Nutrition* 24(5):280-87, September-October 2000.
7. Langer, G., et al.. "Nutritional Interventions for Preventing and Treating Pressure Ulcers," *The Cochrane Database of Systematic Reviews*, 2004.
8. Lee, S., et al. "Pressure Ulcer healing with a Concentrated, Fortified, Collagen Protein Hydrolysate Supplement: A Randomized Controlled Trial," *Advances in Skin and Wound Care* 19(2):92-96, March 2006.
9. Hunt, T.K. "Vitamin A and Wound Healing," *Journal of the American Academy of Dermatology* 15(4 Pt.2):817-21, October 15, 1986.
10. Ehrlich, H.P., and Hunt, T.K. "Effects of Cortisone and Vitamin A on Wound Healing," *Annals of Surgery* 167(3):324-28, March 1968.
11. Levenson, S.M., and Demetriou, A.A. "Metabolic factors," in Cohen, I.K., et al., eds. *Wound Healing: Biochemical and Clinical Aspects.* Philadelphia:W.B. Saunders Co., 248-73 1992.
12. "Wound Healing," in Gottschlich, M.M., et al., eds. *Nutrition Support Dietetics Core Curriculum*, 2nd ed. Silver Spring, Md.: Aspen Pubs., Inc., 1993.
13. Waldorf, H., and Fewkes, J. "Wound Healing," *Advances in Dermatology* 10:77-96, 1995.
14. Clark, S. "The Biochemistry of Antioxidants Revisited," *Nutrition in Clinical Practice* 17(1):5-17, February 2002.
15. Rackett, S.C., et al. "Diet and Dermatology. The Role of Dietary Manipulation in the Prevention and Treatment of Cutaneous Disorders," *Journal of the American Academy of Dermatology* 29(3):447-61, September 1993.
16. Riet, G., et al. "Randomized Clinical Trial of Ascorbic Acid in the Treatment of Pressure Ulcers," *Journal of Clinical Epidemiology* 48(12):1453-60, December 1995.
17. Vilter, R.W. "Nutritional Aspects of Ascorbic Acid: Uses and Abuses," *Western Journal of Medicine* 133(6):485-92, December 1980.
18. Norris, J.R., and Reynolds, R.E. "The Effect of Oral Zinc Sulfate Therapy on Decubitus Ulcers," *Journal of the American Geriatric Society* 19:793, 1971.
19. Goode, P., and Allman, R. "The Prevention and Management of Pressure Ulcers," *Medical Clinics of North America* 73(6):1511-24, November 1989.
20. Thomas, D.R. "The Role of Nutrition in Prevention and Healing of Pressure Ulcers," *Clinics in Geriatric Medicine* 13(3):497-511, August 1997.
21. Reed, B.R., and Clark, R.A.F. "Cutaneous Tissue Repair: Practical Implications of Current Knowledge II," *Journal of the American Academy of Dermatology* 13(6):919-41, December 1985.
22. Gregger, J.L. "Potential for Trace Mineral Deficiencies and Toxicities in the Elderly," in *Mineral Homeostasis in the Elderly.* Edited by Bales, C.W. New York: Marcel Dekker, 1989.
23. Choban, P.S., et al. "Nutrition Support of Obese Hospitalized Patients," *Nutrition in Clinical Practice* 12(4):149-54, August 1997.
24. Ireton-Jones, C.S. "Evaluation of Energy Expenditures in Obese Patients," *Nutrition in Clinical Practice* 4(4):127-29, August 1989.
25. Lacey, K., Pritchett, E. "Nutrition Care Process and Model: ADA adopts road map to quality care and outcomes management," *Journal of the American Dietetic Association* 103(8): 1061-72, August 2003.
26. Wilson, M.M., et al. "Appetite Assessment: Simple Appetite Questionnaire Predicts Weight Loss in Community-dwelling Adults and Nursing Home Residents," *American Journal of Clinical Nutrition* 82(5):1074-81, May 2005.
27. Tariq, S., et al. "The Use of a No-concentrated-sweets Diet in the Management of Type 2 Diabetes in the Nursing Home," *Journal of the American Dietetic Association* 101(12);1463-6, December 2001.
28. Rubinstein, S.A., and Pierce, C.E. Jr. "Rapid Healing of Diabetic Foot Ulcers with Meticulous Blood Glucose Control," *Acta Diabetologica Latina* 25(1):25-32, January 1988.
29. Apelqvist, J. and Agardh,C.D. "The Association between Clinical Risk Factors and Outcome of Diabetic Foot Ulcers," *Diabetes Research and Clinical Practice* 18(1);43-53, January 1992
30. Maklebust, J., and Sieggreen, M. *Pressure Ulcers: Guidelines for Prevention and Management,* 3rd ed. Springhouse, Pa.: Springhouse Corporation, 2001.

31. Report of the Dietary Guidelines Advisory Committee on the Dietary Guidelines for Americans, 2000.

32. Walker, G. "Pocket Resource for Nutrition Assessment," *Consultant Dietitians in Health Care Facilities* Chicago: American Dietetic Association, 2005.

33. Friedman, F.J., et al. "Hypoalbuminemia in the Elderly is Due to Disease not Malnutrition," *Clinical Experimental Gerontol* 7:191-203, 1985.

34. Covinsky, K.E., et al. "Serum Albumin Concentration and Clinical Assessments of Nutritional Status in Hospitalized Older People; Different Sides of Different Coins?" *Journal of the American Geriatric Society* 50:631-63, 2002.

35. Ferguson, R., et al. "Serum Albumin and Pre-Albumin as Predictors of Hospitalized Elderly Nursing Home Patients," *Journal of the American Geriatric Society*, 41:545-49, 1993.

36. Morley, J.E., and Kraenzle, D. "Causes of Weight Loss in a Community Nursing Home," *Journal of the American Geriatric Society* 42(6):583-85, June 1994.

37. Thomas, D.R. "Nutritional Factors Affecting Wound Healing," *Ostomy/ Wound Management* 42(5):40-49, June 1996.

38. Thomas, D.R. "Improving Outcome of Pressure Ulcers with Nutritional Interventions: A Review of the Evidence," *Nutrition* 17(2):121-25, February 2001.

39. Thomas, D.R, et al. "Hospital Acquired Pressure Ulcers and Risk of Death," *Journal of the American Geriatric Society* 44(12):1435-40, December 1996.

40. Pinchofsky-Devin, G.D., and Kaminski, M.V., Jr. "Correlation of Pressure Sores and Nutritional Status," *Journal of the American Geriatric Society* 34(6):435-40, June 1986.

41. Bergstrom, N., and Braden, B. "A Prospective Study of Pressure Sore Risk Among Institutionalized Elderly," *Journal of the American Geriatric Society* 40(8):747-58, August 1992.

42. Demling, R.H., and DeSanti, L. "Oxandrolone, an Anabolic Steroid, Significantly Increases the Rate of Weight Gain in the Recovery Phase After Major Burns," *Journal of Trauma-Injury Infection & Critical Care* 43(1):47-51, July 1997.

43. A.S.P.E.N. The Clinical Guidelines Task Force, Guidelines for the Use of Parenteral and Enteral Nutrition in Adult and Pediatric Patients. Journal of Parenteral Nutrition. 26 supplement 2002, S1.

44. Thomas D.R. "Distinguishing Starvation from Cachexia," *Geriatric Clinics of North America* 18:883-892, 2002.

45. Rubenstein, L.Z. "An Overview of Aging-demographics, Epidemiology and Health Services," in Morley, J.E., et al., eds. *Geriatric Nutrition: A Comprehensive Review* New York: Raven Press; 1990.

46. Bourdel-Marchasson I., et al. "A Multi-center Trial of the Effects of Oral Nutritional Supplementation in Critically Ill Older Inpatients, GAGE Group, Groupe Aquitain Geriatrique d'"Evaluation," *Nutrition* 16(1):1-5, January 2000.

47. Henderson, C.T., et al. "Prolonged Tube Feeding in Long-term Care: Nutritional Status and Clinical Outcomes," *Journal of the American College of Clinical Nutrition* 11(3):309-25, June 1992.

48. Hartgrink, H.H., et al. "Pressure Sores and Tube Feeding in Patients with a Fracture of the Hip: A Randomized Clinical Trial," *Clinical Nutrition* 17(6):287-92, December 1998.

49. Mitchell, S.L., et al. "The Risk Factors and Impact on Survival of Feeding Tube Placement in Nursing Home Residents with Severe Cognitive Impairment," *Archives of Internal Medicine* 157(3):32732, February 10, 1997.

50. Thompson, M.P., and Merria, L.K. "Unexplained Weight Loss in Ambulatory Elderly," *Journal of the American Geriatric Society* 39(5):497-500, May 1991.

51. Morley, J.E., and Thomas, D.R. "Anorexia and Aging: Pathophysiology," *Nutrition* 15(6):499-503, June 1999.

52. Souba, W.W. "Drug Therapy: Nutritional Support," *New England Journal of Medicine* 336(1):41-48, January 1997.

53. Atkinson, S., et al. "A Prospective, Randomized, Double-blind, Controlled Clinical Trial of Enteral Immunonutrition in the Critically Ill," *Critical Care Medicine* 26(7):1164-72, July 1998.

54. Matsuyama, N., et al. "The Possibility of Acute Inflammatory Reaction Affects the Development of Pressure Ulcers in Bedridden Elderly Patients," *Rinsho Byori-Japanese Journal of Clinical Pathology* 47(11):1039-45, November 1999.

55. Barone, E.J., et al. "Interleukin-1" and Collagenase Activity are Elevated in Chronic Wounds," *Plastic & Reconstructive Surg* 102:1023-27, 1998.

56. Segal, J.L., et al. "Circulating Levels of IL-2R, ICAM-1, and IL-6 in Spinal Cord Injuries," *Archives of Physical Medicine & Rehabilitation* 78(1):44-47, January 1997.

57. Bonnefoy, M., et al. "Implication of Cytokines in the Aggravation of Malnutrition and Hypercatabolism in Elderly Patients with Severe Pressure Sores," *Age & Ageing* 24(1):37-42, January 1995.

58. Thomas, D.R., et al. "Nutritional Management in Long-term Care: Development of a Clinical Guideline. Council for Nutritional Strategies in Long-Term Care" *Journals of Gerontology Series A-Biological Sciences & Medical Sciences* 55(12):M725-34, December 2000.

59. Thomas, D.R. "The Role of Nutrition in Prevention and Healing of Pressure Ulcers," *Clinics in Geriatric Medicine* 13(3):497-511, August 1997.

60. *www.nestlenutrition.com*. Last accessed September 13, 2006.

61. *www.diabetes.org*. Last accessed September 13, 2006.

62. *http://new.cms.hhs.gov/manuals/downloads/som107ap_pp_guidelines_ltcf.pdf*.Last accessed September 13, 2006.

63. Posthauer, M.E. "The value of nutritional screening and assessment," *Advances in Skin and Wound Care* 19(7):388-390, July 2006.

CHAPTER 11

Pressure redistribution: Seating, positioning, and support surfaces

David M. Brienza, PhD
Mary Jo Geyer, PT, PhD, FCCWS, CLT-LANA, C.Ped
Stephen Sprigle, PhD, PT
Karen Zulkowski, DNS, RN, CWS

OBJECTIVES

After completing this chapter, you'll be able to:

- demonstrate an understanding of tissue biomechanical properties, their measurement, and their relationship to soft tissue–loading tolerance

- identify support surface characteristics related to the maintenance of tissue integrity

- demonstrate an understanding of the categories, functions, and limitations of various support surfaces

- outline an assessment process for selecting an appropriate support surface (seat cushion or horizontal support) and related interventions (positioning).

Preventing skin breakdown

Multiple intervention strategies are needed to prevent and treat skin breakdown. Managing loads on the skin and associated soft tissue is one of these strategies. A comprehensive care plan should include tissue load management strategies for individuals both while in bed and when seated. Properly chosen support surfaces; adequate periodic pressure redistribution; protection of especially vulnerable bony prominences, such as the heels; and consideration of special patient needs are all essential components of the care plan.

A support surface is a specialized device for pressure redistribution designed for management of tissue loads, micro-climate, and other therapeutic functions. Types of surfaces include mattresses, integrated bed systems, mattress replacements, mattress overlays, and seat cushions. Unless specifically identified as a mattress or seat cushion, the term "support surface" will refer to both product categories in this chapter. Achieving a good match between the patient's needs and the performance capabilities of the support surface has a profound, positive impact on a patient's health and well being; conversely, a poor match has an equally negative impact. Support surfaces redistribute the body's weight and protect the skin's tissue while providing for proper body alignment, comfort and, as part of a seating system, postural control during functional movement. Because these effects frequently conflict, clinical decision-making requires a compromise between protective and functional goals.

In a perfect world, we would be able to choose the "right" surface by using an algorithm that inputs an individual's characteristics, conditions, environment, and desires, thus producing a prescription for an ideal, personalized support surface. Unfortunately, the research in this area has failed to produce strong evidence to justify the selection of one product over another for any given situation. Some guidance is available, but it's not sufficient enough to replace good clinical decision-making and follow-up evaluations. Furthermore, existing clinical recommendations need to be updated regularly to reflect new research, technology, and treatment strategies as they become available.

Knowledge of a product's composition and contents is a necessary part of the selection process. Although describing the materials and components of support surface technology may be informative, it isn't always instructive. In terms of selecting a product, the information on the function or performance of the surface is most critical, regardless of composition. Krouskop and van Rijswijk focused on performance parameters when they identified nine key support surface characteristics.[1] (See *Support surface performance parameters*.)

Unfortunately, the information from clinical validation studies necessary for function- and performance-based categorization of seat cushions and support surfaces isn't yet available. The best we can do now is to group the devices according to the technologies and materials used in their construction and relate the characteristics of these technologies to the factors believed to have significant effects on the prevention and healing of pressure ulcers.

Soft-tissue biomechanics

Human soft tissues consist of a variety of macrostructures including skin, fat, muscle, vessels, nerves, ligaments, and tendons. The rela-

---

Support surface performance parameters

Nine parameters must be considered when evaluating the characteristics of a support surface for the patient with a wound:
- Redistribution of pressure
- Moisture control
- Temperature control
- Friction control (between patient and product)
- Infection control
- Flammability
- Life expectancy
- Fail safety
- Product reputation

Adapted with permission from Krouskop, T., and van Rijswijk, L. "Standardizing Performance-Based Criteria for Support Surfaces," *Ostomy/Wound Management* 41(1):34-44, January-February 1995.

---

tive amounts and arrangement of tissue macromolecules of the skin and supporting soft tissues are adapted to their specific functions and dictate their biomechanical properties.

In most connective tissue, fibroblasts secrete the macromolecules that make up the extracellular matrix. The matrix is made up of two main classes of macromolecules:
- polysaccharide chains of a class called glycosaminoglycans, which are usually found covalently linked to protein in the form of proteoglycans
- fibrous proteins that are either primarily structural (for example, collagen and elastin) or primarily adhesive (for example, fibronectin and laminin).

Glycosaminoglycans and proteoglycans form a highly hydrated, gel-like "ground substance" in which the proteins are embedded. The ground substance is analogous to glue that fills the lattice of collagen and elastin fibers, providing lubrication and shock absorbing qualities. The polysaccharide gel resists compressive forces on the matrix, while

Stress-relaxation phenomenon

The stress vs. strain curve, shown below, illustrates the stress-relaxation phenomenon. With the compression of tissue (strain) held constant, the force (stress) generated in the tissue as a result of that compression reduces over time. The degree of stress relaxation—that is, the amount of reduction in the holding force—can be determined by measuring the distance along the vertical axis between the time when the load is first applied to the time when it reaches steady-state (downward sloping ends).

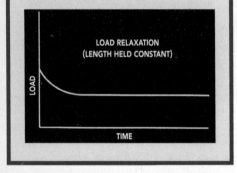

the collagen fibers along with elastin fibers provide tensile strength and resilience.

Tissue mechanical properties

In general, soft tissues are anisotropic, incompressible biosolid, biofluid mixtures.[2] Because soft tissue is largely incompressible, it tends to move slowly from areas of greater pressure to areas of lesser pressure. This slow movement of ground substance and interstitial fluid is responsible for the time-dependent (viscoelastic) behavior of the soft tissue manifested as four phenomena: stress relaxation, creep, hysteresis, and pseudoelasticity (preconditioning).[3]

These phenomena may be graphically represented as stress-strain curves. Stress is represented as the deforming force on the y axis and the tissue strain (deformation) is plotted

on the x axis. When soft tissue is suddenly deformed (strained) and the strain is thereafter kept constant, the corresponding stress induced in the tissue decreases over time. This phenomenon is known as stress relaxation. (See *Stress-relaxation phenomenon*.) Alternatively, creep describes the progressive tissue deformation that occurs over time when stress remains constant. (See *Creep phenomenon*.) During cyclic loading, such as that produced by a dynamic, or alternating pressure, mattress the stress-strain relationship demonstrated during the loading phase is different from that of the recovery, or unloaded, portion of the cycle. This effect is known as hysteresis. Finally, pseudoelasticity is the term associated with an increase in the repeatability and predictability of a tissue's stress-strain relationship following a defined period of repetitive cyclic loading.

Tissue loading and pressure ulcer formation

Body weight resting on bony prominences, such as the scapula, sacrum, greater trochanters, ischial tuberosities, and heels, can cause significant concentrations of pressure at the skin's surface and in the underlying soft tissue. The pressure peaks and the pressure gradients surrounding these peaks can put the soft tissue at risk for breakdown. However, high pressure alone usually isn't an indicator for the development of a pressure ulcer. Research has clearly demonstrated that the damaging effects of pressure are related to both its magnitude and duration. Simply stated, tissues can withstand higher loads for shorter periods of time. (See *Guidelines for sitting duration,* page 206.)

Limitations of interface pressure as a predictor of tissue damage

Tissue interface pressure is the force per unit area that acts perpendicularly between the patient's body and the support surface.[4] It's measured noninvasively by placing a pressure sensor between the patient's skin and the support surface. This measurement is believed to provide an approximation of the pressure on the tissue test site or surrounding area. Single sensors have been used to measure local pressure over a single bony prominence; multiple sensors integrated into a mat may be used to "map" the entire body area in contact with the support surface.

Interface pressure has been used extensively as a tool for predicting the clinical effectiveness of various support surfaces and for comparing products. Many research efforts have been directed toward establishing an interface pressure threshold beyond which pressure ulcers would form. However, what the research has failed to do is to identify a specific threshold at which loads can be deemed harmful across either subject populations or various tissue body sites. This is because a tissue's loading tolerance varies according to its composition, condition, location, age, hydration, and metabolic state. Therefore, while interface pressure may aid in comparing one surface to another based on an individual's relative responses, interface pressure alone isn't sufficient to evaluate the efficacy of a particular device or class of devices.

More recent research has gone beyond assuming that tissue necrosis is a result of ischemia due to external pressure alone. In fact, all of the well-known extrinsic pressure ulcer risk factors (pressure, shear, friction, temperature, and moisture) tend to influence the tissue's ability to withstand loading. Therefore, current investigations are focusing on a variety of physiologic, biochemical, and biomechanical tissue responses to loading.

Clinical implications of aging

The gross morphology of the soft tissues undergoes significant changes due to aging, including decreased moisture content and decreased elasticity manifested as rough, scaly skin with increased wrinkling and laxity. Dry, inelastic skin with larger, more irregular epidermal cells leads to decreased barrier function. These changes are reflected in the tissue biomechanical properties and have been associated with increased risk of tissue injury.

At the microscopic level, flattening of the dermal-epidermal junction (rete ridges) has been observed with the height of the dermal papillae declining by 55% from the third to

Creep phenomenon

Creep reflects the ability of tissue to resist deformation over time when the force causing the deformation remains constant. The creep phenomenon shown here indicates that the tissue progressively deforms over time without any additional force being applied. If creep were zero, the curve would be a flat line, indicating that deformation was constant over time.

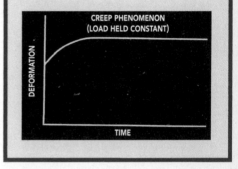

CREEP PHENOMENON (LOAD HELD CONSTANT)

ninth decade of life. As the space between the well-vascularized dermis and epidermis increases, several functional changes occur. Decreases have been reported in the area available for nutrient transfer, the number of cells within the stratum basale, and the skin's resistance to shearing. A 30% to 50% decrease in epidermal turnover during the third to the eighth decade of life has also been reported. This diminution in repair rate has been quantified as both decreased collagen deposition and diminished wound tensile strength. The loss of subcutaneous fat with aging decreases our protection from injury due to pressure and shearing forces between the bony prominences and the support surface. Moreover, decreased sensory perception increases the risk of injury by mechanical forces such as pressure. And, the more rigid, less elastic, drier nature of an elderly person's skin can result in tissue that tears and bleeds more easily.

Guidelines for sitting duration

This graph provides guidelines on sitting tolerance based on the magnitude of localized pressure.

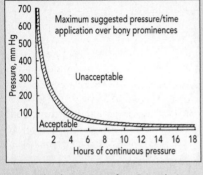

Reprinted with permission from Reswick, J., and Rogers, J. *Experiences at Rancho Los Amigos Hospital with Devices and Techniques to Prevent Pressure Sores. Bedsore Biomechanics.* London: University Park Press, 1976.

Support surface characteristics

Prevention of pressure ulcers is accomplished primarily by managing tissue loads. Support surfaces have been designed to reduce the effects of tissue loading by controlling the intensity and duration of pressure, shear, and friction. Also, attempts have been made to control the physical factors associated with increased risk through elimination of excess moisture and effective dissipation of heat.

Pressure redistribution

Pressure redistribution is the ability of a support surface to distribute load over the contact areas of the human body. (This term replaces prior terminology of pressure reduction and pressure relief surfaces.[5]) The redistribution of pressure reduces the magnitude of pressure and shear forces, both of which can cause excessive tissue distortion and damage soft tissues. Pressure (stress) is defined as force per unit area; the pressure distribution is influenced by mechanical and physical characteristics of the support surface, mechanical properties of the body's tissues, and weight distribution (posture).

Immersion

Immersion is defined as the depth of penetration into a support surface.[5] The fundamental strategy for reducing pressure near a bony prominence is to allow the prominence to be immersed into the support surface. Immersion allows the pressure concentrated beneath a specific bony prominence to be spread out over the surrounding area, including other bony prominences. For example, when a person is sitting on a relatively hard cushion, a disproportionately large portion of his body weight is born by the tissue beneath the ischial tuberosities. On a softer surface, the ischial tuberosities and buttocks may immerse more deeply, even to the level of the greater trochanters. With greater immersion, the body weight divided by a greater surface area results in decreased average pressure. This definition of immersion doesn't distinguish between immersion resulting from compression of the support surface and immersion resulting from the displacement of a support surface's fluid components.

The potential for immersion depends on both the force-deformation characteristics of the cushion and its physical dimensions. For fluid-filled support surfaces, immersion depends on the thickness of the surface and the flexibility of the cover. For elastic and viscoelastic support surfaces, immersion depends on their stiffness and thickness. Consider how the thickness of a seat cushion might limit the potential for immersion. If the seat cushion is 1.5″ (3.8 cm) in depth and the vertical distance between the ischial tuberosities and greater trochanters is 2″ (5 cm), the potential for immersion isn't enough to unload the ischial tuberosities.

Envelopment

Envelopment is the ability of a support surface to conform or mold around irregularities in the body.[5] Good envelopment implies that the surface conforms to the body without a substantial increase in pressure. Examples of irregularities are creases in clothing, bedding, or seat covers, and protrusions of bony prominences. A fluid support medium would envelop perfectly. However, surface tension plays an important role in envelopment. For example, a fluid-filled support surface such as a waterbed doesn't envelop as well as water alone. The membrane containing the water has surface tension, which has a hammocking effect on irregularities of the interface. Poorly enveloping support surfaces may cause high local peak pressures, thereby potentially increasing the risk of tissue breakdown.

Pressure gradient

Pressure gradient, also known *as pressure differential,* is defined as the change in pressure over a distance. Although various distances have been reported in the literature, it's expressed most commonly as a change in millimeters of mercury (mm Hg) per square centimeter or square inch. When the pressure across a surface is plotted on a graph, the slope of the curve is the pressure gradient. Because the skin and other soft tissues at risk for breakdown consist of a mixture of interstitial fluid and ground substance into which structural elements are embedded, a pressure differential between adjacent regions will result in a slowing of the flow of the tissue's fluid elements from a region of high pressure to one of lesser pressure. This flow is analogous to the movement produced when one compresses the surface of a bucket of wet sand with one's hand.

Several investigators have hypothesized that the flow of interstitial fluid caused by pressure gradients is the primary factor in the development of pressure ulcers.[6,7] The flow of ground substance and interstitial fluids from an area of high pressure is believed to increase the likelihood of intercellular contact, resulting in cellular ruptures.[6,7] This theory is consistent with the classic experimental results of several researchers showing a relationship between duration of pressure application and the magnitude of pressure that results in the formation of a pressure ulcer.[8,9]

Pressure gradient is intimately linked to pressure and is affected by immersion and envelopment in a similar manner. Under certain circumstances, it's possible to have pressure gradients without high pressure, and vice versa. For example, the boundary of the contact area on a support surface necessarily demonstrates a significant pressure gradient where the pressure magnitude transitions from zero outside the area of support to a nonzero value in the supported region. Despite these significant gradients, boundary areas are typically areas of lower risk for pressure ulcer development, suggesting that pressure gradient only becomes an important factor when combined with high pressure. Further research is needed to test and investigate this hypothesis.

Shear and friction reduction

Shear is an action or stress resulting from applied forces that causes or tends to cause two contiguous internal parts of the body to deform in the transverse plane. The term shear is commonly used to refer to the effect of a loading condition in which the skin surface remains stuck to a support surface while the underlying bony structure moves in a direction tangential to the surface. For example, when the head of a bed is raised or lowered, if the skin over the sacrum does not slide along the surface of the bed, or the bed does not absorb the resulting shear force by deforming in the horizontal direction, the effect will be a shearing of the soft tissue between the sacrum and the support surface. In engineering terms, the resulting shearing or deformation of the soft tissue would be referred to as "shear strain." The characteristics of the support surface affecting this potentially harmful situation are the coefficient of friction of the surface and the ability of the surface to deform horizontally. Some support surface technologies protect the skin from shear better than others. Shear as a contributing factor for pressure ulcers is currently a topic of international discussion. A task force

Friction and shear forces

This illustration shows the friction and shear forces acting on a person lying in bed.

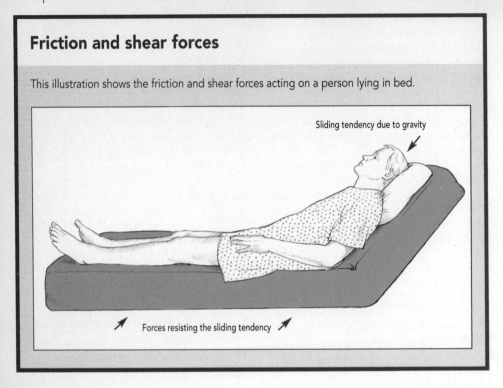

Sliding tendency due to gravity

Forces resisting the sliding tendency

is looking at ways to measure shear and quantify its effects on skin.[5]

Friction is the resistance to motion of the external tissue sliding in a parallel direction relative to the support surface resulting in external tissue damage.[5] Friction refers to the force acting tangential to the interface that opposes shear force. For example, when someone is pulled across a bed sheet during transfer, the frictional force prevents one from sliding off the surface. In a static condition (when a person is not sliding along the surface), the friction force is equivalent to the shear force at the surface. (See *Friction and shear forces*.)

The maximum friction is determined by the coefficient of friction of the support surface and the pressure. This is why surfaces with high coefficients of friction have the potential for producing high shear. Friction and shear are local phenomena and are affected by moisture on the skin. Moist or wet skin usually has a higher coefficient of friction and, as will be discussed below, is more susceptible to damage caused by shearing. Ironically friction is necessary to prevent a

person from simply sliding off the bed surface or wheelchair cushion. For optimal prevention of pressure ulcers, the friction necessary to prevent sliding should be applied in low-risk regions of the support surface and minimized near high-risk areas surrounding bony prominences.

Temperature control

One of the extrinsic factors in pressure ulcer development, temperature, has not been definitively investigated. However, some clinical trials have shown that the application of repetitive surface loading alone induces an elevated skin temperature of 41° F or greater.[10] In addition, peak skin temperatures have been found to be proportional to the magnitude and duration of the applied pressure.[10,11] The conclusions of research vary depending upon the amount and duration of pressure that's simultaneously applied with varying temperatures.[12,13]

In addition, higher ambient temperatures have been shown to cause an increase in tissue metabolism and oxygen consumption on the order of 10% for every 1.8° F increment.[14] Thus, patients with compromised tissue already at risk for pressure ulcers may have increased demands for oxygen in excess of their metabolic capabilities. Any increase in temperature in combination with pressure is believed to increase the susceptibility of the tissue to injury either from ischemia or reperfusion injury when the pressure is relieved.[15]

Also, it has been proven that increased temperature causes an exponential increase in blood perfusion, which has been associated with either an increase in core body temperature or in local skin temperature.[16,17] For example, in a study of operatively acquired pressure ulcers, the single greatest predictor of pressure ulcer development was the use of a warming blanket under the patient.[18] These findings clearly indicate the need for additional studies to definitively determine the effects of skin temperature modulation on the development of pressure ulcers. Therefore, when choosing the right support surface for the patient, its heat transfer rate is an objective performance measurement related to its ability to control temperature effects.

Moisture control

Moisture is another key extrinsic factor in pressure ulcer development. The sources of skin moisture that may predispose the skin to breakdown include perspiration, urine, feces, and fistula or wound drainage. Excessive moisture may lead to maceration of the skin.[19] Increases may be due to the slight increase in friction that occurs with light sweating[20] or to the increase in bacterial load resulting when alkaline sources of moisture neutralize the protection provided by the normal acid mantle of the skin.

The detrimental effect of an increase in moisture adjacent to the skin has been demonstrated by tensile tests on excised skin strips in a controlled humidity environment. In Wildnauer's study, the tensile strength of the strips decreased 75% with an increase in relative humidity from 10% to 98%.[21] Skin with such reduced strength may be more prone to mechanical damage from shear stress and could easily be abraded.[22-24]

Materials and components used in support surface systems

The components and materials described here are the most commonly used in support surface systems and may be used alone or in combination. They include foam, gel and gel pads, fluid-filled bladders, viscous fluid, and elastomers.

Foam

Foam may be elastic or viscoelastic and may be comprised of open or closed cells. Open-cell foam is defined as a permeable structure in which there's no barrier between cells, and gases or liquids can pass through the foam. Closed-cell foam is defined as a nonpermeable structure in which there's a barrier between cells, preventing gases or liquids from passing through the foam.

Elastic foam

Elastic foam is a type of porous polymer material that conforms in proportion to the applied load.[5] Consequently, greater loads result in predictably greater deformations, and vice versa. If time is a factor in the load versus deformation characteristic, the response is considered to be viscoelastic, which is discussed separately. The response of support surfaces made from resilient foam is predominately elastic. Foam is said to have "memory" because of its tendency to return to its nominal shape or thickness.

Foam products typically consist of foam layers of varying densities or combinations of gel and foam. Other products have a series of air-filled chambers covered with a foam structure or are available as multidensity, closed-cell products and may be 4″ to 10″ deep with deflectable tips. For these types of products, "memory" is not total because only the foam components will return to their unloaded shape. Several seat cushion products have this construction. Support surfaces with a combination of fluid-filled bladders and resilient foam provide a degree of postural stability with a resilient shell and improved en-

Elastic foam seat cushions

These photos show four different types of elastic foam seat cushions.

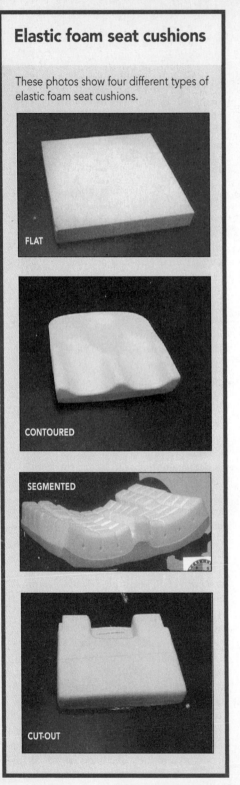

FLAT

CONTOURED

SEGMENTED

CUT-OUT

velopment with a fluid or viscous fluid-filled layer at the interface.

An ideal combination of characteristics for an elastic support surface is resistance that adjusts to the magnitude of compressive forces.[25,26] The support surface should have a high enough compression resistance to fully support the load (prevent bottoming-out) without providing too high a reactive force (memory) so that the interface pressure remains low. Over time and with extended use, foam degrades and loses its resilience. This decreased ability results in higher interface pressures. Krouskop[26] estimates that in approximately 3 years, a foam mattress wears out, and the compressive forces are transferred to the underlying supporting structure used to support the foam. In other words, the mattress "bottoms out."

Foams of varying densities may be combined or cut to relieve or conform to bony landmarks to enhance pressure distribution and even reduce shear forces. For example, multidensity, closed-cell foam products with deflectable tips provide some shear protection. Many pressure-reducing mattresses have loose-fitting covers to reduce friction.

Foam's stiffness and thickness limit its ability to immerse and envelop; soft foams will envelop better than stiffer foams, but will necessarily be thicker to avoid bottoming out. Foam seat cushions are typically contoured to improve their performance. Precontouring the seat cushion to provide a better match between the buttocks and the cushion increases the contact area and immersion, thereby reducing average pressure and pressure peaks.[27-29] (See *Elastic foam seat cushions*.)

Foam tends to increase skin temperature because its materials and the air they entrap are poor heat conductors. Moisture doesn't increase as much on foam products with a porous cover because the open-cell structure of the cover provides a pathway through which moisture can diffuse. Patient movement can also increase transfer rates. Mean temperature increases of 6.1° F (3.4° C) and a 10.4% increase in moisture at the skin surface have been recorded on foam products after 1 hour of contact.[30]

Viscoelastic foam

Viscoelastic foam is a type of porous polymer material that conforms in proportion to the applied load and to the rate of loading.[5] Viscoelastic foam products consist of temperature-sensitive, viscoelastic open-cell foam. At temperatures near that of the human body, the foam becomes softer, allowing the layer of foam nearest to the body to provide improved pressure distribution through envelopment and immersion when compared to high resilient foam. Viscoelastic foam acts like a self-contouring surface because the elastic response diminishes over time, even after the foam is compressed. However, the desirable temperature and time-sensitive responses of viscoelastic foam may not be realized when the ambient temperature is too low. The properties of viscoelastic foam products vary widely and must be chosen according to the specific needs of the patient for both seat and mattress applications. Solid gel products respond similarly to viscoelastic foam products and are included in this category.

Mean temperature increases of 5° F have been reported for viscoelastic foam.[30] Solid gel products tend to maintain a constant skin-contact temperature or may decrease the contact temperature. (See *Viscoelastic gel seat cushion*.)

Gel pads have higher heat flux than foam due to the high specific heat of the gel material. However, in Stewart's study,[30] the heat transfer decreased after 2 hours. This indicates that the heat reservoir was indeed filling, which suggests that the temperature may increase during longer periods—for example, more than 2 hours—of unrelieved sitting. Moisture increased 22.8% over a 1-hour period.[30] The relative humidity of the skin surface increases considerably because of the nonporous nature of the gel pads.

Fluid-filled bladders and compartments

Fluid-filled products may consist of small or large chambers filled with air, water, or other viscous fluid materials, such as silicon elastomer, silicon, or polyvinyl. The fluid flows from chamber to chamber or within a single chamber in response to movement and requires no supplemental power. The term "air-flotation" is sometimes used to describe interconnected multichamber surfaces. (See *Fluid-filled products*, page 212.)

Viscoelastic gel seat cushion

The photo shows a viscoelastic gel seat cushion. Viscoelastic products are also available in other shapes.

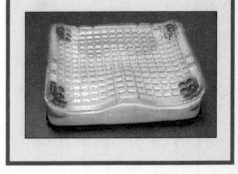

 PRACTICE POINT

Be careful to maintain the correct levels of inflation in air cushions to achieve optimal pressure reduction. Under-inflation causes bottoming out and over-inflation increases the interface pressure. For viscous fluid-filled surfaces, such as seat cushions, it's important to monitor the distribution of viscous material and manually move it back to the areas under bony prominences if it has moved away from these areas.

Most fluid-filled products permit a high degree of immersion, allowing the body to sink into the surface. The surface conforms to bony prominences, effectively increasing the surface-pressure distribution area and lowering the interface pressure by transferring the pressure to adjacent areas. These products are capable of achieving small to modest deformations without large restoring shear forces. In a direct comparison of interface pressures with air-fluidized and low-air-

Fluid-filled products

As the photos demonstrate, fluid-filled products come in a variety of forms.

ROHO CUSHION

RIK MATTRESS

Features of support surfaces

The features covered in this section can be used alone or in combination with other features. They include air-fluidized, low-air-loss, alternating pressure, and lateral rotation products.

Air-fluidized

A support surface with an air-fluidized feature provides pressure redistribution via a fluidlike medium created by forcing air through beads as characterized by immersion and envelopment.[5] These beds were originally developed in the late 1960s for use with burn patients. These products consist of granular materials such as silicon beads encased in a polyester or Gore-Tex sheeting. The granular material takes on the characteristics of a fluid when pressurized air is forced up through them. In some models (such as FluidAir, by KCI), the fluidization feature is variable, permitting individualization based on the patient's needs. These products aid in the reduction of evaporative water loss. Feces and other body fluids flow freely through the sheet; to prevent bacteriologic contamination, the bed must be pressurized at all times and the sheet must be properly disinfected after use by each patient and at least once per week with long-term use by a single patient.[32]

Air-fluidized beds use fluid technology to decrease pressure through the principle of immersion while simultaneously reducing shear. Air-fluidized products permit the highest degree of immersion currently available among support surfaces. The surface conforms to bony prominences by permitting deep immersion into the surface—almost two-thirds of the body may be immersed.[33] The immersion effectively lowers the interface pressure by increasing the surface-pressure distribution area. The greater deformations possible with this technology enable the transfer of pressure to adjacent body areas and other bony prominences. Envelopment and shear force are minimized. A loose but tightly woven polyester or Gore-Tex cover sheet is used to

loss beds, the Rik mattress was shown to relieve pressure as effectively as the air-fluidized and low-air-loss surfaces used in the study.[31]

Skin temperature is affected by the specific heat (ability to conduct heat) of the fluid material contained in the support device. Air has a low specific heat, and water has a high specific heat. The viscous material used in the RIK mattress also has a high specific heat, and skin temperature decreases have been demonstrated with this product.[31]

Given the large variety of materials used as covers in products falling into the fluid-filled category, it's difficult to generalize on the moisture control characteristics of these products. However, the insulating effects of rubber and plastic used in some fluid-filled products have been shown to increase the relative humidity due to perspiration.[30]

Air-fluidized and low-air-loss beds

AIR-FLUIDIZED BED   LOW-AIR-LOSS BED

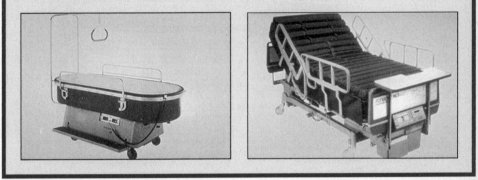

reduce surface tension. Low surface tension enhances envelopment and minimizes shear forces.

The pressurized air in these products is generally warmed to a temperature level of 82.4° to 95° F (28° to 35° C); however, warming may be beneficial or harmful depending on a patient's needs. For example, heat may be harmful to patients with multiple sclerosis, but beneficial for patients in pain. The beneficial effects must be balanced against the increasing metabolic demands of the tissue.

The high degree of moisture-vapor permeability of the air-fluidized system is effective in managing body fluids; in patients with severe burns, air-fluidized beds have been known to cause dehydration. (See *Air-fluidized and low-air-loss beds.*)

 PRACTICE POINT

Air-fluidized beds are advantageous for burn patients due to their effectiveness in managing body fluids.

Low-air-loss

Low-air-loss is a feature of a support surface that provides a flow of air to assist in managing the heat and humidity (microclimate) of the skin.[5] Low-air-loss systems use a series of connected, air-filled cushions or compartments, which are inflated to specific pressures to provide loading resistance based on the patient's height, weight, and distribution of body weight. An air pump circulates a continuous flow of air through the device, replacing air lost through the surface's pores. The inflation pressures of the cushions vary with the patient's weight distribution; some systems have individually adjustable sections for the head, trunk, pelvic, or foot areas.[34] As with other fluid-filled surfaces, the temperature of the skin is affected by the specific heat of the fluid material. However, the constant air circulation and evaporation tend to keep the skin from overheating.

In low-air-loss systems, the patient lies on a loose-fitting, waterproof cover placed over the cushions. The waterproof covers are designed to let air pass through the pores of the fabric and are usually made of a special nylon or polytetrafluoroethylene fabric with high moisture-vapor permeability. Manufacturers have addressed the problem of skin dehydration by altering the number, size, and configuration of the pores in the covers.[34] The material is very smooth, with a low coefficient of friction; in addition, it's impermeable to bacteria and easy to clean.[33] Low-air-loss devices have been shown to prevent build-up of moisture and subsequent skin maceration.[33]

Alternating-pressure integrated cushions

The photo shows the characteristics of alternating-pressure integrated cushions.

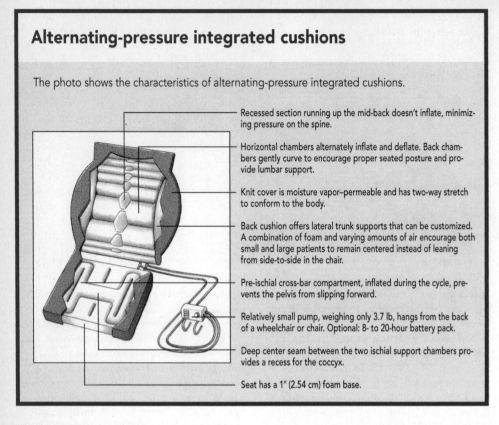

Recessed section running up the mid-back doesn't inflate, minimizing pressure on the spine.

Horizontal chambers alternately inflate and deflate. Back chambers gently curve to encourage proper seated posture and provide lumbar support.

Knit cover is moisture vapor–permeable and has two-way stretch to conform to the body.

Back cushion offers lateral trunk supports that can be customized. A combination of foam and varying amounts of air encourage both small and large patients to remain centered instead of leaning from side-to-side in the chair.

Pre-ischial cross-bar compartment, inflated during the cycle, prevents the pelvis from slipping forward.

Relatively small pump, weighing only 3.7 lb, hangs from the back of a wheelchair or chair. Optional: 8- to 20-hour battery pack.

Deep center seam between the two ischial support chambers provides a recess for the coccyx.

Seat has a 1" (2.54 cm) foam base.

Alternating pressure

Alternating pressure is a feature of a support surface that provides pressure redistribution via cyclic changes in loading and unloading as characterized by frequency, duration, amplitude, and rate of change parameters over the "active area" of the surface.[5] These systems contain air-filled chambers or cylinders arranged lengthwise or in various other patterns. Air or fluid is pumped into the chambers at periodic intervals to inflate and deflate the chambers in opposite phases, thereby changing the pressure distribution. The frequency of the alternating pressure feature can have an effect on its use. For example, very short peak inflation, and the cycling time appears to have a dramatic effect on increasing lymphatic flow.[35]

Rather than increasing the surface area for distribution through immersion and envelopment, alternating pressure devices distribute the pressure by shifting the body weight to a different surface-contact area. This may in-

crease the interface pressure of that area during the inflation phase.

Alternating pressure technology has the same potential as any other fluid-filled support surface to influence temperature at the interface, thus care must be taken to maintain the correct levels of inflation. The skin moisture control and temperature control characteristics of alternating pressure surface also depend on the characteristics of the cover and supporting material. (See *Alternating-pressure integrated cushions*.)

Lateral rotation

Lateral rotation is a feature of a support surface that moves the patient in a regular pattern around a longitudinal axis as characterized by degree of patient turn, duration, and frequency.[5] Although these devices have been used for several decades for other medical purposes, such as pulmonary therapy, research is conflicting on their use for pressure ulcer treatment.[36] Lateral rotation may be continuous (that is, on an automatic timed cycle) or manual, where the bed is rotated and locked in that position. The therapy works by positioning the patient in such a way so that one lung is higher than the other to prevent pneumonia. This therapy is not intended for patients with cervical or spinal fracture, intracranial pressure instability, or long-bone fractures.

Matching support to patient needs

Although widely used, support surfaces have neither performance standards nor criteria for function that can be tested against clinical outcomes. Indeed, the basis for effective function isn't known, or is poorly understood, for such common products as wheelchair seat cushions and horizontal support surfaces intended for skin protection and healing of wounds. Despite this, clinicians must have some basis for decision-making regarding the selection of these products. The following key questions should be used to guide the decision-making process.

What are the patient's specific load management needs?

Regardless of body position, the first step in determining an individualized protective intervention is to perform a general physical assessment and functional evaluation. Much of this information will then be used to assess the patient's risk for pressure ulcer development.

General physical examination and functional evaluation

Patient evaluation is described elsewhere in this text, however, additional items germane to the selection of a support surface include assessing the capability of the patient for specific bed mobility (movement on the surface, ingress and egress, and ability to place supportive devices); the number of available turning surfaces; the time spent in lying in bed or sitting per day; the number of devices or pillows needed for positioning, the patient's body weight and its distribution, and the presence of contractures.

Wheelchair cushion selection

For selection of wheelchair cushions, the evaluation is quite extensive because cushions are part of the total seating system that also includes the wheelchair. Indeed, no cushion can perform effectively in the prevention of pressure ulcers if the wheelchair isn't properly fitted. Therefore, it's recommended that a trained seating specialist perform the seat cushion evaluation and selection.

The seating evaluation should also include a mat examination to determine the functional postural limitations of the spine, pelvis, and extremities and to determine appropriate measurements for wheelchair fitting. An extensive functional examination is also required to consider the seating and mobility needs of the individual in the immediate, intermediate, and community environments.[37-39]

Strategies for maintaining tissue integrity can be extremely complicated for spinal cord-injured patients, elderly people, and other populations with degenerative neuromuscular conditions or diseases. For example, a patient's ability to sit unsupported can be characterized by the amount of external support needed to maintain posture: hands-free, hands-dependent, or prop-sitting with external support only.[39] This capability has significant implications for compensatory functional postures, ability to reposition, and the method used for intermittent pressure relief.

Specialty mattress selection

When selecting a specialty mattress, a patient's weight and the distribution of that weight are important factors. Indeed, each mattress overlay, replacement, or integrated bed unit has weight limits. For heavier patients, bariatric (bari) beds should be used. However, in patients approaching the manufacturer's recommended weight limits, the distribution of the weight should be examined. For example, patients who are heavier in the hip region, but who don't exceed the manufacturer's weight limit, may, in fact, need to be placed on a bariatric product to have effective pressure redistribution. Patients with contractures may have their weight dispersed unevenly. For example, contractures could pull heels into the groin or other body parts together and create special needs for tissue management beyond what a mattress can provide.

Assessing risk

The most commonly used risk assessment scales for prediction of pressure ulcer incidence are the Braden, Norton, and Waterlow scales.[40-42] The sensitivity and specificity of these scales vary depending on the population setting and the position of the patient's body. For example, different Braden cut-off scores are associated with different settings (nursing home versus intensive care unit), and in a recent study of risk assessment scales for general inpatients versus wheelchair users, the Waterlow outperformed the Braden.[43-45] Risk assessment scales specifically designed for wheelchair users are currently being developed.

Bergstrom and colleagues[45] reported that mattress selection based on categorizing patients via a pressure ulcer risk assessment scale produced both efficacious and cost-effective results. Patients of a large tertiary care hospital scoring nine or less on the Braden pressure ulcer risk assessment scale were provided a group 2 support surface (low-air-loss mattress) as a preventive measure. Those scoring above nine were evaluated and provided the most appropriate surface according to patient needs. Results indicated that not only did pressure ulcer incidence and prevalence drop by more than 50%, but costs associated with overlays, replacement mattresses, and low-air-loss beds also decreased.

Similar results have been realized by studies that selected wheelchair cushions from a set of cushion alternatives based upon risk assessment. Krouskop and colleagues[46] described how a seating clinic assigned risk to their clients with spinal cord injury by using such factors as gender, interface pressure, lifestyle, and stability. In 80% to 90% of the clients, cushions were selected from three al-

ternatives, with the remaining clients being provided other cushion types.

When assessing risk, remember that proper follow-up care is necessary to prevent pressure ulcers regardless of the cushion or bed prescribed. Skin redness often occurs because of positioning and use and doesn't necessarily indicate that a poor surface choice was made.

Clinical judgment

Clinicians should know how to evaluate bed or cushion performance, which includes an assessment of how adequately the product provides pressure redistribution, or if the patient is "bottoming out" or actually having soft tissues in close proximity to the hard undersurface. Clinicians should also observe any powered products for loss of power, sensor malfunctions, or disconnected hoses. Frequently checking the product's performance is especially important for patients who are unable to relay their discomfort due to cognitive or communication impairment.

Interface pressure-mapping

Interface pressure-mapping—comparison of a patient's relative responses from one surface to another—can be an effective clinical tool to aid in the selection of a support surface for a specific patient. Pressure-mapping may also be used to determine the relative effectiveness of modifications to the wheelchair and other positioning devices or to obtain information about pressure relief for patients with spinal cord injuries. For example, Henderson and colleagues used a pressure-mapping system to compare three methods of relieving pressure in seated individuals with spinal cord injuries.[47] The positions studied were tilted back 35 degrees, tilted back 65 degrees, and forward-leaning seated posture. The results indicated that the greatest pressure relief over the ischial tuberosities was seen in the forward-leaning position, followed by the 65-degree backward-tilt position. Observing the change in the pressure distribution on the mapping display allows patients without sensation to observe the effects of various weight-shifting methods and learn to consciously integrate them into their seated behavior.

Using clinical practice guidelines

Clinical practice guidelines offer recommendations, based on scientific evidence and the professional judgment of expert panels, about how health care professionals can provide quality care. The two most commonly referenced clinical practice guidelines in regard to support surface selection are:
• AHCPR Clinical Practice Guideline Number 15, "Treatment of Pressure Ulcers"[48]
• Consortium for Spinal Cord Medicine Clinical Practice Guideline, "Pressure Ulcer Prevention and Treatment Following Spinal Cord Injury."[49]

How does the product function and how well does it perform?

Answers to what the product does and how it performs should be sought from a variety of sources. Sources of information for support surfaces include marketing materials, controlled clinical trials, and objective indirect data from laboratory testing or clinical studies (interface pressure and other physiological responses).

Laboratory testing

What a support surface does has been largely determined by studies using laboratory methods to measure variables believed to be clinically relevant in pressure ulcer formation. For example, Krouskop's[50] study of foam mattress overlays provided the following recommended specifications for selection based on the results of independent laboratory testing:
• a thickness of 3″ to 4″ (7.5 to 10 cm)
• a density of 1.3 to 1.6 lb per cubic foot as an indicator of the amount of foam in the product
• a 25% indentation load deflection (ILD) equal to about 30 lb (the amount of force required to compress the foam to 75% of its thickness as an indicator of the foam's compressibility and conformability)
• a modulus of 2.5 or greater (the ratio of 60% ILD to 25% ILD).

Support surface and cushion standards

Standards have been developed for wheelchair seat cushions and are under development for other support surfaces. Publishing national or international standards for support surfaces requires that uniform test methods be developed to quantify clinically relevant characteristics. Simply stated, to make valid comparisons among products, characteristics and properties need to be measured using the same test and under the same conditions. Testing conditions should model clinically relevant parameters as closely as possible. The requirement that the tests be repeatable across laboratories in different countries means that standardized tests typically use models rather than human subjects. Clinicians, therefore, must consider test results as relative measures.

The results of standard tests often don't include pass-fail criteria. Just as there are valid reasons to purchase an automobile with a big engine that only gets 15 mpg over another with a little engine that gets 25 mpg, so are there reasons to purchase support surfaces with, for example, a lower pressure distribution characteristic but higher moisture dissipation ability over a product with a higher pressure distribution characteristic but lower moisture dissipation ability. The primary objectives of the standard tests are to characterize their different functional properties and to permit comparisons of performance among products with similar functions.

The range of products on the market places a heavy burden on clinicians to keep abreast of new technology; therefore, patients, clinicians, vendors, manufacturers, third-party payers, and researchers all benefit from standard terminology, definitions, and test methods. Clinicians benefit from a mechanism to objectively match a seat cushion or support surface's characteristics to the needs of their patients.[21] Vendors benefit by being able to clearly describe products from different manufacturers in a manner understood by clinicians and patients. Testing standards aid manufacturers by guiding new product development and assisting in the redesign of existing products. In addition, standards promote quality assurance within manufacturing processes. The final potential beneficiaries of standards are third-party payers because the seat cushion and support surface market is a payer's market; that is, payer reimbursement drives the market. A validated system to test and objectively characterize support surfaces will give funding agencies an objective means for funding decisions. In fact, standards form the basis for certain tests used by funding agencies to classify or categorize products.

Seat cushion standards

Standards for seat cushions are being developed by the International Standards Organization (ISO). In the United States, the effort is organized through the Rehabilitation Engineering and Assistive Technology Society of North America as an accredited standards organization for the American National Standards Institute.[23,24] One of the four interrelated working groups focuses on tissue integrity management and has developed test methods that address key performance features of cushions, including load deflection and hysteresis, frictional properties, lateral and forward stiffness, sliding resistance, impact damping, recovery, loaded contour depth and overload deflection, water spillage, and biocompatibility.[51] Additional tests are being developed that measure heat and water vapor transmissibility and stability of properties with use (fatigue). Although all these tests have clinical relevance, a subset is described below. And, even though tests have been designed for seat cushions, the constructs are described in relation to both cushions and horizontal support surfaces to illustrate key concepts.

Load deflection

Materials used in mattresses and cushions support the body by compression (foam and air), deflection (gel and viscous fluid), or tension (bladder material and fabric). Material stiffness impacts how materials deform to accommodate the body. Load deflection tests typically involve loading a cushion or support surface with a standardized indentor that mimics a part(s) of the body. Deflection into the support surface is measured as the weight on the indentor is increased.

Clinically, materials can be too stiff or too soft. When too stiff, the body does not immerse, and high pressures or instability can result. When too soft, materials can "bottom-out," leading to poor support and high pressures. Foams are made with different stiffness ratings, called Indentation Force Deflection. Many products use a combination of foam with a softer material positioned on top of a more stiff material. This configuration permits deflection of the top surface while protecting against bottoming-out through the use of the stiffer bottom layer.

Because the amount of air impacts the stiffness of a support surface or cushion, products that use air are often adjustable. Too much air leads to an overly stiff surface, and too little air can lead to bottoming-out. In addition to body weight, the amount of tissue, the type of tissue (hypotonic, normal, hypertonic), and a person's posture or position all influence how stiff a surface must be to adequately support a person.[52]

Frictional properties

Friction is the result of a relationship between materials; so standardized tests for friction measure the sliding forces of one material on another. In terms of cushions and support surfaces, these standardized tests concentrate on cover materials, such as fabrics and bed linens.

Sliding resistance

Unlike friction tests, which focus on cover material, sliding resistance tests measure the influence of the entire system, including the cover and all support materials. All users of support surfaces and cushions have to transfer onto and off the bed or wheelchair. For people who can't fully transfer, certain materials and designs facilitate easier transfers. However, if a support is too easy to slide upon, stability on that surface can be compromised. Standardized tests of sliding resistance involve loading the surface with an indentor modeled on the human body or buttocks and pulling it forward or sideways. The force required to slide the indentor on the surface is measured and reflects sliding resistance.

Loaded contour depth and overload test
This test measures the immersion of a standardized indentor into a cushion surface. Clinically, this test provides two key pieces of information about seat cushions: the initial contour of a cushion and the amount of deflection that may occur when someone sits upon it. The overload portion of the test adds 33% more weight and measures additional immersion of the indentor. A cushion that has "bottomed-out" will not deflect further under the additional weight. A support surface should maintain a margin of safety that allows additional cushioning during overload conditions. Certain functional movements and postural adjustments, such as leaning and reaching, impart an overload condition on the surface.

As noted, several standardized tests have been developed for wheelchair cushions by the ISO. A similar approach focusing on horizontal support surfaces began a few years ago by the National Pressure Ulcer Advisory Panel (NPUAP). Most of these tests are or will be voluntary. Therefore, all stakeholders should request test results as a means to compare performance across products and also to encourage this voluntary testing and disclosure.

Product effectiveness

The effectiveness of a support service product is measured by two methods: its efficacy in use by patients and in comparison to similar products. Several articles provide an overview of support surface research.[53-56] Rather than basing comparisons on functional classification, most studies compared classes of products based on the product's ability to redistribute pressure.

Considering the limitations ascribed to interface pressure measurement, it may be more useful to categorize devices according to their ability to evenly distribute pressure over the contact surface area rather than ascribe any significance to the magnitude of pressure measured at a particular location.[57] However, the most common comparison has been the use of interface pressure to compare a product against a "standard" hospital bed or mattress. When reviewing this literature,

remember that the "standard" support surface probably varies from study to study. Most studies also vary in the patient population (for example, orthopedic or neurologic) and setting studied (for example, acute care, intensive care, long-term care, and home care). All three independent variables (products compared, subject population, setting) affect both outcomes and the interpretation of results. Finally, when comparing performance studies, remember that treatment studies, in which subjects already have ulcers, are fundamentally different from prevention studies.

Prevention effectiveness

Generally, studies have shown that nonpowered, constant low-pressure supports (foam, air, gel, and combinations of these materials) are more effective in preventing pressure ulcers than a "standard" hospital mattress. Generalization of the results of studies comparing different pressure redistribution products is difficult. Most comparative studies of various constant low-force products demonstrated no differences in the prevention of pressure ulcers.[58,59]

Conclusions from research investigating the more complex technology, including low-air-loss and alternating-pressure products, are similar. Evidence suggests that both low-air-loss and alternating-pressure surfaces are more effective than "standard" mattresses, but comparative studies of the performance of low-air-loss and alternating-pressure products are inconsistent regarding the clinical superiority of one over the other. Moreover, comparisons of alternating-pressure to constant low-pressure products have not produced definitive differences.

Because the evidence is not definitive, clinicians must carefully read the original study to generalize the results to a specific clinical situation. The characteristics of the population, setting, and products must closely match one's clinical situation and the limitations of the study must be known when considering its clinical applicability. For example, consider the design of alternating-pressure products where such variables as cell height or bladder thickness and cycle timing and frequency can significantly affect product performance. One can't necessarily generalize the performance of one alternating-pressure product to another. Similarly, the results of a support surface study within acute care might not produce similar results within home care using the same support surfaces.

Evidence about specific cushions and their respective effectiveness is insufficient. Contradictions also exist in the literature regarding the clinical benefits of cushions designed to reduce the risk of sitting-acquired pressure ulcers. Most research has used indirect outcomes, such as interface pressure or blood flow. Relatively few studies have measured direct outcomes related to specific types of cushions,[22,60-62] but these have not resulted in definitive findings of efficacy of one product over another. One facility performed two studies targeting elderly wheelchair users. The first study found no difference in the incidence of pressure ulcers in users of flat foam compared to custom-contoured foam cushions, and a subsequent study found more users of flat foam (41%) developed ulcers compared to users of a contoured foam-viscous fluid cushion (25%), but this difference did not reach statistical significance. In a study tracking interface pressure and wheelchair cushions in elderly users, Brienza and colleagues[62] found interface pressures were higher for subjects who developed sitting-acquired pressure ulcers compared to those who didn't develop ulcers. No definitive relationship was found between interface pressures and cushion types across these subjects.

Treatment effectiveness

Widely varying subject populations and care settings have complicated the ability to compare results across studies investigating the effectiveness of support surfaces in the treatment for pressure ulcers. Furthermore, a number of treatment outcome measures have been used to judge effectiveness, such as the relative or actual reduction in ulcer size (area or volume), the percentage of ulcers healed within a specified time period, and the time until wound closure. Different operational definitions have also been used for wound

status, such as "healed" and "closure," making it difficult to compare equitably.

Generally, studies targeting support surfaces for ulcer treatment have produced results similar to those targeting prevention. Low-air-loss and air-fluidized surfaces have been shown to improve treatment outcomes more effectively compared to "conventional" treatment[63,64] and nonpowered foam alternatives.[54,55] Results of alternating pressure surfaces studies are inconsistent with some studies showing a treatment effect and others showing none. No clinically significant treatment differences have been shown among similar products.

What other patient needs must be met?

While load management and product function are critical areas to consider in matching patient support needs, we must also consider pressure relief. This can be done through turning and repositioning, heel protection and managing heel pressure.

Turning and repositioning schedules

The frequency of repositioning required to prevent ischemia is variable and unknown, yet regular repositioning is believed to help deter the deleterious effects of pressure by decreasing the duration of exposure. Through the process of repositioning, the body's weight is redistributed, and new pressure areas are introduced. To provide effective pressure relief, both pressure and time must be considered. For example, in 1961, Kosiak recommended that repositioning be done in intervals of 1 to 2 hours based on the interface readings from healthy subjects.[65] This view has also been endorsed by the Agency for Health Care Research and Quality (AHRQ), in its clinical practice guideline.[4]

Turning schedules have been studied empirically and experimentally. Bliss[66] studied turning schedules in a spinal injury ward and found that 2 hours was adequate for some, whereas others required more frequent, and some, less frequent, turning. An important aspect of these findings is that some patients exhibited redness after 2 hours, and that many patients disliked frequent turning.

In an experimental study by Knox and colleagues,[67] variables such as temperature, pressure, and redness were monitored while people rested on a mattress for 60, 90, and 120 minutes. Some subjects exhibited redness after each of the intervals, leading the researchers to conclude that a 2-hour turning schedule might not be sufficient.

Such theoretical evidence points directly to the duration of loading as the way to maintain tissue integrity. If, however, the above experiment is only one example of patients experiencing redness after less than a 2-hour turning schedule, then it cannot be construed as the answer for all clinical practices.

In addition, no knowledge exists as to how turning schedule should be affected by support services. Therefore, the best approach is to evaluate and reevaluate each patient to best determine an appropriate turning schedule.

Positioning

In addition to the AHRQ guidelines for repositioning and turning, a number of recommendations exist in regard to positioning for management of tissue loads. (See *AHRQ positioning guidelines.*)

The following eight positions are commonly used to reposition patients on horizontal surfaces:
• a prone position with rotation of 30 degrees to the right or left
• a supine position with 30 degrees of rotation to the right or left
• a supine position with slight right or left sacral relief[68]
• a supine position with the head of the bed elevated 30 degrees or less and the feet blocked
• a supine position with the head of the bed elevated 30 degrees or less and the knees flexed with the bed. (See *Horizontal positioning,* page 222.)

In all of these positions, the heels must be elevated with pillows or other devices. Note the use of pillows and towels to separate and protect bony prominences. Additional posi-

> ## AHRQ positioning guidelines
>
> The Agency for Health Care Research and Quality (AHRQ) 1992 guidelines for positioning include the following:
> • Keep the patient's heels protected and elevated off the surface of the bed.
> • Maintain the elevation of the head of the bed at 30 degrees or less if medical status permits.
> • Turn or reposition the patient's body at least every 2 hours.
> • Note that the use of pressure reducing surfaces doesn't replace turning schedules.
> • Limit the patient's lateral rotation to 30 degrees from the supine or prone position to avoid direct loading of the greater trochanter.
> • Position the patient's body to avoid loading over an existing ulcer or wound.
> • Eliminate the use of "donut" type devices.
> • Use pillows or wedges to separate bony prominences.

tioning technique includes blocking the feet and knees in a flexed position to prevent shear forces created when the patient slides down in bed.

Small shifts in weight can also be accomplished by positioning. For instance, foam wedges or pillows, used to position the patient on his side, can be altered slightly every 15 minutes. Pulling them out gradually over 1 to 1½ hours shifts the weight slightly. If the patient is in a wheelchair, he still requires shifts in his body weight. If possible, this patient should be taught to shift his weight every 15 minutes with repositioning every hour.

Horizontal positioning

The following illustrations show how to position patients properly on horizontal surfaces.

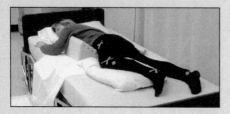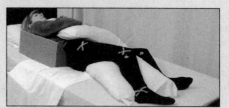

30-degree rotation from prone and supine positions, respectively

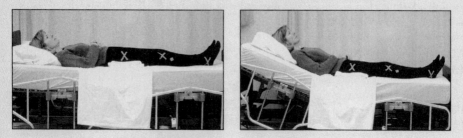

Head of the bed elevated 30 degrees or less with unilateral sacral relief and feet blocked, respectively

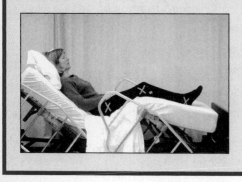

Head of the bed elevated 30 degrees with knees flexed to prevent shearing at the sacrum

Heel protection

The heel presents unique challenges for pressure-reducing interventions due to its small radius of curvature and its thin layer of subcutaneous tissue between the skin and calcaneal structures.[71] This small contact area affords minimal protection from the pressure exerted by the weight of the foot and, frequently, a portion of the lower limb. The lower limb is approximately one-sixth of the total body weight, so, even if a small proportion of this rests on the heel, high interface pressure may result, even on air support systems. Therefore, the AHRQ guideline[4] recommends using additional pressure-reducing devices for immobile patients' heels.

In addition, heel ulcers are especially painful and are among the most difficult to heal.[70] Indeed, the sequelae of heel pressure ulcers can be devastating, possibly resulting in infection and, in extreme cases, amputation of the foot. Also, the costs associated with heel pressure ulcers increase proportionally with morbidity and length of hospital stay, underscoring the importance of prevention in high-risk patients.

Existing clinical practice guidelines recommend the use of pillows to suspend the heels.[4,71] However, pillows don't protect against footdrop and, due to patient movement, pillows require time and diligent positioning to maintain proper suspension. To provide continuous heel suspension via heel protective devices, clinicians must consider proper fit, turning schedules and number of turning surfaces, patient position, the presence of additional equipment, as well as the performance characteristics of the product. Clinical requirements for pressure-reducing heel protection include:

• reducing pressure, friction, and shear
• separating and protecting the ankles
• maintaining heel suspension
• permitting repositioning without increasing pressure in other areas
• preventing footdrop
• enhancing patient comfort
• increasing nursing time-efficiency.

Evidence for managing heel pressure

Relatively few studies of heel protection devices have been completed in the past decade. However, of those studies that have been explored, the majority of them have examined the pressure distribution capabilities of heel wraps, heel dressings, pillows, water-filled gloves, and various specialty heel products using interface pressure or pressure ulcer incidence as the primary outcomes, which we will examine here.[72]

As with other support surfaces, most products consist of a combination of materials and incorporate multiple strategies to optimize their therapeutic function. The distribution of pressure on a heel support surface depends on the relative fit between the heel and the surface, the mechanical properties of the heel tissue and the device, and the distribution of weight in the body part (heel). An ideal pressure distribution is one in which soft-tissue shape isn't altered relative to its unloaded condition.[73]

In a study designed to investigate the efficacy of clinically "familiar" heel devices, the preventive use of routine nursing care, hydro-

colloid dressings, egg-crate foam, polyester-filled heel boots, and foam footdrop splints were compared in geriatric, orthopedic patients at risk for pressure ulcers.[74,75] In a similar study, 4" × 4" gauze pads, in combination with an absorbent pad and gauze roll and a laminated foam boot (Lunax Boot by Bio-Sonics), were compared in at-risk intensive care patients with heel redness.[76] Although both studies lacked various aspects of statistical analyses limiting their interpretation, the egg-crate boot and laminated foam boot were more effective in preventing pressure ulcers, whereas other methods either increased incidence or, as in the case of the footdrop splints, were uncomfortable despite their ability to effectively suspend the heel. What's notable about this study is that despite routine nursing care, consisting of heel observation every 2 to 3 hours with subsequent pressure ulcer care, as needed, (direct pressure relief and repositioning of patients heels), deterioration of the heel tissue still ensued. However, a similar study's simultaneous use of heel elevation with a pillow or bath blanket under the calf, the Spenco Silicore quilted heel protector, and prompt reporting of heel discomfort by patients to the nursing staff resulted in zero incidence of pressure ulcers in 30 hip replacement patients.[77]

In an additional survey on the use of water-filled examination gloves, it would appear that they are an inexpensive method of decreasing heel pressure and a fairly common practice as 79.4% of nurses surveyed reported routine use of this method.[78] This same study found significantly higher heel interface pressures using a water-filled glove method as compared to a conventional mattress (144.6 mm Hg; 126.5 mm Hg). Thus, nursing staff may need to reevaluate the efficacy of their heel protection interventions if they are only using a conventional mattress.

Flemister[79] also examined heel interface pressures with use of both a foam and polyester heel protector in seven patients assessed at moderate to high risk for pressure ulcer development. The foam heel protector marginally reduced heel interface pressures (1.3 mm Hg), whereas the polyester protector actually resulted in a significant increase in interface pressure.

While there are a variety of heel protective devices commercially available, the results seem to vary across the board. The few studies that have been performed suggest that while matching the device to the patient may be challenging, with careful consideration of patient needs and characteristics, it can be done

What's available in this setting?

A patient's needs can change over the course of his illness. A product that's appropriate for acute care use may not work in the patient's home. Clinical judgment should examine therapy goals (ease of getting into or out of the bed for therapy or mobility), ability of the patient to move himself in the bed, other complications (heel breakdown, pulmonary complications), and body weight/weight distribution.

What's practical?

The issue of practicality relates to the overall care plan, the goals of load management (prevention versus treatment), how complicated the product is to use, and whether it will be operated by a health care professional, family member, or the patient. Many hospitals, long-term care facilities, and home care agencies have developed product selection guidelines that are usually presented as an algorithm[4] or graph. These guidelines are typically based on the availability of equipment from previous purchases in accordance with other published guidelines. Another common method used in selection and purchasing decisions is the subjective assessment of equipment based on a trial use in the clinical setting. This gives the staff a chance to use the equipment in a variety of situations and judge its performance.

How easy is the product to use?

Equipment that's easy to use has been associated with successful compliance. Awkward design or difficult assembly may cause the patient and his family to abandon using the equipment or increase the likelihood of misuse. Directions must be clear and obvious. For example, if the product is powered, it should have a battery back-up to facilitate transferring patients to other locations as needed.

What service and maintenance is available?

A 24-hour call service with on-site repair or replacement is essential.

What type of alarm system does the product have?

Visual alarms are rarely sufficient, especially if the alarm is obscured under the bed. In the home-care setting, visible alarms are of little value unless there's constant attendance.

Is the equipment easily maintained?

If the equipment must be deflated for storage, reinflation time may be critical as well as the ability to deflate the equipment in the event of a cardiac arrest. Additionally, if the product isn't a personal use item, one must consider how long it takes to clean and ready the item for subsequent use.

What operating mechanism and space requirements does the product have?

If the product has some form of movement, is cessation possible to facilitate such procedures as bedpan usage and hygiene care? Is the product the correct size for the home or setting where it will be used? Is the floor structure sound and capable of holding the weight of the bed? Will the bed fit through the door?

How much does the product cost?

Technology has produced some innovative treatment products, but costs are high for patients, insurance companies, and hospitals. Prevention is more cost-effective than any other treatment. Available technology (support surfaces) may provide solutions when used correctly by properly educated staff. Indeed, one recent study demonstrated that educated staff can reduce the number of pressure ulcers better than noneducated staff. The same study indicated that the cost of care is significantly less under the supervision of educated staff.[69]

The cost of support surfaces varies. Third-party reimbursement (Medicare may provide coverage), rental versus purchase, and cost-benefit issues need to be carefully evaluated. Some devices are only available on a rental basis. Although reimbursement is an issue in any setting, operational costs are of particular importance if the product is used in the home care setting where costs will be absorbed by the patient.

Consideration should also be given to the projected number of days that a support surface will be in use. More patients are being placed on advanced technology surfaces for considerably longer periods of time. Cost-effectiveness may be measured by relating the cost of the product to its efficacy.

PRACTICE POINT

Consider these patient factors before purchasing support surfaces:

- Ease of use
- Operational costs of the equipment
- Service contracts and back-up service
- Alarm systems
- Daily maintenance
- Operating mechanisms and space requirements

When managing the allocation of specialty mattress and bed systems, a continuous process of evaluation and reevaluation should be employed to ensure that the patient's needs are reassessed on a regular basis.

Summary

Understanding the nature of pressure ulcer etiology, the factors affecting pressure redistribution, and other physical factors associated with the use of specific support surface products and heel protection products is a necessity for nursing and other health care personnel involved with tissue integrity management. As standardized test methods are developed for support surface products, the clinical validation of specialized protective devices and the development of clinical practice guidelines will be possible. Until then, matching products to patient needs is a challenging process and must be based on the available evidence regarding the performance characteristics of existing support surfaces. Continued research in heel protection is needed.

Heels in patients at risk for pressure ulcers require additional protection beyond the use of specialty beds and mattress overlays. Although existing clinical practice guidelines recommend the use of pillows to suspend the heels, pillows don't protect against footdrop, require time and attention to positioning details, and can't protect the heels continuously due to patient movement. To provide continuous heel suspension via heel protective devices, clinicians must consider proper fit, turning schedules and number of turning surfaces, patient position, the presence of additional equipment, and the performance characteristics of the product when selecting heel protection devices.

Show what you know

1. The feature of a support surface primarily indicated for pulmonary therapy that provides rotation about a longitudinal axis as characterized by degree of patient turn, duration, and frequency is called:

A. low-air-loss.
B. alternating pressure.
C. air-fluidized.
D. lateral rotation.

ANSWER: D. Lateral rotation moves side to side to aid pulmonary function, but unless a second feature is present such as low-air-loss, it's not appropriate for pressure ulcer prevention.

2. The selection of an appropriate support surface depends on:

A. the clinical condition of the patient.
B. the characteristics of the support surface.
C. the characteristics of the care setting.
D. all of the above.

ANSWER: D. All are important considerations. A patient at home may have different needs than one in an acute care setting.

3. *Support surfaces are designed to:*

A. lower pressure.
B. eliminate pressure.
C. redistribute pressure.
D. relieve pressure.

ANSWER: C. Support surfaces redistribute pressure.

4. *The ability of a support surface to distribute load over the contact areas of the human body is:*

A. immersion.
B. envelopment.
C. pressure gradient.
D. pressure redistribution.

ANSWER: D. This is the newly revised National Pressure Ulcer Advisory Panel definition of pressure redistribution. Immersion is the depth of penetration into a support surface. Envelopment is the ability of a support surface to conform to the body irregularities. Pressure gradient is a change in pressure over a distance.

References

1. Krouskop, T., and van Rijswijk, L. "Standardizing Performance-Based Criteria for Support Surfaces," *Ostomy/Wound Management* 41(1):34-44, January-February 1995.
2. Cochran, G. "Identification and Control of Biophysical Factors Responsible for Soft Tissue Breakdown," *RSA Progress Report*, 1979.
3. Silver-Thorn, M. "In Vivo Indentation of Lower Extremity Limb Soft Tissues," *IEEE Transactions on Rehabilitation Engineering* 7(3):268-77, September 1999.
4. AHCPR. *Pressure Ulcers in Adults: Prediction and Prevention.* AHCPR Clinical Practice Guideline No. 3. Rockville, Md.: Agency for Health Care Policy and Research, Public Health Service, U.S. Department of Health and Human Services. Publication No. 92-0047, 1992.
5. National Pressure Ulcer Advisory Panel (NPUAP). Support Surface Initiative. NPUAP, Support Surface Standards Initiative—Terms and Definitions, March 2006. Available at: *www.npuap.org.* Accessed June 11, 2006.
6. Krouskop, T.A. "A Synthesis of the Factors That Contribute to Pressure Sore Formation," *Medical Hypotheses* 11(2):255-67, June 1983.
7. Reddy, N.G., et al. "Interstitial Fluid Flow as a Factor in Decubitus Ulcer Formation," *Journal of Biomechanics* 14(12):879-81, December 1981.
8. Daniel, R.D., et al. "Etiologic Factors in Pressure Sores: An Experimental Model," *Archives of Physical Medicine and Rehabilitation* 62(10):492-98, October 1981.
9. Reswick, J., and Rogers, J. *Experiences at Rancho Los Amigos Hospital with Devices and Techniques to Prevent Pressure Sores. Bedsore Biomechanics.* London: University Park Press, 1976.
10. Vistnes, L. "Pressure Sores: Etiology and Prevention," *Bulletin of Prosthetic Research* 17:123-25, 1980.
11. Verhonick, P.D., et al. "Thermography in the Study of Decubitus Ulcers," *Nursing Research* 21:233-37, May-June 1972.
12. Patel, S.C., et al. "Temperature Effects on Surface Pressure-Induced Changes in Rat Skin Perfusion: Implications in Pressure Ulcer Development," *Journal of Rehabilitation Research and Development* 36(3):189-201, May-June 1999.
13. Kokate, J.K., et al. "Temperature-Modulated Pressure Ulcers: A Porcine Model," *Archives of Physical Medicine and Rehabilitation* 76(7):666-73, July 1995.
14. Brown, A., and Brengelmann, G. *Energy Metabolism. Physiology and Biophysics.* Philadelphia: W.B. Saunders Co., 1965.
15. Fisher, S.T., et al. "Wheelchair Cushion Effect on Skin Temperature," *Archives of Physical Medicine and Rehabilitation* 59(2):68-72, February 1978.
16. Johnson, J.M., and Park, M. "Reflex Control of Skin Blood Flow by Skin Temperature: Role of Core Temperature," *Journal of Applied Physiology* 47(6):1188-93, December 1979.
17. Johnson, J.M., et al. "Reflex Regulation of Sweat Rate by Skin Temperature in Exercising Humans," *Journal of Applied Physiology* 56(5):1283-88, May 1984.
18. Aronovitch, S. "A Comparative Study of an Alternating Air Mattress for the Prevention of Pressure Ulcers in Surgical Patients," *Ostomy/Wound Management* 45(3):34-44, March 1999.
19. Yarkony, G. "Pressure Ulcers: A Review," *Archives of Physical Medicine and Rehabilitation* 75(8):908-17, August 1994.
20. Sulzberger, M., et al. "Studies on Blisters Produced by Friction: Results of Linear Rubbing and Twisting Techniques," *Journal of Investigational Dermatology* 47(5):456-65, November 1966.
21. Wildnauer, R.H., et al. "Stratum Corneum Biomechanical Properties: Influence of Relative Humidity on Normal and Extracted Human Stratum Corneum," *Journal of Investigational Dermatology* 56(1):72-78, January 1971.
22. Geyer, M.J., et al. "A Randomized Control Trial to Evaluate Pressure-Reducing Seat Cushion for Elderly Wheelchair Users," *Advances in Skin & Wound Care* 14(3):120-29, May-June 2001.
23. Cochran, G.V., and Palmieri, V. "Development of Test Methods for Evaluation of Wheelchair Cushions," *Bulletin of Prosthetics Research* 33:9-30, Spring 1980.
24. Sprigle, S.L., et al. "Development of Uniform Terminology and Procedures to Describe Wheelchair Cushion Characteristics," *Journal of Rehabilitation Research and Development* 38(4):449-61, July-August 2001.
25. Noble, P.C., et al. "The Influence of Environmental Aging Upon the Load-Bearing Properties of Polyurethane Foams," *Journal of Rehabilitation Research and Development* 21(2):31-38, July 1984.
26. Krouskop, T., et al. "Evaluating the Long-Term Performance of a Foam-Core Hospital Replacement Mattress," *Journal of Wound, Ostomy, and Continence Nursing* 21(6):241-46, November 1994.
27. Sprigle, S., et al. "Reduction of Sitting Pressures with Custom Contoured Cushions," *Journal of*

Rehabilitation Research and Development 27(2):135-40, Spring 1990.

28. Brienza, D.M., et al. "A System for the Analysis of Seat Support Surfaces Using Surface Shape Control and Simultaneous Measurement of Applied Pressures," *IEEE Transactions on Rehabilitation Engineering* 4(2):103-13, June 1996.

29. Brienza, D.M., and Karg, P.E. "Seat Cushion Optimization: A Comparison of Interface Pressure and Tissue Stiffness Characteristics for Spinal Cord Injured and Elderly Patients," *Archives of Physical Medicine and Rehabilitation* 79(4):388-94, April 1998.

30. Stewart, S., et al. "Wheelchair Cushion Effect on Skin Temperature, Heat Flux and Relative Humidity," *Archives of Physical Medicine and Rehabilitation* 61(5):229-33, May 1980.

31. Wells, J., and Karr, D. "Interface Pressure, Wound Healing and Satisfaction in the Evaluation of a Non-Powered Fluid Mattress," *Ostomy/Wound Management* 44(2):38-54, February 1998.

32. Peltier, G., et al. "Controlled Air Suspension: An Advantage in Burn Care," *Journal of Burn Care Research* 8(6):558-60, November-December 1987.

33. Holzapfel, S. "Support Surfaces and their Use in the Prevention and Treatment of Pressure Ulcers," *Journal of Enterostomal Nursing* 20(6):251-60, November-December 1993.

34. Weaver, V., and Jester, J. "A Clinical Tool: Updated Readings on Tissue Interface Pressure," *Ostomy/Wound Management* 40(5):34-43, June 1994.

35. Gunther, R., and Brofeldt, B. "Increased Lymphatic Flow: Effect of a Pulsating Air Suspension Bed System," *Wounds: A Compendium of Clinical Research and Practice* 8(4):134-40, 1996.

36. Anderson, C., and Rappl, L. "Lateral Rotation Mattress for Wound Healing," *Ostomy/Wound Management* 50(4): 50-4, 56, 58, April 2004.

37. Engstrom, B. Seating for Independence. *Ergonomic Seating and Propulsion Improves Performance.* Presentation, Pittsburgh, Pa., August 1997.

38. Waugh, K. *Therapeutic Seating I: Principles and Assessment.* Pittsburgh, Pa: RESNA, 1997.

39. Minkel, J. "Seating and Mobility Considerations for People with Spinal Cord Injuries," *Physical Therapy* 80(7):701-709, July 2000.

40. Braden, B.J. and Bergstrom, N. "Clinical Utility of the Braden Scale for Predicting Pressure Sore Risk," *Decubitus* 2(3):44-46, 50-51, August 1989.

41. Norton, D. "Norton Scale for Decubitus Prevention," [German] *Krankenpflege* 34(1):16, 1980.

42. Waterlow, J. "Pressure Sores: A Risk Assessment Card," *Nursing Times* 81(48):49-55, November 27-December 3, 1985.

43. Braden, B., and Bergstrom, N. "Predictive Validity of the Braden Scale for Pressure Sore Risk in a Nursing Home Population," *Research in Nursing and Health* 17(6):459-70, December 1994.

44. Anthony, D., et al. "An Evaluation of Current Risk Assessment Scales for Decubitus Ulcer in General Inpatients and Wheelchair Users," *Clinical Rehabilitation* 12(2):136-42, April 1998.

45. Bergstrom, N., et al. "Using a Research-Based Assessment Scale in Clinical Practice," *Nursing Clinics of North America* 30(3):539-50, September 1995.

46. Krouskop, T.A., et al. "Custom Selection of Support Surfaces for Wheelchairs and Beds: One Size Doesn't Fit All," *Dermatology Nursing* 4(3):191-94, 204, June 1992.

47. Henderson, J.L., et al. "Efficacy of Three Measures to Relieve Pressure in Seated Persons with Spinal Cord Injury," *Archives of Physical Medicine and Rehabilitation* 75(5):535-39, May 1994.

48. Agency for Healthcare, Policy and Research. "Treatment of Pressure Ulcers," Publication No. 95-0652, 1994.

49. Consortium for Spinal Cord Medicine. Pressure Ulcer Prevention and Treatment Following Spinal Cord Injury: A Clinical Practice Guideline for Health-Care Professionals. Washington, D.C.: Paralyzed Veterans of America, 2000.

50. Krouskop, T. "Scientific Aspects of Pressure Relief." IAET Annual Conference, Washington, D.C., 1989.

51. ISO/CD 16840-3: *Wheelchair Seating-Part 3: Postural Support Devices.* Committee Draft, International Organization for Standardization, June 2002.

52. National Pressure Ulcer Advisory Panel (NPUAP). NPUAP's Support Surface Standards Initiative (S31), April 2003. Available at: *www.npuap.org*

53. Whittemore, R. "Pressure-Reduction Support Surfaces: A Review of the Literature," *Journal of Wound, Ostomy, and Continence Nursing* 25(1):6-25, January 1998.

54. Cullum, N. "Evaluation of Studies of Treatment or Prevention Interventions. Part 2: Applying the Results of Studies to Your Patients," *Evidence Based Nursing* 4(1):7-8, January 2001.

55. Cullum, N., et al. "Beds, Mattresses, and Cushions for Pressure Sore Prevention and Treatment," *Nursing Times* 97(19):41, May 10-16, 2001.

56. Thomas, D.R. "Issues and Dilemmas in the Prevention and Treatment of Pressure Ulcers: A Review," *Journals of Gerontology, Series A, Biological Sciences and Medical Sciences* 56(6):328-40, 2001.

57. Rithalia, S.V., and Kenney, L. "Mattresses and Beds: Reducing and Relieving Pressure," *Nursing Times* 96(36 Suppl):9-10, September 7, 2000.

58. Cullum, N., et al. "Preventing and Treating Pressure Sores," *Quality in Health Care* 4(4):289-297, December 1995.

59. Lazzara, D.J., and Buschmann, M.T. "Prevention of Pressure Ulcers in Elderly Nursing Home Residents: Are Special Support Surfaces the Answer?" *Decubitus* 4(4):42-48, November 1991.

60. Lim, R., et al. "Clinical Trial of Foam Cushions in the Prevention of Decubitus Ulcers in Elderly Patients," *Journal of Rehabilitation Research and Development* 25(2):19-26, Spring 1988.

61. Conine, T., et al. "Pressure Ulcer Prophylaxis in Elderly Patients Using Polyurethane Foam or Jay Wheelchair Cushions," *International Journal of Rehabilitation Research* 17(2):123-37, June 1994.

62. Brienza, D.M., et al. "The Relationship Between Pressure Ulcer Incidence and Buttock-Seat Cushion Interface Pressure in At-Risk Elderly Wheelchair Users," *Archives of Physical Medicine and Rehabilitation* 82(4):529-33, April 2001.

63. Allen, V. et al. "Air-Fluidized Beds and Their Ability to Distribute Interface Pressures Generated Between the Subject and the Bed Surface," *Physiological Measurement* 14(3):359-64, August 1993.

64. Munro, B.H., et al. "Pressure Ulcers: One Bed or Another?" *Geriatric Nursing* 10(4):190-92, July-August 1989.

65. Kosiak, M. "Etiology of Decubitus Ulcers," *Archives of Physical Medicine and Rehabilitation* 42(1):19-28, January 1961.

66. Bliss, M.R. "Pressure Sore Management and Prevention," in Brocklehurst, J.C., et al., eds. *Textbook of Geriatric Medicine and Gerontology,* 4th ed. London: Churchill Livingstone, 1992.

67. Knox, D.M., et al. "Effects of Different Turn Intervals on Skin of Healthy Older Adults," *Advances in Wound Care* 7(1):48-56, January 1994.

68. Rappl, L., and Sears, M. "Choosing and Using Seat Support Surfaces for Skin and Wound Management," Symposium on Advanced Wound Care, New Orleans, La., 1997.

69. Moody, B., et al. "Impact of Staff Education on Pressure Sore Development in Elderly Hospitalized Patients," *Archives of Internal Medicine* 148(10):2241-243, October 1988.

70. Versluyen, M. "Pressure Sores: Causes and Prevention," *Nursing* 33(6):216-18, June 1986.

71. Wound Ostomy and Continence Nurses Society (WOCN) *Guideline for Prevention and Management of Pressure Ulcers.* WOCN: Glenview, Ill., 2003.

72. Abu-Own, A., et al. "Effects of Compression and Type of Bed Surface on the Microcirculation of the Heel," *European Journal of Vascular and Endovascular Surgery* 9(3):327-34, April 1995.

73. Petrie, L.A., and Hummel, R.S. III. "A Study of Interface Pressure for Pressure Reduction and Relief Mattresses," *Journal of Enterostomal Therapy* 17(5):212-16, September-October 1990.

74. Zernike, W. "Preventing Heel Pressure Sores: A Comparison of Heel Pressure Relieving Devices," *Journal of Clinical Nursing* 3(6):375-80, November 1994.

75. Zernike, W. "Heel Pressure Relieving Devices: How Effective Are They?" *Australian Journal of Advanced Nursing* 14(4):12-19, June-August 1997.

76. Cheneworth, C.C., et al. "Portrait of Practice: Healing Heel Ulcers," *Advances in Wound Care* 7(2):44-48, March 1994.

77. Cheney, A.M. "Portrait of Practice: A Successful Approach to Preventing Heel Pressure Ulcers After Surgery," *Decubitus* 6(4):39-40, July 1993.

78. Williams, C. "Using Water-Filled Gloves for Pressure Relief on Heels," *Journal of Wound Care* 2(6):345-48, 1993.

79. Flemister, B.G. "A Pilot Study of Interface Pressure with Heel Protectors Used for Pressure Reduction," *Journal of ET Nursing* 18(5):158-61, September-October 1991.

CHAPTER 12

Pain management and wounds

Linda E. Dallam, MS, APRN,BC, CWCN, GNP
Christine Barkauskas, RN, BA, CWOCN, APN
Elizabeth A. Ayello, PhD, RN, APRN,BC, CWOCN, FAPWCA, FAAN
Sharon Baranoski, MSN, RN, CWOCN, APN, DAPWCA, FAAN
R. Gary Sibbald, BSc, MD, FRCPC (Med)(Derm), FAPWCA, MEd

OBJECTIVES

After completing this chapter, you'll be able to:

- define and identify the components of wound-associated pain

- describe the similarities and differences of pain associated with various types of chronic wounds

- utilize two validated tools for your patients to rate their chronic wound associated pain

- assess the advantages and disadvantages of wound pain treatment modalities.

Etiology and definitions of pain

"Pain has an element of blank;
It cannot recollect
When it began, or if there were
A day when it was not."

—Emily Dickinson

As clinicians, we have a tendency to identify certain types of wounds as having a specific type or amount of pain. However, pain is what the patient states it is—not what we believe it to be. Our responsibility as clinicians is to accurately assess the patient's pain and treat it adequately, without judging the patient or doubting that the pain is as de-

scribed. Pain is often more important to patients than clinicians with surveys indicating that pain is the most important parameter for many patients, but is often only the 3rd or 4th priority for clinicians.

There are several definitions of pain in the literature. Both the 1979 International Association for the Study of Pain (IASP) Subcommittee on Taxonomy[1] and the Agency for Healthcare Research and Quality (AHRQ, formerly the Agency for Healthcare Policy and Research, or AHCPR)[2] support a common definition of pain. They have defined pain as "an unpleasant sensory and emotional experience associated with actual or potential tissue damage or described in terms of such damage."[1,2]

Another commonly used pain definition is that of McCaffery,[3,51] who states that "pain is whatever the experiencing person says it is and exists whenever he says it does." McCaffery's definition of pain encompasses the subjective component and acknowledges the patient as the best judge of his own pain experience. Experts in the field of pain have come to accept that the patient's self-reporting of pain, its characteristics, and its intensity encompass the most reliable assessment. This belief that the patient in pain is his own best judge is also accepted as the basis for pain assessment and management by such regulatory agencies as the Joint Commission on Accreditation of Healthcare Organizations (JCAHO)[4] as well as such professional organizations as the American Pain Society.[5]

PRACTICE POINT

Pain is what the person says it is and exists whenever he says it does. The true etiology of pain isn't known. More research is needed to learn the true cause of the individual patient's pain.

Types of pain

Pain can be nociceptive or neuropathic. Nociceptive pain can result from ongoing activation of primary afferent neurons by noxious stimuli, with an intact nervous system. Neuropathic pain is initiated or caused by a primary lesion or dysfunction of the nervous system.[6]

The two types of nociceptive pain are somatic and visceral. Somatic pain arises from bone, skin, muscle, or connective tissue. It's usually aching, throbbing, and well-localized. Pressure ulcer pain is usually somatic in nature. Visceral pain arises from the visceral organs such as the gut, or from an obstruction of a hollow viscous organ, as occurs with a blockage of the small bowel. Visceral pain is poorly localized and is commonly described as cramping. Both types of nociceptive pain respond well to non-opioids and opioids.

In neuropathic pain, there's abnormal processing of the sensory input by the peripheral or central nervous system. The pain is typically described as burning, stabbing, or electrical. Diabetic ulcer pain and the pain of shingles are examples of neuropathic pain. Neuropathic pain responds more readily to an adjuvant, such as tricyclic antidepressants or anticonvulsant therapy. Tricyclic antidepressants, such as amitriptylene nortriptylene or desipramine are good choices because of their high antinoradrenalin activity. Amitriptylene is a first generation tricyclic with almost equal anti-noradrenalin, anti-histamine, anti-seritonin and anti-adrenergic actions. Nortriptylene is a second generation tricyclic that has a higher antinoradrenalin activity at a lower dose, with less side effects such as double vision, dry mouth, and urinary retention. Desipramine has the same advantages as noradrenalin with less drowsiness. If tricyclics don't provide relief of neuropathic pain at reasonable dosages, then anticonvulsants, such as gabapentin and its derivative pregabalin should be considered. Indeed, gabapentin has been shown to be useful in treating neuropathic pain.[7] Pregabalin has also proved to be useful in the treatment of neuropathic pain with studies demonstrating a benefit in painful postherpetic neuropathy[8] and painful diabetic neuropathy. [9]

Pain can also be acute or persistent (chronic). Acute pain has a distinct onset, with an obvious cause and short duration and is usually associated with chronic wounds, subsiding as healing takes place. Chronic pain can be from a chronic wound or other long-term diseases, such as cancer. If it persists for 3 months or more, chronic pain is usually associated with functional and psychological impairment. Chronic pain can fluctuate in character and intensity.

The American Geriatric Society (AGS)[10] supports the use of "persistent" pain rather than "chronic" pain to circumvent the negative stereotypes that have been associated with the word "chronic." The AGS Clinical Practice Guideline, "The Management of Persistent Pain in Older Persons" states: "Unfortunately, for many elderly persons, chronic pain has become a label associated with negative images and stereotypes commonly associated with long-standing psychi-

PRACTICE POINT

Interventions for noncyclic wound pain

- Administer topical or local anesthetics.
- Consider operating room procedure under general anesthesia rather than bedside debridement for large, deep ulcers.
- Administer opioids and nonsteroidal anti-inflammatory drugs before and after procedures.

- Assess and reassess for pain during and after procedures.
- Avoid using wet-to-dry dressings.
- Consider alternatives to surgical/sharp debridement, such as transparent dressings, hydrogels, hydrocolloids, hypertonic saline solutions, or enzymatic agents.[28]

---

atric problems, futility in treatment, malingering, or drug-seeking behavior. Persistent pain may foster a more positive attitude by patients and professionals for the many effective treatments that are available to help alleviate suffering."[10]

Persistent pain and acute pain can occur at the same time; similarly, nociceptive and neuropathic pain may also occur at the same time. All types of pain can be associated with functional or psychosocial losses and can affect the quality of life, or the quality of spiritual, social, emotional, and physical decline associated with dying. Pain can be debilitating and can also cause suffering beyond its physical component.

PRACTICE POINT

Reframing the phrase "patient complains of pain" to "patient reports pain" may help to foster a more positive and objective way for practitioners and caregivers to connect with the patient's experience of pain. Use the term persistent pain rather than chronic pain.

The persistent (chronic) pain experience

Krasner[11-13] has conceptualized pain in chronic wounds as the chronic wound pain experience. Within this model, pain is divided into three subconcepts: noncyclic, cyclic, and chronic pain. *Noncyclic* or *incident* pain is defined as a single episode of pain that might occur, for example, after wound debride-

ment. *Cyclic* or *episodic* pain recurs as the result of repeated treatments, such as dressing changes or turning and repositioning. *Chronic* or *continuous* pain is persistent and occurs without manipulation of the patient or the wound. For example, the patient may feel that the wound is throbbing even when he's lying still in bed and with no treatment occurring at the local wound site. (See *Interventions for noncyclic wound pain.* See also *Interventions for cyclic wound pain,* page 232, and *Interventions for persistent [chronic] wound pain,* page 233.)

Pain and wound types

The type of pain a patient experiences depends largely on the type of wound. Various wound types, and the types of pain that accompany them, are discussed throughout this section.

Pressure ulcer pain

Pain at the site of a pressure ulcer is supported by pressure ulcer experts and anecdotal reports by clinicians, although few studies have been published concerning pressure ulcer pain. The National Pressure Ulcer Advisory Panel (NPUAP) stated at its first conference in 1989 that "pressure ulcers are serious wounds that cause considerable pain, suffering, disability, and even death."[14] Van Rijswijk and Braden[15] reevaluated the Agency for Health Care Policy and Research (AHCPR) Treatment of Pressure Ulcer Guidelines in light of studies published after

PRACTICE POINT
Interventions for cyclic wound pain

- Perform interventions at a time of day when the patient is less fatigued.
- Provide analgesia 30 minutes prior to dressing change.
- Assess the patient for pain during and after dressing changes.
- Provide analgesia 30 minutes prior to whirlpool.
- If the patient's dressing has dried out, thoroughly soak the dressing—especially the edges.
- Observe the wound for signs of local infection.
- Gently and thoroughly irrigate the wound to remove debris and reduce the bacterial bioburden, which can cause contaminated wounds to become infected. Infection will increase the inflammation and pain at the wound site.

- Avoid using cytotoxic topical agents.
- Avoid aggressive packing.
- Avoid drying out the wound bed and wound edges.
- Protect the periwound area with sealants, ointments, or moisture barriers.
- Minimize the number of daily dressing changes.
- Select pain-reducing dressings.
- Avoid using tape on fragile skin.
- Splint or immobilize the wounded area as needed.
- Utilize pressure-reducing devices in bed or chair.
- Provide analgesia as needed to allow positioning of patient.
- Avoid trauma (shearing and tear injuries) to fragile skin when transferring, positioning, or holding a patient.

release of the 1994 Guidelines.[16] They reaffirmed the AHCPR panel's first recommendation about assessing pressure ulcer patients for pain. Based on the additional evidence from studies supporting reduction of pain with the use of moisture-retentive dressings, van Rijswijk and Braden[15] proposed that the 1994 AHCPR recommendations about pain and pressure ulcers be rewritten.

The etiology of pain in patients with pressure ulcers isn't known. Pieper[17] quotes the work of Rook,[18] and suggests that the common sources of pressure ulcer pain are from the "release of noxious chemicals from damaged tissue, erosion of tissue planes with destruction of nerve terminals, regeneration of nociceptive nerve terminals, infection, dressing changes, and debridement."

According to a study by Szors and Bourguignon,[19] pressure ulcer pain depends not only on the stage of the pressure ulcer but also on whether a dressing change is taking place at the time the assessment is made. The majority of the patients reported pressure ulcer pain with dressing changes; a lower number had persistent pain at rest. They stated that the pain ranged from sore to excruciating. Seventy-five percent rated their pain as mild, discomforting, or distressing; 18% rated their pain as horrible or excruciating. Clinicians need to ensure adequate pain control for persistent pain with long- acting pain and breakthrough medication as well as to time the breakthrough medication for the pain experienced at dressing change. In addition, appropriate cleansing and debridement methods and dressings need to be chosen that will minimize pain and trauma at the time of removal and reapplication.

Arterial ulcer pain
Pain associated with peripheral vascular disease can be caused by intermittent claudication; it may occur at night, when the patient's legs are elevated, or at other periods of rest. Intermittent claudication pain results from exercise or activity and has been described as

---

PRACTICE POINT ▬▬▬▬▬

Interventions for persistent (chronic) wound pain

- Utilize all of the interventions listed for noncyclic and cyclic wound pain.
- Control edema.
- Control infection.
- Monitor wound pain while the patient is at rest (at times when no dressing change is taking place).
- Control pain to allow healing and positioning.
- Provide regularly scheduled analgesia, including opioids, patient-controlled analgesia, and topical preparations such as lidocaine gel 2%, depending on the severity of pain.

- Attend to nonwound pain from comorbid pain syndromes such as contractures and diabetes, and iatrogenically induced pain from central lines, venipunctures, catheters, feeding tubes, blood gas drawing, or other equipment or procedures.
- Address the emotional component of the pain or the patient's suffering. For example, find out what the wound represents to him, what the pain means, whether he has associated losses of function, and whether the wound has altered his body image. In addition, determine whether his mental status or behavior has changed related to unrelieved pain.

---

cramping, burning, or aching. Blood flow with exertion is inadequate to meet the needs of tissues; the resultant lack of circulation causes intermittent claudication.

Nocturnal pain may have the same symptoms but usually precedes the occurrence of rest pain. Rest pain occurs—even without activity—when blood flow is inadequate to meet the needs of tissues in the extremities. It's described as a sensation of burning or numbness aggravated by leg elevation. It's a constant, intense pain that isn't easily relieved by using pain medications. Pain can sometimes be alleviated by stopping the activity or exercise, and placing legs in a dangling or dependent position.

Venous ulcer pain

The range of venous ulcer pain is extensive; the patient may report mildly annoying pain, a dull ache, or sharp, deep muscle pain. Pain is more intense at the end of the day secondary to edema resulting from the legs being in a dependent position, often aggravated by standing, sitting, or crossing the legs. The pathophysiology of venous disease is related to reduction or occlusion of blood return to

the heart. Incompetent superficial, perforating, or deep veins can cause pooling of fluid in the legs leading to pitting edema and resultant pain. To minimize pain, patients should be instructed to elevate the legs when sitting and to encourage the appropriate use of support stockings. Stocking selection is based on accurate individualized measurement and putting them on before the legs are placed on the floor in the morning. Other clinical management goals that help to minimize venous disease-related edema include the avoidance of prolonged sitting, weight reduction, and smoking cessation.

Thrombus formation in the deep veins can lead to leg swelling and pain, mimicking an infection or superficial phlebitis. The patient may report localized tenderness and pain over the long and short saphenous veins. Increased bacterial burden in the superficial wound bed can lead to delayed healing and localized pain. Clinicians should look for non-healing, increased exudate, red-friable granulation tissue, new debris or slough on the surface, and an unpleasant smell or odor (See NERDS© in chapter 7, Wound bioburden). When venous disease has been present for a long period of time, the veins become leaky to fibrin (woody fibrosis). In addition, red blood cells can leak into the tissue causing staining that's often referred to as hemosiderin and hyperpigmentation. The woody fibrosis does not go away at the end of the day and patients can have acute and chronic inflammatory changes within the woody fibrosis, leading to acute and chronic lipodermatosclerosis-type pain.

Neuropathic ulcer pain

Neuropathy is the most common complication of diabetes. The amount of pain present depends on the severity of the neuropathy. The patient may state that the pain interferes with his entire life—especially his ability to sleep. The affected extremity may feel like it's asleep or have the "pins and needles" pain that occurs after a part of the body has "fallen asleep" and starts to wake up. The quality of pain can be aching, burning, stinging, stabbing, or shooting and may include increased skin sensitivity (allodynia) and itching. True pain relief is primarily accomplished with pharmacologic intervention. All pain needs to be adequately assessed to ascertain the most effective treatment modality. If a patient reports excessive pain in a neuropathic limb that hasn't had pain before, an infection may be developing.

Patients with diabetes lose protective sensation after 10 to 15 years. This loss of protective sensation allows these individuals to undergo sharp surgical debridement without nociceptive pain although they may have referred pain in the leg or foot. If persistent nociceptive pain develops in a neuropathic limb, it usually means there's disruption of the deeper structures. In a person with a foot ulcer, clinicians should check for underlying osteomyelitis. If a patient has a tender, swollen foot without ulceration and an increase in skin surface temperature, there's a strong possibility of a Charcot joint.

PRACTICE POINT

Determining whether pain results from neuropathy or is associated with peripheral vascular disease is extremely important because patients with diabetes have a high incidence of peripheral vascular disease. In addition, pain in a painless foot usually indicates disruption of the deeper structures and a strong possibility of associated osteomyelitis, Charcot foot or even both conditions co-existing.

Understanding wound pain

Most of our understanding of wound pain comes from literature about other diseases.[20] Clinicians are increasingly acknowledging that pain is a major issue for patients suffering from many different types of wounds.[20] (See *Pain: What we know, what we don't know.*)

The European Wound Management Association (EWMA)[21] has developed a position document on wound pain titled "Pain at wound dressing changes." Of the 3,918 respondents from the United States and 10 countries in western and eastern Europe, pain prevention was the second highest ranking consideration at dressing change, with prevention of trauma being first.[21] Pain from leg ulcers was ranked as the most severe pain compared to other wound types, and dressing removal caused the greatest pain.[21]

The EWMA Pain at wound dressing changes position document is subdivided into three sub-topics as follows:
• Understanding wound pain and trauma from an international perspective [22]
• The theory of pain[23]
• Pain at wound dressing changes: A guide to management [24]

A copy of this EWMA document can be found on the Internet and is available in Dutch, English, French, German, Italian and Spanish.[22-24] (See *EWMA suggestions for preparing the wound pain environment*, page 236.)

Another international consensus document (statement) found on the Internet was developed by the World Union of Wound Healing Societies (WUWHS).[25] This document entitled, "Principles of best practice: Minimizing pain at wound dressing related procedures," outlines challenges, several pain myths, and common misunderstandings as part that are useful for improved clinical practice. (See

---

PRACTICE POINT
Pain: What we know, what we don't know

McCaffery and Robinson[51] reported on the self-evaluation of nurses about pain.

- Observable changes in vital signs must be relied upon to verify a patient's report of severe pain: False (answered correctly by 88.4%).
- Pain intensity should be rated by the clinician, not the patient: False (answered correctly by 99.1%).
- A patient may sleep in spite of moderate or severe pain: True (answered correctly by 90.6%).
- Intramuscular (I.M.) meperidine is the drug of choice for prolonged pain: False (answered correctly by 85.6%).
- Analgesics for chronic pain are more effective when administered as needed rather than around the clock: False (answered correctly by 92.7%).
- If the patient can be distracted from the pain, he has less pain than he reports: False (answered correctly by 94.7%).
- The patient in pain should be encouraged to endure as much pain as possible before resorting to a pain relief measure: False (answered correctly by 98.4%).
- Respiratory depression (less than 7 breaths per minute) probably occurs in at least 10% of patients who receive one or more doses of an opioid for relief of pain: False (answered correctly by 60.5%; clinicians tend to exaggerate the risk of respiratory depression with opioid use; according to McCaffery and Robinson, the risk is less than 1%).
- Vicodin (hydrocodone 5 mg and acetaminophen 500 mg) is approximately equal to the analgesia of one-half of a dose of meperidine 75 mg I.M.: False (correctly answered by 48.3%).
- If a patient's pain is relieved by a placebo, the pain isn't real: False (answered correctly by 86.1%).
- Beyond a certain dose, increasing the dosage of an opioid such as morphine won't increase pain relief: False (answered correctly by 57.2%).
- Research shows that promethazine reliably potentiates opioid analgesics: False (correctly answered by 35.1%).
- When opioids are used for pain relief under the following circumstances, what percentage of patients is likely to develop opioid addiction:
  - Patients who receive opioids for 1 to 3 days: Answer is less than 1% (correctly answered by 82.8%).
  - Patients who receive opioids for 3 to 6 months: Answer is less than 1% (correctly answered by 26.7%).

Wound pain myths, page 237.) There are also helpful suggestions for care planning and treatment interventions. (See *WUWHS procedural wound pain interventions,* page 238.)

Lastly, a third international document (not a consensus statement), addresses the management of pain associated with burns. This document is titled, "The management of pain associated with dressing changes in patients with burns," and can be found on the World Wide Wounds website. [26]

Pressure ulcer-related pain was investigated in five qualitative studies. Hollingworth[20] determined that nurses' assessment, management, and documentation of pain after doing wound dressings was inadequate. A qualitative study by Krasner[27] examined the reflections of 42 general and advanced practice nurses after they cared for patients with pressure ulcers and pain. Three patterns—nursing expertly, denying the pain, and confronting the challenge of pain—with eight subsequent themes were identified. They were:

- Nursing expertly
- Reading the pain
- Attending to the pain

EWMA suggestions for preparing the wound pain environment [21-24]

Preparing the environment: Prepare, plan, prevent

- Choose an appropriate non-stressful environment, close windows, turn off mobile phones, etc.
- Explain to the patient in simple terms what will be done and the method used.
- Assess the need for skilled or unskilled assistance, such as help with simple hand holding.
- Be thoughtful in positioning the patient to minimize discomfort and avoid unnecessary contact or exposure.
- Avoid prolonged exposure of the wound, (e.g., waiting for specialist advice).
- Avoid any unnecessary stimulus to the wound and handle wounds gently, being aware that any slight touch can cause pain.
- Involve the patient throughout; frequent verbal checks and use of pain tools offer real-time feedback.
- Consider preventative analgesia.

– Acknowledging and empathizing with the patient
- Denying the pain
– Assuming that it doesn't exist
– Not hearing the cries
– Avoiding failure
- Confronting the challenge of pain
– Coping with frustration
– Being with the patient.[27]

Krasner[12,13,27] suggested that clinicians use this information to provide more patient-centered sensitive care for patients with pressure ulcer pain.

Few studies (four quantitative and five qualitative) have been published concerning the pain experience of patients with pressure ulcers. The first study to quantify pain by pressure ulcer stage was completed by Dallam and colleagues.[28] They studied the perceived intensity and patterns of pressure ulcer pain in hospitalized patients. The study population was diverse, with 66% being white (non-Hispanic) and the remainder being Black (non-Hispanic), Hispanic, or Asian. Of the 132 patients, 44 (33.3%) were respondents and 88 (66.7%) were nonrespondents as they couldn't communicate responses to the instruments. Two different scales were used to measure pain intensity: the Visual Analog Scale and the Faces Pain Rating Scale (FRS). (See the next section for additional discussion of these pain scales.) The authors found a high degree of agreement between the two pain scales. They also noted that the FRS scale was easier to use for patients who were cognitively impaired or if English was a second language.

The major findings of this important study by Dallam and colleagues[28] include the following:
- majority of patients with pressure ulcers had pain (68% of respondents reported some type of pain)
- most patients didn't receive analgesics for pain relief; only 2% ($n = 3$) in this population were given analgesics for pressure ulcer pain within 4 hours of the pain measurement
- patients who couldn't express or respond to pain scales may still have had pain
- patients with deeper pressure ulcer stages (stages III and IV) had more pain.

Some procedures, such as surgical debridement or wet-to-dry dressings, may increase pain. While the study[28] didn't identify the interventions that might be most effective in controlling pain, patients whose beds had static air mattresses rather than regular hospital bed mattresses, and those whose wounds were dressed with hydrocolloid dressings, had significantly less pain. The study[28] also demonstrated that patients are able to differentiate between ulcer site pain, generalized pain, and other local pain sites such as I.V. and catheter sites. Cognitively impaired patients are able to indicate the presence of pain and respond to pain intensity scales.

Wound pain myths[25]

- **Myth 1:** Wet to dry dressing are still the gold standard for wound care. Adherent gauze can disrupt delicate healing tissue and provoke severe pain.
- **Myth 2:** Transparent films are the best dressing for treating and reducing the pain of skin tears and other minor acute wounds. The misuse of transparent films is a common cause of skin tears.
- **Myth 3:** Using paper tape is the least painful way to secure a dressing. Heightened nerve sensation in a wide area around a wound can make adhesive tape painful to remove.
- **Myth 4:** Pulling a dressing off faster than slower reduces pain at dressing changes. This method has the potential to inflict tissue damage and traumatic pain.
- **Myth 5:** Using a skin sealant on peri-wound skin reduces the risk of pain and trauma. Skin sealants only create a thin topical layer and do not protect deeper dermal layers.
- **Myth 6:** People with diabetic foot wounds do not experience pain. There may some loss of peripheral nerve sensation but also heightened sensitivity.
- **Myth 7:** Pain comes from the wound. The surrounding tissue nerves play little role. Spinal-cord responses to incoming pain signals can give rise to abnormal sensitivity in the surrounding area (allodynia).
- **Myth 8:** The only way to treat wound pain is by oral analgesic 30-60 minutes before dressing changes. Oral analgesic can give some relief but should not be seen as a single solution. A full pain assessment must be used to evaluate and fine-tune any prescribed therapy.

In another quantitative study, Szors and Bourguignon[19] selected a cross-sectional method to examine the pain experience of 32 patients with stage II, III, and IV pressure ulcers at rest and during dressing changes. This study demonstrated that a majority of patients had pressure ulcer-related pain. Twenty-eight (87.5%) reported pain at dressing change and 27 (84.4%) reported pain at rest (when dressing changes or other treatments weren't being carried out). Of the nearly 85% of patients reporting pain during dressing changes, 21 (75%) rated their pain as mild, discomforting, or distressing and 5 (18%) described their pain as horrible or excruciating. Twelve (42%) reported their pain as continuous, occurring both at rest and at dressing changes.

Despite the number of patients experiencing pressure ulcer pain at rest and at dressing changes, the study showed that only 6.3% (n = 2) received analgesia for their pressure ulcer pain.[19]

Both quantitative studies by Dallam et al.[28] and Szors and Bourguinon[19] found that many patients suffer with untreated or under-treated pressure ulcer pain. The first study determined that only 2% of patients with pressure ulcer pain received analgesia, while the second study, 4 years later, found little improvement in the administration of pain-relieving medication. Only 6% of patients with pressure ulcer pain had analgesics prescribed to address their pain.

Both studies reflect the need for clinicians to realize the potential for pain from pressure ulcers. Because only 44 of the 132 patients with pressure ulcer pain could respond to pain scales, Dallam and colleagues[28] recommend that pressure ulcer pain should be suspected even when the patient can't report pain. Both studies recommend further research to identify interventions that can relieve pressure ulcer pain and the associated suffering.

Franks and Collier[29] conducted the Riverside Pressure ulcer study where they compared 75 home- care patients in the United Kingdom who had pressure ulcers with 100 home-care patients without pres-

WUWHS procedural wound pain interventions[25]

- Be aware of current status of pain.
- Know and avoid, where possible, pain triggers.
- Know and use, where possible, pain reducers.
- Avoid unnecessary manipulation of the wound.
- Explore with the patient simple distraction techniques, such as counting up and down, focusing on the breath entering and leaving the lungs, or listening to music.
- Reconsider management choices if pain becomes intolerable and document as an adverse event.
- Observe the wound and surrounding skin for evidence of infection, necrosis, or maceration.
- Consider the temperature of the product before applying it to the wound.
- Avoid excessive pressure from a dressing, bandage, or tape.
- Follow the manufacturer's instructions when using a dressing or technology.
- Assess comfort of intervention and/or dressing/bandages applied after the procedure.

Ongoing evaluation and modification of the management plan and treatment intervention is essential as wounds change over time. More advanced non-pharmacological techniques that require specialist training or skilled personnel, such as the use of hypnosis or therapeutic touch, may be considered.

An alternative explanation is that the home-care patients with pressure ulcers did not have the same co-morbid conditions as previously reported in hospital populations.

In a quantitative study of pain documentation among 128 patients with chronic wounds, of the patients whose pain assessment was recorded, over half of the patients with venous ulcer had pain (54%), almost a third with diabetic ulcers had pain (30%), and one quarter of those with pressure ulcers (25%) had pain.[35]

Langemo and colleagues[30] published a qualitative phenomenological study about pain and pressure ulcer patients. They interviewed eight adults, half with active pressure ulcers at the time of the study and the other half with healed pressure ulcers. Seven themes were identified:

1. perceived etiology of the pressure ulcer
2. life impact and changes
3. psychospiritual impact
4. extreme painfulness associated with the pressure ulcer
5. need for knowledge and understanding
6. need for and effect of numerous, stressful treatments
7. the grieving process.

The fourth theme—extreme pain—was subdivided into three categories: intensity of pain, duration of pain, and analgesic use. Patients commonly referred to the intensity of pain from pressure ulcers with descriptors such as "it burned," "feeling like being stabbed," "sitting on a bunch of needles," or "stinging." Some examples of statements by actual study respondents include a woman with a stage II pressure ulcer who said, "I felt like somebody was getting a knife and really digging in there good and hard." In the words of another male respondent, "They [pressure ulcers] are very painful because no matter what way you put your bottom, it hurts."[30]

Respondents also commented on the duration of the pain, with statements such as "the majority of the time, even when I was lying down, it hurt." Pain continued to be a problem even after the pressure ulcer had healed. As one respondent stated, "Every now and again, it still hurts. But there is nothing there. This time there is nothing really there." The fear of addiction resulting from analgesic use was expressed by some respondents. One re-

sure ulcers. An interesting finding of this study was that patients with pressure ulcers had less pain than the comparison group. The authors speculated that perhaps pressure ulcer pain might not be the problem, as previously presumed, or that pain control was somehow more effective for these patients.

spondent with a stage IV pressure ulcer on the buttock commented, "I was constantly in pain and was taking morphine and other types of painkillers to try and ease the pain."

Another qualitative study reported about the pain of 10 pressure ulcer patients.[31] Although Rastinehad identified 22 themes, lack of communication and painful treatment interventions were the two most common complaints.[31] Some patients related accounts of communication failures that contributed to stress, tension, and anxiety.[31]

In the phenomenological European Pressure Ulcer Advisory Panel (EPUAP) funded study by Hopkins et al.,[52] endless pain was one of the three main themes identified in older people living with pressure ulcers. The eight patients were all over age 65 and had stage III or IV pressure ulcers for more than one month. None had spinal cord injuries as suggested by Langemo for future qualitative pressure ulcer pain studies.[30] The four sub-themes of endless pain were: constant presence, keeping still, equipment pain, and treatment pain. For some patients, keeping still reduced their pain. For others, pain was exacerbated by pressure relieving equipment as well as during dressing change. All but one of the patients described their endless pain in a graphic way. "You put a bit of weight on your heel and (it) feels as though it's burst open." Patients also described how not moving reduced pain. "I don't dare move because everything then gets worse. I lie very still."[52]

These [28-31] and other studies[32-35, 52] continue to underscore the need for assessment of pain in patients with pressure ulcers and other chronic wounds and the importance of adequate pain management.

Pain assessment

Despite the American Pain Society's identification of pain as "the fifth vital sign,"[5] it isn't always included in the assessment of a patient's pressure ulcer. Dallam and colleagues[28] urged that pain be added to the assessment of pressure ulcers and that a patient's pain status be assessed during dressing changes as well as when the patient is at rest. (See *Essential pain assessment elements*.)

Essential pain assessment elements

Use the PQRST mnemonic (shown below) to assess your patient's pain.

P = Palliative/provocative factors
- What makes the pain worse?
- What makes it better?

Q = Quality of pain
- What kind of pain are you experiencing?
- Would you describe it as sore, aching, deep, cramping, burning, shooting, or sensitive (or any combination thereof)?
- Do you have other symptoms with the pain, such as fever, chills, nausea, or vomiting?

R = Region and radiation of pain
- Where is the pain?
- Where does it radiate?

S = Severity of pain
- Would you describe your pain as none, mild, moderate, severe, or excruciating?
- Rate your pain on a scale from 0 to 10, with 0 representing "no pain" and 10 being "the worst imaginable pain."
- What is the pain intensity at its worst, best, and now?

T = Temporal aspects of pain
- Is the pain better or worse at any particular time of the day or night?
- When does it start or when does it stop?
- Is it intermittent or constant, or does it occur only when you're moving?

Additional pain assessment elements

Include the following additional elements in your initial assessment plan and treatment:
- detailed history consisting of:
  - medication usage
  - treatment history
  - previous surgeries and injuries
  - impact on quality of life and activities of daily living.
- physical examination, emphasizing the body system involved in the pain complaint (for example, the musculoskeletal or neurologic system)
- psychosocial assessment, including family history of depression or chronic pain
- appropriate diagnostic workup to determine the cause of pain and to rule out any contributing, treatable causes.

A thorough pain assessment enables the clinician to develop an effective pain treatment regimen and evaluate its effectiveness.

They also cautioned clinicians to remember that absence of response or expression of pain doesn't mean that the patient doesn't have pain. Despite research about the pain experience,[28,30-34] assessment of pain in persons with pressure ulcers continues to be under reported.[35] Documentation of pain assessment may vary by chronic wound type, as patients with venous ulcers (63%) and diabetic ulcers (53%) were more likely to have their pain assessment recorded compared to those with pressure ulcers (45%).[35]

Two assessment guides include pain as part of pressure ulcer assessment. The AHCPR[16] treatment guidelines include an example of a sample pressure ulcer pain assessment guide in Attachment A. There's a place to check either yes or no regarding pain. Ayello's[36,37] ASSESSMENT mnemonic asks the clinician to quantify the patient's pain experience including the presence of pain, when the pain occurs (for example, is it episodic or constant), and if the patient is receiving measures for pain relief. The caregiver completes the following boxes under t = tenderness to touch or pain:
- no pain
- pain present on touch, anytime
- pain only when performing ulcer care.[36,37]

The mnemonic PQRST, which outlines the specific questions to ask the patient, is another useful tool for assessing a patient's pain.

A complete and thorough pain assessment enables the clinician to develop an effective pain treatment regimen and evaluate its effectiveness. (See *Additional pain assessment elements*.) The American Society for Pain Management Nursing recently released its position statement and clinical practice recommendations for pain assessment in specific patient populations—groups that clinicians may not always identify as needing pain assessment. These groups include patients with advanced dementia, infants and preverbal toddlers, and intubated and/or unconscious patients.[53] The Hartford Institute for Geriatric Nursing has produced a series on pain assessment called "Try This." These one-page (front and back) documents provide a succinct summary that covers the important points on pain assessment in the older adult and in patients with dementia.[38]

PRACTICE POINT

Pain is the fifth vital sign.

Pain intensity scales

Pain intensity scales are used to determine how much pain the patient is having by utilizing a simple verbal, visual, or numeric measure. The gold standard for assessing pain intensity is self-report and the utilization of standard pain intensity instruments.[39, 40] Pain intensity scales are unidimensional, quantitative measures designed to measure the sensory aspect of a patient's pain and to

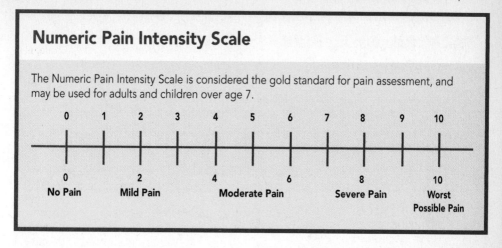

Numeric Pain Intensity Scale

The Numeric Pain Intensity Scale is considered the gold standard for pain assessment, and may be used for adults and children over age 7.

0 1 2 3 4 5 6 7 8 9 10

0	2	4	6	8	10
No Pain	**Mild Pain**	**Moderate Pain**		**Severe Pain**	**Worst Possible Pain**

obtain a more objective approximation of his pain by minimizing inaccuracies.[40]

The use of pain intensity scales to quantify pain levels and determine patients' responses to pain treatments has been mandated in all hospitals by JCAHO.[4] Two of the most widely accepted and utilized pain assessment scales are the Numeric Pain Intensity Scale and the FACES Pain Rating Scale.[41] Another scale is the Visual Analog Scale (VAS), which consists of a 10-cm line that has no numbers on it. At one end is the term "no pain," and at the other end is the phrase "pain as bad as it could possibly be."[2]

Numeric Pain Intensity Scale

In particular, the Numeric Pain Intensity Scale is commonly known as the gold standard for pain assessment for adults and children over age 7.[2,41] The scale is a 10-cm line with the words "no pain" at one end, "worst possible pain" at the other end, and the numbers zero to ten (0 to 10) running from one end of the scale to the other. (See *Numeric Pain Intensity Scale*.) The patient is asked to select a number on the scale, which represents the level of pain he's experiencing. Zero indicates no pain, 5 indicates moderate pain, and 10 indicates the worst possible pain.[2] The Numeric Pain Intensity Scale is sometimes presented verbally;[2,41] however, visual presentation may help to standardize the process of pain assessment and assist hearing

impaired patients. In addition, the scale has been translated into many languages.[6]

The pain intensity rating scale aids in the adequate assessment and treatment of pain. It also helps clinicians choose the appropriate classification of pain medication recommendations based on any given patient response.[14,41,42] Whether the patient has a response to the interventions can also be determined by using the scale if the numbers show a downward trend on repeated assessments.

FACES Pain Rating Scale

A third option is the FACES Pain Rating Scale (FPRS),[43] which consists of six faces that range from a happy, smiling face (no pain) to a crying, frowning face (worst pain). The first Face, which is number 0 indicates an absence of pain, the next face on the scale, number 2, indicates very little pain, and so forth. The last face on the scale, indicates extreme/worst pain. The patient is asked to choose the face that most closely reflects his own pain at that point in time. (See *FACES Pain Rating Scale*, page 242.) The FPRS is preferred for use with children when compared with other pain intensity scales.[41] The validity and reliability in adult patients hasn't been established, although the FPRS has been used in studies with a geriatric population and a high degree of agreement was found between the FPRS and the VAS ($r = 92$, $p < 0.5$).[44] It has been used with cognitively impaired patients and those for whom English

FACES Pain Rating Scale

The FACES Pain Rating Scale may be used for children ages 3 and older, for cognitively impaired patients, and for non-native speakers of English.

Do you have:

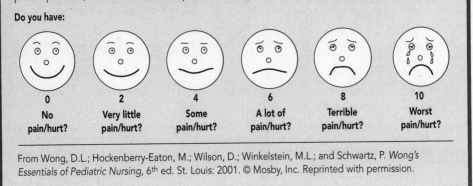

0	2	4	6	8	10
No pain/hurt?	Very little pain/hurt?	Some pain/hurt?	A lot of pain/hurt?	Terrible pain/hurt?	Worst pain/hurt?

From Wong, D.L.; Hockenberry-Eaton, M.; Wilson, D.; Winkelstein, M.L.; and Schwartz, P. *Wong's Essentials of Pediatric Nursing*, 6th ed. St. Louis: 2001. © Mosby, Inc. Reprinted with permission.

is the second language. A high consistency between the two scales was noted when utilized on any population.

After the initial pain assessment has been completed, reassessment should be performed at regular intervals. Reassess the patient after administration of pain medication or non-drug pain-relieving interventions to ensure that optimal pain relief has been achieved.

Pain management

Accurate and continuous pain assessment is the foundation of successful pain management.[6,39] However, evidence supports that pain is poorly assessed. Seventy-six percent of physicians with patient care responsibilities in oncology rated poor pain assessment as the number one barrier to adequate pain management.[7] Donovan et al.[45] found that of the 58% of hospitalized patients reporting excruciating pain, fewer than half had a member of the health care team ask them about their pain or note the pain in their records. The use of pain assessment measures has been shown to improve pain management for patients.[44,46] However, problems using the pain assessment scales in everyday practice persist. One problem includes the

lack of clinicians knowledge and familiarity in the use of pain rating scales. Training is required for clinicians to administer pain scales with adequate patient instructions on the possible responses to the pain scale questions.

After pain has been identified, its cause should be determined and treated. "The goal of pain management in the pressure ulcer patient is to eliminate the cause of pain, to provide analgesia, or both."[15] Practical ways of treating pain after the specific chronic wound etiology have been described by Freedman and colleagues.[47,51]

Dressing changes, debridement, wound edema, infection, turning, and positioning are some of the factors that can cause wound-associated pain. An appropriate plan of action can be implemented after the specific cause has been identified. For example, if the pain results from dressing changes, medication prior to dressing changes or switching to a different dressing may be indicated. "Besides medications, pain may be treated with physical and occupational therapy to decrease muscle spasms, decrease contractures, and aid in selecting less painful methods of wound debridement and cleaning. Proper seating, positioning, and adaptive equipment may also help to decrease pain."[16] The optimal way to treat the pain associated with

Skin: An essential organ

The Payne-Martin Classification System for Skin Tears divides skin tears into three categories based on whether tissue is lost in the tear.

Category I
Skin tears without tissue loss

Category I linear-type skin tear

In this Category I, linear-type skin tear, note areas of senile purpura.

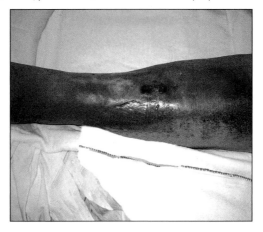

Category I flap-type skin tear

This Category I, flap-type skin tear has an epidermal flap covering the dermis to within 1 mm of the wound margin.

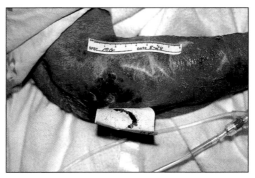

(continued)

Skin: An essential organ (continued)

Category II
Skin tears with partial tissue loss

Category II scant tissue loss–type skin tear

Less than 25% of the epidermal flap has been lost in this Category II, scant tissue loss–type skin tear.

Category II moderate to large tissue loss–type skin tear

More than 25% of the epidermal flap has been lost in this Category II, moderate to large tissue loss–type skin tear.

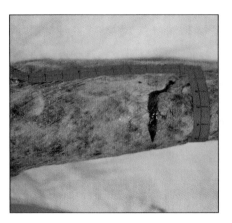

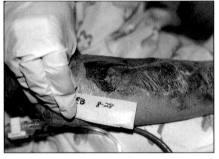

Category II scant tissue loss–type skin tear

Note other vulnerable areas of skin discoloration to the side and below the skin tear on this 90-year-old male.

Category III
Skin tears with complete tissue loss

The epidermal flap is absent in this Category III skin tear (skin tear with complete tissue loss).

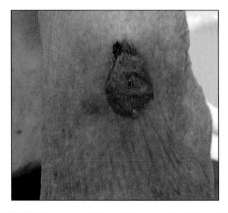

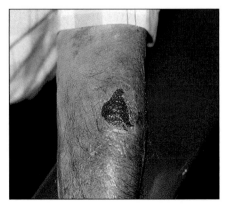

Wound assessment

Maceration

This photograph shows maceration of the surrounding skin caused by an overwhelmed dressing.

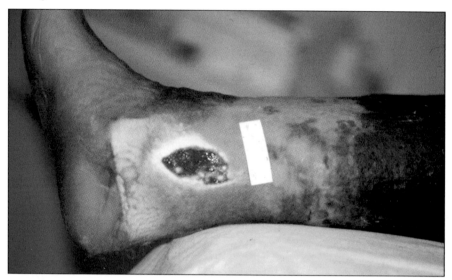

Wound edges with epithelialization

In this photograph, wound edges are attached and epithelialization present.

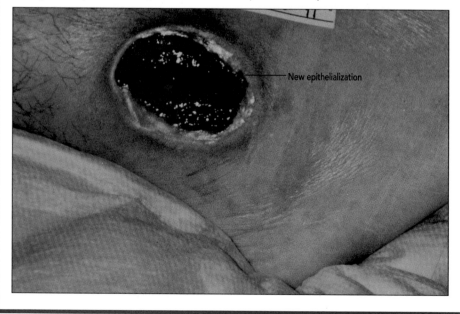

New epithelialization

Wound assessment (continued)

Geography of chronic wounds: Location, location, location
A + B + C + = the total wound

A is the wound bed; B is the wound edge; and C is the surrounding skin.

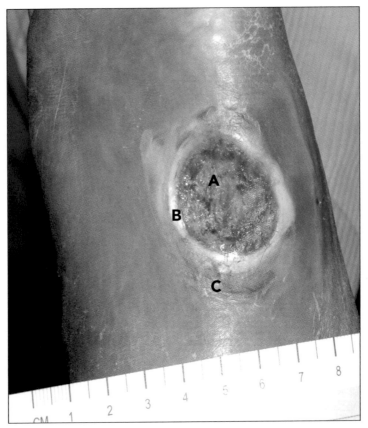

Photo: M. Tomic-Canic. Used with permission.

Wound assessment *(continued)*

Wound terminology

Using current terminology is imperative for an accurate assessment. The photograph below labels this wound's characteristics as well as its length and width.

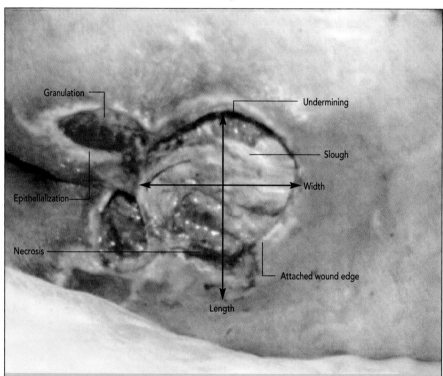

Diagnosing infection

Progression of bacterial balance to bacterial damage in a chronic wound

CONTAMINATED OR COLONIZED

Bacteria are present on the wound surface (contaminated). A steady state of replicating organisms are attaching to the wound tissue and multiplying, but they aren't associated with tissue damage or delayed healing (colonization).

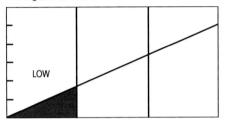
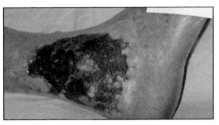

CRITICALLY COLONIZED
(LOCAL INFECTION, COVERT INFECTION, INCREASED BACTERIAL BURDEN)

- The bacterial burden in the wound bed is increasing, initiating an immune response (inflammation).
- The wound is no longer healing at the expected rate: wound size isn't decreasing
- Look for the signs outlined in the enabler NERDS©.

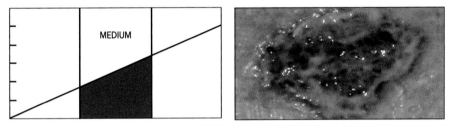

INFECTED

- Bacteria are present within the wound and have spread to the deeper and surrounding tissue; they're multiplying and causing tissue damage.
- There's an associated host inflammatory response that has now spread to the deeper tissue and surrounding skin.
- The wound is painful and may increase in size with potential satellite areas of breakdown.
- Look for the signs outlined in the enabler STONES©.

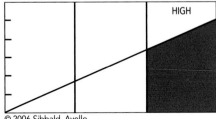
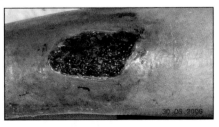

Diagnosing infection (continued)

NERDS©: Superficial increased bacterial burden

Letter	Key information to know	Comments
NONHEALING WOUND	• The wound is nonhealing despite appropriate interventions (healable wound with the cause treated and patient-centered concerns addressed). • Bacterial damage has caused an increased metabolic load in the chronic wound creating a proinflammatory wound environment that delays healing.	• To determine a healing trajectory, the wound size should decrease 20% to 40% after 4 weeks of appropriate treatment to heal by week 12. • If the wound does not respond to topical antimicrobial therapy, consider a biopsy after 4 to 12 weeks to rule out an unsuspected diagnosis, such as vasculitis, *Pyoderma gangrenosum*, or malignancy
EXUDATIVE WOUND	• An increase in wound exudates can be indicative of bacterial imbalance and leads to periwound maceration. • Exudate is often clear before it becomes purulent or sanguineous.	• Increased exudates needs to trigger the clinician to assess for subtle signs of infections. • Protect periwound area using the LOWE© memory jogger (Liquid film-forming acrylate; Ointments; Windowed dressings; External collection devices) for skin barrier to wound margins.
RED AND BLEEDING WOUND	• When the wound bed tissue is bright red with exuberant granulation tissues and bleeds easily, bacterial imbalance can be suspected.	• Granulation tissue should be pink and firm the exuberant granulation tissue that is loose and bleeds easily reflects bacterial damage to the forming collagen matrix and an increased vasculature of the tissue.
DEBRIS IN THE WOUND	• Necrotic tissue and debris in the wound is a food source for bacteria and can encourage a bacterial imbalance.	• Necrotic tissue in the wound bed will require debridement in the presence of adequate circulation. • Debridement choice needs to be determined based on wound type, clinician skill, and resources.
SMELL FROM THE WOUND	• Smell from bacterial byproducts caused by tissue necrosis associated with the inflammatory response is indicative of wound related bacterial damage. *Pseudomonas* has a sweet characteristic smell/green color; anaerobes have a putrid odor due to the breakdown of tissue.	• Clinicians need to differentiate the smell of bacterial damage from the odor associated with the interaction of exudates with different dressing materials, particularly some hydrocolloids. Odor may come from superficial or deep tissue damage, and this should not be relied on along with exudates alone as the only signs of increased superficial bacterial burden.

Diagnosing infection (continued)

STONES©: Deep compartment infection

Letter	Key information to know
SIZE IS BIGGER 	• Size as measured by the longest length and widest width at right angles to the longest length. Only very deep wounds need to have depth measured with a probe. • An increased size may be due to deeper and surrounding tissue damage by bacteria or alternately because the cause has not been treated or there is a systemic or local host factor impairing healing.
TEMPERATURE INCREASED 	• With surrounding tissue infection, temperature is increased. This may be performed crudely by touch with a gloved hand or by using an infrared thermometer or scanning device. There should be a high index of suspicion for infection if > 3° F difference in temperature exists between 2 mirror-image sites.
OS (PROBES TO OR EXPOSED BONE) 	• There is a high incidence of osteomyelitis if bone is exposed or if the clinician can probe to the bone in a person with a neurotrophic foot ulcer. • An MRI is probably the most discriminating diagnostic test when available and considered necessary for diagnostic dilemmas.
NEW AREAS OF BREAKDOWN 	• Note the satellite areas of skin breakdown that are separated from the main ulcer. • It is important to remember this may be due to the cause of the wound, infection, or local damage being left uncorrected.
EXUDATE, ERYTHEMA, EDEMA 	• All of the features here are due to the inflammatory response. With increased bacterial burden, exudates often increases in quantity and transforms a clear or serous texture to frank purulence and may have a hemorrhagic component. The inflammation leads to vasodilatation (erythema), and the leakage of fluid into the tissue will result in edema.
SMELL 	• Bacteria that invade tissue have a "foul" odor. There is an unpleasant sweet odor from *Pseudomonas* Gram-negative organisms and anaerobe organisms can cause a putrid smell from the associated tissue damage.

Comments

- Clinicians need to have a consistent approach to measurement.
- An increased size from bacterial damage is due to the bacteria spreading from the surface to the surrounding skin and the deeper compartment. This indicates that the combination of bacterial number and virulence has overwhelmed the host resistance.

It is important to distinguish between infection and the other 2 potential causes of temperature change:
- A difference in vascular skin supply (decreased circulation; is colder)
- Inflammatory conditions are not usually as warm, but they can demonstrate a marked increase temperature with extensive deep tissue destruction (acute Charcot joint).

- Radiographs and bone scans are less reliable for diagnosis of osteomyelitis with loss of bone mass that occurs with neuropathy. Radiographs of well-calcified bone, such as pressure ulcers of the pelvis, may be more reliable. The majority of ulcers that probe to bone in other locations are less likely to be associated with osteomyelitis

- Search for the cause of the satellite areas of breakdown and the need to correct the cause.
- Check for local damage and consider infection, increased exudates, or other sources of trauma.

- For exudates control, determine the cause and then match the absorbency of the dressing (non, low, moderate, heavy) to the amount of exudates from the wound.
- Assess surrounding skin to evaluate for maceration. Again, use the LOWE© memory jogger (Liquid film-forming acrylate; Ointments; Windowed dressings; External collection devices) for skin barrier for wound margins.
- For erythema and edema control, the cause or the tissue infection needs to be treated.

- Make sure the smell is from organisms and not from the normal distinct odor from the interaction of exudates with some of the dressing material.
- Systemic antimicrobial agents are indicated that will treat the causative organisms, and devitalized tissue should be aggressively debrided in wounds with the ability to heal.

Wound debridement

Slough

Necrotic tissue that's moist, stringy, and yellow (devitalized issue) is referred to as *slough*.

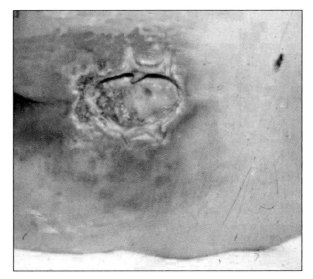

Eschar

In a wound that has become dehydrated, necrotic tissue turns thick, leathery, and black. This tissue is referred to as *eschar*.

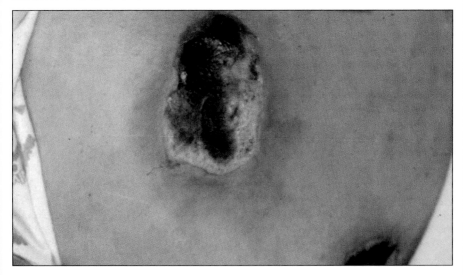

Wound debridement *(continued)*

Differentiating tendon from slough

Performing debridement requires knowing where and what to cut. For example, tendon and slough both are yellow, and the clinician must be able to distinguish between them.

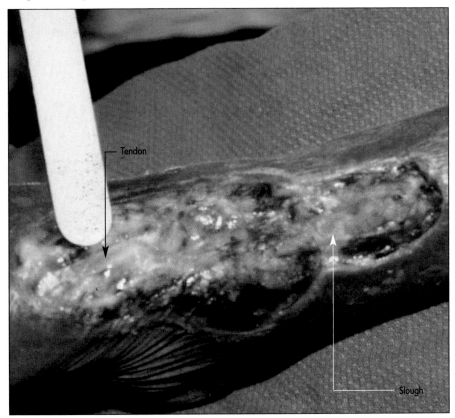

(continued)

Wound debridement (continued)

Surgical debridement case series

This pressure ulcer with slough and eschar requires surgical debridement due to advancing cellulitis.

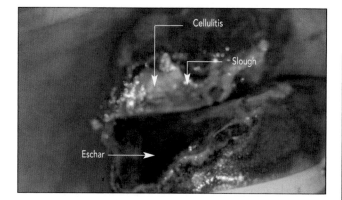

This photograph shows the same pressure ulcer after surgical debridement. Note the absence of eschar. Cellulitis is still present.

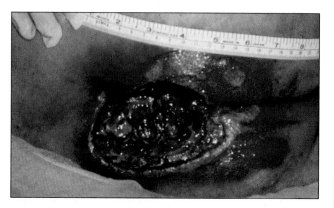

The same pressure ulcer after 7 days of treatment shows minimal necrotic tissue and significant amounts of granulation tissue. Note the change in the cellulitis surrounding the wound.

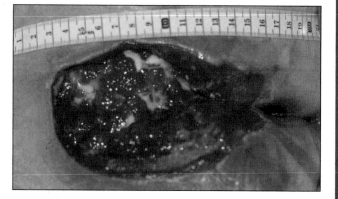

Wound debridement (continued)

Sharp debridement at the bedside

Small wounds may be debrided at the bedside, as shown below.

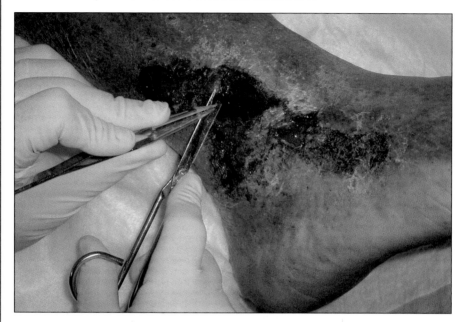

Notice the increased size of this ulcer after debridement.

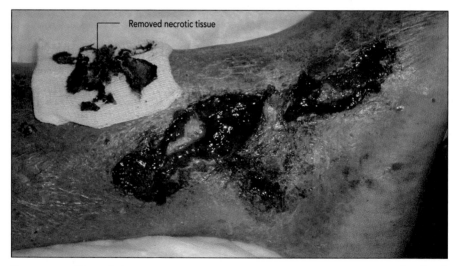

Removed necrotic tissue

Photos courtesy of Steven Black, MD

(continued)

Wound debridement (continued)

Maggot therapy

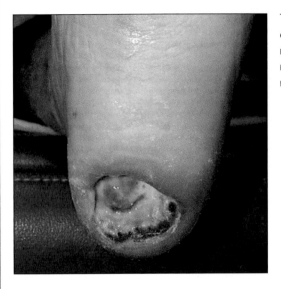

This photo shows a heel ulcer with osteomyelitis on a middle-aged female with diabetes, who was on immunosuppressants following a kidney transplant 27 years ago.

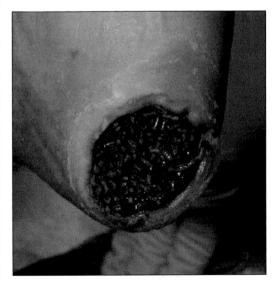

This photo shows the same ulcer with sterile maggots placed in the wound for the purpose of debridement.

Wound debridement *(continued)*

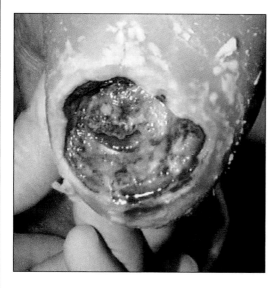

This photo shows the same ulcer after removal of the first application of maggots.

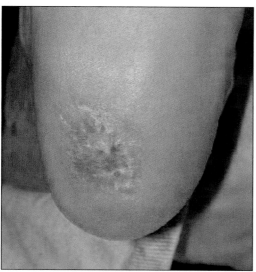

This final photo shows the same ulcer healed.

Photos courtesy of Pamela Mitchell, BTER Foundation

Seating, positioning, and support surfaces

Multiple sensors integrated into a mat may be used to "map" the entire body area that comes in contact with the support surface. This pressure map of a patient lying face up on a horizontal support surface shows varying degrees of pressure exerted by the patient's heels, calves, thighs, buttocks, shoulders, and head.

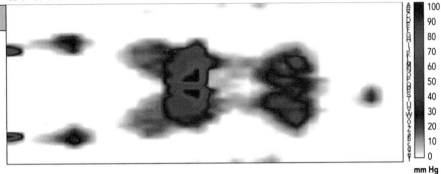

Pressure ulcers

Pressure ulcers are commonly staged using the National Pressure Ulcer Advisory Panel (NPUAP) classification system described briefly here. For the further NPUAP descriptions that accompany these revised definitions (not included here due to space limitations), see chapter 13, pages 256 and 257.

Suspected deep tissue injury

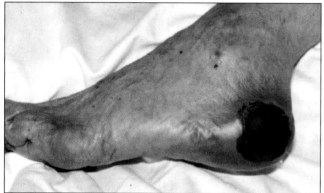

© J.M. Levine, MD

Purple or maroon localized area of discolored intact skin or blood-filled blister due to damage of underlying soft tissue from pressure and/or shear. The area may be preceded by tissue that is painful, firm, mushy, boggy, warmer or cooler as compared to adjacent tissue.

Unstageable pressure ulcer

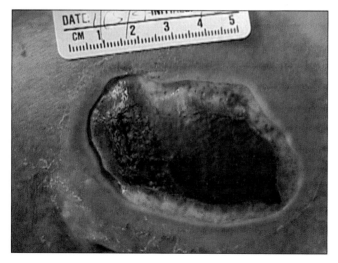

Full thickness tissue loss in which the base of the ulcer is covered by slough (yellow, tan, gray, green or brown) and/or eschar (tan, brown or black) in the wound bed.

(continued)

Pressure ulcers *(continued)*

Stage I

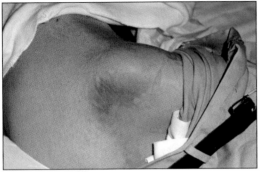

© 2006 J.M. Levine, MD

Intact skin with non-blanchable redness of a localized area usually over a bony prominence. Darkly pigmented skin may not have visible blanching; its color may differ from the surrounding area.

Stage II

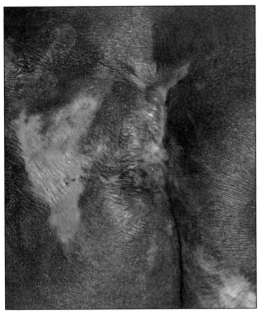

© 2007 H. Brem, MD

Partial thickness loss of dermis presenting as a shallow open ulcer with a red pink wound bed, without slough. May also present as an intact or open/ruptured serum-filled blister.

Pressure ulcers (continued)

Stage III

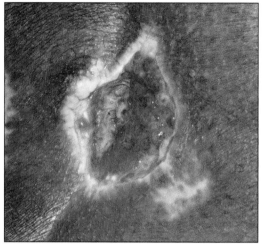

© 2007 H. Brem, MD

Fulll thickness tissue loss. Subcutaneous fat may be visible but bone, tendon or muscle are not exposed. Slough may be present but does not obscure the depth of tissue loss. May include undermining and tunneling.

Stage IV

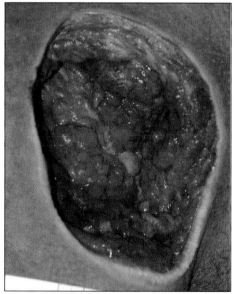

© 2007 H. Brem, MD

Full thickness tissue loss with exposed bone, tendon or muscle. Slough or eschar may be present on some parts of the wound bed. Often includes undermining or tunneling.

Vascular ulcers

Vascular ulcers include wounds resulting from arterial, venous, and lymphatic conditions.

Arterial ulcer

This photograph shows a necrotic great toe with blisters on the toes and foot, representing arterial insufficiency.

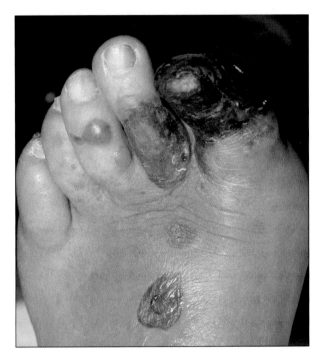

Venous ulcer

This photograph shows a venous ulcer. Venous ulcers are typically moist with irregular edges and firm, fibrotic, and indurated surrounding skin.

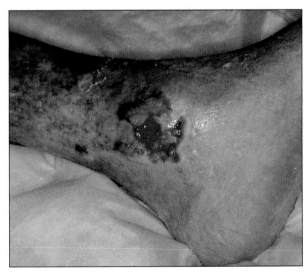

Vascular ulcers *(continued)*

Lymphedema

This photograph shows lymphedema with fibrosis and scarring.

- Aplasia/dysplasia or damage to lymphatic vessels or nodes
- Proliferation of fibroblasts
- Disturbance of local metabolism, chronic inflammation
- Increased infections (cellulitis)

Failure to identify lymphedema→improper treatment

- Pain
- Further damage to lymphatics
- Increased risk of complications
- Functional limitations > disability

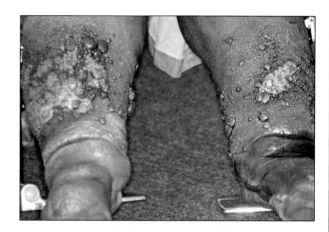

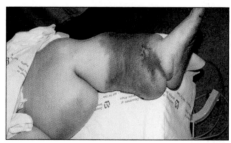

© 2007 Mary Jo Geyer

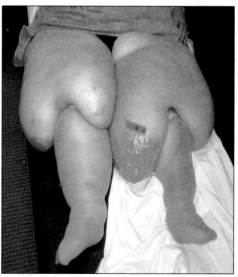

© 2007 Mary Jo Geyer

Diabetic foot ulcers

Ulcer on the sole

Repetitive, moderate pressure can cause skin breakdown and ulcers in the neuropathic foot, as shown here.

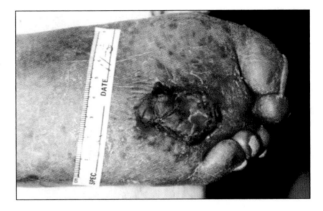

Charcot's foot with infection

This photograph shows Charcot's foot with infection present. Treatment of such wounds may include administration of parenteral antibiotics and surgical debridement of necrotic and infected tissue.

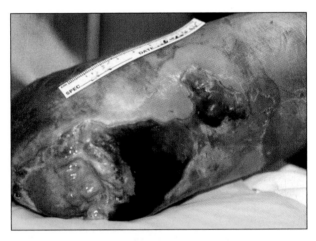

Callus with thick rim of tissue

Diabetic ulcers typically have a thick rim of keratinized tissue surrounding the wound, as shown here.

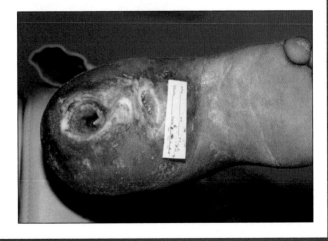

Ulcers in sickle cell disease

Sickle cell ulcer

Sickle cell ulcer with fibrinous material covering the ulcer bed

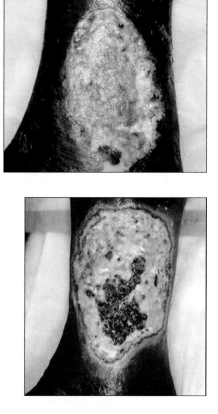

Predebridement

Postdebridement

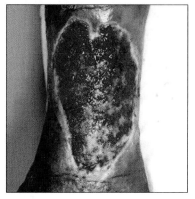

Used with permission of T. Treadwell, MD

(continued)

Ulcers in sickle cell disease (continued)

Recurrent sickle cell ulcer

Recurrent sickle cell ulcer treated with tissue-engineered skin

Healed 8 weeks post application

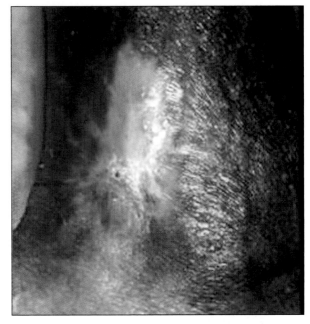

Ulcer remains healed 8 months later—note improved scar

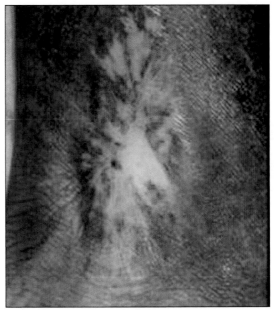

Used with permission of T. Treadwell, MD

Surgical wounds

Surgical closure of a pressure ulcer

This photograph shows markings made for gluteal fasciocutaneous flaps for surgical closure of a stage III pressure ulcer.

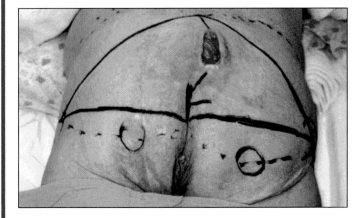

Shown here is surgical closure of the same ulcer.

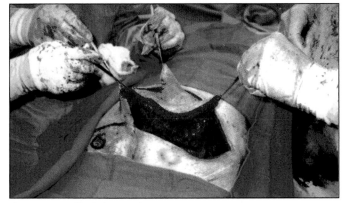

Photos courtesy of S. Black, MD

Atypical wounds

Wounds with uncommon etiologies are called *atypical wounds.*

Pyoderma gangrenosum

In a patient with inflammatory bowel disease and pyoderma gangrenosum, this ulcer on the lateral leg shows areas of cribriform scarring.

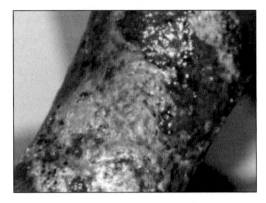

Peristomal pyoderma gangrenosum in a patient with Crohn's disease

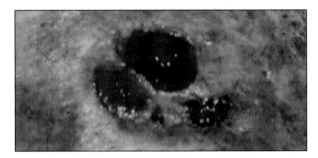

Infectious cause

Shown here is the leg and foot of a patient with Hansen's disease due to *Mycobacteria leprae.* In addition to neuropathic changes of the toes and plantar aspect of the foot, this patient has a large lateral leg ulcer as well.

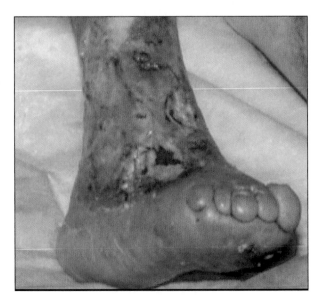

Atypical wounds *(continued)*

Buruli ulcer

This photo shows extensive sloughing and massive ulceration, typically leading to contractures and extensive disability and disfigurement.

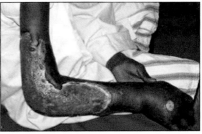

© 2007 E. Ampadu, MD

Cryofibrinogenemia

This patient has painful punctate ulcers on the feet and legs secondary to cryofibrinogenemia.

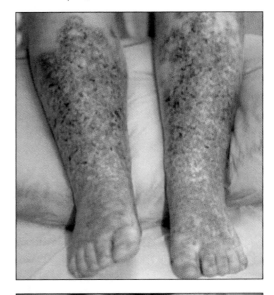

Vasculitis

This photograph shows reticulated erythema and necrotic ulcers on the thighs of a patient with vasculitis.

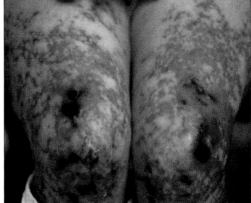

(continued)

Atypical wounds *(continued)*

Calciphylaxis

Shown here is necrotic plaque with livedo reticularis in a dialysis patient with end-stage renal disease and calciphylaxis.

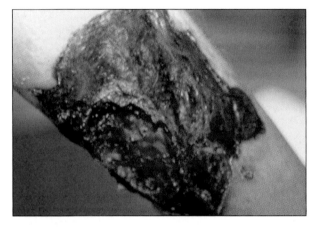

This photograph shows calciphylaxis of both extremities in a patient with end-stage renal failure. Despite aggressive local wound care, the wounds never healed, and the patient died of sepsis.

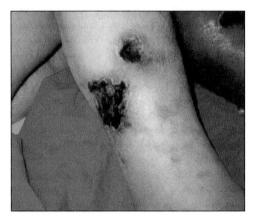

Necrotizing fasciitis

Necrotizing fasciitis of the abdomen

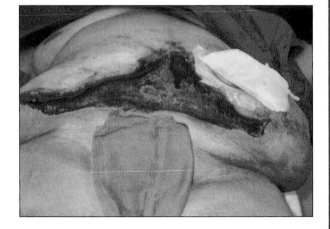

Atypical wounds (continued)

Malignancies

Shown here is a right medial leg ulcer in a venous distribution secondary to T cell lymphoma.

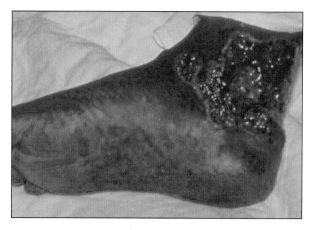

Marjolin ulcer

Shown here is a chronic wound that developed malignant changes (squamous cell carcinoma).

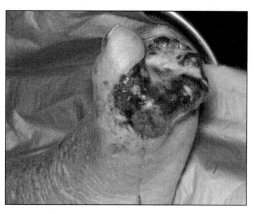

Factitial dermatitis

This photograph shows an angulated factitial ulcer on the breast. The term *factitial dermatitis* denotes a self-imposed injury.

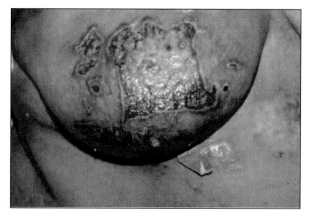

(continued)

Atypical wounds (continued)

Extravasation

Extravasation can cause tissue loss that may evolve into extensive wounds, as shown in this I.V. site 24 hours after infiltration of calcium chloride.

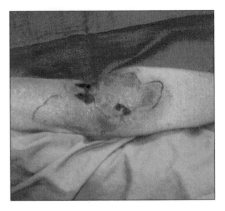

Shown here is the same site 48 hours later after wound debridement.

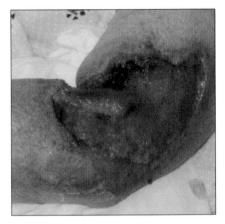

This photograph shows the same site after surgical debridement down to viable tissue.

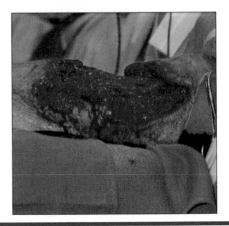

Special populations

Bariatric patients: Skin assessment

Pannus

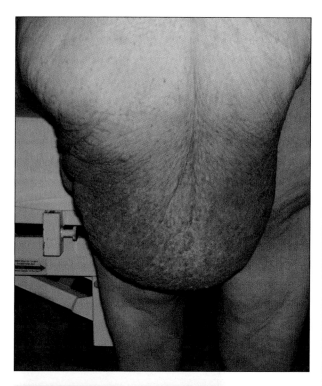

Skinfolds on back of neck

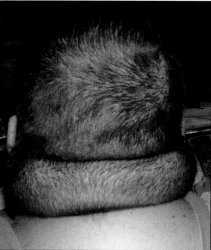

Photos © 2006 Coloplast Corp. Used with permission.
Photographer: K.L. Kennedy-Evans, RN, CS, FNP

(continued)

Special populations *(continued)*

Candidiasis in skin fold

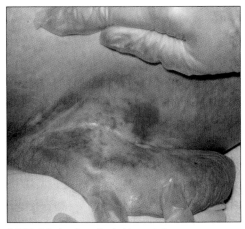

© 2006 Coloplast Corp. Used with permission.
Photographer: K.L. Kennedy-Evans, RN, CS, FNP

Intertrigo

- Fissure at the base of a skin fold, which is macerated and moist.
- Breast in female patient with a body mass index of 60.

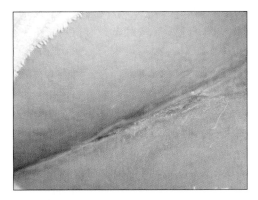

Intertrigo with erythema, erosion, and denudation

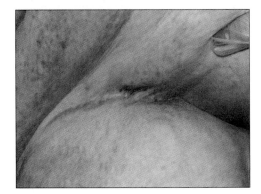

© 2006 Coloplast Corp. Used with permission
Photographer: K.L. Kennedy-Evans, RN, CS, FNP

pressure ulcers requires more research, but clinicians can look at the cause of the ulcer, patient-centered concerns, and all the components of local wound care to minimize pain at each step in their care plan.

PRACTICE POINT

Pain management should include interventions that:
• treat the cause
• address patient-centered concerns
• educate the patient
• improve activities of daily living (ADLs) and quality of life
• select local wound care measures for cleansing, debridement, and moist interactive dressings that minimize pain and trauma
• provide palliation to the dying patient
• decrease or eliminate pain with minimal adverse effects
• minimize patient's dependency on health care workers and family members.

Pain medication

The World Health Organization[48] (WHO) developed a three-step analgesic ladder for the treatment of cancer pain that has been accepted for use in patients with nonmalignant pain.[7] (See *WHO analgesic ladder*.) The WHO approach advises clinicians to match the patient's reported pain intensity of 0 to 10 with the potency of the analgesic to be prescribed, starting with non-opioid analgesics and progressing to stronger medications (if pain isn't relieved). For example, a patient who reports a pain score of 1 to 3 (mild pain) should receive a non-opioid with or without an adjuvant. If he reports a score of 4 to 6 (moderate pain), a weak opioid with or without an adjuvant should be administered. If the patient's pain score is from 7 to 10 (severe pain), he should be given a strong opioid with or without an adjuvant.

An adjuvant medication is a drug that has a primary indication other than pain but is analgesic for some painful conditions.[6] Examples of adjuvant medications are anticonvulsants or tricyclic antidepressants. (See *Adjuvant agents*, page 244.) Adding an adjuvant medication is most useful in addressing

WHO analgesic ladder

This analgesic ladder, developed by the World Health Organization (WHO)[48] for pain management in patients with cancer, may be used as a guideline to manage mild through severe wound pain.

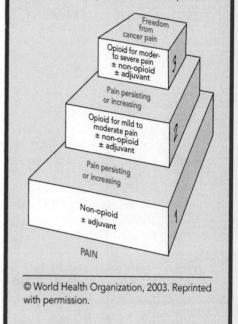

© World Health Organization, 2003. Reprinted with permission.

the burning, stinging, shooting or stabbing symptoms of neuropathic pain. Using a combination of drugs such as an opioid and a non-opioid can enhance pain relief because the two drugs work synergistically. The opioid works on the CNS to alter the perception of pain and the non-opioid works on the periphery to block painful impulses. Using a combination method may decrease the need for higher doses of opioids.

Step 1: Non-opioid analgesics

Acetaminophen or nonsteroidal anti-inflammatory drugs (NSAIDs) should be initiated as first-line therapy. They should be administered on a regular rather than an as-needed basis to increase their effectiveness and main-

Adjuvant agents

Drug class	Name	Indications
Tricyclic antidepressants	Amitriptyline Desipramine Nortriptyline	• Multi-purpose • Any chronic pain • Neuropathic pain
Anticonvulsants	Carbamazepine Clonazepam Gabapentin Pregabalin Valproic acid	• Burning, neuropathic, lancinating pain
Systemic local anesthetics	Lidocaine Mexiletene	• Burning pain
Topical anesthetics	Capsaicin EMLA cream Lidocaine gel Lidocaine 1% Lidocaine 4% Lidocaine patch 5%	• Analgesic for intact skin (use on wound periphery prior to dressing changes) • Before changing vacuum-assisted-closure (VAC) dressing (instill solution through the VAC tubing, with the VAC at 50 mmHg and clamp tubing for 15 to 20 minutes)* • Saturate gauze for 15 to 20 minutes prior to dressing change • Post-herpetic neuralgia, stump pain

*Systemic absorption and toxicity can occur in large wounds. Lidocaine products should not be used in patients who are on class 1 antiarrhythmic drugs such as tocaine or mexiletine.

tain a constant level of the medication in the blood. When using NSAIDS, if one group doesn't work, try another group. (See *Non-opioid analgesics*.)

NSAID groups include:
• salicylates: aspirin, diflunisal, choline magnesium trisalicylate, salsalate
• propionic acids: naproxen, ibuprofen, fenoprofen, ketoprofen, flurbiprofen, suprofen
• acetic acids: indomethacin, tolmetin, sulindac, diclofenac, ketorolac
• oxicams: piroxicam.

Ketorolac tromethamine may provide increased analgesia in comparison to oral NSAIDs and is available for administration both I.V. and I.M., but is limited to a five-day period of utilization and may not be useful in the management of persistent (chronic) pain. Clinicians must remember that the NSAIDs have increased side effects in elderly people, especially GI bleeding, and may be associated with a decrease in renal function. These agents should be used with caution in persons over age 65; mild opioids may be safer for pain relief in this population.

Although studies are limited, some researchers are exploring the effects of topical opioids in the treatment of painful skin ulcers. Twillman and colleagues[49] used nine case studies to report decreased pain at the site of an open ulcer when a morphine-infused gel dressing was utilized in persons with painful skin ulcers due to a variety of medical conditions. The researchers report remarkable efficacy in eight out of the nine patients studied and felt there should be further research in this area as so many patients stand to gain pain relief.

Tricyclic antidepressants, such as amitriptyline, imipramine, nortriptyline, and desipramine have been shown to relieve neuropathy and post-hepatic neuralgia, but are contraindicated in patients with coronary disease (may be taken cautiously at low doses of 10 to 30 mg in a daily night-time dosage).[7] Hydroxyzine (Vistaril, Atarax) has analgesic, antiemetic, and mild sedative activity as well as antihistamine effects. These drugs may help to induce sleep in patients with chronic pain. Diabetic patients with neuropathic pain or other patients with conditions arising from peripheral nerve syndromes may benefit from the use of certain anticonvulsants, such as gabapentin, pregabalin [8,9] phenytoin, carbamazepine, sodium valproate, or clonazepam.[7]

Opioids vary in strength from mild to very strong and are available in different forms such as oral, oral-transmucosal, rectal, transdermal, subcutaneous, I.V., and I.M. forms. The oral form is preferred for long-term use. However, in the case of preprocedural or postprocedural pain, such as debridement, it may be better to use an I.V. route to allow for better pain control and faster ability to increase the dosage as needed. Whether an oral or I.V. route is used, doses should be scheduled on a regular basis to avoid breakthrough pain. If breakthrough pain occurs when the patient is on a long-acting (sustained-release) opioid regimen, a short-acting (immediate-release) opioid may be taken and used together with the long-acting opioid to provide pain relief. Breakthrough pain is most likely to occur when the patient is moved, if a dressing change is required, if tubes are being manipulated, or if the patient has an increase in activity.

Constipation can be one of the most common adverse reactions with the use of opioid analgesics. This adverse effect can be easily remedied by taking stool softeners, laxatives, and increasing fiber and fluids (especially water). It's better to anticipate constipation and treat it before it happens. The best agent to use is a 15 to 30 g dose of lactulose.

Other common adverse effects of opioids include sedation, nausea, vomiting, itching, urinary retention, and sensory or motor deficits. Many clinicians fear respiratory depression and subsequently undertreat pain. Respiratory depression may occur with the use of opioids but is uncommon except for patients with advanced lung disease, particu-

> ## Non-opioid analgesics
>
> - Acetaminophen
> - Aspirin
> - Tramadol
> - Nonsteroidal anti-inflammatory drugs
>   - Celecoxib
>   - Ibuprofen
>   - Ketorolac
>   - Rofecoxib
>   - Salsalate

larly COPD. This side effect can be decreased or eliminated with the use of lower doses at first that are increased gradually while monitoring the patient's respiratory status.

Meperidine (Demerol) is not recommended for the management of persistent (chronic) pain. Disadvantages include the hazards of normeperidine, a metabolite of meperidine. Repeated doses of meperidine can cause an accumulation of normeperidine, which causes central nervous system excitability and toxicity. This toxicity will be manifested in the patient by twitching, numbness, seizures, and hallucinations.[2] Coma and death are also possible. According to the 1999 APS Principles of Analgesic Use in the Treatment of Acute and Cancer Pain,[7] "although the oral doses of meperidine have about one quarter of the analgesic effectiveness of similar parenteral doses, they produce just as much of this toxic metabolite." The American Pain Society also warns that patients with compromised renal function are particularly at risk for the accumulation of this toxic metabolite.

 EVIDENCE-BASED PRACTICE

Caretakers tend to underutilize opioid analgesics because of the fear of addiction. Caretaker education is very important, especially in the home-care setting where the caregiver is the one deciding when to give the patient pain medication.

Combination or weak opioids

- Acetaminophen with codeine
- Hydrocodone with acetaminophen
- Hydrocodone with ibuprofen
- Oxycodone with acetaminophen
- Propoxyphene
- Propoxyphene with acetaminophen

Opioids: Morphine and morphine-like agents

- Morphine
- Dolophine
- Fentanyl patch
- Levorphanol
- Oxycodone

Addiction to opioids should be a concern, but the fear of addiction has been greatly exaggerated. Studies have shown that when a patient takes an opioid for pain relief the incidence of addiction is about 1%. And, the length of time on the analgesic or the amount given is irrelevant for addiction.[18] However, although the incidence of addiction is low, the potential for abuse does exist. Therefore, clinicians should remain diligent in monitoring the patient who's taking opioids. An indication that abuse is developing is if the patient begins to use the drug for reasons other than pain relief.

Step 2: Opioid for mild to moderate pain

Weak opioids, or opioids combined with NSAIDs, may be used if step 1 is ineffective. (See *Combination or weak opioids.*)

Propoxyphene and combined propoxyphene drugs are step 2 drugs, but these agents should be avoided in elderly patients because the drug metabolite may cause CNS and cardiac toxicity. Codeine may cause excessive constipation, nausea, and vomiting.[50]

Step 3: Opioid for moderate to severe pain

Such opioids as morphine and morphine-like agents may be used when steps 1 and 2 are ineffective. (See *Opioids: Morphine and morphine-like agents.*)

Morphine is the drug of choice for chronic pain and is more cost-effective than meperidine, available for many different routes, and is easily titratable. It has fewer, easily treatable adverse effects. The adverse effects of constipation and nausea are usually treated with antiemetic drugs and laxatives. Other adverse effects are usually dose-related and can be resolved with dose adjustments.[6]

 PRACTICE POINT

Helpful hints for using opioids:
- Oral-transmucosal fentanyl citrate works in 10 minutes (good for dressing changes). Oral-transmucosal fentanyl should only be used in patients who are opioid tolerant (patients whose total dose of opioids are equal to 60 mg of morphine a day, for a total of one week or longer).
- Fentanyl patches should be started at the lowest dose for patients who are opioid naïve (have never used opioids).

It will take 2 to 3 days for the first patch to reach maximum effect. If immediate pain relief is required, a short-acting opioid can be used along with the patch and then discontinued when the patch begins to work.
- Use short-acting agents (at 10% to 15% of total daily dose) for breakthrough pain.
- Titrate up to long-acting agents if patient needs more than two breakthrough doses on a normal day.
- Don't wait for constipation to begin. Start patient on stool softeners and laxatives to avoid this common adverse effect.

- To taper or discontinue opioid analgesics, decrease the dose by 25% every 2 to 3 days. Monitor for pain or withdrawal symptoms, as these would indicate that the tapering is too rapid.

PRACTICE POINT

Symptoms of withdrawal or abstinence from opioids include:
- tachycardia
- hypertension
- diaphoresis
- piloerection
- nausea and diarrhea
- abdominal pain
- body aches
- psychosis.

The presence of these symptoms may indicate that the opioid medication is being tapered too quickly, and not that the patient is addicted to it.

Some researchers are exploring the effects of topical opioids in the treatment of painful skin ulcers.[49] One study reported decreased pain at the site of an open ulcer when a morphine-infused gel dressing was used in patients with painful skin ulcers due to a variety of medical conditions. The researchers report remarkable efficacy in eight out of the nine patients studied.[49]

Nonpharmacologic treatment modalities

Management of pain from wounds can require a combination of pharmacologic and nonpharmacologic treatments; the latter may include the use of music, massage, and relaxation techniques. Pain associated with dressing changes and debridement can be minimized by allowing patients to call time outs. Many other nonpharmacologic treatments can also be used prior to, and in conjunction with, medications. These include physical and occupational therapy, repositioning the patient, support surfaces, and optimizing local wound care with materials that minimize pain.

Physical and occupational therapy

Physical and occupational therapy services may be a valuable asset to utilize in conjunction with pharmacologic therapy. Passive and active range-of-motion exercises should be taught to the patient and his caregivers. Additional measures include the following:
- Patients with peripheral vascular disease may benefit from a walking program to facilitate development of collateral circulation in the lower extremities.
- Application of a transcutaneous electrical nerve stimulation unit may help to decrease pain, particularly in patients with chronic or acute wounds. It's believed that the electrical stimulation provided by the unit helps to inhibit pain transmission cells.
- Hot or cold packs can be applied to decrease spasms in the affected area.
- Stretching exercises help to decrease contractures.
- Exercise helps to decrease muscle spasms with massage.

Local pain management

The use of appropriate dressings and dressing techniques can help to relieve pain during and between dressing changes. Findings from the international study by Moffatt et al.[21] reveal the importance of pain-free dressing changes. All respondents agreed that gauze dressings caused the most pain, while pain was noticeably less severe with the use of hydrogels, hydrofiber, alignates, and soft silicone dressings.

Dressing types
When providing wound care, choose products carefully to provide the patient with a pain-free experience. (See chapter 9, Wound treatment options.) Patients who express discomfort despite careful product selection should be given medication prior to dressing changes.

All of the moist-wound dressings can be left on wounds for a longer period of time than wet-to-dry dressings. This decreases the frequency of dressing changes, thereby decreasing the opportunities for the patient to experience pain associated with dressing changes.

The following interventions will ease the dressing change process for your patients:

Treating the cause/aggravating factors

• Provide pressure redistribution for your patients.
• Keep the patient's heels off the bed at all times.
• Control edema to avoid decreased blood flow to the wound, which may lead to additional pain.
• Eliminate or decrease pain from other possible pain sources.

Addressing patient-centered concerns

• Keep in mind that pharmacologic management is the gold standard for moderate to severe pain. Give pain medication around the clock, if necessary, to keep the pain under control.
• Instruct the patient and his family regarding pain management to alleviate fear of addiction with the use of opioids.
• Explain the role that pain control plays in improved wound healing.
• Explain dressing change procedures to the patient before dressing changes.
• Allow the patient to select the time for dressing changes, if appropriate.
• Assess for pain and medicate the patient before and after dressing changes or debridement.
• Allow the patient or his family members to participate in dressing changes, as indicated.
• Offer the patient distraction techniques, such as conversation, TV, and videos during dressing changes.
• Inform the patient that he may call a "time-out" if pain is present during dressing changes.
• Ensure that the patient has adequate rest and sleep. Lack of rest and sleep will decrease the patient's pain threshold, decrease his mental performance, and increase his emotional response to pain.
• Teach the patient to substitute tapping, rubbing, and gentle slapping for scratching.
• Instruct the patient in relaxation techniques and the use of visual imagery when encountering a potentially pain-provoking situation.
• Reevaluate the pain management plan when needed. Document the effectiveness of the analgesic or other treatments for pain relief with a pain score. This will help to assess if the pain management program is working.
• Address other factors, such as loss of function, inability to perform acts of daily living (ADLs), and possible changes in body image to help the patient deal with ancillary problems that might contribute to his pain.

PRACTICE POINT

Wet-to-dry dressings can desiccate a wound, thus causing pain on removal. (Remove viable stuck tissue from the wound surface leading to bleeding, trauma, pain and delayed wound healing). Avoid these dressings in favor of moisture-retentive dressings to promote a healing environment and patient comfort.

Cleansing and debridement

• Assess pain when the patient is at rest to provide adequate pain control.
• Use warm normal saline solution or noncytotoxic wound cleaners to clean wounds.

Don't use cytotoxic solutions such as betadine or hydrogen peroxide to clean wounds. They not only deter wound healing, they may cause burning, adding to the patient's discomfort.

Use moist wound therapy to enhance autolytic debridement as an alternative to surgical or sharp debridement to eliminate pain associated with sharp debridement.

Change dressings in a timely manner. Excess exudate on periwound skin or dressings allowed to dry on a wound may increase the patient's pain.

Protect the periwound skin with skin barrier wipes, film-forming liquid acrylates, or ointment (petrolatum or zinc oxide) to prevent excoriation, trauma, maceration, or dermatitis that can delay wound healing, increase wound size, and increase patient discomfort. Avoid using strong adhesive tape on elderly patients or patients with fragile skin.

Alternative pain management methods

There are many natural pain control methods and therapies that may be implemented to ease pain, stress, and anxiety. These methods can improve one's outlook, attitude, and quality of life. Alternative therapies, when used in conjunction with pain medications, may enhance the beneficial effects of pain medication.

Laughter

Laughter helps you breathe deeper, lower your blood pressure, and change your mood.

Acupuncture

The application of needles to specific areas of the body may decrease or eliminate pain and has been used for more than 2,500 years.

Environment

Having the room at a comfortable temperature, avoiding bright lights, and keeping the room quiet may help to decrease pain.

Distraction

Playing cards, watching television, visiting with friends, petting an animal, and writing about his feelings can help the patient and focus his attention on something else other than the pain.

Music

Music increases blood flow to the brain and increases energy which, in turn, causes an increase in the production of endorphins (a natural body chemical similar to morphine) that work to decrease or eliminate pain and anxiety.

Magnets

Dating back to the ancient Egyptians and Greeks, the theory is that magnets may effect changes in cells or body chemistry that can produce pain relief. The use of magnets is popular with athletes who report their effectiveness in controlling pain.

Capsaicin

Capsaicin is a chemical that's found in chili peppers and is the primary ingredient in many pain-relieving creams for the treatment of neuropathic pain. It produces a burning sensation locally that replaces the pain sensation.

Summary

Patient completed pain scores from validated pain assessment scales can be useful as the basis for treating chronic wound-associated pain. The scales enable the clinician to accurately assess the patient's pain, thereby facilitating effective treatment modalities to help decrease the wound-associated pain. Pain is detrimental for patients because it can exhaust them, affect their ability to perform their ADLs, add to feelings of decreased worth as a person, affect their interactions with loved ones and friends, deter wound healing and, overall, diminish their quality of life and the quality of death for patients who are in the process of dying. As clinicians, we are obligated to provide adequate pain relief for our patients by using an appropriate selection of the treatment modalities available to us.

Show what you know

1. *Which of the statements listed below most accurately defines pain? Pain is:*

A. an objective finding based on prolonged elevation of the patient's blood pressure and pulse rate.
B. a state of discomfort evidenced by the person being unable to sleep.
C. a physical consequence of wound care.
D. whatever the experiencing person says it is.

ANSWER: D. McCaffery's classic definition of pain is that it's whatever the experiencing person says it is.[6] A is incorrect as research has shown that sudden severe pain may elevate vital signs, but this only occurs for a short time.[6] B is incorrect as research has shown that patients can sleep even though they have moderate or severe pain.[6] C is incorrect because, although pain may be a consequence of wound care, this isn't a definition of pain.

2. Which of the following statements best describes the Numeric Pain Intensity Scale? It's a:

A. 10-cm line with the words "no pain" at one end and the "worst possible pain" at the other end.
B. series of faces ranging from smiling to frowning.
C. rainbow of colors starting with green and ending with red.
D. a decision tree for determining which medications to give to a person experiencing pain.

ANSWER: A. The Numeric Pain Intensity Scale is a 10-cm line with the words "no pain" at one end and "worst possible pain" at the other end. B refers to the Faces Pain Rating Scale. C doesn't describe a pain scale. D refers to the WHO analgesic ladder.

3. According to the WHO analgesic ladder, which medications should you use initially for relief of mild pain?

A. None
B. Non-opioid with or without an adjuvant
C. Opioid with or without an adjuvant
D. Opioid

ANSWER: B. A non-opioid is the drug recommended to use for mild pain. An adjuvant can be added to the non-opioid if there is neuropathic pain, as well as nociceptive pain. A is wrong as drugs are part of the WHO analgesic ladder. C and D are incorrect as they are part of step 2 in the ladder.

References

1. "Pain Terms. A List with Definitions and Notes on Usage Recommended by the IASP Subcommittee on Taxonomy," *Pain* 6(3):249-252, June 1979.
2. Acute Pain Management Guideline Panel. *Acute Pain Management: Operative or Medical Procedures and Trauma, Clinical Practice Guideline*, No.3. Rockville, Md.: AHCPR, 1992.
3. McCaffery, M., and Beebe, A. *Pain: A Clinical Manual for Nursing Practice.* St. Louis: Mosby–Year Book, Inc., 1989.
4. Dahl, J.L., and Gordon, D.B. "Joint Commission Pain Standards: A Progress Report," *APS Bulletin* 12(6), 2002.
5. American Pain Society. *Pain: The Fifth Vital Sign.* Available at *www.ampainsoc.org/advocacy/fifth.htm.* November 1995.
6. McCaffery, M., and Passero, C. *Pain: Clinical Manual,* 2nd ed. St. Louis: Mosby–Year Book, Inc.1999.
7. *Principles of Analgesic Use in the Treatment of Acute Pain and Cancer Pain,* 4th ed. Glenview, Ill.: American Pain Society, 1999.
8. Lesser, H., et al. "Pregabalin relieves symptoms of painful diabetic neuropathy: a randomized controlled trial," *Neurology* 63(11):2104-10, December 14, 2004.
9. Dworkin, R.H., et al. "Pregabalin for the Treatment of Postherpetic Neuralgia: a Randomized, Placebo-controlled Trial," *Neurology* 60(8):1274-83, April 2003.
10. American Geriatric Society. "The Management of Persistent Pain in Older Persons," *AGS Panel on Persistent Pain in Older Persons* 50(6 Suppl):S205-S224, June 2002.
11. Krasner, D. "The Chronic Wound Pain Experience: A Conceptual Model," *Ostomy/Wound Management* 41(3):20-29, April 1995.
12. Krasner, D. "Caring for the Person Experiencing Chronic Wound Pain," in *Chronic Wound Care: A Clinical Source Book for Healthcare Professionals,* 3rd ed. Edited by Krasner, D.L. Wayne, Pa.: HMP Communications, 2001.
13. Krasner, D. "Managing Wound Pain in Patients with Vacuum-Assisted Closure Devices," *Ostomy/Wound Management* 48(5):38-43, May 2002.
14. National Pressure Ulcer Advisory Panel, "Pressure Ulcer Prevalence, Cost, and Risk Assessment: Consensus Development Conference Statement," *Decubitus* 2(2):24-28, May 1989.
15. Van Rijswijk, L., and Braden, B.J. "Pressure Ulcer Patient and Wound Assessment: An AHCPR Clinical Practice Guideline Update," *Ostomy/Wound Management* 45(1A Suppl):56S-67S, January 1999.
16. Bergstrom, N., et al. "Pressure Ulcer Treatment," Clinical Practice Guideline #15. Rockville, Md.: AHCPR, 1994.
17. Pieper, B. "Mechanical Forces: Pressure, Shear and Friction," in *Acute and Chronic Wounds: Nursing Management,* 2nd ed. Edited by Bryant, R.A. St. Louis: Mosby–Year Book, Inc., 2000.
18. Rook, J.L. "Wound Care Pain Management," *Advances in Wound Care* 9(6):24-31, November-December 1996.
19. Szors, J.K., and Bourguignon, C. "Description of Pressure Ulcer Pain at Rest and Dressing Change," *Journal of Wound, Ostomy, and Continence Nurses* 26(3):115-20, May 1999.
20. Hollingworth, H. "Nurse's Assessment and Management of Pain at Wound Dressing Changes," *Journal of Wound Care* 4(2):77-83, February 1995.
21. Moffatt, C.J., et al. "Understanding Wound Pain and Trauma: An International Perspective," *EWMA Position Document: Pain at Wound Dressing Changes* 2-7, 2002.
22. Moffatt, C., et al. "Understanding Wound Pain and Trauma: An International Perspective," *EWMA Position Document: Pain at Wound Dressing Changes* (Electronic version) 2-7, 2002.
23. Wulf, H & Baron, R. "The Theory of Pain" *EWMA Position Document: Pain at Wound Dressing Changes* (Electronic version) 8-11, 2002.
24. Briggs, M., et al. "Pain at Wound Dressing Changes: a Guide to Management," *EWMA Position Document: Pain at Wound Dressing Changes* (Electronic version) 12-17, 2002.
25. Briggs, M., and Ferris, F.D., et al. "Principles of Best Practice. Minimising pain at wound dressing-related procedures: A consensus document," *A World Union of Wound Healing Societies' Initiative* (Electronic version) 1-10, 2004.

26. Latarjet, J. "The management of pain associated with dressing changes in patients with burns," *World Wide Wounds* (Electronic version) 1-10, Nov 2002.

27. Krasner, D. "Using a Gentler Hand: Reflections on Patients with Pressure Ulcers Who Experience Pain," *Ostomy/ Wound Management* 42(3):20-29, April 1996.

28. Dallam, L., et al. "Pressure Ulcer Pain: Assessment and Quantification," Journal of Wound, Ostomy, and Continence Nursing 22(5):211-17, September 1995.

29. Franks, P.J., and Collier, M.E. "Quality of Life: The Cost to the Individual," in *The Prevention of Pressure Ulcers.* Edited by Morrison, M.J. St. Louis: Mosby–Year Book, Inc., 2001.

30. Langemo, D.K., et al. "The Lived Experience of Having a Pressure Ulcer: A Qualitative Analysis," *Advances in Skin & Wound Care* 13(5):225-35, September-October 2000.

31. Rastinehad, D. "Pressure ulcer pain," *JWOCN* 33(3):252-57, May/June 2006

32. Fox, C. "Living With a Pressure Ulcer: A Descriptive Study of Patients' Experiences," *Br J Community Nurs* 7:10-22, July 2002.

33. Roth, R.S., Lowery, J.C., Hamill, J.B. "Assessing Persistent Pain and its Relation to Affective Distress, Depressive Symptoms, and Pain Catastrophizing in Patients with Chronic Wounds: A Pilot Study," *Am J Phys Med Rehabil* 83(11):827-34, November 2004.

34. Shukla, D; Tripathi, AK; et al. Pain in acute and chronic wounds: A descriptive study. *Ostomy Wound Mgmt,* 51(11):47-51. November 2005.

35. Ayello, E.A., et al. "Is Pressure Ulcer Pain Documented? Submitted for publication, 2006.

36. Ayello, E.A. "Teaching the Assessment of Patients with Pressure Ulcers," *Decubitus* 5(4):53-54, July 1992.

37. Ayello, E.A. "A Pressure Ulcer ASSESSMENT Tool," *Advances in Skin & Wound Care* 13(5):247, September-October 2000.

38. Hartford Institute for Geriatric Nursing, Try This. www.hartfordign.org. last accessed June 11,2006

39. Fink, R., and Gates, R. "Pain Assessment," in *Textbook of Palliative Nursing.* Edited by Ferrell, B.R., and Coyle, N. Oxford University Press, 2001.

40. Keele, K.D. "The Pain Chart," *Lancet* 48(2):6-8, February 1948.

41. Wong, D.L., and Baker, C.M. "Pain in Children: Comparison of Assessment Scales," *Pediatric Nursing* 14(1):9-17, January-February 1988.

42. Flaherty, S.A. "Pain Measurement Tools for Clinical Practice and Research," *Journal of the American Association of Nurse Anesthetists* 64(2):133-140, April 1996.

43. Wong, D.L., et al. *Wong's Essentials of Pediatric Nursing,* 6th ed. St. Louis: Mosby, 2001.

44. Simon, W., and Malabar, R. "Assessing Pain in Elderly Patients Who Can't Respond Verbally," *Journal of Advanced Nursing* 22(4):663-669, October 1995.

45. Donovan, M., et al. "Incidence and Characteristics of Pain in a Sample of Medical-Surgical Patients," *Pain* 30(1):69-78, July 1987.

46. Faires, J.E., et al. "Systematic Pain Records and Their Impact on Pain Control: A Pilot Study," *Cancer Nursing* 12(6):306-13, December 1991.

47. Freedman, G., et al. "Practical Treatment of Pain Inpatients with Chronic Wounds: Pathogenesis-guided Management," *The American Journal of Surgery* 188(suppl):31S-35S, July 2004.

48. *Cancer Pain Relief,* 2nd ed., Geneva: World Health Organization, 1996.

49. Twillman, R.K., et al. "Treatment of Painful Skin Ulcer with Topical Opioids," *Journal of Pain and Symptom Management* 17(4):288-92, April 1999.

50. Derby, S., and O'Mahony, S. "Elderly Patients," *In* Ferrell, B.R., and Coyles, N (eds.) *Textbook of Palliative Nursing.* New York: Oxford University Press USA, 2001

51. McCaffery, M., and Robinson, E.S. "Your Patient is in Pain, Here's How You Respond," *Nursing* 32(10):36-45, October 2002.

52. Hopkins, A., et al. "Patient Stories of Living with a Pressure Ulcer," *Journal of Advanced Nursing* 56(4):1-9, April 2006.

53. Herr, K., et al. "Pain Assessment in the Nonverbal Patient: Position Statement with Clinical Practice Recommendations," *Pain Management Nursing* 7(2) 6:44-52, June 2006.

Part Two

Wound classifications and management strategies

CHAPTER 13

Pressure ulcers

Elizabeth A. Ayello, PhD, RN, APRN,BC, CWOCN, FAPWCA, FAAN
Sharon Baranoski, MSN, RN, CWOCN, APN, DAPWCA, FAAN
Courtney H. Lyder, ND, GNP, FAAN
Janet Cuddigan, PhD, RN, CWCN, CCCN

OBJECTIVES

After completing this chapter, you'll be able to:

- discuss the significance of pressure ulcers as a health care problem
- state the prevalence and incidence of pressure ulcers around the world
- describe the etiology of a pressure ulcer
- define pressure ulcer classification systems
- state how to complete a risk assessment tool
- discuss strategies for pressure ulcer prevention
- discuss strategies for treating a patient with pressure ulcers.

Pressure ulcers as a health care problem

Pressure ulcers have been seen as a nursing problem throughout time. The reality is that pressure ulcers are a global health care concern and more than a nursing issue. All clinicians need to be responsible for the prevention and treatment of pressure ulcers.

Over the centuries, pressure ulcers have been referred to as decubitus ulcers, bedsores, and pressure sores. The term *pressure ulcer* has become the preferred name of choice because it most closely describes the etiology and resultant ulcer. The National Pressure Ulcer Advisory Panel (NPUAP) re-

vised its definition of pressure ulcers at its 2007 consensus conference to read: "localized injury to the skin and/or underlying tissue usually over a bony prominence, as a result of pressure, or pressure in combination with shear and/or friction. A number of contributing factors are also associated with pressure ulcers; the significance of these factors is yet to be elucidated."[9] Pressure ulcers are usually located over bony prominences (such as the sacrum, coccyx, hips, heels) and are staged according to the extent of observable tissue damage.[1] (See *NPUAP pressure ulcer staging definitions*, pages 256 and 257.)

Treatment interventions have varied along with the terminology. Wax, honey, feathers, leaves, bugs, ointments, and magic potions survived for centuries as caregivers searched for the right answer. Today, research supports using moist wound therapy to promote a microenvironment conducive to healing. Numerous products and dressing choices are available for clinicians to utilize in their practice. (See chapter 9, Wound treatment options.)

The incidence and prevalence of pressure ulcers is truly an enigma. Pressure ulcers aren't a reportable event in all health care settings, so data is speculative at best. We do know, however, that the numbers are significant enough to warrant a national health care initiative in the United States. As early as 1989, the federal government focused their attention on pressure ulcers with the appointment of a panel charged with the development of the Agency for Health Care Policy and Research (AHCPR) guidelines. Another federal initiative that supports the fact that many individuals get pressure ulcers is Healthy People 2010. The objective is to reduce the incidence of pressure ulcers in the long-term care population by 50%.[2] In addition, the Centers for Medicare and Medicaid Services (CMS, formerly the Health Care Financing Administration) considers a pressure ulcer to be a sentinel event in a resident of a long-term care facility who has been assessed as being at low risk for a pressure ulcer. According to CMS, the only residents who are at high risk are those who have impaired transfer or bed mobility, are comatose, malnourished, or have end-stage disease; other patients are at low risk.[3] In 2004, the CMS revised its guidance for surveyors in long-term care facilities regarding Tag F-314 pressure ulcers. The revision now states that these facilities will incur monetary fines for level 2 through 4 pressure ulcers in residents who get pressure ulcers or when the stage of an existing pressure ulcer worsens.[4] New Jersey also requires hospitals to report the occurrence of stage III or IV pressure ulcers.[5] In addition, the Agency for Healthcare Research and Quality (AHRQ) noted in its 2006 statistical brief report that there was a 63% increase in hospital stays in which pressure ulcers were noted ,even though the total number of hospitalizations for this time period (1993-2003) increased by only 11%.[6] The Institute for Healthcare Improvement (IHI)

has made pressure ulcers 1 of the 12 improvements in patient care included in its "Protecting 5 million lives from harm" initiative for U.S. hospitals to reduce incidents of medical harm.[7] Moreover, CMS is studying pressure ulcers as 1 of 17 patient safety issues for hospitals.[8] Given the attention that regulatory and quality improvement agencies have shown to pressure ulcer occurrence, pressure ulcer risk assessment should be a priority of patient care across all care settings.

The financial cost to all institutions and facilities isn't precisely known. AHRQ reports the average cost of pressure ulcers for hospitalized patients is $37,800.[6] Published estimates of treatment costs vary by hospital, long-term care, and home care settings; the one certainty is that pressure ulcers do create a financial burden for the facility, patient, and family. Pressure ulcers cost institutions valuable staff time, supplies, and reputation.

Pressure ulcer practices should be supported by scientific, evidence-based practice, not anecdotal success stories. This presents a problem. We don't have adequate research-based, randomized clinical studies to support all of our current practices. Wound care interventions and modalities have often been based on "it works for me." We need to encourage health care providers to participate in research studies so that we'll have the evidence in the future to direct and improve our clinical decision process, thereby improving patient outcomes.

Wound etiology

Pressure ulcers have long been believed to be localized wounds that develop over bony prominences due to excessive pressure eventually resulting in tissue ulceration. What we do know is that the primary factor causing pressure ulcers is pressure. Maklebust[10] defined pressure as "a perpendicular load or force exerted on a unit of area." The correlation between tissue compression and ischemia is supported in the literature. The amount of pressure and the duration of that pressure are inversely proportional.[11] Low amounts of pressure over long periods of

NPUAP pressure ulcer staging definitions

Pressure ulcer stage	Previous NPUAP staging definitions
Suspected deep tissue injury	A pressure-related injury to subcutaneous tissues under intact skin; initially, these lesions appearing as a deep bruise and may herald the development of subsequent development of a Stage III-IV pressure ulcer even with optimal treatment
Stage I	An observable pressure-related alteration of intact skin whose indicators as compared to an adjacent or opposite area on the body may include changes in one or more of the following parameters: skin temperature (warmth or coolness), tissue consistency (firm or boggy feel), sensation (pain, itching) and or a defined area of persistent redness in lightly pigmented skin, whereas in darker skin tones, the ulcer may appear with persistent red, blue, or purple hues
Stage II	Partial-thickness skin loss involving the epidermis and or dermis; ulcer is superficial and presents clinically as an abrasion, blister, or shallow crater
Stage III	Full-thickness skin loss involving damage or necrosis of subcutaneous tissue which may extend down to, but not through, underlying fascia; ulcer presents clinically as a deep crater with or without undermining of adjacent tissue
Stage IV	Full-thickness skin loss with extensive destruction, tissue necrosis, or damage to muscle, bone, or supporting structure (such as a tendon or joint capsule)
Unstageable	(No previous definition)

© 2007 National Pressure Ulcer Advisory Panel. Used with permission.

time can be just as detrimental to tissue as high amounts of pressure over short periods of time. The long-held standard of 32 mm Hg as a critical closing pressure is being revisited. Continued research is needed in the areas of capillary pressure, the application of uniform pressure, and the application of localized pressure. (See chapter 11, Pressure redistribution: Seating, positioning, and support surfaces.)

Current (2007) NPUAP staging definitions	Proposed 2007 NPUAP descriptions to accompany revised definitions
Purple or maroon localized area of discolored intact skin or blood-filled blister due to damage of underlying soft tissue from pressure and/or shear. The area may be preceded by tissue that is painful, firm, mushy, boggy, warmer or cooler as compared to adjacent tissue.	Deep tissue injury may be difficult to detect in individuals with dark skin tones. Evolution may include a thin blister over a dark wound bed. The wound may further evolve and become covered by thin eschar. Evolution may be rapid exposing additional layers of tissue even with optimal treatment.
Intact skin with non-blanchable redness of a localized area usually over a bony prominence. Darkly pigmented skin may not have visible blanching; its color may differ from the surrounding area.	The area may be painful, firm, soft, warmer or cooler as compared to adjacent tissue. Stage I may be difficult to detect in individuals with dark skin tones. May indicate "at risk" persons (a heralding sign of risk).
Partial thickness loss of dermis presenting as a shallow open ulcer with a red pink wound bed, without slough. May also present as an intact or open/ruptured serum-filled blister.	Presents as a shiny or dry shallow ulcer without slough or bruising.* This stage should not be used to describe skin tears, tape burns, perineal dermatitis, maceration or excoriation. *Bruising indicates suspected deep tissue injury.
Full thickness tissue loss. Subcutaneous fat may be visible but bone, tendon or muscle are *not* exposed. Slough may be present but does not obscure the depth of tissue loss. May include undermining and tunneling.	The depth of a stage III pressure ulcer varies by anatomical location. The bridge of the nose, ear, occiput and malleolus do not have subcutaneous tissue and stage III ulcers can be shallow. In contrast, areas of significant adiposity can develop extremely deep stage III pressure ulcers. Bone/tendon is not visible or directly palpable.
Full thickness tissue loss with exposed bone, tendon or muscle. Slough or eschar may be present on some parts of the wound bed. Often includes undermining or tunneling.	The depth of a stage IV pressure ulcer varies by anatomical location. The bridge of the nose, ear, occiput and malleolus do not have subcutaneous tissue and these ulcers can be shallow. Stage IV ulcers can extend into muscle and/or supporting structures (e.g., fascia, tendon or joint capsule) making osteomyelitis possible. Exposed bone/tendon is visible or directly palpable.
Full thickness tissue loss in which the base of the ulcer is covered by slough (yellow, tan, gray, green or brown) and/or eschar (tan, brown or black) in the wound bed.	Until enough slough and/or eschar is removed to expose the base of the wound, the true depth, and therefore stage, cannot be determined. Stable (dry, adherent, intact without erythema or fluctance) eschar on the heels serves as the "the body's natural (biological) cover" and should not be removed.

Body tissues differ in their ability to tolerate pressure. The blood supply to the skin originates in the underlying muscle. Muscle is more sensitive to pressure damage than skin.[12] Tissue tolerance is further compromised by extrinsic and intrinsic factors. Examples of extrinsic factors are moisture, friction, and irritants. Intrinsic factors that affect the ability of the skin and supporting structures to respond to pressure and shear

Pressure gradient

In the illustration to the right, the V-shaped pressure gradient results from the upward force (upward arrows) exerted by the supporting surface against downward force (downward arrows) exerted by the bony prominence. Pressure is greatest on tissues at the apex of the gradient and lessens to the right and left of this point.

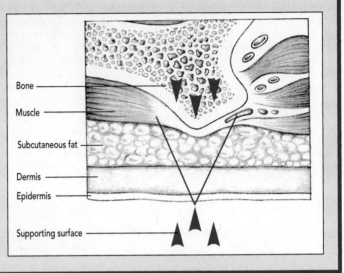

Bone
Muscle
Subcutaneous fat
Dermis
Epidermis
Supporting surface

forces are numerous. They include age, spinal cord injury, nutrition, and steroid administration that are believed to affect collagen synthesis and degradation.[13] Other intrinsic factors that affect tissue perfusion are systemic blood pressure, extra corporeal circulation, serum protein, smoking, hemoglobin and hematocrit, vascular disease, diabetes mellitus, vasoactive drugs, and increase in body temperature.[13]

PRACTICE POINT

Muscle tissue dies first from pressure. Look at a variety of extrinsic and intrinsic factors that could put your patient at risk for pressure ulcers.

How do pressure ulcers occur? This is an interesting and challenging question. Literature reviews demonstrate only that the etiology of pressure ulcers continues to remain largely unclear. One theory of how pressure ulcers occur is that they begin from the bone outward. Deep tissue injury near the bone occurs first, and it isn't until later when the tissue death continues and reaches the outer layer of the skin (the epidermis) that the skin breaks.[14] The pressure gradient

model[14] has been used to explain how pressure translates into tissue death. (See *Pressure gradient*.) External pressure is transmitted from the epidermis inward toward the bone as well as counter-pressure from the bone. Pressure is transmitted from the body surface to the underlying bone, compressing all of the tissue in between. The greatest pressure occurs over the bone, gradually decreasing at the skin level. Blood vessels, fascia and muscle, subcutaneous fat, and the skin are compressed between these two counter pressures. Muscle and subcutaneous fat have a low tolerance for decreased blood flow, making them less resilient than skin to pressure. Destruction of tissue below the skin level isn't seen until surface damage is evident. Unless there's an impairment in the nervous system resulting in loss of sensation, a patient will normally shift his weight by changing position when pressure is exerted against the skin for a period of time.[10]

PRACTICE POINT

Patients with altered sensation are at risk for the development of pressure ulcers.

Shearing force

Shear injury is a mechanical force parallel, rather than perpendicular, to an area of tissue. In the illustration below, gravity pulls the body down the incline of the bed. The skeleton and attached deep fascia slide within the skin, while the skin and superficial fascia, attached to the dermis, remain stationary, held in place by friction between the skin and the bed linen. This internal slide compromises blood supply to the area.

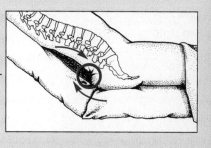

Effects of shear on tissue

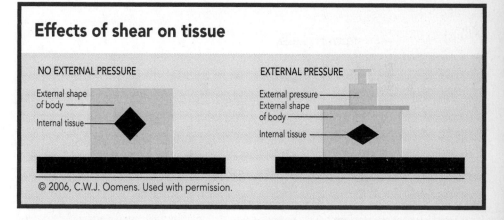

NO EXTERNAL PRESSURE

External shape of body
Internal tissue

EXTERNAL PRESSURE

External pressure
External shape of body
Internal tissue

© 2006, C.W.J. Oomens. Used with permission.

The second theory of how pressure ulcers form is that skin destruction occurs at the epidermis and proceeds downward to the deeper tissues. Maklebust and Sieggreen[14] call this theory the "top to bottom model." The injury is seen as intact skin with blanchable erythema. This is the least-favored model of pressure ulcer development, given its limited evidence base.

Friction and shear are also mechanical forces contributing to pressure ulcer formation. The tissue injury resulting from these forces may look like a superficial skin insult. Shear and friction are two separate phenomenon, yet often work together to create tissue ischemia and ulcer development.

Shear is a "mechanical force that acts on an area of skin in a direction parallel to the body's surface. It's affected by the amount of pressure exerted, the coefficient of friction between the materials contacting each other,

and the extent to which the body makes contact with the support surface."[15] The NPUAP[16] has posted new definitions of shear stress and shear strain on their Web site. You can think of shear stress and strain as pulling the bones of the pelvis in one direction and the skin in the opposite direction. (See *Shearing force*. See also *Effects of shear on tissue*.) The deeper fascia slides downward with the bone and the superficial fascia remains attached to the dermis. This insult and compromise to the blood supply creates ischemia and leads to cellular death and tissue necrosis. Shear and friction go hand in hand—you'll rarely see one without the other.

PRACTICE POINT

You won't see shear injury at the skin level because it occurs underneath the skin. You will see friction injury. Elevation of the head

Pressure ulcer sites

Shown in the illustration to the right are the most common sites where pressure ulcers develop.

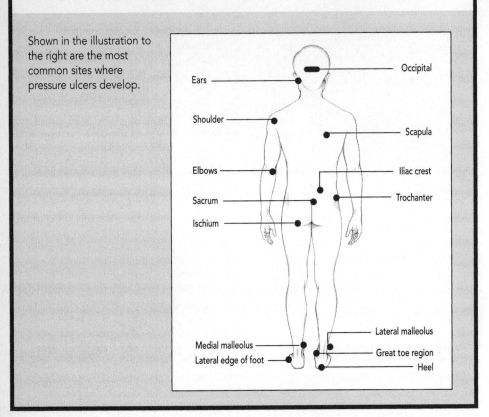

of the bed increases shear injury in the deep tissue, and may account for the number of sacral ulcers we see in practice.

Friction was originally defined by the AHRQ as the "mechanical force exerted when skin is dragged across a coarse surface such as bed linens."[15] NPUAP defines friction or frictional force as "the resistance to motion in a parallel direction relative to the common boundary of two surfaces."[16] Simply stated, friction or frictional force results when two surfaces move across one another. A skin insult caused by friction looks like an abrasion or superficial laceration. Friction, however, isn't a primary factor in the development of pressure ulcers. It can contribute to an insult or stripping of the epidermal layer of the skin, creating an environment conducive to further insult. An alter-

ation in the coefficient of friction increases the skin's adherence to the outside surface (for example, the bed). Friction then combines with shearing forces and the ultimate outcome may be a pressure ulcer. Tissues subjected to friction are more susceptible to pressure ulcer damage.[17] The three mechanical forces (pressure, friction, and shear) may act in concert to create tissue damage. Other patients at risk for pressure ulcers from friction are elderly people, those with uncontrollable movements such as spastic movements, and those who use braces or appliances that rub against the skin.[14]

Exactly what causes pressure ulcers remains controversial.[18] Theories on the etiology of a pressure ulcer need continued research. Those described here may be correct, but additional research and basic science hold the answers to many unanswered questions.

Most pressure ulcers occur in the lower part of the body over bony prominences such as the sacrum, coccyx, ischial tuberosities, greater trochanters, elbows, heels, scapulae, iliac crests, and lateral and medial malleoli.[14] (See *Pressure ulcer sites*.) Other areas, where pressure ulcers may be overlooked, include the occiput (especially in infants and toddlers, see Neonates/pediatrics section of chapter 20), ears (especially in patients using nasal oxygen cannulas), and the great toe region. Several national surveys demonstrated that the most common site for pressure ulcers among patients in acute care facilities is the sacrum, with the heels being second.[19-21] The incidence of heel ulcers has increased incrementally over the past decade, creating a need for prevention protocols targeting the heels. The HEELS© mnemonic (See *HEELS© mnemonic*.) can be used to care for heels at risk for pressure ulcers.

PRACTICE POINT

Careful observation of the sacrum and the heels is warranted because these are the most frequent sites of pressure ulcers.

Prevention

Preventing pressure ulcers is of vital importance. Elements of pressure ulcer prevention include identifying individuals at risk for developing pressure ulcers, preserving skin integrity, treating the underlying causes of the ulcer, relieving pressure, paying attention to the total state of the patient to correct any deficiencies, and educating the patient and his family.

Risk factors and risk assessment

Risk assessment is used to identify:
- patients at risk
- the level of risk
- the type of risk.

Identifying individuals at risk for pressure ulcers enables clinicians to make decisions

---

HEELS© mnemonic

H ave the foot or leg movement?
E valuate sensation.
E liminate friction & foot drop risk.
L ook at heels!
S uspend heels with devices as needed.

© 2005, Ayello, Cuddigan, and Black

---

about when to begin using preventive measures. This is important for the most effective use of resources because the level of risk guides the intensity and cost of preventive interventions. We tend to prescribe preventive protocols based on total scores, often ignoring the type of risk—and missing the point of a risk-based protocol. We should custom design protocols according to which pressure ulcer risk assessment subscale scores are low (that is, which risk factors are high). So, for example, if your patient has low subscores on activity, mobility, and moisture, and high scores for nutrition, you should customize interventions to prevent pressure and control moisture, but you don't need a big nutritional intervention, maybe just maintenance.

The clinical practice guidelines on pressure ulcer prevention from the Agency for Health Care Policy and Research (AHCPR; now the AHRQ) are considered an important starting point for identifying at-risk patients and determining the need for prevention interventions. For example, the AHCPR Panel for Prediction and Prevention of Pressure Ulcers[22] suggests that bedridden patients and those with impaired ability to change position are at risk for pressure ulcers because of immobility. The guideline also suggests that these individuals should be assessed for additional factors that increase risk for developing pressure ulcers, which include incontinence, nutritional factors such as inadequate dietary intake or impaired nutritional status, and altered level of consciousness.[22] All risk assessments should be documented using a validated tool.

The many pressure ulcer risk assessment tools include the Norton Scale,[23] the Gosnell

Scale,[24] the Braden Scale,[25] the Knoll Scale,[26] and the Waterlow Scale.[27] Deciding which scale to use can be challenging. Reviewing the reliability (consistency) and validity (accuracy) of each validated risk assessment scale should always be the first step in the decision-making process. Reliability for risk assessment scales is usually described by inter-rater reliability. "A common measure of inter-rater reliability for a risk assessment tool is percentage agreement, which looks at the percentage of instances in which different raters assign the same score to the same patients. Validity, or accuracy, is measured by the ability of the tool to correctly predict who will or won't develop a pressure ulcer."[28]

Predictive validity is dependent on the sensitivity and specificity of the tool. Sensitivity "is the percentage of individuals who develop a pressure ulcer who were assessed as being at risk for a pressure ulcer. A tool has good sensitivity if it correctly identifies true positives while minimizing false negatives. Specificity is the percentage of individuals who don't develop a pressure ulcer who were assessed as being not at risk for developing an ulcer. A tool has good specificity if it identifies true negatives and minimizes false positives."[28,29] Because of the amount of clinical research supporting their reliability and validity, the Norton and the Braden Scales are mentioned in the AHCPR guidelines as appropriate to use to determine pressure ulcer risk assessment. One study that compared four of the risk assessment scales found that the Gosnell Scale was the most appropriate for patients with neurologic and orthopedic conditions.[30]

Braden Scale

The Braden Scale is the most commonly used pressure ulcer assessment scale in the United States. Available in many languages and used world wide, this copyrighted tool, created in 1987 by Barbara Braden and Nancy Bergstrom, is available at http://www.braden scale.com.braden.pdf. The Braden Scale has six subscales: sensory perception, moisture, activity, mobility, nutrition, and friction/shear.[25] (See *Braden Scale: Predicting pres-*

sure ulcer risk, pages 264 and 265.) The scale is based on the two primary etiologic factors of pressure ulcer development—intensity and duration of pressure and tissue tolerance for pressure. "Sensory perception, mobility, and activity address clinical situations that predispose a patient to intense and prolonged pressure, while moisture, nutrition, and friction/shear address clinical situations that alter tissue tolerance for pressure."[28]

Each subscale contains a numerical range of scores, with 1 being the lowest score possible. The sensory perception, moisture, activity, mobility, and nutrition subscales have scores ranging from 1 to 4. Friction/shear is the only subscale where scores range from 1 to 3. Definitions of each subscale as to what patient characteristics to evaluate are given for each numerical ranking. The Braden Scale score is derived from totaling the numerical ratings from each of the six subscales. Six is the lowest possible score and 23 is the highest.

A low numerical score means the patient is at high risk for developing pressure ulcers. The original risk score was 16.[25] Subsequent research is the basis for the recommendation to use 18 as the risk score for elderly,[31] Black, and Hispanic patients.[32,33] Although Braden and Bergstrom[28,29] suggest the following levels of risk based on total Braden Scale scores: 15 to 18, at risk; 13 to 14, moderate risk; 10 to 12, high risk; and 9 or below, very high risk; in practice, many clinicians have only two categories—patients who are at risk for pressure ulcers and those who aren't. It's important that nurses accurately perform ulcer risk assessments. Recent research found that 75.6% of hospital nurses correctly rated a patient's level of risk after having computer-based testing on the use of the Braden Scale.[34] Nurses were best at identifying patients at either extreme, high, or low levels of risk. Persons at "mild risk" were least likely to have correct nurse ratings.[34] Determining the risk level is helpful in deciding on appropriate prevention strategies. Clinical judgment should play a part in interpreting the total Braden Scale score because not all risk factors are quantified on the scale.

After the total Braden Scale score is computed, a patient's risk and need for preventive protocols can be determined. Because each health care facility may differ in terms of staffing patterns, access to clinicians who specialize in wound care, and the preventive products utilized, it's difficult to prescribe a set of protocols that will fit all circumstances; however, a broad outline of protocol development has been developed. More specific protocols should be written by each facility, and staff education for use of these protocols must be provided prior to their implementation.[28,29] (See *Braden score interventions,* page 266.)

Questions have surfaced regarding when to assess patients and when to do risk reassessment. These two aspects of care are both very important. The AHCPR clinical practice guideline on pressure ulcer prevention recommends that initial pressure ulcer risk assessment be done upon admission as well as reassessments at periodic intervals.[22] However, the guideline doesn't provide time frames for reassessments. Reassessment intervals should be based on the acuity of the individual for whom the pressure ulcer risk is being calculated. Studies by Bergstrom and Braden[31,35] found that in a skilled nursing facility, 80% of pressure ulcers develop within 2 weeks of admission and 96% develop within 3 weeks of admission. The following recommendations for assessment and reassessment are based on this research.[28,29,35]

• Acute care—Initial assessment on admission, reassess at least every 48 hours or whenever the patient's condition changes for general care units, and every 24 hours for critical care units. Due to the short lengths of stay and acuity of all hospitalized patients, the recent *Prevent Pressure Ulcers How-to Guide* by the IHI recommends that pressure ulcer risk assessment be done every 24 hours.[7]

• Long-term care—Initial assessment on admission, then reassess weekly for the first 4 weeks, monthly to quarterly after that, and whenever the resident's condition changes.

• Home health care—On admission, then reassess with every RN visit.

As far as what time of day a pressure ulcer risk assessment should be done, research demonstrates that no particular time of day is better than another to do a pressure ulcer risk assessment. Outside of home care, patient care activities can vary from shift to shift. Risk assessment can be scheduled on either the day or evening shift, according to when it will best fit with staffing patterns and be performed most consistently.[28,29]

Importance of risk assessment

Some clinicians believe that an informal pressure ulcer risk assessment is sufficient and that a formal risk assessment is unnecessary. On the contrary, an informal risk assessment can't take the place of a formal risk assessment like one conducted using the Braden Scale. Research has shown that in the absence of formal risk assessment, clinicians tended to intervene consistently only at the highest levels of risk. In some studies, for example, turning—considered an important part of pressure ulcer prevention—was prescribed for fewer than 50% of patients at mild or moderate risk for developing pressure ulcers. Pressure reduction was prescribed more than turning, but not with adequate consistency.[36]

In a study that introduced formal risk assessment and linked levels of risk to preventive protocols, the incidence of pressure ulcers dropped by 60%; severity of pressure ulcers and cost of care decreased as well.[36] This could be due to better identification of patients at mild and moderate risk and a more consistent use of preventive interventions for patients in all risk categories.

Patient care to prevent pressure ulcers

Preventing pressure ulcers can best be accomplished by using a multidisciplinary approach.[25,28,37,38] Several pressure ulcer prevention protocols and guidelines exist in the literature.[22,37-47] Most advocate taking a holistic approach to pressure ulcer prevention. Any good prevention program begins with assessing the patient's skin. The skin should be assessed and its condition documented daily in acute and long-term care set-

(Text continues on page 266.)

Braden Scale: Predicting pressure ulcer risk

SENSORY PERCEPTION
Ability to respond meaningfully to pressure-related discomfort

1. Completely limited:
Unresponsive (doesn't moan, flinch, or grasp) to painful stimuli due to diminished level of consciousness or sedation
OR
limited ability to feel pain over most of body surface.

2. Very limited:
Responds only to painful stimuli. Can't communicate discomfort except by moaning or restlessness
OR
has a sensory impairment that limits the ability to feel pain or discomfort over half of body.

MOISTURE
Degree to which skin is exposed to moisture

1. Constantly moist:
Skin is kept moist almost constantly by perspiration or urine. Dampness is detected every time patient is moved or turned.

2. Often moist:
Skin is often but not always moist. Linen must be changed at least once per shift.

ACTIVITY
Degree of physical activity

1. Bedfast:
Confined to bed.

2. Confined to chair:
Ability to walk severely limited or nonexistent. Can't bear own weight and must be assisted into chair or wheelchair.

MOBILITY
Ability to change and control body position

1. Completely immobile:
Doesn't make even slight changes in body or extremity position without assistance.

2. Very limited:
Makes occasional slight changes in body or extremity position but unable to make frequent or significant changes independently.

NUTRITION
Usual food intake pattern
NPO: Nothing by mouth
IV: Intravenously
TPN: Total parenteral nutrition

1. Very poor:
Never eats a complete meal. Rarely eats more than one-third of any food offered. Eats two servings or less of protein (meat or dairy products) per day. Takes fluids poorly. Doesn't take a liquid dietary supplement
OR
is NPO or maintained on clear liquids or I.V. fluids for more than 5 days.

2. Probably inadequate:
Rarely eats a complete meal and generally eats only about half of any food offered. Protein intake includes only three servings of meat or dairy products per day. Occasionally will take a dietary supplement
OR
receives less than optimum amount of liquid diet or tube feeding.

FRICTION AND SHEAR

1. Problem:
Requires moderate to maximum assistance in moving. Complete lifting without sliding against sheets is impossible. Frequently slides down in bed or chair, requiring frequent repositioning with maximum assistance. Spasticity, contractures, or agitation leads to almost constant friction.

2. Potential problem:
Moves feebly or requires minimum assistance. During a move, skin probably slides to some extent against sheets, chair, restraints, or other devices. Maintains relatively good position in chair or bed most of the time but occasionally slides down.

Used with permission from Barbara Braden, PhD, RN, FAAN, and Nancy Bergstrom, PhD, RN, FAAN. © 1988.

3. Slightly limited:
Responds to verbal commands but can't always communicate discomfort or need to be turned
OR
has some sensory impairment that limits ability to feel pain or discomfort in one or two extremities.

4. No impairment:
Responds to verbal commands. Has no sensory deficit that would limit ability to feel or voice pain or discomfort.

3. Occasionally moist:
Skin is occasionally moist, requiring an extra linen change approximately once per day.

4. Rarely moist:
Skin is usually dry; linen only requires changing at routine intervals.

3. Walks occasionally:
Walks occasionally during day, but for very short distances, with or without assistance; spends majority of each shift in bed or chair.

4. Walks frequently:
Walks outside the room at least twice per day and inside room at least once every 2 hours during waking hours.

3. Slightly limited:
Makes frequent though slight changes in body or extremity position independently.

4. No limitations:
Makes major and frequent changes in position without assistance.

3. Adequate:
Eats over half of most meals. Eats a total of four servings of protein (meat, dairy products) each day. Occasionally will refuse a meal, but will usually take a supplement if offered
OR
is on a tube feeding or TPN regimen that probably meets most nutritional needs.

4. Excellent:
Eats most of every meal and never refuses a meal. Usually eats a total of four servings of meat and dairy products. Occasionally eats between meals. Doesn't require supplementation.

3. No apparent problem:
Moves in bed and in chair independently and has sufficient muscle strength to lift up completely during move. Maintains good position in bed or chair at all times.

Braden score interventions

- At risk: 15 to 18—Consider a protocol of frequent turning, facilitating maximal re-mobilization, protecting the patient's heels, providing a pressure-reducing support surface if the patient is bedridden or confined to a chair, and managing moisture, nutrition, and friction and shear. If other major risk factors are present (advanced age, fever, poor dietary intake of protein, diastolic blood pressure below 60 mm Hg, or hemodynamic instability), advance to the next level of risk.

- Moderate risk: 13 to 14—Consider a protocol of frequent turning, facilitating maximal remobilization, protecting the patient's heels, providing a pressure-reducing support surface, providing foam wedges for 30-degree lateral positioning, and managing moisture, nutrition, and friction and shear. If other major risk factors are present, advance to the next level of risk.

- High risk: 10 to 12—Consider a protocol that increases the frequency of turning, supplements turning with small shifts in position, facilitates maximal remobilization, protects the patient's heels, provides a pressure-reducing support surface, provides foam wedges for 30-degree lateral positioning, and manages moisture, nutrition, and friction and shear.

- Very high risk: 9 or below—Consider a protocol that incorporates the points for high-risk patients. Add a pressure-relieving surface if the patient has intractable pain, severe pain exacerbated by turning, or additional risk factors such as immobility and malnutrition. A low-air-loss bed is no substitute for a turning schedule.

- Managing moisture—Use a commercial moisture barrier, and use absorbent pads or diapers that wick and hold moisture. Address the cause of the moisture if possible, and offer a bedpan or urinal and a glass of water in conjunction with turning schedules.

- Managing nutrition—Consult a dietitian and act quickly to alleviate nutritional deficits. Increase the patient's protein intake and increase his calorie intake if needed. Provide a multivitamin containing vitamins A, C, and E.

- Managing friction and shear—Elevate the head of the bed no more than 30 degrees and have the patient use a trapeze when indicated. Use a lift sheet to move the patient. Protect the patient's elbows, heels, sacrum, and back of head if he's exposed to friction.

- Other general care issues—Don't massage reddened bony prominences and don't use donut-type devices. Maintain good hydration and avoid drying out the patient's skin.

Adapted with permission from Ayello, E.A., and Braden, B. "How and Why to Do a Pressure Ulcer Risk Assessment," *Advances in Skin & Wound Care* 15(3):125-32, May-June 2002.

tings and at each home care visit. Careful attention to preventing skin injury during performance of activities of daily living is paramount. The bathing schedule should be individualized based on the patient's age, skin texture, and dryness or excessive oiliness of the skin. Use of nondrying products to clean the skin is recommended. One study found that the incidence of stage I and II pressure ulcers could be reduced by educating the staff about using body wash and skin protectant products.[48] Avoid excessive friction and hot water when cleaning. Use nonalcoholic moisturizers after bathing. A daily bath may not be needed for all patients; elderly patients, for example, may benefit from "lotion" baths.

For the incontinent patient, moist barriers and ointments should be considered as treatment options. Soiled skin should be cleaned immediately and products to protect the skin applied. If containment products are used, follow the correct methods of application. Reasons for incontinence should always be determined and appropriate measures to address the cause of the incontinence should be implemented.

The skin should be protected from injury. Pad bony prominences using dressings, such as films, hydrocolloids, foams, stockinettes, or roller gauze. Although a recent review of the literature suggests that one type of massage may be beneficial for at risk patients[49] most clinical guidelines recommend not to massage reddened bony prominences because this can lead to further tissue damage.[22,46] Keep the patient's heels off the bed; use pillows, wedges, and foot elevation devices as indicated. (See *HEELS© mnemonic,* page 261.) A folded bath blanket under the calves can "float the heels," completely relieving heel pressure in a bedridden patient.

PRACTICE POINT

Keep the patient's heels off the mattress!

Be careful not to drag your patient during transfers or position changes. Use appropriate devices, such as a turn sheet or mechanical lifting device, to prevent friction injuries to the patient's skin. Use the 30-degree lateral position for patients in bed. Keep the head of the bed below 30 degrees to prevent shearing injuries, unless contraindicated due to the patient's clinical condition.

Although no random clinical studies have documented the effects of specific nutritional interventions in preventing pressure ulcers, a large prospective cohort study by Bergstrom and Braden[31] found that nursing home residents who developed pressure ulcers had a significantly lower intake of protein. Clinicians need to ensure that a patient's caloric, protein, and vitamin and minerals needs are met. Recommendations from the dietitian can be an important source of assistance in helping patients to get their required nutrients. The European Pressure Ulcer Advisory Panel (EPUAP) has specific guidelines for nutrition in the care of pressure ulcers.[50]

Physical and occupational therapists are important members of the pressure ulcer team, a valuable resource for maximizing the patient's mobility. Their expertise in selecting appropriate size wheelchairs and evaluating seating angles and postural alignment can't be over emphasized. Patients who are confined to a chair should be repositioned every hour, with small shifts in weight made every 15 minutes. Although most clinicians consider turning and repositioning a bedridden patient every 2 hours a standard of care, the appropriate turning interval for all patients has yet to be determined by research. For some, 2 hours may be too long, whereas for others every 2 hours may not be necessary, as for palliative care patients, where frequent repositioning would cause more pain and suffering than benefit. Turning and repositioning needs to be customized for each patient. Brown cautions about having a rigid "turn Q 2 hours check box" on flow sheets and provides support for flexibility in documentation of turning and repositioning schedules in the patient's record.[51]

PRACTICE POINT

Turning schedules should be developed based on the individual patient's needs and care goals.

Appropriate pressure relieving devices and surfaces need to be used. See the NPUAP Web site (www.npuap.org) to review the latest definitions of physical concepts related to support surfaces as developed by the NPUAP Support Surface Standards Initiative.[16] (Also see chapter 11, Pressure redistribution: Seating, positioning, and support surfaces.) Devices such as "donuts" shouldn't be used.

Ongoing monitoring and documentation is essential. Communication of the prevention plan to all members of the health care team, including the patient and his family, is imperative. Supplement your verbal teaching with one of the prevention booklets designed for use by the consumer, such as pamphlets available from wound care companies as well as the AHRQ. The AHRQ also has a consumer version available in Spanish.

Pressure ulcer staging

A comprehensive wound assessment includes many parameters, one of which is staging. (See chapter 6, Wound assessment.) Once the wound etiology is known, the correct classification system to describe the wound can be selected. For example, arterial and venous ulcers are described by their characteristics. Diabetic or neuropathic ulcers are now being classified by the American Diabetes Association, Wagner Grading System for Vascular Wounds, or San Antonio Diabetic Wound Classification System. The NPUAP staging system was designed specifically for pressure ulcers. An outcome of the first NPUAP consensus conference[52] was the NPUAP staging system for pressure ulcers, which was based on Shea's[53] and the International Association of Enterostomal Therapists[54] (now called WOCN) staging systems. In February 2007, NPUAP once again revised the staging system. Pressure ulcer staging is a system to describe the level of tissue destroyed. It provides practitioners with a common language to communicate with each other what the pressure ulcer looks like clinically. Staging is only part of the total assessment of the ulcer, which includes other factors such as surrounding skin and presence of infection, to name a few. (See chapter 6, Wound assessment.) Among the staging systems used, Shea's[53] is the earliest to be used in the United States, with the NPUAP staging system[52] being the most widely used. In Europe, the EPUAP grading system is more commonly used.[41]

Pressure ulcers should be staged by determining the deepest area of tissue insult. Necrotic wounds can't be numerically staged since visualization of the wound bed is necessary to determine the level of tissue involvement. Staging of necrotic wounds should be done after the necrotic tissue is removed. (See chapter 8, Wound debridement.) The wound should be described and you should note that it's unstageable at this time. Be sure to offload the area and begin other appropriate treatments. In the long-term care setting, the CMS mandates that necrotic pressure ulcers be documented as a stage IV.[4]

PRACTICE POINT

Even though you can't "stage" an unstageable ulcer in acute care, remember that the tissue damage could worsen and still needs to be treated.

NPUAP classification of pressure ulcers staging definitions

The most widely used pressure ulcer staging tool, the NPUAP classification system for staging pressure ulcers is described below. (See color photos of staging, pages C18 and C19.)

Stage I

The original definition of a stage I pressure ulcer was "nonblanchable erythema of intact skin, the heralding lesion of skin ulceration."[52] Given the diversity of people with different skin pigmentation, detecting stage I pressure ulcers can be a challenge if clinicians only use color as an indicator. To provide a more culturally sensitive definition, in 1997 NPUAP revised the definition to include indicators that went beyond color: "An observable pressure-related alteration of intact skin whose indicators, as compared with the adjacent or opposite area on the body, may include changes in 1 or more of the following: skin temperature (warmth or coolness), tissue consistency (firm or boggy feel), and/or sensations (pain, itching). The ulcer appears as a defined area of persistent redness in lightly pigmented skin, whereas, in darker skin tones, the ulcer may appear with persistent red, blue, or purple tones."[55] NPUAP continued to refine this stage I definition due to the emerging concept of deep tissue injury and the difficulties this category posed as to where it should fit in the existing staging system.[56-60] After a presentation at its 2005 national conference, an on-line survey, and feedback from published articles, the new NPUAP staging system recommendations were presented at the February 2007 consensus conference.[9] After input from consensus conference participants, NPUAP modified the

NPUAP position statement on reverse staging

What is staging?

Staging is an assessment system that classifies pressure ulcers based on anatomic depth of soft tissue damage.[69] This assessment system only describes the anatomic status of the ulcer at the time of assessment. Staging of pressure ulcers can only occur after necrotic tissue has been removed, allowing complete visualization of the ulcer bed. Pressure ulcer staging is only appropriate for defining the maximum anatomic depth of tissue damage.

What is reverse staging?

In 1989, due to a lack of research-validated tools to measure pressure ulcer healing, clinicians resorted to using pressure ulcer staging systems in reverse order to describe improvement in an ulcer

Why not reverse stage?

Pressure ulcers heal to progressively more shallow depth; they do not replace lost muscle, subcutaneous fat, or dermis before they re-epithelialize.[80] Instead, the ulcer is filled with granulation (scar) tissue composed primarily of endothelial cells, fibroblasts, collagen, and extracellular matrix. A stage IV pressure ulcer cannot become a stage III, stage II, and/or subsequently stage I ulcer. When a stage IV ulcer has healed, it should be classified as a healed stage IV pressure ulcer, not a stage 0 pressure ulcer. Therefore, reverse staging does not accurately characterize what is physiologically occurring in the ulcer. The progress of a healing pressure ulcer can only be documented using ulcer characteristics or by improvement in wound characteristics using a validated pressure ulcer healing tool.[80]

How should you document a healing pressure ulcer?

NPUAP does recognize that federal regulations require long-term care facilities to reverse stage at the present time; however, long-term care facilities are encouraged to also document in the medical record appropriate healing using either descriptive characteristics of the wound (such as depth, width, and presence of granulation tissue) or using a validated pressure ulcer healing tool. If a pressure ulcer reopens in the same anatomical site, the ulcer resumes the previous staging diagnosis (once a stage IV, always a stage IV).

What is NPUAP doing to replace reverse staging?

Since 1996, NPUAP has developed and validated the Pressure Ulcer Scale for Healing (PUSH) tool.[152] This tool documents pressure ulcer healing. Presently, this tool is being pilot tested for adoption by the U.S. Health Care Financing Administration Minimum Data Set Post Acute Care system.

Reprinted with permission from "NPUAP Position Statement on Reverse Staging: The Facts about Reverse Staging in 2000." Available at *http://www.npuap.org/*

stage I pressure ulcer definition to be "intact skin with non-blanchable redness of a localized area usually over a bony prominence." In darkly pigmented skin, it may not have visible blanching and its color may differ from surrounding skin. (See *NPUAP pressure ulcer staging definitions*, pages 256 and 257, and color photos on pages C18 and C19.) In revising the staging system, NPUAP developed descriptors to accompany the succinct definitions as well as added two new categories to the four stages that include unstageable and suspected deep tissue injury.[9]

Ayello and Lyder[61] reported that people with darkly pigmented skin had the lowest prevalence of stage I pressure ulcers, but the highest prevalence of stage II to IV ulcers. The incidence of pressure ulcers was higher in people with darkly pigmented skin in several studies conducted by Lyder and colleagues.[32,33] In unpublished data, Lyder found a higher accuracy of 78% versus 58% when the new revised stage I definition was used.[62] One study[63] provided evidence to support skin temperature (warmth or coolness) as part of the revised stage I definition. Sprigle and colleagues[63] also found that warmth or coolness was present in 85% of patients with stage I pressure ulcers.

Staging concepts

Staging competency

Accuracy of staging pressure ulcers is a challenge. Nurses have reported being less confident in identifying stage III ulcers.[64-67] Clinicians can test their ability to classify pressure ulcers by taking the staging test on the EPUAP Web site (www.epuap.org).[68]

Staging healing ulcers—Reverse staging controversy

Pressure ulcer staging is only appropriate to use to define the maximum depth of tissue "wounded." Some clinicians have erroneously used it in reverse order to describe improvement in the ulcer.[69] Use of the NPUAP staging system to describe healing is physiologically inaccurate and shouldn't be done. (See *NPUAP position statement on reverse staging,* page 269.) When stage IV pressure ulcers heal to progressively more shallow depth, they don't replace lost muscle, subcutaneous fat, and dermis before they re-epithelialize. Instead, the wound is filled with granulation tissue. Thus, the ulcer doesn't heal from a stage IV to III, II to I. More information on why clinicians shouldn't follow this inaccurate practice of "reverse staging" can be found in the NPUAP position statement on reverse staging or on the NPUAP Web site (www.npuap.org).[16] Despite this physiologic understanding, clinicians in long-term care must follow the CMS guidance for Tag F-314 pressure ulcers that requires reverse staging of the pressure ulcer as it heals.[4]

Deep tissue injury

Pressure ulcer staging concepts may not address all forms of pressure ulcers. Clinicians often struggle with the concept of deep tissue injury (DTI) that presents as a purplish color, most often seen in the heel area. Typically, these wounds appear as dusky, boggy, or discolored areas of purple ecchymosis. (See color photo on page C17.) Sometimes they appear a few days after surgery as a discolored area on the sacrum and may be misidentified as a burn.[70] Often these areas deteriorate rapidly from intact skin to deep open wounds. The belief is that these ulcers aren't true stage I or II ulcers.

What do we call these ulcers? Are they "deep tissue injury"? How should they be staged? Are they—stage I, stage III, or stage IV? Can these pressure ulcers be prevented, and, if so, how? What is the best treatment for these pressure ulcers? Clinicians have sought guidance about this particular type of pressure ulcer. Their concerns have been addressed by the NPUAP Task Force on unstageable DTI ulcers to review what's known about these ulcers and how they should be classified.[56-60] The proposed definition of DTI was "a pressure-related injury to subcutaneous tissues under intact skin." Initially, these lesions have the appearance of a deep bruise and may herald the subsequent development of a stage III or IV pressure ulcer even with optimal management. This proposed NPUAP definition was modified and finalized as a separate stage at the 2007 consensus conference. It's now defined as "purple or maroon localized area of discolored intact skin or blood-filled blister due to damage of underlying soft tissue from pressure and/or shear."[9] See *NPUAP pressure ulcer staging definitions,* pages 256 and 257, for the descriptors for this new stage.

Early detection of DTI

The staging system relies on visual inspection of the skin. Newer technologies may hold the promise of early detection for pressure ulcer injury *before* visible signs of tissue destruction can be seen. One study reports on the pre-ulcerative changes in long-term residents using diagnostic ultrasound.[71]

Pressure ulcer treatment

Although the debate continues as to whether all pressure ulcers are avoidable[16,72], several guidelines are now available for clinicians to use in planning treatment.[11,37-47,50,74] The AHCPR, now known as the AHRQ, developed the first evidence-based guidelines called "Treatment of Pressure Ulcers" in December 1994.[15] The guidelines provide the foundation for evidence-based pressure ulcer management.

A pressure ulcer won't heal unless the underlying causes are effectively managed. A general assessment should include identifying and effectively managing the medical diseases, health problems (such as urinary incontinence), nutritional status, pain level, and psychosocial health that may have placed the patient at risk for pressure ulcer development. Unless these major areas are effectively addressed, the probability of the pressure ulcer healing is unlikely.

The comprehensive management of pressure ulcers includes cleaning, controlling infections, debridement, dressings that promote a moist wound environment, nutritional support, and redistributory pressure (turning and use of support surfaces). (See chapter 11, Pressure redistribution: Seating, positioning, and support surfaces.) The use of adjunctive therapies to heal pressure ulcers should be considered for recalcitrant pressure ulcers.

Pressure ulcer assessment

As discussed above, no universal system for pressure ulcer classification exists—and until staging of the pressure ulcer occurs, effective treatment can't commence. Staging alone, however, doesn't determine the seriousness of the ulcer. In the United States, the NPUAP staging system is the most commonly used. (See *NPUAP pressure ulcer staging definitions,* pages 256 and 257, for more detailed information about unstageable ulcers.)

PRACTICE POINT

Unstageable pressure ulcers are those covered with necrotic (slough and eschar) tissue. Until the tissue is removed, the ulcer can't be accurately visualized and is therefore unstageable in patients in the acute and home care settings. Necrotic ulcers must be documented as stage IV in long-term care patients.[4]

Monitoring healing

Because reverse staging of pressure ulcers to monitor healing is inappropriate, several instruments have been developed and validated to assess the healing of pressure ulcers.

Tools that measure healing

The two most widely used tools are the Pressure Sore Status Tool (PSST)[74] and the Pressure Ulcer Scale for Healing (PUSH).[75] The PSST is comprised of 13 variables used to provide a numerical indicator of the status of the pressure ulcer (healing or deteriorating).[74] The score ranges from 1, which indicates tissue health (or healed), to 65, which indicates wound degeneration. The variables that comprise the PSST score include: size (length and width), depth, edges, undermining, necrotic tissue type, necrotic tissue amount, exudate type, exudate amount, skin color of surrounding wound, peripheral tissue edema, peripheral tissue induration, granulation tissue, and epithelialization. The PSST provides a comprehensive assessment of the pressure ulcer.[74] This tool is currently being evaluated for use with other wound types.

The PUSH tool[75] is comprised of only three variables: surface area (length and width), exudate amount, and tissue appearance to derive a numerical indicator of the status of the pressure ulcer. (See *NPUAP PUSH tool,* page 272.) A score of 0 would indicate that the pressure ulcer has healed, with the highest score of 17 indicating wound degeneration. The PUSH tool intentionally took a "minimalist approach." Using research databases on its development, the PUSH tool seeks to select the minimal number of assessment parameters needed to monitor healing or deterioration of the ulcer. This makes it ideal for quality assurance monitoring of large groups of patients and identify-

NPUAP PUSH tool

PATIENT NAME: PATIENT ID. #

ULCER LOCATION: DATE:

Directions

Observe and measure the pressure ulcer. Categorize the ulcer with respect to surface area, exudate, and type of wound tissue. Record a subscore for each of the ulcer characteristics. Add the subscores to obtain the total score. A comparison of total scores measured over time provides an indication of the improvement or deterioration in pressure ulcer healing.

LENGTH	0	1	2	3	4	5	Blank
	$0\ cm^2$	$<0.3\ cm^2$	$0.3-0.6\ cm^2$	$0.7-1.0\ cm^2$	$1.1-2.0\ cm^2$	$2.1-3.0\ cm^2$	
$\times$ WIDTH		6	7	8	9	10	Sub-score
		$3.1-4.0\ cm^2$	$4.1-8.0\ cm^2$	$8.1-12.0\ cm^2$	$12.1-24.0\ cm^2$	$>24.0\ cm^2$	
EXUDATE AMOUNT	0 None	1 Light	2 Moderate	3 Heavy			Sub-score
TISSUE TYPE	0 Closed	1 Epithelial Tissue	2 Granulation Tissue	3 Slough	4 Necrotic Tissue		Sub-score
							Total score

LENGTH $\times$ WIDTH
Measure the greatest length (head to toe) and the greatest width (side to side) using a centimeter ruler. Multiply these two measurements (length $\times$ width) to obtain an estimate of surface area in square centimeters (cm^2). Do not guess! Always use a centimeter ruler and always use the same method each time the ulcer is measured.

EXUDATE AMOUNT
Estimate the amount of exudate (drainage) present after removal of the dressing and before applying any topical agent to the ulcer. Estimate the exudate as none, light, moderate, or heavy.

TISSUE TYPE
This refers to the types of tissue that are present in the wound (ulcer) bed. Score as a "4" if any necrotic tissue is present. Score as a "3" if any amount of slough is present and necrotic tissue is absent. Score as a "2" if the wound is clean and contains granulation tissue. Score as a "1" if the wound is superficial and reepithelializing. Score as a "0" if the wound is closed.
  4–Necrotic tissue (eschar): Black, brown, or tan tissue that adheres firmly to the wound bed or ulcer edges and may be either firmer or softer than surrounding tissue.
  3–Slough: Yellow or white tissue that adheres to the ulcer bed in strings or thick clumps or is mucinous.
  2–Granulation tissue: Pink or beefy-red tissue with a shiny, moist, granular appearance.
  1–Epithelial tissue: For superficial ulcers, new pink or shiny tissue (skin) that grows in from the edges or as islands on the ulcer surface.
  0–Closed/resurfaced: The wound is completely covered with epithelium (new skin).

ing patients who are deteriorating and require reassessment and possibly treatment changes. Its brevity, combined with its accuracy in monitoring, makes it ideal for incorporation in the Minimum Data Set–Post Acute Care (MDS-PAC). The PUSH tool isn't intended to provide a comprehensive assessment of pressure ulcers and hasn't yet been validated for other types of wounds, although it's being tested in research studies and clinical use. A survey of 103 respondents found the PUSH tool reliable and easy to use.[76]

Although tools exist for measuring pressure ulcer healing, more evidence is needed to determine pressure ulcer healing rates.[77-80] Among chronic wounds, pressure ulcers have the slowest healing rate at 0.077 mm/day with 2.156 mm of healing expected at 4 weeks.[79]

Recently, the use of high-frequency portable ultrasound to measure wound healing has been introduced. The use of this technology, which can capture three-dimensional measurements, has been shown to be quite beneficial in objectively monitoring healing. Ultrasound is also "color blind"; that is, it can detect stage I pressure ulcers in darkly pigmented skin.[81]

Cleaning

Cleaning the pressure ulcer to remove devitalized tissue and decrease bacterial burden is often recommended. Pressure ulcers exhibit delayed healing in the presence of high levels of bacteria.[82] Solutions that don't traumatize the ulcer should be used.[83] Normal saline solution (0.9%) is usually recommended because it isn't cytotoxic to healthy tissue.[15] Although the active ingredients in newer wound cleaners may be noncytotoxic (surfactants), the inert carrier may be cytotoxic to healthy granulation tissue. Review of all ingredients is warranted. Hellewell et al.[84] found that antiseptic cleaners were the most cytotoxic to granulation tissue. An in vitro study found relative toxicity indexes ranging from 0 to 100,000 with Saline and Shur-clens to be least toxic to fibroblasts, while Dial antibacterial soap and Ivory Liqui-gel were most toxic.[85] Least toxic to keratinocytes were Biolex, Shur-clens, and Techni-Care while hydrogen peroxide, modified Dakin's solution, and povidone (10%) were most toxic.[85]

The mechanical method used to deliver the cleaning agent must provide enough pressure to remove debris without presenting trauma to the ulcer bed. Optimal pressure to clean an ulcer is between 4 to 15 pounds per square inch (psi).[86] A 35-ml syringe with a 19 gauge needle creates an 8 psi irrigation pressure stream,[15] which was found to be more effective in removing bacteria than other irrigation pressures.[87] It should be noted that irrigation pressures exceeding 15 psi can cause trauma to the ulcer bed and may drive bacteria into the tissue.[88] New technology such as battery-powered, disposable irrigation devices can provide an alternative to loosen wound debris from the syringe and needle system.

Debridement

The presence of necrotic devitalized tissue promotes the growth of pathologic organisms and prevents wounds from healing.[89] Therefore, debridement is a very important step in the management of pressure ulcers. There's no optimal debridement method; therefore, selection of the debridement method should be based on the goals of the patient, absence or presence of infection, amount of necrotic tissue present, and economic considerations for the patient and the facility.

Many types of debridement, including surgical, autolytic, enzymatic, mechanical, biological, and laser, are available. (See chapter 8, Wound debridement.) However, surgical (or sharp laser) debridement is considered by many the most quick and effective type of debridement because it involves the cutting away (with a scalpel) of necrotic tissue.[90] In addition, surgical debridement is relatively quick and can be done at the bedside. Surgical debridement is essential when cellulitis or sepsis is suspected.[91] Autolytic debridement involves the use of a semi-occlusive or occlusive dressing (hydrocolloids, hydrogels). This type of debridement uses the body's own natural enzymes to digest necrotic tissue. It's relatively painless, but takes much longer than sharp debridement. Watch closely for signs and symptoms of infection. Enzymatic debridement uses proteolytic enzymes (such as papain and urea, collagenase, and trypsin) to remove necrotic tissue. Mechanical debridement uses wet-to-dry gauze to adhere to the necrotic tissue, which is then removed. Upon removal of the gauze dressing, necrotic tissue and wound debris are removed. However, healthy granulation tissue is also removed. This can delay wound healing.[90]

Pressure redistribution

The use of support surfaces is an important consideration in redistributing pressure. (See chapter 11, Pressure redistribution, seating, positioning, and support surfaces.) The NPUAP Support Surface Standards Initiative redefined terms about the physical concepts related to support surfaces that can be obtained on their Web site.[16] The use of dynamic support surfaces in high-risk patients has lead to improved outcomes and cost savings. The CMS has divided support surfaces into three categories for reimbursement purposes. Group one devices are those support surfaces that are static; they don't require electricity. Static devices include air, foam (convoluted and solid), gel, and water-overlay mattresses. These devices are ideal when a patient is at low to moderate risk for pressure ulcer development. They redistribute pressure, may decrease shearing, and are relatively inexpensive. If foam is used, it should weigh 1.3 lb per cubic foot and be more than 3" (7.5 cm) thick.

Group two devices are powered by electricity or a pump and are considered dynamic in nature. These devices include alternating and low-air-loss mattresses. These mattresses are good for patients that are at moderate to high risk for pressure ulcers or have full-thickness pressure ulcers. The advantages of alternating air mattresses include portability, redistribution of pressure, reduced shearing, and moderate cost. The disadvantage of some of these mattresses is their inability to reduce heat accumulation on the patient's body. The advantages of low-air-loss mattresses are pressure reduction, low moisture retention and reduction of heat accumulation. The dis-

advantage of low-air-loss beds is that they can be expensive.

Group three devices are also considered dynamic in nature. This classification comprises only air-fluidized beds. These beds are electric and contain silicone-coated beads. They're used for patients at very high risk for pressure ulcers, and after flap or graft surgery. They're often used for patients with nonhealing full-thickness pressure ulcers or those with numerous truncal full-thickness pressure ulcers. The advantages of air-fluidized beds are that they redistribute pressure and reduce heat accumulation, moisture retention, and shearing forces. The patient's ability to move in a fluidized bed is hampered and considered a disadvantage of the product. Few studies demonstrate significant differences within the support surface classifications and preventing or healing pressure ulcers. Therefore, the level and type of risk factors should guide the level and type of support surface selected.

Dressings

The use of moist wound therapy dressings is a major component in managing a pressure ulcer. (See chapter 9, Wound treatment options.) At present, it's conservatively estimated that there are thousands of different dressings available for pressure ulcer management. Dressings can be broken down into several classifications: gauze, nonadherent gauze, transparent films, hydrocolloids, foams, alginates, hydrogels, collagens, antimicrobials, composites, and combinations. Matching the dressing to the wound bed characteristics is essential. A guiding principle is to maintain a moist environment.

Although nongauze dressings are usually more expensive than gauze dressing, less frequent dressing changes, faster healing rates, and decreased rates of infection can make nongauze-based dressing more cost-effective over time.[92-95] It's also important to note that wet-to-dry gauze dressings are a form of debridement and shouldn't be used on ulcers with good granulation tissue. CMS specifically states that use of wet-to-dry dressings should be limited in long-term care patients.[4] No specific dressing heals all pressure ulcers within an ulcer classification. Consequently, a careful assessment of the pressure ulcer, the patient's needs, and environmental factors (frequency of dressing changes to increase adherence) must be considered. (See chapter 9, Wound treatment options.)

Nutrition

Nutrition is important to maintain the body in positive nitrogen balance, thereby increasing wound healing.[50] It's important to increase protein stores for patients with pressure ulcers who are malnourished. In the absence of deficiency, however, little empirical evidence exist showing that vitamins and mineral supplements aid in pressure ulcer healing or prevention.[96-99] Therefore, providing supplements to patients without protein, vitamin, or mineral deficiencies should be avoided.[100-102] The use of enteral and parental nutritional support should always be considered when the patient is unable to meet his caloric needs.

Control of infections

All pressure ulcers will become colonized with both aerobic and anaerobic bacteria; therefore, pressure ulcers aren't sterile wounds. (See chapter 7, Wound bioburden.) Because all pressure ulcers will be colonized, avoid swab-culturing the surface of a pressure ulcer. Clean technique is customarily used when treating pressure ulcers. If an ulcer may be infected (independent of a puncture biopsy), most experts assess for the amount of drainage and odor and examine the surrounding tissue for cellulitis. It should be noted that some infected ulcers may not demonstrate the typical signs and symptoms associated with infection; rather, they may appear as nonhealing ulcers.

Until the pressure ulcer infection is controlled, the ulcer won't heal. The use of topical agents such as sulfa silvadene and oral antibiotics for a 1- or 2-week period may be useful. A few studies have noted that cleaning an infected wound with 1% povidone-iodine has been demonstrated to reduce the bacterial load and increase healing. Clearly, additional research is needed to examine the role of topical antibiotics in decreasing bacterial loads in pressure ulcers. Systemic antibiotics should only be used when a systemic infection is suspected.

Adjunctive therapies

The use of adjunctive therapies is the fastest growing area in pressure ulcer management. Adjunctive therapies include electrical stimulation, hyperbaric oxygen, radiant heat, growth factors, and skin equivalents. Except for electrical stimulation, published research substantiating the effectiveness of adjunctive therapies in healing pressure ulcers is scarce.

Electrical stimulation is the use of electrical current to stimulate a number of cellular processes, such as increasing fibroblasts, neutrophil macrophage collagen, DNA synthesis, and increasing the number of receptor sites for specific growth factors.[103] Electrical stimulation appears to be most effective on stage III and IV pressure ulcers that were unresponsive to traditional methods of healing. Although there's much data to suggest that electrical stimulation is effective in healing pressure ulcers, the optimal electrical charge needed to stimulate pressure ulcer healing remains unclear. The literature suggests an optimal electrical charge of 300 to 500 uA/sec produces positive effects on the pressure ulcer.[104] However, additional research is needed to determine the optimal electrical charge based on the characteristics of pressure ulcers (for example, stage, depth, and amount of drainage).

Hyperbaric oxygen is believed to promote wound healing by stimulating fibroblast, collagen synthesis, epithelialization, and control of infection.[105] However, controlled clinical studies couldn't be found regarding the association of hyperbaric oxygen and the healing of pressure ulcers. The limited literature that does exist suggests that topical hyperbaric oxygen doesn't increase tissue oxygenation beyond the superficial dermis.[106]

Research into radiant heat (normothermia) as an adjunctive therapy to heal pressure ulcers is being conducted. It's believed that increasing the thermal wound environment not only increases blood flow, but promotes fibroblasts and other factors associated with pressure ulcer healing as well.[107] Mustoe et al.[108] investigated the role of radiant heat in healing pressure ulcers; their findings suggest that radiant heat is beneficial to pressure ulcer healing. Additional research is needed to increase knowledge about the benefits of radiant heat in pressure ulcer healing.

The use of growth factors and skin equivalents in healing pressure ulcers is emerging. The use of cytokine growth factors (for example, recombinant platelet-derived growth factor-BB [rhPDGF-BB]) and fibroblast growth factors (bFGF) and skin equivalents are currently being studied. Only one multicenter, randomized double-blind study was found.[108] This study enrolled 45 patients with stage III or IV pressure ulcers who were randomized to either treatment group 1 (300 ug/ml of rhPDGF), treatment group 2 (100 ug/ml rhPDGF) or treatment group 3 (placebo). After 4 weeks of treatment, patients in group 1 had a 40% reduction in ulcer area, group 2 had a 71% reduction in ulcer area and group 3 had a 17% reduction in pressure ulcer area. Clearly, the use of growth factors may have a crucial impact on the future of wound healing. However, additional research is needed to evaluate the efficacy of specific growth factors in healing pressure ulcers.

Prevalence and incidence

It has been said, "what can be measured can be managed." To improve pressure ulcer care, the number of patients with pressure ulcers must be accurately determined. Doing so will require careful attention to prevalence and incidence data. The data represent the percentage of patients with pressure ulcers among all those surveyed in a setting (prevalence) and the percentage of patients who developed pressure ulcers after admission to the setting (incidence).

In 1989, at its first consensus conference, NPUAP brought attention to the pressure ulcer problem in the United States by reporting prevalence and incidence data.[52] (See *Incidence and prevalence, 1999 to 2000.*) They set a national goal to reduce the incidence of pressure ulcers by 50% by the year 2000.[52] During the next decade, NPUAP engaged in an active program to improve pressure ulcer practice through education, research, and public policy.

At the close of the 20th century, NPUAP assessed the progress toward this goal through its Pressure Ulcers Challenge 2000 project. This 2-year project included a Medline database search for all articles on pressure ulcer incidence and prevalence published and indexed between January 1, 1990 and December 31, 2000. More than 300 studies on pressure ulcer incidence and prevalence were found. Pressure ulcer incidence and prevalence data were analyzed across care settings and in specific populations such as people with spinal cord injuries, elderly patients, infants and children, patients with hip fractures, people of color, and those at the end of life receiving palliative or hospice care.[1,109]

Study data presented in the NPUAP monograph[1] detailing the results of the project indicate a wide variation in the range of incidence rates (acute care, 0.4% to 38%; long-term care, 2.2% to 23.9%; and home care, 0% to 17%).[1,109] Inconsistencies in methodology used and the populations studied contribute to these differences and make comparisons and analyses of trends problematic. However, many positive developments in the prevention and treatment of pressure ulcers have occurred over the past decade, including development of evidence-based practice guidelines, standardization of risk assessment, and improved technologies for prevention and treatment.[1,109] NPUAP estimates that pressure ulcer prevalence in acute care is 15%, with incidence of 7%.[1,109] Although methodological issues require caution in interpreting the data, the estimates are based on several large studies conducted from 1990 to 2000. (See *Incidence and prevalence, 1990 to 2000,* page 278.)

Prevalence

Due to the variations in the range of prevalence rates, sample characteristics, and study methodologies, these results should be interpreted cautiously. Prevalence rates over the last decade ranged from 10% to 18% in general acute care,[1,110] 2.3% to 28% in long-

Incidence and prevalence, 1999 to 2000

The chart below shows pressure ulcer incidence and prevalence data collected by the National Pressure Ulcer Advisory Panel (NPUAP) for 1999 and 2000.

PRESSURE ULCER INCIDENCE

	1999 to 2000	Pre -1990
Acute care	0.4% to 38% Best estimate: 7%	5% to 11%
Long-term care	2.2% to 23.9%	No data
Home care	0% to 17%	No data

PRESSURE ULCER PREVALENCE

Acute care	10% to 17% Best estimate: 15%	3% to 14%
Long-term care	2.3% to 28%	15% to 25%
Home care	0% to 29%	7% to 12%

Adapted with permission from the National Pressure Ulcer Advisory Panel (NPUAP), Cuddigan, J., et al., eds. *Pressure Ulcers in America: Prevalence, Incidence, and Implications for the Future.* Reston, Va.: NPUAP, 2001.

term care,[1,111-112] and 0% to 29% in home care.[1,112-113] Because of population and methodological differences, valid comparisons can't be made among these studies or to pre-1990 prevalence ranges (for example, 3% to 14% in acute care, 15% to 25% in long-term care, and 7% to 12% in home care).[1,109] Reported prevalence rates in other countries are:

- Netherlands: 10.1%,[114] 20.4%[115]
- United Kingdom: 1.9%,[116] 7.32%,[117] 9.5%,[118] 14%,[119]
- Canada: 29.7%[120]
- Australia: 11.1%[121]
- Iceland: 8.9%[122]
- Sweden: 63.6%[123]
- Japan: 5.1%[124]
- France: 5.2%[125]
- Germany: 28.3%.[126]

Three large multisite clinical studies in acute care reported prevalence rates of 14.8%, 15%, and 15% at the end of the 1990s; these studies provide the most accurate and current estimate of prevalence rates in acute care.[127-129] Most pressure ulcers, regardless of setting, are partial-thickness (stages I and II) and are located on the sacrum or coccyx. Heels are the second most frequently occurring location.

Incidence

Use caution when analyzing the reported NPUAP incidence rates of 0.4% to 38% in general acute care,[31,130] 2.2% to 23.9% in long-term care,[34,131] and 0% to 17% in home care.[113,132] Because there was no data from long-term care or home care reported at the original NPUAP 1989 consensus conference, no comparison to the 2001 incidence data can be made. Although the reported range in acute care prior to 1990 was 5% to

Incidence and prevalence, 1990 to 2000

These tables summarize pressure ulcer incidence and prevalence data* collected by the National Pressure Ulcer Advisory Panel (NPUAP) from 1990 to 2000.

INCIDENCE

CLINICAL SETTING	STAGES I TO IV		STAGES II TO IV	
	Database	**Clinical**	**Database**	**Clinical**
Acute care	17.6% to 19.1%	7% to 38%	0.4%	12.9%
Critical care	—	8% to 40%	—	—
Operating room	—	4% to 21.5%	—	—
Long-term care	—	7% to 23.9%	2.2% to 12.9%	—
Rehabilitation	4% to 6%	0%	—	—
Home care	0% to 6.3%	16.5% to 17%	3.2%	—

SPECIAL POPULATIONS

Hip fracture	19.1%	—	—	—
End of life	0% to 85%			
Spinal cord injury	7.5% to 23.7%	—	—	31%
Infants and children	8% to 19%			

PREVALENCE

CLINICAL SETTING	STAGES I TO IV		STAGES II TO IV	
	Database	**Clinical**	**Database**	**Clinical**
Acute care		10% to18%	—	—
Critical care	—	—	—	—
Operating room	—	8.5%	—	—
Long-term care	2.3% to 12%	23% to 28%	11.2%	—
Rehabilitation	12% to 27%	0% to 25%	—	—
Home care	—	0% to 29%	—	—

SPECIAL POPULATIONS:

Hip fracture	—	—		—
End of life	14% to 28%		—	
Spinal cord injury	15.2% to 30%	10.2%	7.4%	32%
Infants and children	—			

* Incidence and prevalence data are reported according to the methodology used. Data were obtained from existing databases (for example, MDS, medical records) or through clinical observations of the investigator(s). Some investigators considered stages I to IV pressure ulcers, whereas others excluded stage I ulcers from study. Due to differences in methodologies and sample characteristics among studies, valid comparisons between pre-1990 and post-1990 rates can't be made. The reader should be cautioned against using these incidence and prevalence rates to benchmark or determine an "acceptable" pressure ulcer rate for a given setting, facility, agency, or population.

Used with permission from National Pressure Ulcer Advisory Panel (NPUAP). Cuddigan, J., et al., eds. *Pressure Ulcers in America: Prevalence, Incidence, and Implications for the Future.* Reston, Va.: NPUAP, 2001.

11%,[52] NPUAP believes that the difference in the reported ranges doesn't reflect a change in incidence rates over time. This may be due to several factors including differences in incidence rates among studies, staging definitions, incidence rate formulas, populations, and various data sources. Reported incidence rates around the world are as follows:
- United Kingdom: 4.03%[133]
- Canada: 9.7%[134]
- Sweden: 55%[123]
- Japan: 4.4%.[124]

Prevalence and incidence definitions and formulas

Lack of clarity and consistency in definitions and calculation formulas impedes our understanding of pressure ulcer prevalence and incidence. Standardization of definitions and formulas will enhance comparability of data among future studies. NPUAP recommends the adoption of consistent definitions and formulas for determining pressure ulcer prevalence and incidence.[1,135] Similarly, the European Pressure Ulcer Advisory Panel (EPUAP) has published a draft statement on prevalence and incidence monitoring.[136]

NPUAP suggests that prevalence should be defined as a "cross-sectional count of the number of cases at a specific point in time, or the number of people with pressure ulcers who exist in a patient population at a given point in time. In assessing prevalence, it doesn't matter in what setting the pressure ulcer was acquired."[1,135] Suggested standard formulas for obtaining prevalence are:
- Pressure ulcer point prevalence

$$\frac{\text{Number of people with a pressure ulcer} \times 100}{\begin{array}{c}\text{Number of people in a population} \\ \text{at a particular point in time}\end{array}}$$

- Pressure ulcer period prevalence

$$\frac{\text{Number of people with a pressure ulcer} \times 100}{\begin{array}{c}\text{Number of people in a population} \\ \text{at a particular period in time}\end{array}}$$

- Pressure ulcer period prevalence

NPUAP recommends using the following definition of incidence: "the number of new cas-

---

Pitfalls to calculating prevalence and incidence

Be sure to avoid the following pitfalls when calculating pressure ulcer prevalence and incidence for your facility.
- Define the population and apply the definition consistently throughout the study.
- Count the number of patients with pressure ulcers — not the number of pressure ulcers.
- Count only pressure ulcers, not other wounds.
- Define the stages of the pressure ulcers you count to include and assess them accurately.

Adapted with permission from Ayello, E.A., et al. "Methods for Determining Pressure Ulcer Prevalence and Incidence," in *Pressure Ulcers in America: Prevalence, Incidence, and Implications for the Future*, edited by Cuddigan, J., et al. Reston, Va.: National Pressure Ulcer Advisory Panel, 2001.

---

es appearing in a population indicates the rate at which new disease occurs in a population previously without disease."[1,22,136,137] Several approaches to measuring incidence have been used. NPUAP defines "cumulative incidence" as "the rate of new pressure ulcers in a group of patients of fixed size, all of whom are observed over a period of time."[1,137] The formula is as follows:
- Pressure ulcer cumulative incidence

$$\frac{\begin{array}{c}\text{Number of people developing a} \\ \text{new pressure ulcer} \times 100\end{array}}{\begin{array}{c}\text{Total number of people in a population} \\ \text{at beginning of time period}\end{array}}$$

A problem with using this approach is that it doesn't count pressure ulcers that occur in people admitted to the setting after the study population has been defined. Therefore, it may not be the true incidence of new ulcers in that setting.

Another way is to calculate prevalence is to measure the number of new cases of pressure ulcers that occur in a changing population. In this case, the people who are being studied have varying lengths of stay. Incidence is calculated as the number of people developing pressure ulcers per 1,000 patient-days, and is called incidence density. Calculate this by using the following suggested formula:

- Pressure ulcer incidence density

$$\frac{\text{Number of people developing a new pressure ulcer} \times 1000}{\text{Total patient days free of pressure ulcers}}$$

$$=$$

$$\frac{\text{Number of people developing a pressure ulcer}}{1000 \text{ patient-days}}$$

Using the NPUAP recommended standard formulas alone may not be enough to avoid errors in prevalence and incidence calculations. (See *Pitfalls to calculating prevalence and incidence,* page 279.)

Competencies and curriculum

Accurate and current knowledge is essential for clinicians to prevent and treat pressure ulcers. Pressure ulcer knowledge varies among members of the wound care team. For example, in two studies, physicians were found to have low levels of pressure ulcer knowledge.[138,139] In addition, some nurses believe that their basic education is insufficient regarding wound care.[64-67] What's more, high pressure ulcer prevalence rates have been linked to poor knowledge.[140-143] Several initiatives are under way to decrease pressure ulcers by increasing the knowledge level of clinicians including the IHI[7] and the New Jersey Hospital Association's "No Ulcers" project.[144] As knowledge about pressure ulcers has increased, their occurrence has decreased across care settings. Certification has made a difference in pressure ulcer knowledge. In a recent study, nurses who had any wound care certification either from the Wound Ostomy Continence Nurses Society (WOCN), the American Academy of Wound Management (AAWM), or the National Alliance of Wound Care (NAWC) had higher scores on a standardized 47-item pressure ulcer test.[145]

NPUAP has approved a competency-based curriculum on pressure ulcer prevention[16,146] and treatment[16,147] for registered nurses. Other curriculum components include competencies, content outline, a case study with answers, and references. Twelve essential pressure ulcer prevention competencies and eight essential pressure ulcer treatment competencies are recommended. The entire copyrighted registered nurse curriculum document is available free on the NPUAP Web site.[16] The NPUAP competency-based curriculum is an important contribution to nursing practice.[146,147]

Building knowledge about pressure ulcer care is vital. While many experts believe that all pressure ulcers cannot be prevented,[148] it's been shown that education can reduce pressure ulcers and expedite their treatment.[149] A variety of continuing education programs, symposiums, and national conferences exist in this knowledge building as well as company-sponsored online learning programs. For example, the interactive computer-based testing on pressure ulcer risk assessment using the Braden Scale as described by Maklebust and colleagues[34] as well as the EPUAP pressure ulcer staging module[68] are just some of the resources available. The John A. Hartford Institute for Geriatric Nursing also has several one-page quick references in their "Try This" series, one of which is using the Braden Scale.[150] The National Database of Nursing Quality Indicators (NDNQI) has 4 modules on several aspects of pressure ulcer care that can be accessed from their Web site where clinicians can acquire knowledge as well as measure their learning by using the interactive testing available online.[151]

Summary

Pressure ulcers are a common health care problem throughout the world. Intensity and duration of pressure as well as tissue tolerance are the etiologic factors that lead to pressure ulcer development. Results of a pressure ulcer risk assessment using a validated tool can serve as the foundation for developing a pressure ulcer prevention protocol based on the level and type of risk the individual demonstrates. After determining the pressure ulcer stage and other wound factors, a comprehensive plan to treat the pressure ulcer that uses a combination of local wound care, debridement, moist wound healing, cleaning, and pressure relief needs to be implemented. A multidisciplinary approach to patient care that includes patient and family education as well as staff education is essential. Use of the standardized formulas as proposed by NPUAP will provide a basis for universal comparison of prevalence and incidence data. Many educational resources are available to clinicians to increase their knowledge level so as to decrease pressure ulcer incidence and enhance treatment.

Show what you know

1. *A pressure ulcer is a lesion caused by:*

   A. incontinence.
   B. unrelieved pressure.
   C. heat.
   D. diabetes mellitus.

ANSWER: B. Unrelieved pressure is the cause of tissue death in pressure ulcers. Incontinence and diabetes mellitus may be other patient characteristics that may put a patient at risk for pressure ulcers, but in and of themselves don't cause the pressure ulcer. Heat causes burns not pressure ulcers.

2. *A patient is dragged across the bed when transferring to a stretcher. Which one of the following forces that contribute to pressure ulcer development has occurred?*

   A. Electrical stimulation
   B. Shear
   C. Friction
   D. Maceration

ANSWER: C. Electrical stimulation is an adjunct therapy used to heal pressure ulcers. Shear is a mechanical trauma caused by tissue layers sliding against each other. Maceration is not a mechanical force caused by dragging the skin across a surface.

3. *A patient has a 2 by 3 cm sacral pressure ulcer that has some depth and extends into the subcutaneous tissue with some undermining; no bone is palpable nor visible. There's a small amount of slough seen in one corner of the wound. Using the NPUAP staging classification system, this pressure ulcer is:*

   A. stage I.
   B. stage II.
   C. stage III.
   D. stage IV.

ANSWER: C. In this ulcer the tissue destroyed is into the subcutaneous tissue. The newly revised NPUAP staging system now includes that stage III pressure ulcers are full thickness wounds that may have some slough and undermining/tunneling, but bone or muscle is not visible or palpable. The ulcer isn't a stage I because the epidermis is no longer intact. It isn't a stage II because the tissue destroyed is deeper than superficial level (partial thickness) and is well into the subcutaneous tissue. It isn't a stage IV because in this ulcer muscle or bone is not palpable or visible.

4. *Which of the following Braden Scale scores for an elderly black male would indicate pressure ulcer risk?*

   A. 23
   B. 21
   C. 19
   D. 17

ANSWER: D. The research-based cutscore for onset of pressure ulcer risk for older patients and blacks is 18. With the Braden Scale, scores at or lower than the cutoff score indicate risk for pressure ulcer development. Options A, B, and C are all wrong answers because they're higher than the cutoff score of 18. With the Braden Scale, low numerical scores indicate a risk for pressure ulcers.

5. *Which one of the following should be included in a care plan to prevent pressure ulcers?*

   A. Turn and reposition every 4 hours.
   B. Clean skin daily using hot water and soap.
   C. Encourage the patient who's confined to a chair to relieve pressure every hour.
   D. Limit fluids to 10 cc per kg of body weight daily.

ANSWER: C. (See AHCPR 1992 prevention guidelines in chapter 11, Pressure redistribution.) Turn the patient at least every 2 hours. Don't use hot water, but rather warm water, and use lanolin-based soaps to avoid drying the skin. There's no need to limit the patient's fluids.

6. *Which one of the following parameters is NOT part of the NPUAP PUSH tool?*

   A. Depth
   B. Exudate
   C. Tissue type
   D. Length × width

ANSWER: A. Depth is not on the PUSH tool to measure pressure ulcer healing. Exudate, tissue type, and length × width are the three variables measured.

7. The best current estimate for pressure ulcer prevalence in acute care in the United States is:

A. 20%.

B. 15%.

C. 7%.

D. 0.8%.

ANSWER: B. Seven percent is the best estimate of incidence, and 0.8% is the target number as identified in the initiative, Healthy People 2010.

References

1. National Pressure Ulcer Advisory Panel (NPUAP). Cuddigan, J., et al., eds. *Pressure Ulcers in America: Prevalence, Incidence and Implications for the Future.* Reston, VA: NPUAP, 2001.

2. U.S. Department of Health and Human Services. *Healthy People 2010: Understanding and Improving Health,* 2nd ed. Washington, DC: U.S. Government Printing Office, November, 2000.

3. Health Care Financing Administration. *Survey Procedures for Long Term Care Facilities. Investigative Protocol: Pressure Sore/ulcer.* Baltimore, MD: Health Care Financing Administration, 1999.

4. Centers for Medicare and Medicaid Services (CMS) Tag F-314 Pressure Ulcers. Revised guidance for surveyors in long term care. Issued Nov 12, 2004. Available at: http//new.cms.hhs.gov/manuals/download/som107ap_pp_guidelines_ltcf.pdf Accessed December 13, 2006.

5. Interim mandatory patient safety reporting requirements for general hospitals. Patient safety reporting initiative. Health Care Quality Assessment. New Jersey Department of Health and Senior Services. December 6, 2004.

6. Russo, C.A., Elixhauser, A. Hospitalizations Related to Pressure Sores, 2003, Healthcare Cost and Utilization Project, Agency for Healthcare Research and Quality, Rockville, MD. April 2006. Available at: http://www.hcup-us.ahrq.gov/reports/statbriefs/sb3.pdf. Accessed December 19, 2006.

7. The Institute for Healthcare Improvement. Available at: http://www.ihi.org/IHI/Programs/Campaign/. Accessed December 23, 2006.

8. www.qualigigm.org/Professionals/Topic/Patient Safety/Monitoring.aspx. Accessed on January 30, 2007.

9. Black, J., Baharestan, M.M., Cuddigan, J., Dorner, B., Edsberg, L., Lengemo, D., Postheauer, M.E., Ratliff, C., Taler, G., and the National Pressure Ulcer Advisory Panel's updated pressure ulcer staging system. "2007 Staging System," *Advances in Skin & Wound Care* 20(5):269-274, May 2007.

10. Maklebust, J. "Pressure Ulcers: Etiology and Prevention," *Nursing Clinics of North America* 22(2):359-77, June 1987.

11. Kosiak, M. "Etiology and Pathology of Ischemic Ulcers," *Archives of Physical Medicine and Rehabilitation* 40(2):62, February 1959.

12. Parish, L.C., et al. *The Decubitus Ulcers.* New York: Masson Publishing, 1983.

13. Dyson, M., and Lyder, C. Wound management-physical modalities. In: Morison, M., ed., *The Prevention and Treatment of Pressure Ulcers.* Edinburgh: Harcourt Brace/Mosby International, 2001.

14. Maklebust, J., and Sieggreen, M. *Pressure Ulcers: Guidelines for Prevention and Management,* 3rd ed. Philadelphia: Lippincott Williams & Wilkins, 2001.

15. Bergstrom, N., et al. *Treatment of Pressure Ulcers in Adults.* Clinical practice guideline, Number 15. Rockville, MD: Public Health Service, U.S. Department of Health and Human Services; Agency for Health Care Policy and Research publication 95-0652, December 1994.

16. National Pressure Ulcer Advisory Panel (NPUAP) web page. Available at: http://www.npuap.org. Accessed January 2007.

17. Dinsdale, S.M. "Decubitus Ulcers: Role or Pressure and Friction in Causation," *Archives of Physical Medicine and Rehabilitation* 55(4):147-52, April 1974.

18. Maklebust, J. "Pressure ulcers: The great insult." *Nursing Clinics of North America* 40(2):365-389, 2005.

19. Barczak, C.A., et al. "Fourth National Pressure Ulcer Prevalence Survey," *Advances in Wound Care* 10(4):18-26, July-August 1997.

20. Meehan, M. "Multisite Pressure Ulcer Prevalence Survey," *Decubitus* 3(4):14-7, November 1990.

21. Meehan, M. "National Pressure Ulcer Prevalence Survey," *Advances in Wound Care* 7(3):27-30, 34, May 1994.

22. Panel on the Prediction and Prevention of Pressure Ulcers in Adults. *Pressure Ulcers in Adults: Prediction and Prevention.* Clinical Practice Guideline No. 3. AHCPR Publication No. 92-0047. Rockville, Md.: Agency for Health Care Policy and Research, 1992.

23. Norton, D., et al. *An Investigation of Geriatric Nursing Problems in Hospital.* London: National Corporation for the Care of Old People, 1962.

24. Gosnell, D.J. "An Assessment Tool to Identify Pressure Sores," *Nursing Research* 22(1):55-59, January-February 1973.

25. Bergstrom, N., et al. "The Braden Scale for Predicting Pressure Sore Risk," *Nursing Research* 36(4):205-10, July-August 1987.

26. Abruzzese, R.S. "Early Assessment and Prevention of Pressure Sores," in Lee, B.Y., ed. *Chronic Ulcers of the Skin.* New York: McGraw-Hill Book Co., 1985.

27. Waterlow, J. "Pressure Sores: A Risk Assessment Card," *Nursing Times* 81(48):49-55, November 27-December 3, 1985.

28. Ayello, E.A., and Braden, B. "How and Why to do Pressure Ulcer Risk Assessment," *Advances in Skin and Wound Care* 15(3):125-32, May-June 2002.

29. Ayello, E.A., and Braden, B. "Why is pressure ulcer risk assessment so important?" *Nursing* 31(11):75-79, November 2001.

30. Jalali, R., Rezaie, M. Predicting pressure ulcer risk: Comparing the predictive validity of 4 scales. *Advances in Skin and Wound Care* 18(2):92-97, 2005.

31. Bergstrom, N., and Braden, B. "A Prospective Study of Pressure Sore Risk Among Institutionalized Elderly," *Journal of the American Geriatric Society* 40(8):747-58, August 1992.

32. Lyder, C.H., et al. "Validating the Braden Scale for the Prediction of Pressure Ulcer Risk in Blacks and Latino/Hispanic Elders: A Pilot Study," *Ostomy/Wound Management* 44(suppl 3A):42S-49S, March 1998.

33. Lyder, C.H., et al. "The Braden Scale for Pressure Ulcer Risk: Evaluating the Predictive Validity in Black and Latino/Hispanic Elders," *Applied Nursing Research* 12(2):60-68, May 1999.

34. Maklebust, J., Sieggreen, M.Y., Sidor, D., Gerlach, M.A., Bauer, C. Anderson, C. "Computer-based testing of the Braden Scale for predicting pressure sore risk," *Ostomy/Wound Management* 51(4):40-52, 2005.

35. Bergstrom, N., et al. "Predicting Pressure Ulcer Risk: A Multisite Study of the Predictive Validity of the Braden Scale," *Nursing Research* 47(5):261-69, September-October 1998.

36. Braden, B., and Bergstrom, N. "Clinical Utility of the Braden Scale for Predicting Pressure Sore Risk," *Decubitus* 2(3):44, August 1989.

37. Brem, H., Lyder, C. Protocol for the successful treatment of pressure ulcers. *The American Journal of Surgery* 188:1A (Suppl to July), 9S-17S, 2004.

38. Baranoski, S. Raising awareness of pressure ulcer prevention and treatment. *Advances in Skin and Wound Care* 19(7):398-405, 2006.

39. Ratliff, C.R. WOCN's evidence-based pressure ulcer guideline. *Advances in Skin and Wound Care* 18:4:204-209, 2005.

40. Whitney, J., Phillips, L., Aslam, R., et al. "Guidelines for the treatment of pressure ulcers," *Wound Repair and Regeneration.* 14:663-679, 2006.

41. European Pressure Ulcer Advisory Panel. Pressure Ulcer Prevention Guidelines. Oxford, UK, 1998. Available at: http://www.epuap.org. Accessed December 23, 2006.

42. Ministry of Health, Prediction and Prevention of Pressure Ulcers in Adults. *Ministry of Health Nursing Clinical Practice Guidelines* January 2001 Singapore. Available at: http://www.gov.sg/moh/newmoh/pdf/abo/clinic2001/Book.pdf. Accessed December 23, 2006.

43. Paralyzed Veterans of America. Pressure Ulcer Prevention and Treatment Following Spinal Cord Injury: A Clinical Practice Guideline for Health-Care Professionals. Washington, DC; 2000. Available at: www.pva.org Accessed December 23, 2006.

44. National Collaborating Centre for Nursing and Supportive Care, National Institute for Clinical Excellence (NCCNSC/NICE). Pressure ulcer risk assessment and prevention, including the use of pressure-relieving devices (beds, mattresses and overlays) for the prevention of pressure ulcers in primary and secondary care. London (UK): National Institute for Clinical Excellence (NICE), 2003.

45. Registered Nurses Association of Ontario (RNAO). Risk assessment & prevention of pressure ulcers. Toronto (ON): Registered Nurses Association of Ontario (RNAO), 2005.

46. Wound, Ostomy and Continence Nurses Society. Guideline for prevention and management of pressure ulcers. WOCN: Mount Laurel, NJ, 2003.

47. Keast, D.H., Parslow, N., Hughton, P.E., Norton, L., Fraser, C. "Best practice recommendations for the prevention and treatment of pressure ulcers: Update 2006," *Wound Care Canada* 4(1):R19-R29, 2006.

48. Thompson, P., Langemo, D., Anderson, J., Hanson, D., Hunter, S. "Skin care protocols for pressure ulcers and incontinence in long-term care: a quasi-experimental study," *Advances in Skin and Wound Care* 18(8):422-9, 2005.

49. Duimel-Peeters, I.G.P., Halfens, R.J.G., Berger, M.P.F., Snoeckx, L.H. The effects of massage as a method to prevent pressure ulcers. "A review of the literature," *Ostomy/Wound Management* 51(4):70-80, 2005.

50. European Pressure Ulcer Advisory Panel. Nutrition and Pressure Ulcer Guidelines. Oxford, UK. Available at http://www.epuap.org. Accessed January 2007

51. Brown, G. "Wound documentation: Managing risk," *Advances in Skin and Wound Care* 19(3):155-165; quiz 166-7, 2006.

52. National Pressure Ulcer Advisory Panel. "Pressure Ulcers Prevalence, Cost, and Risk Assessment: Consensus Development Conference Statement," *Decubitus* 2(2):24-28, May 1989.

53. Shea, J.D. "Pressure Sores: Classification and Management," *Clinical Orthopaedics and Related Research* 112:89-100, October 1975.

54. International Association of Enterostomal Therapy (IAET). "Dermal Wounds: Pressure Sores. Philosophy of the IAET," *Journal of Enterostomal Therapy* 15(1):9-15, January-February 1988.

55. Henderson, C.T., et al. "Draft Definition of Stage I Pressure Ulcers: Inclusion of Persons with Darkly Pigmented Skin. NPUAP Task Force on Stage I Definition and Darkly Pigmented Skin," *Advances in Skin & Wound Care* 10(5):16-19, September 1997.

56. Ankrom, M.A., Bennett, R.G., Sprigle, S., Langemo, D., Black, J.M., Berlowitz, DR, Lyder, CH, and the NPUAP. "Pressure-related deep tissue injury under intact skin and the current pressure ulcer staging system," *Advances in Skin and Wound Care.* 18(1):35-42, 2005.

57. Black, J.M., and NPUAP. "Moving towards consensus on deep tissue injury and pressure ulcer staging," *Advances in Skin and Wound Care.* 18(8):415-421, 2005.

58. Donnelly, J. "Should we include deep tissue injury in pressure ulcer staging system? The NPUAP debate," *J Wound Care* 14(5):207-10, 2005.

59. Doughty, D., Ramundo, J., Bonham, P., et al. "Issues and challenges in staging of pressure ulcers," *JWOCN* 33(2):125-132, 2006.

60. Zulkowski, K., Langemo, D., Posthauer, M.E. "Coming to consensus on deep tissue injury," *Advances in Skin and Wound Care.* 18(1):28-29, 2005.

61. Ayello, E.A., and Lyder, C.H. "Pressure Ulcers in Persons of Color: Race and Ethnicity," in *Pressure Ulcers in America: Prevalence, Incidence, and Implications for the Future*, edited by Cuddigan, J., et al. Reston, Va.: National Pressure Ulcer Advisory Panel, 2001.

62. Lyder, C.H. Accuracy of Stage I Pressure Ulcer Definitions in Dark Skinned Individuals. Unpublished data.

63. Sprigle, S., et al. "Clinical Skin Temperature Measurement to Predict Incipient Pressure Ulcers," *Advances in Skin & Wound Care* 14(3):133-37, May-June 2001.

64. Ayello, E.A. , Baranoski, S., Salati, D.S. "Best practices in wound care prevention and treatment," *Nursing Management* 37(9): 42-48, 2006.

65. Zulkowski, K. Ayello, E.A. "Urban and rural nurses' knowledge of pressure ulcers in the USA," *WCET Journal* 25(3): 24-30, 2005.

66. Ayello, E.A., Baranoski, S., Salati, D.S. "A survey of nurses' wound care knowledge," *Advances in Skin and Wound Care* 18(5):268-75, 2005.

67. Ayello, E.A., Baranoski, S., Salati, D.S. "Wound care survey report," *Nursing2005* 35(6):36-45, 2005.

68. European Pressure Ulcer Advisory Panel (EPUAP). Available at: www.epuap.org. Last accessed December 23, 2006.

69. Maklebust, J. "Policy Implications of Using Reverse Staging to Monitor Pressure Ulcer Status," *Advances in Wound Care* 10(5):32-35, 1997.

70. Stewart T.P., Magnano, S.J. "Burns or pressure ulcers in the surgical patient?" *Decubitus* 1988;1(1):36-40.

71. Quintavalle, P.R., Lyder, C.H., Mertz, P.J., Phillips-Jones, C., Dyson, M. "Use of high-resolution, high-frequency diagnostic ultrasound to investigate the pathogenesis of pressure ulcer development," *Advances in Skin and Wound Care* 19(9):498-505, 2006.

72. Langemo, D.K., Brown, G. "Skin Fails too: Acute, Chronic, and end-stage skin failure," *Advances in Skin and Wound Care* 19(4):206-11, 2006.

73. European Pressure Ulcer Advisory Panel. (EPUAP) Treatment Guidelines. Available at http://www.epuap.org. Accessed January 2007.

74. Bates-Jensen, B.M. "The Pressure Sore Status Tool a Few Thousand Assessments Later," *Advances in Wound Care* 10(5):65-73, September-October 1997.

75. NPUAP PUSH Task Force. "Pressure Ulcer Scale for Healing: Derivation and Validation of the PUSH Tool," *Advances in Wound Care* 10(5):96, September-October 1997.

76. Berlowitz, D.R., Ratliff, C, Cuddigan, J., Rodeheaver, G.T., and the National Pressure Ulcer Advisory Panel. The PUSH Tool: A survey to determine its perceived usefulness. *Advances in Skin and Wound Care.* 18(9):480-483, 2005.

77. Wallenstein, S., Brem, H. Statistical analysis of wound-healing rates for pressure ulcers. *The American Journal of Surgery.* 188(1A)(Suppl):73S-78S, July 2004.

78. Jessup, R.L. "What is the best method for assessing the rate of wound healing? A comparison of 3 mathematical formulas," *Advances in Skin and Wound Care* 19(3):138, 140-142, 145-146, 2006.

79. Schubert, V., Zander, M. "Analysis of the measurement of four wound variables in elderly patients with pressure ulcers," *Advances in Wound Care* 9(4):29-36, 1996.

80. Xakellis, G., and Frantz, R.A. "Pressure Ulcer Healing: What Is It? What Influences It? How Is It Measured?" *Advances in Wound Care* 10(5):20-26, 1997.

81. Dyson, M., Lyder, C. Wound management physical modalities. In Morison, M, ed., *The Prevention and Treatment of Pressure Ulcers.* Edinburgh: Harcourt Brace/Mosby International, 2001.

82. Robson, M.C., and Heggers, J.P. "Bacterial Quantification of Open Wounds," *Military Medicine* 134(1):19-24, February 1969.

83. Barr, J.E. "Principles of Wound Cleansing," *Ostomy/Wound Management* 41(Suppl 7A):15S-22S, August 1995.

84. Hellewell, T.B., et al. "A Cytotoxicity Evaluation of Antimicrobial Wound Cleansers," *Wounds* 9(1):15-20, 1997.

85. Wilson, J.R., Mills, J.G., Prather, I.D., Dimitrijevich, S.D. "A toxicity index of skin and wound cleansers used on in vitro fibroblasts and keratinocytes," *Advances in Skin and Wound Care* 18(7):373-78, 2005.

86. Rodeheaver, G.T., et al. "Wound Cleansing by High Pressure Irrigation," *Surgery Gynecology and Obstetrics* 141(3):357-62, September 1975.

87. Stevenson, T.R., et al. "Cleansing the Traumatic Wound by High Pressure Syringe Irrigation," *Journal of the American College of Emergency Physicians* 5(1):17-21, January 1976.

88. Bhaskar, S.N., et al. "Effect of Water Lavage on Infected Wounds in the Rat," *Journal of Periodontology* 40(11):671-72, November 1969.

89. Yarkony, G.M. "Pressure Ulcers: Medical Management," in *Spinal Cord Injury Medical Management and Rehabilitation.* Gaithersburg, MD: Aspen, 1994.

90. Dolychuck, K.N. "Debridement," in Krasner, D., et al., eds. *Chronic Wound Care: A Clinical Source Book for Health Care Professionals,* 3rd ed. Wayne, Pa: HMP Communications, 2001.

91. Galpin, J.E., et al. Sepsis Associated with Decubitus Ulcers," *American Journal of Medicine* 61(3):346-50, September 1976.

92. Kim, Y.C., et al. "Efficacy of Hydrocolloid Occlusive Dressing Technique in Decubitus Ulcer Treatment: A Comparative Study," *Yonsei Medical Journal* 37(3):181-85, June 1996.

93. Bolton, L.L., et al. "Quality Wound Care Equals Cost-effective Wound Care: A Clinical Model," *Advances in Wound Care* 10(4):33-38, July-August 1997.

94 Saydak, S. "A Pilot of Two Methods for the Treatment of Pressure Ulcers," *Journal of Enterostomal Therapy* 7(3):139-42, May-June 1990.

95. Lyder, C.H., et al. "Examining the Cost-effectiveness of Two Methods for Healing Stage II Pressure Ulcers in Long-term Care," Under review.

96. ter Riet, G., et al. "Randomized Clinical Trial of Ascorbic Acid in the Treatment of Pressure Ulcers," *Journal of Clinical Epidemiology* 48(12):1452-1460, December 1995.

97. Rackett, S.C., et al. "The Role of Dietary Manipulation in the Prevention and Treatment of Cutaneous Disorders," *Journal of the American Academy of Dermatology* 29(3):447-53, September 1993.

98. Waldorf, H., and Fewkes, J. "Wound Healing," *Advances in Dermatology* 10:77-81, 1995.

99. Erlich, H.P., and Hunt, T.K. "Effects of Cortisone and Vitamin A on Wound Healing," *Annals of Surgery* 167(3):324-28, March 1968.

100. Houwing, R., Rozendaal, M., Woutrs-Wesseling, W., Beulens, J.W.J., Bukens, E., Haalboom, J. "A randomized, double-bind assessment of the effect of nutritional supplementation on the prevention of pressure ulcers in hip-fracture patients," *Clin Nutr* 22(4):401-405, 2003.

101. Langer, G., Schloemer, G., Kneer, A., Kuss, O., Behrens, J. "Nutritional interventions for preventing and treating pressure ulcers," *The Cochrane Database of Systematic Reviews* Issue 4. No:CD003216. 2003.

102. Thomas, DR. "Improving the outcome of pressure ulcers with nutritional intervention: a review of the evidence," *Nutrition* 17:121-25, 2001.

103. Kloth, L.C., and McCulloch, J. "Promotion of Wound Healing with Electrical Stimulation," *Advances in Wound Care* 9(5):42-45, September-October 1996.

104. Gardner, S.E., et al. "Effect of Electrical Stimulation on Chronic Wound Healing: A Meta-analysis," *Wound Repair Regeneration* 7(6):495-503, November-December 1999.

105. Courville, S. "Hyperbaric Oxygen Therapy: Its Role in Healing Problem Wounds," *Canadian Association of Enterostomal Journal* 17(4):7-11, 1998.

106. Gruber, R. P., et al. "Skin Permeability of Oxygen and Hyperbaric Oxygen," *Archives of Surgery* 101(1):69-70, July 1970.

107. Xia, Z., et al. "Stimulation of Fibroblast Growth In Vitro by Intermittent Radiant Warming," *Wound Repair Regeneration* 8(2):138-44, March-April 2000.

108. Mustoe, T.A., et al. "A Phase II Study to Evaluate Recombinant Platelet-derived Growth Factor-BB in the Treatment of Stage 3 and 4 Pressure Ulcers," *Archives of Surgery* 129(2):213-19, February 1994.

109. Ayello, E.A., et al. "Methods for Determining Pressure Ulcer Prevalence and Incidence," in Cuddigan, J., et al., eds. *Pressure Ulcers in America: Prevalence, Incidence, and Implications for the Future*. Reston, VA: NPUAP, 2001.

110. O'Brien, S.P., et al. "Sequential Biannual Prevalence Studies of Pressure Ulcers at Allegheny-Hahnemann University Hospital," *Ostomy/Wound Management* 44(suppl 3A):78s-88s, March 1998.

111. Baker, J. "Medicaid Claims History of Florida Long-term Care Facility Residents Hospitalized for Pressure Ulcers," *Journal of Wound, Ostomy, and Continence Nursing* 23(1):23-25, January 1996.

112. Langemo, D.K., et al. "Incidence and Prediction of Pressure Ulcers in Five Patient Care Settings," *Decubitus* 4(3):25- 30, August 1991.

113. Oot Giromini, B.A. "Pressure Ulcer Prevalence, Incidence and Associated Risk Factors in the Community," *Decubitus* 6(5):24-32, September 1993.

114. Bours, G.J., et al. "The Development of a National Registration Form to Measure the Prevalence of Pressure Ulcers in the Netherlands," *Ostomy/Wound Management* 45(11):28-40, November 1999.

115. Wendte, J.F. "Monitoring the Prevalence of Pressure Ulcers: Does it Support Implementation Projects?" *European Pressure Ulcer Advisory Panel Review* 4(1):22, 2002.

116. Healey, F. "Wound Care. Waterlow Revisited," *Nursing Times* 92(11):80-84, March 13-19, 1996.

117. Dealey, C. "The Size of the Pressure-sore Problem in a Teaching Hospital," *Journal of Advanced Nursing* 16(6):663-70, June 1991.

118. Hanson, R. "Sore Points Sorted," *Nursing Times* 93(7):66-72, February 12-18, 1997.

119. O'Dea, K. "Pressure Sores. Damage Limitation," *Nursing Times* 92(15):46-47, April 10-16, 1996.

120. Harrison, M.B., et al. "Practice Guidelines for the Prediction and Prevention of Pressure Ulcers: Evaluating the Evidence," *Applied Nursing Research* 9(1):9-17, February 1996.

121. Gruen, R.L., et al. "The Point Prevalence of Wounds in a Teaching Hospital," *Australia and New Zealand Journal of Surgery* 67(10):686-88, 1997.

122. Thoroddsen, A. "Pressure Sore Prevalence: A national Survey," *Journal of Clinical Nursing* 8(2):170-79, March 1999.

123. Gunningberg, L., et al. "The Development of Pressure Ulcers in Patients with Hip Fractures: Inadequate Nursing Documentation is Still a Problem," *Journal of Advanced Nursing* 31(5):1155-64, May 2000.

124. Hagisawa, S., and Barbenel, J. "The Limits of Pressure Sore Prevention," *Journal of the Royal Society of Medicine* 92(11):576-78, November 1999.

125. Barrois, B., et al. "A Survey of Pressure Sore Prevalence in Hospitals in the Greater Paris Region," *Journal of Wound Care* 4(5):234-35, May 1995.

126. Lahmann, N., and Dassen, T. "Prevalence of Pressure Ulcers in Eleven German Hospitals in April 2001," *European Pressure Ulcer Advisory Panel Review* 4(1):17, 2002.

127. Amlung, S., et al. "National Prevalence Pressure Ulcer Survey: A Benchmarking Approach," in *14th Annual Clinical Symposium on Wound Care*. The Quest for Quality Wound Care: Solutions for Clinical Practice; September 30, 1999 to October 4, 1999. Denver, CO: Sponsored by the Wound Care Communications Network and University of Pennsylvania Medical Center, 1999.

128. CalNOC. A Statewide Nursing Outcomes Database. Linking Patient Outcomes to Hospital Nursing Care: California Nursing Outcomes Coalition: January 18, 2000.

129. Whittington, K., et al. "A National Study of Pressure Ulcer Prevalence and Incidence in Acute Care Hospitals," *Journal of Wound, Ostomy, and Continence Nursing* 27(4):209-15, July 2000.

130. O'Sullivan, K.L., et al. "Pressure Sores in the Acute Trauma Patient: Incidence and Causes," *Journal of Trauma* 42(2):276-78, February 1997.

131. Berlowitz, D.R., et al. "Are We Improving the Quality of Nursing Home Care: The Case of Pressure Ulcers," *Journal of the American Geriatric Society* 48(1):59-62, January 2000.

132. Ramundo, J.M. "Reliability and Validity of the Braden Scale in the Home Care Setting," *Journal of Wound, Ostomy, and Continence Nursing* 22(3):28-34, March 1995.

133. Clark, M., and Watts, S. "The Incidence of Pressure Sores Within a National Health Service Trust Hospital During 1991," *Journal of Advanced Nursing* 20(1):33-36, July 1994.

134. Goodridge, D.M., et al. "Risk Assessment Scores, Prevention Strategies, and the Incidence of Pressure Ulcers Among the Elderly in Four Canadian Health Care Facilities," *Canadian Journal of Nursing Research* 30(2):23-44, Summer 1998.

135. National Pressure Ulcer Advisory Panel (NPUAP) Board of Directors. "An Executive Summary of the NPUAP Monograph Pressure Ulcers in America: Prevalence, Incidence and Implications for the Future," *Advances in Skin & Wound Care* 14(4):208-215, July-August 2001.

136. Defloor, T., et al. "Draft EPUAP Statement on Prevalence and Incidence Monitoring," *European Pressure Ulcer Advisory Panel Review* 4(1):13-15, 2002.

137. Armitage, P., and Berry, G. *Statistical Methods in Medical Research*. Cambridge, Mass.: Blackwell Scientific Pubs., 1987.

138. Odierna, E., Zeleznik, J. "Pressure ulcer education: A pilot study of the knowledge and clinical confidence of geriatric fellows," *Advances in Skin and Wound Care* 16:26-30, 2003.

139. Garcia, A.D., Perkins, C., Click, C., Bergstrom, N., Taffet, G. *Pressure ulcers education in primary care residencies*. In Ayello, E.A., Baranoski, Research Forum: Examining the problem of pressure ulcers. *Advances in Skin and Wound Care* 18(4): 193-194, 2005.

140. Boxer, E., Maynard, C. "The management of chronic wounds: Factors that affect nurses' decision making," *Journal of Wound Care* 8(8):409-412, 1999.

141. Lamond, D., Farnell, S. "The treatment of pressure sores: A comparison of novice and expert nurses' knowledge, information use and decision accuracy," *Journal of Advanced Nursing* 27:280-286, 1998.

142. Maylor, M., Torrance, C. "Pressure sore survey part 2: Nurses knowledge," *Journal of Wound Care* 8(2):49-52, 1999.

143. Springett, J., Cowell, J., Heanet, M. "Using care pathways in pressure area management: A pilot study," *Journal of Wound Care* 8(5):227-230, 1999.

144. Ayello, E.A., Zulkowski, K., Holmes, A.M., Edelstein, T. "A collaborative statewide across care setting initiative reduces pressure ulcers," *Advances in Skin and Wound Care* In press.

145. Zulkowski, K., Ayello, E.A., Wexler, S. Certification and Education: Do they affect pressure ulcer knowledge in nursing? *Advances in Skin and Wound Care* 20(1): 34-8, 2007.

146. Ayello, E.A., Frantz, R.A. "A competency-based pressure ulcer curriculum for registered nurses in America. Part I, Pressure ulcer prevention," *WCET Journal* 25(1):8-12, 2005.

147. Ayello, E.A., Frantz, R.A. "A competency-based pressure ulcer curriculum for registered nurses in America. Part 2, Pressure ulcer treatment," *WCET Journal* 25(2):8-14, 2005.

148. Brandeis, G.H., Berlowitz, D.R., Katz, P. "Are pressure ulcers preventable? A survey of experts," *Advances in Skin and Wound Care* 14:244, 2001.

149. Carasa, M., Polycarpe, M. "Caring for the chronically critically ill patient: Establishing a wound healing program in a respiratory care unit," *The American Journal of Surgery* 188(1A) Supplement: 18S-21S, July 2004.

150. The John A. Hartford Institute for Geriatric Nursing. *Try This* Series. Available at www.hartfordign.org. Accessed December 23, 2006.

151. National Database of Nursing Quality Indicators (NDNQI) Pressure Ulcer Modules. Available at: www.nursingquality.org. Accessed on December 23, 2006.

152. Thomas, D.R., et al. "Pressure Ulcer Scale for Healing: Derivation and Validation of the PUSH Tool," *Advances in Skin & Wound Care* 10(5):96-101, May 1997.

CHAPTER 14

Venous ulcers, lymphedema, and compression therapy

Mary Y. Sieggreen, MSN, APRN, CS, CVN, APN
Ronald A. Kline, MD, FACS, FAHA
Mary Jo Geyer, PT, PhD, FCCWS, CLT-LANA, C.Ped

OBJECTIVES

After completing this chapter, you'll be able to:

* describe the anatomy and physiology of the venous system

* explain the pathophysiology of lower extremity venous ulcers

* describe the epidemiology of lymphedema

* describe the physiology of edema formation

* describe systems for classifying venous disease

* state the signs and symptoms that comprise a venous assessment

* discuss vascular laboratory tests performed for patients with venous disease

* describe the components of local wound care for a patient with a venous ulcer

* describe surgical treatment for patients with a venous ulcer

* identify education needs for patients with venous disease and lymphedema.

Scope of the problem

"Peripheral vascular disease" is a term commonly used in reference to an arterial problem, even though it includes diseases and conditions of the venous and lymphatic systems as well as the arterial system. Patients with leg ulcers may present with a combination of arterial, venous, and lymphatic disease. This chapter describes venous anatomy and physiology and examines the causes and treatment of lower extremity venous and lymphatic ulcers.

Approximately 10% to 35% of the population has some form of venous disease.[1] It's estimated that between 1% and 22% of the population over age 60 suffers from lower extremity skin ulcers.[2-5] One study found the problem to be underestimated when a self-report survey indicated high numbers of patients cared for their own ulcers without consulting a health care provider.[6] The principal leg ulcer etiology in most patients is some type of peripheral vascular disease. Chronic venous disease is the seventh most common chronic disease. It's the underlying cause in 95% of leg ulcers.[1,7-9] In a U.S. community health survey, 5% of adults had skin changes in the leg and more than 500,000 suffered from venous ulcers. Over 2,000,000 work days are lost in the United States per year due to the associated morbidity of postphlebitic syndrome.[9] Although it's understood that chronic wounds have physical, financial, and psychological affects, it's difficult to measure their effects on a patient's quality of life.[10] It's also difficult to obtain accurate etiological information about leg ulcers and, in about one-third of medical records, no ulcer etiology might be documented.

Epidemiology of lymphedema

The epidemiology of lymphedema is fraught with uncertainty. Many of the problems inherent in determining prevalence and incidence rates have been previously described by Logan[11] and, more recently, by Williams et al.[12] Key issues include the lack of a repeatable and valid definition of lymphedema and methodological inconsistencies in quantifying the presence and/or severity of edema and in assessing skin and tissue changes. Chronic lower extremity edema manifests itself as lymphedema when interstitial fluid, proteins, other cellular components, and foreign debris that would normally drain via an intact lymphatic system accumulate in the subcutaneous tissue. Primary lymphedema may arise from congenital or developmental defects of the lymphatic system and is relatively uncommon. Secondary lymphedema, the most common form, is acquired due to trauma, chronic inflammation/infection (including parasitic), lymph node dissection and irradiation, or surgical interventions unrelated to cancer. Lymphedema usually affects one or more limbs, most commonly the lower limbs and, if untreated, may lead to gross disfigurement described as elephantiasis. Lymphedema is a chronic disorder that can be managed suc-

cessfully with psychosocial support, lifelong adherence to a maintenance protocol (skin care, compression garments, exercise), and attention to precautions.

Lymphedema due to parasitic infection (filariasis) is a significant problem in tropical areas of the world including India, Africa, Haiti, and Malaysia. It's estimated to afflict 2% of the global population or approximately 119 million.[13] However, a discussion of filariatic lymphedema is beyond the scope of this chapter. In developed nations, lymphedema is considered a serious complication following cancer treatment and is most commonly associated with surgery and/or irradiation of the lymph nodes. Breast cancer-related lymphedema has been studied extensively to identify predisposing factors, which include irradiation, the extent of axillary node dissection, combined axillary dissection and irradiation, obesity, surgical wound infection, tumor stage and extent of surgery.[12,14,-16] Despite improvements in surgical interventions, reductions in incidence for this population remain in excess of 30% of women treated, but this data may also reflect improved detection.[12,16] The incidence of lower extremity cancer-related lymphedema is largely unknown but can coexist with other forms of lower extremity edema and venous disease. Reports of incidence vary widely (40% following groin dissection; 55% following ilioinguinal dissection; 6% to 20% following combined pelvic and lymph node dissection for stage III melanoma).[17-19] Tumor location and other factors similar to those identified in breast cancer also impact incidence.

In developed nations, interest in lymphedema of the lower extremities unrelated to cancer treatment has been limited. For example, despite the knowledge that chronic inflammation and ulceration are likely to damage the lymphatic system,[20-23] many clinicians don't recognize the lymphatic component in venous disease and have difficulty in distinguishing lymphedema from edema due to other causes. In addition to venous disease, other non-cancer related factors including trauma, infection, and/or arthritis may contribute to the development of lymphedema.[2,20,24] Failure to recognize lymphatic insufficiency may lead to ineffective treatment and increased morbidity.

A recent prevalence study conducted in southwest London addressed some of the previously mentioned epidemiologic issues by using a broad operational definition of chronic edema/lymphedema and setting specific clinical criteria to identify cases. The population included only those individuals known to, or being treated by, health professionals. The clinical criteria included persistent edema of more than 3 months duration, a minimal response to overnight elevation or diuretics, and the presence of skin changes (thickened skin, hyperkeratosis, and papillomatosis). Individuals with systemic disorders likely to cause edema were excluded (congestive heart failure, hypoalbuminemia, nephrotic syndrome). The authors acknowledged that due to the broad definition, inclusion of cases with mixed etiologies was probable. However, because a sufficient lymphatic system should compensate for an increase in capillary filtration by increasing lymph drainage, they proposed that any chronic edema identified using their clinical criteria represented some form of lymphatic insufficiency[21,25]

This study reported a crude prevalence of 1.33/1,000 with age-related increases reaching 5.4/1,000 in those over age 65 and 10.3/1,000 for those over age 85.[26] Based on current population estimates, this translates into a range of approximately 100,000 to 618,000 cases in the U.K. or approximately 395,000 to 896,000 in the United States. The data were considered to be underestimated as not all patients with chronic edema/lymphedema were likely to be receiving treatment at the time of the study. These estimates are supported by a similar 1.44/1,000 crude prevalence of chronic edema in Norway reported by Petlund.[27] Additional key findings characterized the impact of chronic edema/lymphedema on patients' lives. Nearly a third had experienced an acute infection in the preceding year with 25% requiring hospitalization. Edema also caused time off work in more than 80% of cases and employment status was affected in 9%. Despite the popular belief that lymphedema is not painful, 50% of patients reported pain or discomfort

from their edema. Quality of life also suffered with clear deficits in many domains of the well-validated SF-36 questionnaire.[26] In conclusion, it would appear that chronic edema/lymphedema is a frequently unreported condition associated with significant morbidity that occurs with prevalence similar to that of leg ulceration.

Venous and lymphatic anatomy and physiology

Venous system

The venous system begins at the postcapillary level. Venules begin to coalesce, forming small veins, which again coalesce into larger veins from the periphery to a more central location. The venous system mimics the arterial system in many respects, but has a greater anatomic variability than the arterial tree. In the leg, the veins that course with the tibial and peroneal arteries are usually paired with numerous cross-linking branches, resulting in a retie appearance in some patients. These branches ascend along the respective arteries to form the popliteal vein, which is the first vein of significant size in the lower leg. The popliteal vein proceeds toward the head and becomes the femoral vein, commonly called the superficial femoral vein—a name that causes confusion because the vein in question is actually a deep vein. The superficial femoral vein joins the deep femoral vein to form the common femoral vein. The deep femoral vein is the deep drainage system of the thigh. (See *Deep and superficial venous systems,* page 290.)

Dual venous system

The leg has a dual venous system—the deep system just described and the superficial system represented by the saphenous veins. The greater saphenous vein courses along the medial aspect of the leg. The dorsal digital veins in the foot coalesce to form the greater saphenous vein. The greater saphenous vein is found medial and anterior to the medial malleolus. It ascends in the leg through a variable course and may be bifurcated or even trifurcated. At knee level, its course be-

Deep and superficial venous systems

This illustration shows deep and superficial veins of the lower extremities.

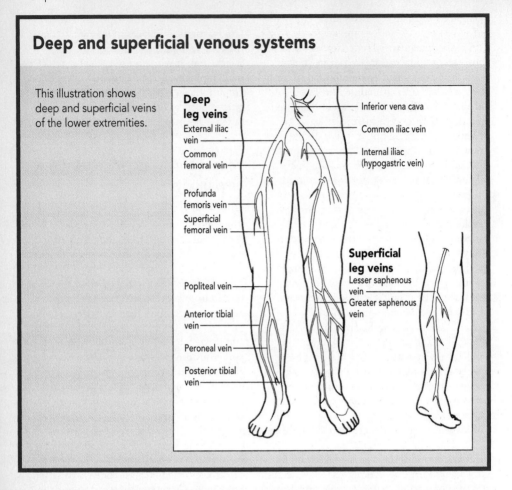

Deep leg veins

External iliac vein

Common femoral vein

Profunda femoris vein

Superficial femoral vein

Popliteal vein

Anterior tibial vein

Peroneal vein

Posterior tibial vein

Inferior vena cava

Common iliac vein

Internal iliac (hypogastric vein)

Superficial leg veins

Lesser saphenous vein

Greater saphenous vein

comes deeper in relationship to the skin. As it ascends the leg, it joins the common femoral vein at the fossa ovale. The lesser saphenous vein drains the posterior aspect of the calf. It perforates into the deep compartment of the calf at the level of the popliteal fossa to join the popliteal vein. As the common femoral vein ascends behind the inguinal ligament it becomes the external iliac vein and joins the internal iliac vein to become the common iliac vein. The common iliac veins join at the level of the umbilicus and to the right of the aorta to become the inferior vena cava. The renal veins drain into the vena cava. More cephalad, the hepatic veins join the vena cava, which then empties into the right heart chamber.

The saphenous system is connected to the deep venous system through numerous perforator veins. Perforator veins shunt blood from the subcutaneous tissue and the greater saphenous system into the deep veins of the leg. They cross through the superficial fascia of the leg, hence their name. The location of perforator veins is somewhat variable and some are ascribed proper names. The lowest perforator connecting the saphenous system with the deep venous system is just above the medial malleolus.

Valve anatomy

Unidirectional valves are present in the deep and superficial venous systems and in the perforator veins. These valves are located just before bifurcation points. The greater saphenous vein contains approximately six to eight valves. With rare exception, a valve is always present just below the insertion of the greater saphenous vein into the common femoral vein at the fossa ovale. The orientation of the valves allows venous blood to flow from distal to proximal. Perforator veins' valves are oriented to shunt blood from the lesser saphenous vein and the greater saphenous system into the deep veins of the leg.

Valve anatomy is that of a bileaflet with valve sinuses present on the lateral bases of each valve leaflet. These sinuses represent a dilation in the normal contour of the vein wall. Their function is to assist in valve closure, a passive act caused by the retrograde flow of venous blood into the sinus thereby coapting (fitting together) the two valve leaflets. The valve leaflets are oriented parallel to the surface of the skin. It's the loss of valve function at various levels that results in varying degrees of venous insufficiency. Valve function is lost under a number of disease states. Inability of the valve to coapt can also occur with over-distention of the venous segment. This effectively stretches the valves apart so that they no longer come in direct contact, thereby allowing blood to reflux into the more dependent portion of the vein. Disease states that cause loss of valve function include:

- congenital valve absence
- deep vein thrombosis
- ectasia
- phlebitis
- valve atresia
- venous hypertension
- venous engorgement.

Venous wall architecture

Venous wall anatomy is similar to arterial wall anatomy except that the respective lamina are thinner. The outermost layer of a vein is the adventitia. The media varies most from the arterial media. The media within a vein contains both elastic and muscular fibers, but to a much lesser degree than the arterial media. Nonetheless, a vein can contract and adjust its size to correspond to the degree of venous blood flow. The intima layer is a delicate single layer of endothelial cells.

The relatively thin media accounts for the lack of venous compliance at increased pressures. At low pressures, the venous system is fairly compliant, but once arterial pressure is reached, the venous wall becomes distended and rigid. Vasoconstriction occurs in both the superficial and deep veins; the more peripheral the vein, the more readily it contracts. This reactivity is under sympathetic adrenergic control. Peripheral veins are more sensitive to this sympathetic drive than central veins. The ability of veins to relax and dilate enables the venous system to hold 75% of the total blood volume.

PRACTICE POINT

Loss of consciousness can occur from venous pooling in motionless lower extremities—a fate not unknown to young military recruits who must stand at attention for prolonged periods of time.

The upward flow of lower extremity venous blood, although aided by unidirectional valves and arterial pressure, is mostly dependent upon the "muscular pump." Pedal dorsal vein pressure in the supine position should approximate that of central venous pressure. Upon assuming an erect posture, this pressure can approach 100 mm Hg. With active muscle contraction, intra-compartmental pressure markedly increases, thereby causing deep veins of the leg to compress and push venous blood upward. This pressure then approaches 200 mm Hg. This is possible because the muscular compartments of the leg are enclosed by relatively rigid fascial encasement. Back-flush of blood is reduced when valves are competent and reflux into the saphenous system is prevented by the unidirectional perforator valves.

Lymphatic system

The lymphatic system is the least understood of the three vascular systems in the leg. The embryologic development of the lymphatic system is still largely unknown.

Lymphatic vessels are divided into three categories:

- initial or terminal lymphatic capillaries
- collecting vessels

• lymph nodes.

Initial or terminal lymphatic capillaries originate in the superficial dermis. At this level they are valveless—the epidermis doesn't contain lymphatic vessels. From the superficial dermis, the valveless system drains into the deep dermal and subdermal system where valved lymphatic vessels can be identified. Lymphatic valves are similar to venous valves, ascending the leg to drain both the dermis and the muscular beds into lymph nodes, routinely found at the popliteal fossa and the inguinal ligament. The lymphatic chain generally parallels the larger veins in the proximal leg above the knee.

Dissection around the deep femoral artery can disrupt the lymphatic system, resulting in surgically induced lymphedema. Above the level of the inguinal ligament, the lymphatic system drains through series of iliac lymph nodes coalescing into peri-aortic nodes, then into the cisterna chyli and more cephalad into the thoracic duct. The thoracic duct ascends along the thoracic aorta on the right side of the chest and drains into the left jugular vein just above the jugulo-subclavian junction. In addition to the thoracic duct, some patients have an accessory right lymphatic duct, which drains into the right jugular venous system. The thoracic duct traditionally has been considered the main lympho-venous drainage, although other methods of drainage exist, including lympho-venous communications within the various muscle compartments and peripheral lympho-venous communications.

Lymphatic vessel anatomy is similar to, but smaller than, either arterial or venous anatomy. The outer adventitial layer, in particular, is quite minimal. The media contains, in addition to a few elastin fibers, some stria of smooth muscle, which is used to help propel lymphatic flow cephalad via contraction. A single layer of endothelium comprises the intima. The relative size of a lymphatic vessel is between one-seventh and one-tenth the size of a major artery or vein.

Aspects of lymphatic flow

Lymphatic flow occurs as the consequence of four distinct etiologies: capillary blood pressure, osmotic pressure, interstitial fluid pressure (hydrostatic), and oncotic pressure. Intrinsic contractility of the lymphatic vessel wall, as previously stated, aids in cephalad lymphatic flow. The muscular pump aids in flow as it does in the venous system. Positive abdominal pressure, negative thoracic pressure, and pulsatile blood flow aid in cephalic flow of lymph.

The lymphatic system provides a drainage mechanism for acellular interstitial fluid. White blood cells are capable of entering the interstitial space and one of their mechanisms of reentry into the vascular space is by way of the lymphatic channels. Lymph is functionally filtered at the node level. The nodes act as a repository for lymphatic cells. Normal lymphatic circulation requires an intact lymphatic system with essentially normal architecture. Whenever a disruption occurs within the lymphatic drainage system, lymphedema ensues.

The lymphatic system also complements the blood vascular system. It forms a one-way drainage and filtration system composed of lymphatic vessels and lymphoid organs arranged in a tree-like hierarchical network. This extravascular system transports fluid, plasma proteins, specific cells critical to immune function (antigen-presenting cells, T lymphocytes), and other macromolecules that have leaked from tissues into the interstitial space back to the blood vascular system. The organs, for example, bone marrow, the thymus, lymph nodes, the spleen, and the tonsils each function to produce, maintain, and distribute lymphocytes. Therefore, the lymphatic system is essential for interstitial tissue fluid balance (volume and pressure), immune surveillance, and fat absorption.[21,28-30] Conversely, lymphatic insufficiency may directly influence the body's response to inflammation or infection by disturbing cellular and cytokine circulation in a particular drainage area.[20] For the purpose of this chapter, only the structures and mechanisms specific to lymphatic circulation of the lower limb will be discussed.

In general, the anatomy of the lymphatic system mirrors that of the venous system. The two systems share similarities in structure and function, but the lymphatics have lymph nodes at various intervals, thinner walls, and more valves than their venous counterparts. While the embryonic origin of the lymphatic system remains largely unknown, its close development with the venous system has been well-documented. Lymphatic vessels originate from lymph sacs (jugular, iliac, retroperitoneal, and cisterna chyli), which lie close to developing veins. In recent years, the venous origin of the lymphatic vessels has been further supported by the presence of a gene (tyrosine kinase 4) specific to venous and lymphatic endothelia (but not arterial endothelia) early in development that subsequently demonstrates sole expression on lymphatic endothelia.[20,31,32]

Lower limb lymphatic anatomy

There are essentially two types of contiguous lymphatic vessels: 1) the small, non-contractile initial lymphatics (also known as *capillaries*), where interstitial fluid absorption begins, and 2) progressively larger, contractile conducting vessels (known as *collectors*) into which the initial lymphatics empty. The lymphatic capillaries, which are blind-ended, have a single layer of endothelial cells with overlapping regions that form one-way valves thus allowing interstitial fluid to enter and preventing lymph from escaping.[29,33,34] Additional anatomical features of the initial lymphatics include the absence of valves and smooth muscle cells and the presence of anchoring filaments that attach the vessels to collagen fibers in the extracellular matrix. Vessels known as precollectors have some segments with capillary-like walls as well as valves and provide a functional transition between the absorbing and conducting elements of the system. Larger contractile conducting vessels (known as *collectors* or *trunks*) have valves and inter-valve segments known as lymphangions that undergo spontaneous smooth muscle contractions initiated by pacemaker cells but can also respond to sympathetic activation.[33,34]

 PRACTICE POINT

Smooth muscle contraction in the lymphangions is dependent on the influx of cal-

cium ions. Therefore, calcium channel blocking agents are likely to have some negative effect on lymphatic contractility that contributes to peripheral edema.[21]

Like the main veins of the leg, the lymphatics are divided by the deep fascia into a deep (subfascial) and superficial (suprafascial) network, connected by perforating vessels. The superficial capillaries originate in the dermis and drain into subcutaneous collectors that organize into larger bundles. The superficial system drains both the dermis and subcutaneous tissue. Skin areas drained by one collector form topographical strips known as *skin zones* where the lymph vessels communicate freely. The skin zones associated with all collectors from a lymph vessel bundle form distinct territories that are separated by watersheds where few vessels communicate.[35]

 PRACTICE POINT

The communication lines (anastomoses) between the lymphatic capillaries in different areas provides an anatomical basis for manual lymph drainage—one component of the definitive therapeutic intervention for lymphedema. Manual lymph drainage consists of specific manual techniques designed to increase lymph flow and to move excess tissue fluid from a congested area across watersheds via the lymphatic capillaries into adjacent areas where alternate routes for drainage remain intact.

The deep (subfascial) lymphatic collectors share the same perivascular sheath with companion arteries and veins and drain the muscles, bones, and joints. Unlike the veins in which blood flows from the superficial veins through the perforating veins into the deep veins, lymph is propelled in the opposite direction, from the deep into the superficial system.[36]

Lymph flow in the leg

The process of lymph drainage begins with the net plasma filtrate from the blood circulation that along with other materials (prelymph) diffuses across the interstitial space and is absorbed by lymphatic capillaries and precollectors. The filling of lymphatic capillaries is passive in response to changes in local tissue pressure originating primarily from rhythmic muscle contraction and aided by arterial pulsation, external pressure, and manual lymph drainage. Lymph flows into the sequentially larger collectors, the more proximal of which are known as *trunks*.

Distention of the vessel wall provides the stimulus for lymphangion contraction. Lymphangions provide the primary propulsive force for lymph flow and contract at a rate of approximately 6 to 10 beats per minute. They function as miniature hearts in series,[20] and are capable of cardiac-like inotropic and chronotropic responses.[20,28,36] Lymph flow can increase as much as 10 times its baseline level in the presence of an increased volume of filtrate, enhanced uptake by the lymphatic capillaries, and increased rate of lymphangion contraction.[25]

PRACTICE POINT

Inducing alternating changes in interstitial fluid pressure via exercise or passive movement increases lymphatic capillary filling. This induction promotes flow in the collectors whose contractility has failed thereby increasing lymph flow. The addition of a bandage or other form of compression enhances the effect of movement.

Afferent collectors pump lymph proximally toward nodes routinely found in the popliteal fossa and at the inguinal ligament where the lymph is filtered. From 7 to 15 collecting trunks ultimately drain the leg to the inguinal lymph nodes via an anteromedial route that follows the course of the great saphenous vein.[20,21] Efferent collectors drain lymph from inguinal nodes through a series of iliac lymph nodes coalescing into peri-aortic nodes and trunks, then into the cisterna chyli, and move cephalad into the thoracic duct. The thoracic duct ascends along the thoracic aorta on the right side of the chest and drains into the left jugular vein just above the jugulo-subclavian junction. In addition to the thoracic duct, an accessory right lymphatic duct may be present, which drains into the right jugular venous system. Centrally, cephalic flow is augmented by breathing and local arterial pulsation. The thoracic duct traditionally has been considered the main lympho-venous drainage route. Other methods of drainage exist including lympho-venous communications within the various muscle compartments and peripheral lympho-venous communications, but they may not be functional unless there's chronic obstruction of the lymphatic vessels or nodes.[37]

PRACTICE POINT

Deep breathing, exercise, and manual lymph drainage all increase lymph flow and are essential components of the definitive treatment for chronic edema/lymphedema.

Tissue edema
Pathophysiology of edema in venous disease

All forms of edema, regardless of the underlying cause, result from an imbalance between capillary filtration and lymph drainage. Therefore, an understanding of edema requires a working knowledge of the physiological principles associated with interstitial fluid balance. Capillary filtration is governed by the Starling fluid exchange principle, which is described by the Starling equation for flow across a semi-permeable membrane. Simply stated, filtration of plasma fluid from the capillary into the interstitium is driven by the water pressure gradient across the capillary wall and is opposed by the colloidal osmotic pressure gradient (oncotic) that provides the force that retains the fluid in circulation.

Filtration is also affected by other factors including 1) the ease with which fluid can cross the capillary wall, 2) the surface area for filtration, and 3) the ability of the capillary wall to prevent leakage of plasma protein into the interstitium. Normally, the sum of all Starling forces favors filtration and accumulation of capillary filtrate in the tissue spaces is avoided mainly through lymph drainage and not, as was previously thought, through reabsorption by the venous capillaries.[21,38,39] The evidence for the lymphatic system providing the primary mechanism for sustained drainage of interstitial fluid has been demonstrated for 12 tissues to date[39] and emphasizes its importance in tissue volume homeostasis. The lymphatics return approximately 2 to 3 liters of fluid and plasma proteins per day into the blood circulation. Without this essential circulation, cardiovascular collapse, and ultimately death, would rapidly ensue.

Edema due to increased filtration
Most forms of edema develop when the capillary filtration rate exceeds lymph drainage for a sufficient period. Also known as *high volume lymphatic insufficiency,* this type of edema is analogous to flooding that occurs when heavy rain falls in a short period of time overwhelming the capacity of watershed tributaries. An increase in capillary filtration may occur in response to 1) increased capillary pressure, 2) a reduction in plasma colloid osmotic pressure, or 3) an increase in capillary wall permeability. Usually, increased capillary pressure is due to chronic elevation of venous pressure from heart failure, fluid overload, or venous disease. Reduced plasma colloid osmotic pressure results essentially from hypoalbuminemia secondary to nephrotic syndrome or failure of hepatic synthesis. Lastly, increased capillary permeability to water and proteins usually results from inflammation, a common factor in venous disease. Inflammation also increases blood flow causing mean capillary pressure to rise with resultant increased capillary filtration. In venous disease where edema is due to high volume lymphatic insufficiency, a gradual functional deterioration of the lymphatics may lead to lymphedema.[30]

Edema due to reduced lymphatic transport
In lymphedema, the edema produced is due to mechanical failure of the lymphatic system and lymph transport function falls below the capacity needed to drain even the normal load of capillary filtrate.[35] This is also known as *low volume lymphatic insufficiency* and is analogous to the flooding that would

occur during a light rain due to a rock slide permanently blocking a stream that functions as a primary watershed. This failure can be due to an inability of the lymphatic capillaries and precollectors to absorb filtrate, dysfunction of some portion of the network in conducting or filtering the normal lymphatic load, or both.

Mechanisms limiting edema formation
The venous hypertension that exists in venous disease inevitably increases capillary filtration as a result of increased capillary pressure. Several mechanisms are important in limiting the edema associated with increased capillary filtration rate and include: 1) increased interstitial pressure due to increased stiffness of the skin and soft tissues; 2) reduction in interstitial colloidal osmotic pressure; 3) increased lymph flow; 4) postural vasoconstriction in a dependent leg via the veni-arteriolar reflex; and 5) activation of the calf muscle pump. These mechanisms provide the physiologic basis for therapeutic interventions.

Increased interstitial fluid pressure
A tissue's ability to resist swelling is proportional to its stiffness (reduced compliance). In such stiffer tissues as muscle or fibrotic interstitial tissue a small increase in interstitial fluid volume will cause a relatively large increase in interstitial pressure, which then opposes filtration. Conversely, in loose and compliant tissue, such as that over the eyelid, the increase in interstitial pressure per unit of interstitial fluid volume will be much less. In these tissues, large volumes of fluid may accumulate before the rise in interstitial pressure effectively opposes filtration and tissue expansion stops. The vasoconstriction that occurs in a dependent leg due to the veni-arteriolar reflex also acts to oppose filtration by decreasing capillary pressure.

 PRACTICE POINT

Using a bandage or non-compliant compression stocking on the leg increases tissue stiffness thereby increasing interstitial pressure, opposing filtration, and consequently reducing edema formation or preventing its reaccumulation. A short stretch bandage will generate high interstitial pressure during muscle contraction, enhancing venous and lymphatic flow but will conversely exert low pressure during muscle relaxation allowing lymph vessels to refill.

Reduced interstitial colloidal osmotic pressure

An increase in filtration rate dilutes the local interstitial protein concentration. This consequently reduces the osmotic filtration force while simultaneously increasing the osmotic absorptive force and aids in retention of plasma fluid within the blood microcirculation. This mechanism is of major importance in protection against both pulmonary and peripheral edema.

Increased lymph flow

In venous disease, elevated venous pressure results in an increased filtration rate. In addition to the osmotic effects mentioned, the increased filtrate drained by the lymphatic capillaries is a stimulus for increased force of lymphangion contraction. Increased filtration can increase lymph transport several times and is presumed to be the major mechanism preventing edema formation. The ability to dramatically increase transport capacity in response to increased lymphatic load is also known as the *lymphatic safety valve function*. Lymphatic capillary filling and contractility is augmented by intermittent changes in tissue pressure resulting from movement (active or passive exercise), manual lymph drainage, arterial pulsation and, in more central tissues, breathing. Activation of the calf muscle pump not only decreases venous pressure but enhances lymph flow.

PRACTICE POINT

Bandaging and stockings enhance the pumping effect of exercise by providing a noncompliant shell against which the foot and calf muscles can press during contraction. Greater evacuation of venous blood leads to a decrease in venous capillary pressure and filtration. Intermittent changes in tissue pressure from walking and other rhythmic exercise increase lymphatic capillary filling and lymphangion contractility thereby increasing lymph flow.[39,40]

Venous disease without accompanying edema indicates that the compensatory mechanisms are working effectively. Conversely, the presence of edema means that either the rise in capillary pressure exceeds the forces opposing filtration or there's failure of the compensatory mechanisms. Inflammation, which may spread within each division or travel via the perivascular perforating sheath, is likely to be a major contributing factor to that failure.[20,36,40]

Lymphatic failure in venous disease

In the early stages of venous disease, lymph flow is increased. In later stages, when lipodermatosclerosis and venous ulcers are present, lymphatic drainage becomes compromised. Both blood and lymph vessels are affected in venous disease. Just as many mechanisms have been proposed regarding the etiology of venous ulcers, there are a number of theories regarding how chronic venous disease affects the lymphatics over time. First, there may be fewer lymph vessels or existing vessels may be smaller either due to a preexisting congenital defect or the acquired obliteration of vessels. Recent electron microscopy studies show lymphatic capillary obliteration in the superficial fibrin/cell and granulation tissue of venous ulcers with evidence of significant lymphatic morphologic changes in lipodermatosclerotic skin suggestive of both decreased absorption and flow.[41] Fluorescent microlymphography has also shown obliteration of portions of the superficial network, dilatation of the remaining lymphatics, and an increase in their permeability.[42-45] Subfascial lymphatic drainage has been shown to be grossly reduced in post-thrombotic syndrome as measured during lymphoscintigraphy,[46] which has also been used to demonstrate the reduced lymphatic function in the legs of patients with venous ulcers compared to non-ulcerated legs.[47,48] Obliterative processes resulting in permanent vessel loss probably develop through lymphangiothrombosis or lymphangitis in a manner similar to veins as lymph clots like blood, but not as readily. Lastly, the contractility of the lymphangions may also fail with or without valvular incompetence and associated lymph reflux. Further research is needed to validate these theories, but these changes likely contribute to slow healing and the recurrence of skin ulcers. As tissue fibrosis increases in later stages, tissue stiffness may prevent edema formation or edema may not be easily detected. Whether this condition may be more appropriately termed chronic lymphatic insufficiency rather than lymphedema is controversial.[49,50] According to the 2003 consensus document of the International Society of Lymphology, lymphedema has been defined as an external (or internal) manifestation of lymphatic insufficiency and deranged lymph transport[30] thereby technically including lymphatic failure in later stages of venous disease.

Lymphedema pathology is broadly classified under either obstructive or nonobliterative pathology. Obstructive pathology can result from anything that causes perilymphangitis. Nonobliterative pathology can result from endolymphangitis proliferans, primary thoracic duct pathology, lymph node obstruction, congenital defects, or lymphatic thrombosis.

Tumors are the most common form of lymph node obstruction in the United States. Primary thoracic duct disease is either congenital or surgically acquired. Endolymphangitis can be the result of repeated intraluminal injury due to a host of noxious agents causing repeated injury. Lymphangiectasis is atrophy of the lymphatic channel; this is true atrophy and not a developmental problem. Congenital factors, which cause a nonobliterative disorder, result in either agenesis or hypoplasia. One type of congenital nonobliterative disorder is congenital familial lymphedema, or *Milroy disease,* which represents approximately 3% of all cases of lymphedema. Milroy disease has a female predominance with a variable age of onset, although it typically occurs later in life.[51]

PRACTICE POINT

Unilateral manifestation of edema is unique to Milroy disease, although the disease can be bilateral.

Lymphatic thrombosis accounts for another form of nonobliterative disease, for which anticoagulants are ineffective. Recent studies on benzopyrones such as warfarin demonstrated a reduction in lymphedema by stimulating macrophage activity,[52,53] thereby causing increased degradation of protein in lymph fluid with a resulting decrease in edema.

Three classes of lymphedema

Traditional classification divides lymphedema into three categories: congenital, lymphedema precox, and lymphedema tarda. The diagnosis of congenital lymphedema is usually made at or near birth. Lymphedema precox occurs sometime after birth, usually in the peripubital age. However, any lymphedema occurring before age 35 can be grouped under lymphedema precox. Lymphedema tarda merely implies that the age at onset of symptoms is after age 35. Although this classification has been used for many years, a newer classification of lymphedema more accurately describes the disorder. Under this new classification lymphedema is described as primary or secondary.

Primary lymphedema can either be obstructive or hyperplastic. Obstructive pathologies are usually described according to their anatomic location. They're divided into distal obliterative or pelvic obliterative. Primary hyperplastic lymphedema is classified as bilateral hyperplasia or megalymphatics Bilateral hyperplasia is characterized by capillary angiomata on the sides of the feet. An obstructive process is usually present at the level of the cisterna chyli or thoracic duct and the valves can be visualized when examined. Megalymphatics are large valveless lymphatic ducts similar to varicosities. The patient may exhibit little or no leg edema, but chylous reflux is present.

Tumor, surgical intervention, or infection may cause secondary lymphatic obstructions. The infectious group can be bacterial or filarial. The most common cause of lymphatic obstruction outside of the United States is from the filarial infection of *Wuchereria bancrofti.* Toxic exposure may also cause a secondary lymphatic obstruction and is typically grouped under the infectious category.

Differentiating a venous disorder from a lymphatic disorder in a swollen extremity with or without tissue loss is a common dilemma. This is the primary clinical issue for wound care clinicians and guidelines for differential diagnosis can be included here. The reason differentiating a venous disorder from a lymphatic disorder is so important is that the effective treatment for lymphedema is different from the treatment of other edemas. This differentiation should be expanded to enhance clinical decision-making. Many disease processes can mimic lymphedema and they need to be excluded in order to make a diagnosis. Arterial venous malformations, lipedema (an abnormal accumulation of fat in the tissues of the leg), erythrocyanosis frigid (bluish discoloration of extremities secondary to cold exposure), factitious edema, and gigantism can also mimic lymphedema.

Differential diagnosis of edema
General principles
In assessing peripheral edema, the first step is to rule out serious systemic causes, such as heart failure or hepatic insufficiency. Unfortunately, patients commonly present with a number of contributing factors requiring additional investigations to obtain a comprehensive perspective of the underlying causes. For example, in advanced cancer many factors may be present including both venous and lymphatic obstruction, hypoalbuminemia, and limb dependency secondary to immobility. However, the following general principles may initially help guide clinical decision-making. Lower extremity edema that's equal between the right and left legs (symmetrical) is more likely to be systemic, that is, from heart failure or hypoproteinemia. Edema that's greater in one leg than the other (asymmetrical) is more likely to be attributed to local venous or lymphatic disease, such as venous obstruction or chronic venous disease. Edema that affects only one leg (unilateral) is likely to result from disease within the limb or the adjacent quadrant of the trunk. Such contributing factors as prolonged dependency and the use of certain medications should also be considered. Although peripheral edema seldom presents with cancer unless advanced at the time of diagnosis, recurrent cancer may frequently cause peripheral edema. Therefore, cancer should always be considered and investigated appropriately.

Characteristic features of lymphedema
It's important to distinguish lymphedema from other forms of peripheral edema to provide appropriate treatment. (See color photos on page C21.) In most patients, the results of the clinical history and physical examination make this distinction possible. Response to diuretic therapy provides a clear illustration of this point. Diuretics increase excretion of salt and water thereby decreasing plasma volume, venous capillary pressure, and filtration. Thus, diuretics have a significant effect on filtration edema but don't improve lymph drainage over the long term.[20] The response to elevation may also assist in differentiating lymphedema from filtration edema. Because most filtration edemas result from higher venous pressures, they tend to improve by 90% or more with overnight elevation while lymphedema will improve by 10% to 20% or not at all.[21] Therefore, failure to achieve limb volume reduction in response to diuretic therapy or elevation would indicate a lymphatic insufficiency. The time until onset of observable edema may also aid in the diagnosis. A slow onset is more typical of lymphedema than edema due to other causes. The appearance of distinctive skin thickening with fissures and other soft tissue changes (such as hyperkeratosis or papillomatosis) that occur in response to chronic congestion of the lymphatics help to further differentiate lymphedema from filtration edema. Regardless of the common belief that lymphedema doesn't pit, pitting does occur if sustained pressure is applied for a longer period of time to accommodate for the increase in fibrosis and skin thickness. Thickness is particularly apparent at the base of the toes, a sign first noted by Kaposi. Although lacking in specificity, the Kaposi-Stemmer sign consists of an inability to pinch and pick up a fold of skin at the base of the second toe and is predictive of lymphatic insufficiency.[35] Lastly, an increase in swelling of more proximal segments of the affected limb, the contralateral limb and/or the adjacent trunk quadrant in response to

compression (bandaging, garments or pneumatic compression) is an indication of lymphatic insufficiency proximal to the limb segment undergoing compression.

Unfortunately, failure to make this observation along with continuation of inappropriate compression therapy frequently leads to further congestion of the more proximal segment with associated damage to the lymphatic system. This condition is commonly observed in individuals with later stages of venous disease who have effectively decongested the leg, but have developed lymphedema of the thigh, buttock, or genital area. Individuals with this response should be referred to a certified lymphedema therapist as appropriate treatment will require complex decongestive therapy including manual lymph drainage and may require treatment of the trunk and/or contralateral limb. (In the United States, refer to www.lymphnet.org for a list of Lymphology Association of North America certified therapists by state.)

Lymphatic failure in venous disease: Implications for management

Because all edema is caused by either increased capillary filtration overwhelming the safety valve capacity of an intact lymphatic system or by mechanical failure of the lymphatics, improving lymph drainage is a primary therapeutic goal in all forms of peripheral edema. As expected then, there are similarities between the treatment of venous disease and lymphedema. However, failure to recognize lymphatic insufficiency in the later stages of venous disease can lead to improper treatment and further damage to the lymphatics. Management implies prevention as well as treatment and includes the following components: 1) meticulous skin and wound care, 2) interventions to reduce filtration edema, and 3) interventions to increase lymph flow via various forms of compression therapy, exercise, and/or manual lymph drainage.

Skin and wound care

In lymphedema, high protein interstitial content and diminished immune function create an ideal environment for bacterial growth. An increased risk of infection, particularly

cellulitis, has been associated with lymphatic insufficiency. These infections tend to be recurrent and occur without the presence of venous ulcers.[26] Fibrotic skin changes, such as fissures along with hyperkeratosis, papillomatosis, and increased surface debris and scale, enhance opportunities for fungal and bacterial colonization and invasion. Thus, meticulous skin care and increased vigilance are required to prevent infection. Increased edema leads to a higher volume of wound drainage with attendant concerns over skin maceration, frequency of dressing changes, dressing selection for maximum absorption, and appropriate bandaging. These changes may be particularly evident in the toes and forefoot requiring specific compression wrapping of the toes in order to provide a therapeutic gradient in the foot as well as the leg. The altered size and shape of the leg make bandaging techniques more complex and may require different approaches to padding and the use of multiple layers of short-stretch bandages to adequately increase tissue pressure. Bandaging may limit mobility and patients may need assistive devices and training to permit functional ambulation, which is a crucial component of effective treatment. In some cases, additional adjunctive techniques, such as deep breathing and manual lymph drainage, may be needed to enhance healing. The direct effect of edema on wound healing remains unclear. However, the presence of edema in both post-thrombotic syndrome and venous ulcers is indicative of suboptimal treatment and conveys a poorer prognosis.[20] Individuals with pure lymphedema (mechanical failure of the lymphatic system without venous disease) rarely develop ulcers because they do not present with the associated microangiopathy of venous disease. In later stages of venous disease, lymphatic insufficiency is superimposed on the existing venous disease that complicates many aspects of wound care.

Decreasing filtration edema

Leg elevation is frequently recommended in lieu of exercise for those individuals who use wheelchairs as their primary form of mobility. Unfortunately, in order to achieve optimum reduction in venous pressure, and thus filtration edema, individuals must lie completely flat with the legs elevated above the level of the heart. This posture doesn't lend itself to functional activities and elevation is generally only partially effective as most individuals adopt a sitting position with their legs elevated and/or elevate their legs only when resting. Another method of decreasing filtration edema is with diuretics without consideration of the underlying disorder. Diuretics should only be prescribed in cases of sodium and fluid retention associated with heart failure or nephrotic syndrome. As stated previously, diuretics decrease venous volume and ultimately filtration rate, but they don't enhance lymph flow and their long-term use in lymphedema is ineffective and may be harmful.

Ulcer pathophysiology

Venous ulcers

Venous ulcers are chronic skin and subcutaneous lesions usually found on the lower extremity at the pretibial and the medial supra malleolar areas of the ankle, where the perforator veins are located. Venous ulcers were formerly known as "venous stasis" ulcers because their development was thought to be caused by blood pooled in the veins. More recent literature indicates that venous hypertension rather than venous stasis is both the cause of these ulcers and the reason they don't heal.[54] It's difficult to restore skin integrity in the presence of chronic venous hypertension because the underlying edema must be controlled in addition to healing the ulcer.

Venous ulceration may be precipitated by deep vein thrombosis (DVT), which can remain undiagnosed for years prior to the onset of the ulcer. (See *Venogram.*) It has long been thought that the natural course of lower-extremity DVT is the eventual development of leg ulcers.[55]

Symptomatic and asymptomatic thrombi may cause long-term complications by scarring the intima and creating valvular incompetence. When the valves are rendered incompetent, blood backs into the distal veins during diastole. With loss of perforator valve

function, the high intracompartmental venous pressure, which can approach 200 mm Hg during active muscle contraction, results in distention of the saphenous system. This in turn causes a cascading effect with dilation of the greater saphenous vein and worsening of already compromised valvular function. The weight of the column of blood increases the pressure inside the capillaries.

Characteristics of venous ulcers

Venous hypertension distends the superficial veins, resulting in vein wall damage and exudation of fluid into the interstitial space, thereby causing edema of venous insufficiency. Over time, an actual leakage of red cells occurs through these compromised veins. As they break down, the red blood cells deposit hemosiderin into the tissues, causing a form of "internal tattooing" of the skin; the coloration is that of a brownish hue noticeable even in black skin. (See *Hemosiderin deposit,* page 302.) The skin loses its normal texture, becomes somewhat shiny and subsequently sclerotic, giving a taut skin appearance in these areas.

Edema and loss of red cells into the subcutaneous tissue occur at the point of greatest gravitational pressure, the ankle. This gives rise to the pathopneumonic features of chronic venous stasis, hyperpigmentation, and stocking distribution induration of the subcutaneous tissues,[56,57] the characteristics of long-standing venous insufficiency called lipodermatosclerosis. These areas are prone to subsequent ulceration or infection; extreme pruritus and excoriation are usually present, potentially aggravating the injured skin. Dermatitis due to endogenous or exogenous sources and severe allergic reactions may complicate the situation. The skin may present as itchy, erythematous, and weeping, or dry and scaly. (See *Venous ulcer with granulating base,* page 302.) Chemical or mechanical factors may be responsible for contact dermatitis surrounding a leg ulcer.[58]

Another sequelae of venous hypertension is irritability of the musculature. Many patients with venous insufficiency—even those in whom the condition is mild—report nocturnal leg cramps. Depolarization may occur due to fluid distention of the muscular cells, causing tetanic-like contractions of various muscle groups. Distention of veins in the sub-dermal plexus results in the varicosities typi-cally seen with venous insufficiency. (See *Varicose veins*, page 303.) The appearance of telangiectasias, more commonly called "spi-der veins," is the result of distention of the smaller subdermal capillary network. (See *Telangiectasias*, page 303.)

In some circumstances, venous aneurysms can occur due to massive dilation of the greater saphenous vein and its tributaries. Further stagnation of flow in these areas in the presence of an abnormal vessel wall can result in thrombophlebitis, which worsens the venous outflow of the leg and aggravates an already deleterious condition. Thrombosis adheres to the wall of the vein and although recanalization occurs eventually, the valves remain incompetent. In an attempt to com-pensate for the reduced venous return, the surrounding collateral veins dilate. Chronic edema occurs in the ankle. Increased venous pressure impedes capillary flow, decreasing oxygen available for transport from the capil-laries to the tissues, and protein and red blood cells leak into the interstitial tissues. The effect is cumulative, eventually leading to tissue damage, scar formation and, ultimate-ly, ulceration.

Endothelium in the normal saphenous vein facilitates contraction in response to nora-drenaline. In varicose veins, the endothelial-enhanced noradrenaline vasoconstriction is decreased. Endothelial damage is thought to be a possible cause of venous dilatation and subsequent varicose veins.[59]

Venous leg ulcers are also correlated with increased ambulatory venous pressures. Nicolaides[60] obtained ambulatory venous pressures on 220 patients admitted with ve-nous problems. The study found that no pa-tients with ambulatory venous pressures (AVP) less than 30 mm Hg had ulcers while 100% of those with AVP greater than 90 mm Hg had leg ulcers. The incidence of ulcera-tion wasn't preferentially associated with ei-ther superficial or deep venous disease.

Venogram

In this venogram, the patient's left venous valve (B) is intact. On the patient's right (A), collateral veins are present due to ve-nous occlusion, possibly from an undiag-nosed deep vein thrombosis.

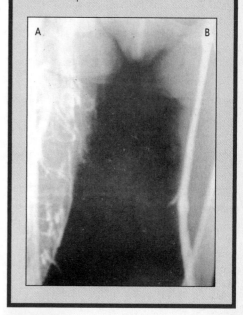

EVIDENCE-BASED PRACTICE

Nicolaides' study[60] suggests that ambulatory ve-nous pressures should be measured in patients with nonhealing venous ulcers to determine whether they may benefit by a procedure such as a venous valve transplant, which reduces the AVP to less than 30 mm Hg.

Pathogenesis of venous ulcers

Several theories have been proposed to ex-plain the mechanism of venous hypertension leading to ulceration. In 1917, Homans sug-gested that stasis of blood in dilated veins in the skin may cause anoxic cell death, leading to ulcers. Blalock[61] found the blood oxygen content to be higher than normal in varicose

Hemosiderin deposit

Hemosiderin deposits caused the discoloration seen here in the patient's right leg.

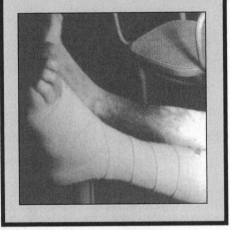

Venous ulcer with granulating base

The venous ulcer shown here has irregular borders and a granulating base with surrounding fibrotic tissue.

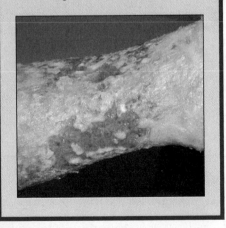

veins, suggesting that arteriovenous communications may be responsible for venous hypertension. In 1972, however, a study using radioactive macro aggregates refuted the arteriovenous shunting hypothesis.[62]

Two current hypotheses—the "fibrin cuff" and "white cell trapping" theories—are more recent attempts to explain venous ulcer formation. The fibrin cuff theory states that sustained venous hypertension causes distention of dermal capillary beds, which allow plasma exudate to leak into the surrounding tissue. Fibrin precipitation in the peripapillary space forms fibrin cuffs, which impair oxygen, nutrient, and growth factor transport. The tissues undergo inflammation and fibrosis.[63] A subsequent study suggests that peripapillary fibrin is present, but doesn't influence healing of lower-extremity ulcers.[64]

The white cell trapping theory states that the neutrophil aggregation in the capillaries causes lipodermatosclerosis. Increasing venous pressure is thought to reduce capillary perfusion pressure and flow rate. Low capillary flow rate initiates white blood cell adherence to the cell wall. Endothelial cells and leukocytes interact and release proteolytic enzymes, oxygen-free radicals, and lipid products. The white cells are then activated, damage the vessel walls, increasing capillary permeability and allowing larger molecules such as fibrinogen to exit the capillaries.[65,66]

The trap hypothesis of venous ulceration was proposed by Falanga and Eaglstein.[67] This hypothesis proposes that fibrin and other macromolecules that leak out bind or trap growth factors and other substances necessary for maintaining normal tissues and healing.

Classifying venous disease

Chronic venous insufficiency has been defined as an abnormally functioning venous system caused by venous valvular incompetence with or without associated venous outflow obstruction, which may affect the superficial venous system, the deep venous system, or both.[68] Chronic venous insufficiency can result in postphlebitic syndrome, which manifests as varicose veins and venous ulcers.

In 1994, the American Venous Forum developed a system based on clinical, etiologic, anatomic, and pathophysiologic (CEAP) data to categorize the key elements in chronic venous disease.[69] The CEAP system provides an objective classification method that clarifies relationships among contributing factors and improves communication regarding venous disease. The system is subdivided into seven categories based on objective signs of chronic venous disease.[70] (See *CEAP classification system*, page 304.)

Diagnosing venous ulcers

Venous disease and ulcer etiology can be determined by obtaining a thorough patient history and performing a physical examination. A focused vascular history includes a clear description of the presenting complaint, past medical history for vascular and related conditions, current and previously taken medications, and risk factors. Signs and symptoms of lower extremity venous disease may include pain, tissue loss, or change in appearance or sensation. It's important to include assessment of the arterial system when evaluating venous and lymphatic disease. Adequate arterial perfusion is essential when using compression therapy for venous and lymphatic ulcers. Noninvasive vascular laboratory testing is used to identify the location of vascular pathology.

Physical examination

Physical examination is important in providing direction for intervention, starting with skin inspection. Skin changes representing venous disease include hyperpigmentation, dermatitis, lipodermatosclerosis, or atrophie blanche, which is a characteristic white patchy scarring at the site of previous ulcers. Because skin color may indicate venous congestion, the color of each toe should be noted and compared to the other foot and toes. In venous insufficiency the skin appears a dusky ruddy color.

Skin should be palpated for temperature changes. The skin over varicose veins is often warmer than the surrounding skin. In chronic venous insufficiency, the skin may become atrophied with scarring from a previous ulcer, or it may have weeping blisters or dry scaly crusts.

Varicose veins

Note the presence of varicose veins in the patient's lower extremities, shown here.

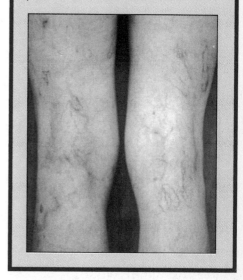

Telangiectasias

Telangiectasias, also known as "spider veins," are shown in the photograph below.

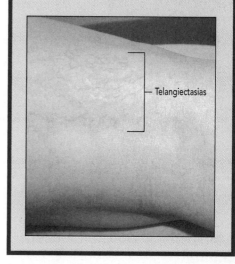

Telangiectasias

CEAP classification system

The CEAP classification system for chronic venous disease consists of four elements:
- **c**linical classification
- **e**tiologic classification
- **a**natomic classification
- **p**athophysiology.

Clinical classification (C0-6)

Class	Description
0	No signs of venous disease
1	Telangiectases or reticular veins
2	Varicose veins
3	Edema
4	Skin changes
5	Healed ulcer
6	Active ulcer

Etiologic classification (E_C, E_P, E_S)
- Congenital (E_C)
- Primary (E_P) — with undetermined cause
- Secondary (E_S) — with known cause

Anatomic distribution classification (A_S, A_D, and A_P)
This element consists of classifications A_S, A_D, and A_P, and segments 1 through 18. See table below for a breakdown.
- Superficial veins (A_S)
- Deep veins (A_D)
- Perforating veins (A_P)

Segment	Classification
1	Superficial veins (A_S) Telangiectases/reticular veins Greater (long) saphenous
2	• Above knee
3	• Below knee
4	• Lesser (short) saphenous
5	• Non-saphenous Deep veins (A_D)
6	Inferior vena cava Iliac
7	• Common
8	• Internal
9	• External
10	Pelvic-gonadal, broad ligament, other Femoral
11	• Common
12	• Deep
13	• Superficial
14	• Popliteal
15	Crural: Anterior tibial, posterior tibial, peroneal (all paired)
16	Muscular: Gastrocnemial, soleal, other Perforating veins (A_P)
17	Thigh
18	Calf

Pathophysiologic classification (P_R, P_O)
- Reflux (P_R)
- Obstruction (P_O)
- Reflux and obstruction (P_R, P_O)

Adapted with permission from Kistner, R.L., and Eklof, B. "Clinical Presentation and Classification of Chronic Venous Disease," in Gloviczki, P., and Bergan, J.J., eds., *Atlas of Endoscopic Perforator Vein Surgery.* New York: Springer-Verlag, 1998.

Patients presenting with foot or leg ulcers should be tested for neuropathy, which is a common finding in the patient with diabetes. Assessment for neuropathy is described in chapter 16, Diabetic foot ulcers.

Edema is commonly found in lower extremity venous disease. Early edema may be observed as a difference in calf circumference between legs and should be confirmed by measurement. After edema has been longstanding, tissue fibrosis occurs making the skin and subcutaneous tissues less resilient to palpation.

Venous signs and symptoms

Patients may report a gradual onset of discomfort associated with venous disease; however, often no symptoms are present initially. Most patients describe general nondescript aching rather than specific pain. Some terms used to describe sensations in the legs include: fullness, swelling, tightness, aching, or heaviness. These symptoms can be reduced with elevation. Venous insufficiency accompanied by acute DVT may be described as sharp, severe, deep, aching pain.[51] Varicose veins occasionally produce a pulling, prickling, or tingling discomfort localized to the area of the varicose vein.[7] In severe cases of venous insufficiency, a form of claudication can occur. The patient may complain of foot edema that makes it difficult to wear shoes.

A venous ulcer is moist and may have a yellow fibrous film covering its surface. This fibrous tissue isn't a sign of infection and doesn't interfere with healing.[52] The ulcer edges are irregular with firm fibrotic and indurated surrounding skin. The surrounding tissue may have brownish rust color, due to the breakdown of the erythrocytes and deposition of hemosiderin. Scar tissue may indicate the site of a previous ulcer. Because of the subcutaneous scarring, there is no allowance for the tissue expansion that occurs with edema in skin of normal elasticity. Scar tissue also prevents blood vessels from transporting oxygen to the skin, further compromising healing.[28]

Vascular testing

Although an experienced vascular clinician can make a vascular diagnosis on history and physical examination, vascular laboratory studies contribute to the accuracy of the diagnosis. The presence, location, and severity of arterial and venous disease are confirmed by vascular laboratory procedures. Information obtained by vascular studies can predict ulcer healing when the cause is arterial insufficiency.[7] Laboratory tests differentiate among conditions contributing to a nonhealing ulcer.

Noninvasive vascular testing is divided into direct tests that image the vessel itself and indirect tests that demonstrate changes distal to the diseased vessel. These tests include Doppler ultrasound, venous duplex ultrasound, ankle-brachial index (ABI), transcutaneous pressure of oxygen ($TCPO_2$), segmental systolic pressures, and plethysmography.

Doppler ultrasound

In a Doppler ultrasound, a transmitting probe sends a signal, which is reflected from an object to the receiving probe. If the signal strikes a moving object such as blood cells, a frequency shift is detected and reflected as sound. The audible signals of venous and arterial flow patterns can be distinguished.

Duplex ultrasound

The venous duplex allows one to evaluate various segments of the venous tree looking for more than 0.5 seconds reflux after either a muscle contraction or manual augmentation of cephalad flow. Another advantage of venous duplex imaging is that it can identify sites of thrombosis with high levels of accuracy. The disadvantage is that it's fairly time-consuming, taking 1 to 2 hours per evaluation for a full leg imaging.

Venous testing

It's possible to perform a crude venous assessment by physical examination using a Doppler ultrasound. By compressing the limb manually, the flow in the veins can be augmented and noted by the audible Doppler signal heard distal to the site of compression. This is a subjective test and reliability is clinician dependent. The introduction of noninvasive vascular testing has provided much anatomic and physiologic information to increase the accuracy of diagnosing venous diseases. Two tests are most commonly used to assess the severity of venous insufficiency. One is the venous photoplethysmography

(PPG) and the other is venous duplex imaging.[53]

Plethysmography

Plethysmography records volume changes in the limb. Several types of plethysmography are available:

- air plethysmography, which uses a pneumatic cuff as a segmental volume sensor
- strain-gauge, which uses a fine bore silicone rubber tube filled with mercury wrapped around the limb to be studied
- impedance plethysmography, which measures the relative change in resistive impedance of the passage of an electrical current through a segment of the body
- PPG, which measures the degree of light attenuation, which is proportional to the quantity of blood present and not actual volume change.[7,71]

Air and PPG are the more common tests for chronic venous disease. A photoplethysmograph consists of infrared light emitting diode and a photo sensor mounted on a probe. The probe is applied to the skin over the area to be tested.[7] The advantage of venous PPG is that it's quick and gives assessment of overall venous refill time. On the other hand, it only evaluates the most dependent portion of the leg in the gator area.

Treating venous ulcers

Treatment goals for all ulcers include:
- providing an environment conducive to new tissue growth
- protecting the wound
- preventing further tissue destruction.

Topical and systemic treatments are addressed simultaneously. It's imperative to consider etiology when deciding treatment because ulcers aren't all alike and treatment for one type may be inappropriate or harmful to another. A vascular specialist consultation is appropriate for ulcers of mixed etiology.

Wound infection

Infected leg ulcers, soft-tissue cellulitis, and osteomyelitis are treated by administering systemic I.V. or oral antibiotics. Topical antibiotics are not indicated for all leg ulcers.[72] Chronic wounds are colonized with normal skin flora and shouldn't be treated with antibiotics. Rigorous and frequent ulcer cleaning assists in removing surface bacteria. Newer silver impregnated dressings have been effective in managing bacteria and promoting healing by keeping the wound surface clean.[73]

Biopsy for a quantitative culture of the inflamed tissue surrounding nonhealing ulcers should be considered if true infection isn't responding to antibiotics. If carcinoma is suspected biopsy of the lesion should be obtained. (See chapter 7, Wound bioburden.)

PRACTICE POINT

Because bone scans are expensive and may give false-positives in the presence of inflammation, their use is indicated when only bone infection, abscess, or fluid collection are suspected.

Skin and wound care

A clean wound, free from dead tissue and wound debris, is necessary for healing to occur. Wound cleaning and debridement are the initial steps in wound care. Many commercial wound cleaners and disinfectants are cytotoxic. Povidone-iodine, hydrogen peroxide, and 0.25% acetic acid have shown evidence of interfering with fibroblast formation and epithelial growth.[74-77] There may be indications for using cidal agents in a wound; however, their use should be time-limited and each caregiver should have a clear understanding of what the goals are and n the goals have been reached.

EVIDENCE-BASED PRACTICE

The advantage of cleaning the wound should be weighed against damaging new tissue growth.[78]

The safest wound cleaner is 0.9% saline solution. Wounds should be cleaned with a force strong enough to dislodge debris but gentle enough to prevent damage to newly growing tissue. The pressure to accomplish this goal ranges from 4 to 15 psi.[79] A 19G needle or 19G angiocatheter distributes approximately 8 psi when used with a 35-cc syringe. A Baxter© cap (shown below) on a saline irrigation bottle is a less expensive

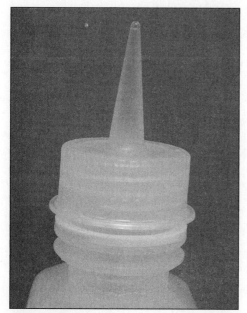

Photo © M.J. Geyer.

method to distribute an adequate amount of pressure. Leg ulcers treated in the home are commonly irrigated with running tap water.

Hydrotherapy or whirlpool has been used to aid in cleaning and debridement of both arterial and venous leg ulcers.[80] A clinical pilot study found that whirlpool followed by vigorous rinsing reduced the bacterial load in venous ulcers more than the whirlpool alone.[81] This may suggest that the vigorous irrigation is the significant factor in cleaning the wound. (See chapter 8, Wound debridement, for more information on wound cleaning.)

Dressings chosen for specific wounds depend on the wound bed condition and the goal for the wound. Many new dressings are designed to support moist wound healing (see chapter 9, Wound treatment options.) Because the skin is fragile in patients with either arterial or venous disease and can be

easily injured, tape and adhesive products should be used with extreme caution. Use other methods of securing dressings that won't injure the skin.

PRACTICE POINT

The preferred attachment device for dressings on vascular leg ulcers is roller gauze, or commercial devices (such as netting or tube gauze) that hold dressings in place without adhesive, which can damage the fragile skin.

Venous ulcers

Venous hypertension and wound care are treated together. Wound care and edema management depend on whether or not the patient can be immobilized. Edema is controlled by conservative means, intermittent elevation, compression bandages, and intermittent pneumatic compression.[82] Studies have demonstrated that moist wound healing combined with compression improves wound-healing rate of venous ulcers.[83] Compression therapy is the mainstay of venous ulcer therapy.[84] Elevating the legs above the heart is recommended whenever the patient can be placed in this position. A compression dressing isn't required when the patient is immobilized with the leg elevated, such as during sleeping hours. Moist gauze dressings with frequent changes can be used instead.

The ambulatory venous patient is best served by semirigid dressings such as the Unna boot, or by multilayered compression wraps. Multilayered compression is more effective than single layer; both 4-layer and short-stretch bandages have higher healing rates than paste plus an outer support. With the discovery of moist wound healing[85] and the advent of hydrocolloid and foam dressings, occlusive dressings may be used under compression wraps to promote growth of granulation tissue, reduce pain from the dressing rubbing against the ulcer, and promote autolytic debridement. One study found ulcers healed twice as fast with the foam dressing under the Unna boot as those ulcers

Compression wrapping

This photograph shows a leg being wrapped with a 4-layer compression therapy dressing.

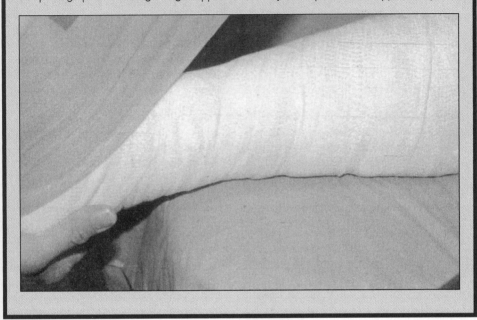

without the foam.[86] (See *Compression wrapping*.)

Compression wraps should be applied starting just below the toes and ending just below the popliteal fossa. A gauze roll or padded gauze dressing is typically used over the wound area. The dressing is covered with an elastic bandage. Stockings reduce ambulatory venous pressure by decreasing venous reflux and improving calf muscle ejection capacity during use.[87] Stockings are graded according to the amount of pressure they exert, from 20 to 60 mm Hg at the ankle. The benefit derived from the stocking is in direct proportion to the fit.

In many cases, patients fail to wear the prescribed compression dressing or stocking because of difficulty donning the stockings or complaints of tightness. The importance of long-term external compression can't be overemphasized. Patients should be taught that the stockings must be replaced every 3 to 6 months. Two pairs should be purchased so that one can be worn while the other is laundered.

PRACTICE POINT

Long-term compression therapy is an essential part of the treatment of venous leg ulcers.

A pneumatic compression pump may be used to reduce lower extremity edema.[91] One study found improved venous ulcer healing when compression pumps were used; however, not all third-party payers agree with the use of these pumps as a treatment method.[88-90] Another study[92] found 4 hours of compression per day improved ulcer healing when used with compression stockings. In yet another study,[93] an intermittent pneumatic compression device provided improved healing when used for 1 hour twice weekly in conjunction with conventional dressings.

Exercise

A graded exercise program may be used to improve the calf muscle pump in those patients with venous diseases associated with abnormalities in pump function. One author[93] determined that a structured exercise program to improve muscle function may have a significant positive outcome in venous disease.[94]

Effective interventions to increase lymph flow include exercise, compression therapy, and manual lymph drainage. Movement of the legs (active and passive) is crucial to increasing the filling of lymphatic capillaries and to augmenting flow in lymphatic collectors that have lost their contractility. Walking also has the beneficial effect of reducing venous pressure via activation of the foot and calf muscle pumps. Increases in the depth of breathing during exercise also aid in proximal venous return and lymphatic flow. Deep breathing can be used alone or with manual resistance and patients with limited mobility can be taught to incorporate deep breathing with lower extremity exercises while in a supine position or sitting in a chair (for example, simple calf pump activation while resting in a supine position, or rocking in a chair).

The addition of short-stretch bandages or an equivalent form of compression will enhance the effect of exercise on lymph flow and reduce venous capillary pressure and filtration. In individuals with heart failure, care must be taken to avoid pulmonary edema as a consequence of a rapid shift in fluid from the interstitium to the circulation.

Appropriate screening for compromised arterial supply and cutaneous sensation must always be completed before application of compression therapy of any kind. As stated previously, care must be taken to observe the response of more proximal segments of the affected limb, the contralateral limb and/or the adjacent trunk quadrant for displacement of edema in response to compression of any kind. Continued compression serves only to displace the fluid to a more proximal segment of the limb unless the fluid is rerouted to an adjacent territory where the routes for drainage remain intact. After these new routes have been established, self-applied manual lymph drainage, deep breathing, exercise, and compression will maintain them. While in theory, pneumatic compression pumps would appear to offer benefits to individuals spending considerable time in a chair, there's currently no evidence that such pumps improve lymph flow and they may simply displace fluid.[30,95-96] Effective removal of edema from the leg reverses much of the associated comorbidity, in particular the skin changes. The achieved limb reduction must be maintained through the use of appropriately fitted compression hosiery or an alternative compression product. The application and removal of such hosiery can be problematic in those with limited hand function or who are unable to see or reach their toes (such as in obese, blind, and arthritic patients). However, application aids are available and instruction in this technique does help. Other strap-type leggings and boot-like devices[75] are available to decrease the functional burden and therapists can be very creative in combining or layering different compressive products to achieve adequate levels of compression. Compliance is crucial to prevent recurrence of edema.

Manual lymph drainage

Manual lymph drainage (MLD) refers to a specific manual technique used by trained therapists to increase lymph flow and to move excess tissue fluid from a congested territory across watersheds via lymphatic capillaries (anastomoses) into adjacent areas where alternate routes for drainage remain intact. Communication is only possible between lymphatic capillaries in the superficial network. Manual lymph drainage is one component of the definitive treatment for lymphedema known as Complex (or Complete) Decongestive Therapy (CDT), which is basically comprised of patient instruction in meticulous skin care, MLD, compression therapy (multi-layer bandaging followed by compression hosiery), and exercise.[30] As in many areas of clinical practice, CDT is supported by extensive experience and has a sound physiologic basis, but research sup-

Complex decongestive therapy

Results of 2 weeks of complex decongestive therapy in a patient with lymphedema of more than 10 years' duration

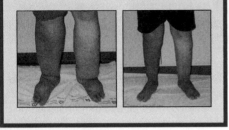

porting its efficacy is somewhat limited.[96,98] (See *Complex decongestive therapy*.)

Surgical treatment for venous ulcers

Surgical treatment for venous ulcers is aimed at correcting the cause of the venous hypertension. Some of these procedures include vein valve transplantation, direct valve repair, and veno-venous bypass. Varicose veins may be treated by excision, ligation, or injection, depending upon the size of the vein.

Surgical treatment for venous insufficiency is still in its infancy compared to the established treatment of arterial occlusive disease. Venous insufficiency can be grouped under two broad categories:

- venous reflux
- venous outflow obstruction.

The net result of both of these disease entities is venous hypertension and the sequelae resulting in venous ulcerations. The mainstay for the treatment of venous insufficiency continues to be good external compression. In many patients, this is all that is required. It acts both as a treatment for various states of venous insufficiency as well as a prophylaxis for the development of the adverse sequelae. In some patients, the use of compression alone is inadequate; for these patients, surgical intervention is usually necessary.

Venous outflow obstruction is usually the result of deep vein thromboses. When it involves isolated segments with normal segments either above or below, the obstruction can result in a cascading event resulting in venous insufficiency. In some patients, the outflow obstruction is the cause of the symptoms. In these patients, bypassing the obstructed segment to relieve the venous outflow obstruction and the corresponding venous hypertension by balloon angioplasty of a sclerotic or stenotic segment with or without stent placement may be necessary.

Other patients require bypass using an autogenous venous conduit. The proximal and distal anastomoses of the venous bypass are dictated by the obstruction site. For example, if a patient has an isolated ilio-femoral thrombosis that has failed to recannulize or has only partially recannulized and the affected leg is symptomatic, a femoral-femoral bypass from the proximal portion of the symptomatic leg to the more distal portion of the contralateral leg can be performed. The saphenous vein is usually used for this but in contrast to arterial bypasses the direction of the valve isn't reversed; rather the valve leaflets are oriented to prevent reflux. Similarly, a bypass from a more proximal vein within a symptomatic leg to the more cephalad iliac vein may be indicated.

In patients with an outflow obstruction, but in whom insufficiency or hypertension is caused by occlusion of the greater saphenous vein, the venous hypertension may be alleviated by isolated partial saphenous vein ligation and stripping. This is usually done at the knee level with stripping of the affected saphenous segment. If, however, the reflux or hypertension is the result of the deep venous system, then stripping the greater saphenous vein wouldn't help and actually may be detrimental due to elimination of one of the venous outflow tracts of the extremity. This information must be known before a surgical procedure is performed to correct venous insufficiency. Three tests are available to evaluate reflux:

- ascending/descending venography
- duplex imaging
- venous PPG.

These tests are all readily available through either a vascular laboratory or a radiology department. Venous PPG can determine whether the deep or superficial system is involved with venous reflux. A better test uses venous duplex, which looks at specific segments of both superficial and deep veins for reflux and can give a more detailed evaluation of the affected extremity. Isolated valve segments of the more proximal venous system can be evaluated using descending venography looking for contrast reflux past the incompetent valve. Venography can also determine sites of stenoses within the venous system as can venous duplex. One of the problems associated with accurate duplex imaging is that it's dependent upon the competence of the technician performing the test. Certain laboratories have more expertise in these areas than do others.

When deep venous insufficiency is due to valvular incompetence, it isn't known how many competent valves are required and in what locations for the deep venous system to become competent again. Research in these areas is ongoing and more attention is now being given to venous insufficiency.

Three techniques are available for surgical correction of venous insufficiency due to valvular incompetence:
• artificial venous valve insertion
• autogenous vein valve transplantation using a segment of vein, usually from the upper extremities or axilla
• direct valvuloplasty.

Autogenous valve transplantation is a procedure in which a segment of vein with a competent valve, usually in the upper extremity or axilla, is identified. This section of vein is rejected and an interposition graft placed at the harvest site. The vein is then transposed into the venous system of the affected extremity maintaining the orientation of the valve to keep the leaflets open in a cephalic direction. Postoperative anticoagulation with heparin and subsequent warfarin is commonly used.

Approximately 75% of the stasis ulcers remain healed at 12-month follow-up after valve transplantation. However, considerable degradation occurs over the course of the second year in these patients, such that only 40% of limbs remain healed.[96] After the second year, results appear to stabilize without further deterioration although the reports on this are limited in both scope and number.

Variations of this procedure using valve segments from other areas or even transposing a deep vein with a competent valve to another deep vein with an incompetent valve can be done. Overall results appeared to be similar to that of transposition of competent vein valve segments.[96]

Direct valvuloplasty is another technique for correcting valvular insufficiency. This is performed by suture approximation of two valve leaflets that don't fully close. It's done either with direct suturing within the areas of the cusps to obtain good apposition, or by external buttressing of an incompetent vein valve sinus. Valve leaflets themselves are brought into apposition by placing the equivalent of a "girdle" around the dilated valve to reduce dilatation and allow the valves to come in apposition in a more normal fashion. This sleeve technique is usually done with prosthetic material. Similarly a transplanted valve that may deteriorate due to dilatation can be made competent again by using this technique.[99]

An external valve repair known as the *Psathakis silastic sling procedure* has been developed.[100] This procedure involves placing a silastic sling around the popliteal vein then attaching it to the two heads of the biceps femoris muscle. When these muscles contract, the sling is intended to occlude the popliteal vein during ambulation. The problem with this procedure is that the sling becomes intimately adherent to the vein and surrounding tissue and over time no longer functions in this fashion.

In patients where no suitable vein valve segment can be found or it's deemed an inadequate operation, the development of a prosthetic valve with its implantation holds some promise. Currently, a prosthetic venous valve comprised of a complex titanium double leaflet system is being developed and may hold promise.

The appropriate use of adequate compression is necessary in conjunction with all the surgical treatments. The application and management of patients with compression hose is dealt elsewhere within this chapter.

Patients with recurrent leg ulcers due to incompetent perforators in the affected area were thought to benefit from a Linton flap. This procedure requires elevation of the skin and fascia at the site of ulceration and a transection with ligation of the incompetent perforator veins feeding the area. Proper application of compression is required afterward to reduce the local venous hypertension. The morbidity associated with this procedure includes tissue slough along the area of incision and the overlying tissue resulting in a prolonged healing period. This was thought to be due to the chronic disease state of the tissue at the ankle. A subfascial ligation of incompetent perforator veins with an endoscope was thought to be an advancement in technique. Using equipment developed for laparoscopic cholecystectomies, the scope is passed from healthy leg tissue into the subfascial space. The fascia is raised, perforator veins are ligated, and then transected through the endoscope. The reason for ligating incompetent perforators is to eliminate the venous hypertension associated with the reflux of venous blood.[101] Long-term follow up for this procedure demonstrates less than satisfactory results. More recently there has been some interest in duplex ultrasound guided foam sclerotherapy that scleroses the perforator veins to achieve the same effect.[102] While this treatment is used extensively in Europe, it's not yet approved in the United States.[103] Further studies are needed to establish the overall effectiveness of this procedure for wound healing.

In some patients, the application of a split-thickness skin graft to an otherwise healthy stasis ulcer may be appropriate. This technique shouldn't be used in patients whose underlying venous problems haven't been addressed. The application of a split-thickness skin graft to an ulcer with persistent venous hypertension will fail, even if the patient is compliant with the use of a compression hose.

PRACTICE POINT

Skin grafting of ulcers should only be done after the underlying venous hypertension is corrected.

Measuring ulcer healing

Calculating healing rates is problematic when no standard measurement for wound healing parameters exists. Following wounds to complete healing is one method, but not satisfactory if changes in therapy are needed. Healing rates can be expressed as percent of ulcer area, measurement of change in ulcer perimeter, or percent of ulcer area healed. However, the perimeter and surface area is much greater in large ulcers. Using these measurements will give erroneously high healing rates for the larger ulcers compared to smaller ulcers. When percent of ulcer healed is used as a measurement, smaller ulcers will appear to heal faster than larger ulcers by comparison.

In another method, ulcers are traced on a celluloid screen, then measured. The area and circumference of the tracing are calculated by a computer program.

Patient education

The patient may inadvertently neglect the ulcer or fail to use prevention measures without understanding the nature of the condition. Be sure to teach your patient ulcer pathology and treatment rationales, and to recognize and report changes that indicate problems with healing. Patient and family education should also include assessment of educational needs and level of understanding. Teaching methods vary and should be chosen to facilitate the most appropriate method for the patient and family.

Summary

Chronic venous insufficiency is a permanent condition. Because of this permanency, patients are given information about the disease process and rationale for intervention. The more information they have, the more likely they are to manage their condition effectively.

Activities that promote venous return are encouraged. Extremity elevation should become a daily routine and external compression is needed for life. Patients must understand the importance of this fact. Protection from trauma to the skin is also essential. A small lesion may progress quickly to a large ulcer due to the edema. It may take years to heal, if at all. In addition, small cuts or bruises should have immediate medical attention. Leg exercises to increase muscle pump activity are taught to the patient. Patients are encouraged to use these exercises during long periods of standing or sitting. When sitting, the legs should be elevated.

Success in managing venous ulcers requires a total patient commitment. Risk factors and ulcer management are dependent upon the patient's activities therefore the patient must have as much information as possible to participate in therapy. An understanding of venous pathophysiology and its contribution to leg ulcers is critical in the management of the ulcers. Venous reconstruction is in its infancy but shows promise to reduce the sequela of postphlebitic syndrome. Venous ulcers always require external compression, ultimately in the form of compression stockings. Ulcers associated with lymphedema usually respond when the edema is reduced. A variety of wound care products are available for leg ulcers, but no research exists showing one product to be more effective than another. Economic concerns make it imperative to choose the appropriate dressings and treatment, but research demonstrates little increased benefit of the newer treatments over the old.

Show what you know

1. *The cause of venous ulcers is:*

   A. venous stasis.
   B. venous hypertension.
   C. embolic phenomenon.
   D. varicose veins.

ANSWER: B. Venous stasis was thought to cause venous ulcers because of pooled blood in the veins. However, current literature reports venous hypertension is responsible for increased pressure along the vein wall and in the subcutaneous tissue.

2. *CEAP is a classification system for venous disease. A patient with C-6, E_S, A_D, A_P, P_R classification would have:*

   A. an active ulcer with a known cause, and reflux disease in the deep and perforating veins.
   B. varicose veins of congenital etiology in the superficial veins, with reflux.
   C. skin changes with undetermined cause, disease in the deep veins with obstruction.
   D. a healed ulcer with known cause and deep venous involvement and reflux and obstruction.

ANSWER: A. The CEAP classification stands for clinical, etiologic, anatomic, and pathophysiologic components to the system. C-6 refers to an active ulcer. E_S means etiology is secondary with a known cause. A_D and A_P refer to anatomic distribution of the deep and perforator veins. And P_R means that reflux is the pathophysiology behind the disease.

3. *The most important treatment component for venous ulcers is:*

   A. moist wound healing.
   B. antibiotics.
   C. compression.
   D. revascularization.

ANSWER: C. Compression is the most important component—the edema must be managed in order for venous and lymphatic ulcers to heal.

4. *The most detrimental activity a patient with any vascular disease can do is:*

   A. walk into the pain.
   B. sleep with legs dependent.
   C. use nicotine.
   D. fail to monitor pulses.

ANSWER: C. Nicotine shouldn't be used in any form. It constricts vessels and contributes to atherosclerosis and venous disease.

References

1. Young, J.R. "Differential Diagnosis of Leg Ulcers," *Cardiovascular Clinics* 13(2):171-93, 1983.
2. Cornwall, J.V., et al. "Leg Ulcers: Epidemiology and Aetiology," *British Journal of Surgery* 73(9):693, September 1986.
3. Coon, W.W., et al. "Venous Thromboembolism and Other Venous Disease in the Tecumseh Community Health Study," *Circulation* 48(4): 839-46, October 1973.
4. Dewolfe, V.G. "The Prevention and Management of Chronic Venous Insufficiency," *Practical Cardiology* 6:197-202, 1980.
5. Callam, M.J., et al. "Chronic Ulcers of the Leg: Clinical History," *British Medical Journal* (Clinical Research Edition) 294(6584):1389-91, May 30, 1987.
6. Nelzen, O., et al. "The Prevalence of Chronic Lower-limb Ulceration has been Underestimated: Results of a Validated Population Questionnaire," *British Journal of Surgery* 83(2):255-58, February 1996.

7. Rutherford, R.B. "The Vascular Consultation" in *Vascular Surgery*, Vol. 1, 4th ed. Philadelphia: W.B. Saunders Co., 1995.

8. Moore, W.S. (ed). *Vascular Surgery: A Comprehensive Review*, Philadelphia: W.B. Saunders Co., 1991.

9. Browse, N.L., et al. Diseases of the Veins: Pathology, Diagnosis, and Treatment. London: Edward Arnold, 1988.

10. Phillips, T.J., and Dover, J.S. "Leg Ulcers," *Journal of the American Academy of Dermatology* 25(6 Pt 1):965-89, December 1991.

11. Logan, V. "Incidence and Prevalence of Lymphoedema: A Literature Review," *J Clin Nurs* 4:213-219, 1995.

12. Williams, A., Franks, P., Moffat, C. "Lymphoedema: Estimating the Size of the Problem," *Palliative Medicine* 19:300-313, 2005.

13. Bundy, M., Grenfell, B. "Reassessing the Global Prevalence and Distribution of Lymphatic Filariasis," *Parasitology* 112(Pt 4):409-428, April 1996.

14. Armer, J. "The Problem of Post-Breast Cancer Lymphedema: Impact and Measurement Issues," *Cancer Investigation* 23(1):76-83, 2005.

15. Petrek, J., Senie, R., Peters, M., Rosen, P. "Lymphedema in a Cohort of Breast Carcinoma Survivors 20 Years after Diagnosis," *Cancer* 92(6):1368-1377, September 2001.

16. Geller, B., Vacek, P., O'Brien, P., Secker-Walker, R. "Factors Associated with Arm Swelling After Breast Cancer Surgery," *J Women's Health* 12:921-930, 2003.

17. Okeke, A., Bates, D., Gillatt, D. "Lymphoedema in Urological Cancer," *European Urology* 45(1):18-25, January 2004.

18. Shaw, J., Rumball, E. "Complications and Local Recurrence Following Lymphadenectomy," *Br J Surg* 77:760-764, 1990.

19. James, J. "Lymphedema Following Ilio-Inguinal Lymph Node Dissection," *Scand J Plast Reconst Surg* 16:167-171, 1982.

20. Mortimer, P. "Implications of the Lymphatic System in CVI-Associated Edema," *Angiology, The Journal of Vascular Diseases* 51(1):3-7, January 2000.

21. Mortimer, P., Levick, R. "Chronic Peripheral Oedema: The Critical Role of the Lymphatic System," *Clinical Medicine* 2004;4(5):448-453, September/October 2004.

22. Duran, W., Pappas, P., Schmid-Schonbein, G. "Microcirculatory Inflammation in Chronic Venous Insufficiency: Current Status and Future Directions," *Microcirculation* 7(6 [Pt 2]):S49-58, 2000.

23. Tiwari, A., Cheng, K., Button, M., Myint, F., Hamilton, G. "Differential Diagnosis, Investigation, and Current Treatment of Lower Limb Lymphedema," *Archives of Surgery* 138(2):152-161, February 2003.

24. Olszewski, W., Pazdur, J., Kubasiewicz, E., Zaleska, M., Cooke, C., Miller, N. "Lymph Draining From Foot Joints in Rheumatoid Arthritis Provides Insight Into Local Cytokine and Chemokine Production and Transport to Lymph Nodes," *Arthritis and Rheumatism* 44(3):541-549, March 2001.

25. Topham, E., Mortimer, P. "Chronic Lower Limb Oedema," *Clinical Medicine* 2(1):28-31, January/February 2002.

26. Moffat, C., Franks, P., Doherty, D., Williams, A., Badger, C. "Lymphoedema: An Underestimated Health Problem," *Q J Med* 96:731-738, 2003.

27. Petlund, C. "Prevalence and Incidence of Chronic Lymphoedema in a Western European Country: Elsevier Science, 1990.

28. Lane, K., Worsley, D., McKenzie, D. "Exercise and the Lymphatic System: Implications for Breast-Cancer Survivors," *Sports Medicine* Volume 35(6):461-471, 2005.

29. Guyton, A., Hall, T. *Textbook of Medical Physiology*: W.B. Saunders; 1999.

30. International Society of Lymphoedema. "The Diagnosis and Treatment of Peripheral Lymphoedema. Consensus Document of the International Society of Lymphology Executive Committee," *Lymphology* 36:84-91, 2003.

31. Kaipainen, A., Korhonen, J., Mustonen, T., et al. "Expression of the FMS-like Tyrosine Kinase 4 Gene Becomes Restricted to Lymphatic Endothelium During Development," *Proc Natl Acad Sci USA* 92(8):3566-3570, April 1995.

32. Saharinen, P., Tammela, T., Karkkainen, M., Alitalo, K. "Lymphatic Vasculature: Development, Molecular Regulation and Role in Tumor Metastasis and Inflammation," *Trends in Immunology* 25(7):387-395, July 2004.

33. Schmid-Schonbein, G. "Microlymphatics and Lymph Flow," *Physiological Reviews* 70(4):987-1028, October 1990.

34. Schmid-Schonbein, G. "Mechanisms Causing Initial Lymphatics to Expand and Compress to Promote Lymph Flow," *Archives of Histology & Cytology* 53(Suppl):107-114, 1990.

35. *Textbook of Lymphology: for Physicians and Lymphedema Therapists*. 5th ed. Munich: Urban & Fischer Verlag; 2003.

36. Foldi, E., Foldi, M., Clodius, L. "The Lymphedema Chaos: A Lancet," *Annals of Plastic Surgery* 22(6):505-515, 1989.

37. Threefoot, S. "The Clinical Significance of Lymphaticovenous Communications," *Ann Intern Med* 72(6):957-958, 1970.

38. Adamson R. *J Physiol* 557:889-907, 2004. 39. Levick, J. "Revision of the Starling Principle: New Views of Tissue Fluid Balance," *J Physiol* 557(3):704, 2004.

39. Levick, J. "Revision of the Starling Principle: New Views of Tissue Fluid Balance," *J Physiol* 557(3):704, 2004.

40. Macdonald, J. "Wound Healing and Lymphedema: A New Look At An Old Problem," *Ostomy Wound Management* 47(4):52-57, 2001.

41. Eliska, O., Eliskova, M. "Morphology of Lymphatics in Human Venous Crural Ulcers with Lipodermatosclerosis," *Lymphology* 34:111-123, 2001.

42. Bollinger, A., Isenring, G., Franzeck, U. "Lymphatic Microangiopathy: A Complication of Severe Chronic Venous Incompetence," *Lymphology* 15:60-65, 1982.

43. Bollinger, A., Leu, A., Hoffmann, U., Franzeck, U. "Microvascular Changes in Venous Disease: An Update," *Angiology* 48(No. 1):27-31, 1997.

44. Leu, A., Leu, H-J., Franzeck, U., Bollinger, A. "Microvascular Changes in Chronic Venous Insufficiency — A Review," *Cardiovascular Surgery* 3(3):237-245, 1995.

45. Junger, M., Steins, A., Hahn, M., Hafner, H.M. "Microcirculatory dysfunction in chronic venous insufficiency (CVI)," *Microcirculation* 7(6 Pt 2):S3-12, 2000.

46. Franzeck, U., Haselbach, P., Speiser, D., Bollinger, A. "Microangiopathy of Cutaneous Blood and Lymphatic Capillaries in Chronic Venous

Insufficiency (CVI)," *The Yale Journal of Biology and Medicine* 66:37-46, 1993.

47. Brautigam, P. "The Importance of the Subfascial Lymphatics in the Diagnosis of Lower Limb Edema: Investigations with Semiquantitative Lymphoscintigraphy," *Angiology* 44:464-470, June 1993.

48. Bull, R., Ansell, G., Stanton, A.W., Levick, J.R., Mortimer, P.S. "Normal cutaneous microcirculation in gaiter zone (ulcer-susceptible skin) versus nearby regions in healthy young adults," *Int J Microcirc Clin Exp* 15(2):65-74, March-April 1995.

49. Bernas, M., Witte, M. "Consensus and Dissent on the ISL Consensus Document on the Diagnosis and Treatment of Peripheral Lymphedema," *Lymphology* 37:165-167, 2004.

50. Foldi, M. "Remarks Concerning the Consensus Document of the ISL 'The Diagnosis and Treatment of Peripheral Lymphedema,'" *Lymphology* 37:168-173, 2004.

51. Fahey, V.A., and White, S.A. "Physical Assessment of the Vascular System" in *Vascular Nursing.* Edited by Fahey, V.A. Philadelphia: W.B. Saunders Co., 1994.

52. Douglas, W.S., and Simpson, N.B. "Guidelines for the Management of Chronic Venous Leg Ulceration: Report of a Multidisciplinary Workshop," *British Journal of Dermatology* 132(3):446-52, March 1995.

53. Belcaro, G., et al. "Noninvasive Tests in Venous Insufficiency," *Journal of Cardiovascular Surgery* 34(1):3-11, February 1993.

54. Browse, N.L., and Burnand, K.G. "The Cause of Venous Ulceration," *Lancet* 2(8292):243-45, July 31, 1982.

55. Dodd, H., and Cockett, F. "The Postthrombotic Syndrome and Venous Ulceration" in *The Pathology and Surgery of the Veins of the Lower Limbs.* Edited by Dodd, H., and Cockett, F. New York: Churchill Livingstone, 1976.

56. Burnand, K., et al. "Venous Lipodermatosclerosis: Treatment with Fibrinolytic Enhancement and Elastic Compression," *British Medical Journal* 280(6206):7-11, January 5, 1980.

57. Nicolaides, A., et al. "Chronic Deep Venous Insufficiency" in *Haimovici's Vascular Surgery,* 4th ed. Edited by Haimovici, H., et al. Oxford: Blackwell Science, 1996.

58. Powell, S. "Contact Dermatitis in Patients with Chronic Leg Ulcers," *Journal of Tissue Viability* 6(4):103-106, October 1996.

59. Owens, J.C. "Management of Postphlebitic Syndrome," *VD&T,* February-March, 1981.

60. Nicolaides, A.N., et al. "The Relation of Venous Ulceration with Ambulatory Venous Pressure Measurements," *Journal of Vascular Surgery* 17(2):414-19, February 1993.

61. Blalock, A. "Oxygen Content of Blood in Patients with Varicose Veins," *Archives of Surgery* 19:898-905, 1929.

62. Lindemayr, W., et al. "Arteriovenous Shunts in Primary Varicosis? A Critical Essay," *Vascular Surgery* 6(1):9-13, January-February 1972.

63. Burnand, K.G., et al. "Peripapillary Fibrin in the Ulcer-bearing Skin of the Leg: The Cause of Lipodermatosclerosis and Venous Ulceration," *British Medical Journal* (Clinical Research Edition) 285(6):1071-72, November-December 1982.

64. Falanga, V., et al. "Pericapillary Fibrin Cuffs in Venous Ulceration: Persistence with Treatment and During Ulcer Healing," *Journal of Dermatology, Surgery, & Oncology* 18(5):409-14, May 1992.

65. Coleridge Smith, P.D., et al. "Causes of Venous Ulceration," *British Journal of Hospital Medicine* (Clinical Research Edition) 296(6638):1726-27, June 18, 1988.

66. Sarin, S., et al. "Disease Mechanisms in Venous Ulceration," *British Journal of Hospital Medicine* 45(5):303-05, May 1991.

67. Falanga, V., and Eaglstein, W.H. "The 'Trap' Hypothesis of Venous Ulceration," *Lancet* 341(8851):1006-08, April 17, 1993.

68. Porter, J.M., et al. "Reporting Standards in Venous Disease," *Journal of Vascular Surgery* 8(2):172-81, August 1988.

69. Ad Hoc Committee of the American Venous Forum. "Classification and Grading of Chronic Venous Disease in the Lower Limbs: A Consensus Statement" in *Handbook of Venous Disorders: Guidelines of the American Venous Forum.* Edited by Gloviczki, P. and Yao, J.S.T. London: Chapman & Hall, 1996.

70. Kistner, R.L., et al. "Diagnosis of Chronic Venous Disease of the Lower Extremities: The CEAP Classification," *Mayo Clinic Proceedings* 71(4):338-45, April 1996.

71. Nicolaides, A.N., and Miles, C. "Photoplethysmography in the Assessment of Venous Insufficiency," *Journal of Vascular Surgery* 5(3):405-12, March 1987.

72. Burton, C., "Venous Ulcers," *American Journal of Surgery* 167(1A Suppl):S37-S41, January 1994.

73. Jones, S.A., Bowler, P.G., Walker, M., Parsons, D. "Controlling wound bioburden with a novel silver containing Hydrofiber dressing," *Wound Repair Regen* 12:288-294, 2004.

74. Lineaweaver, W., et al. "Topical Antimicrobial Toxicity," *Archives of Surgery* 120(3):267-70, March 1985.

75. Lineaweaver, W., et al. "Cellular and Bacteriologic Toxicities of Topical Antimicrobials," *Plastic & Reconstructive Surgery* 75(3): 94-96, March 1985.

76. Cooper, M., et al. "The Cytotoxic Effects of Commonly Used Topical Antimicrobial Agents on Human Fibroblasts and Keratinocytes," *Journal of Trauma* 31(6):775-84, June 991.

77. McCauley, R.L., et al: "In Vitro Toxicity of Topical Antimicrobial Agents to Human Fibroblasts," *Journal of Surgical Research* 46(3):267-74, March 1989.

78. Maklebust, J. "Using Wound Care Products to Promote a Healing Environment," *Critical Care Nursing Clinics of North America* 8(2):141-158, June 1996.

79. Maklebust, J., and Sieggreen, M. *Pressure Ulcers: Guidelines for Prevention and Management,* 3rd ed., Springhouse, Pa.: Springhouse Corp., 2001.

80. Niederhuber, S.S., et al. "Reduction of Skin Bacterial Load with Use of Therapeutic Whirlpool," *Physical Therapy* 55(5):482-86, May 1975.

81. Bohannon, R.W. "Whirlpool versus Whirlpool and Rinse for Removal of Bacteria from a Venous Stasis Ulcer," *Physical Therapy* 62(3):304-308, March 1982.

82. Goldman, M.P., et al. "Diagnosis and Treatment of Varicose Veins: A Review," *Journal of the American Academy of Dermatology* 31(3 PH):393-416, September 1994.

83. Cordts, P.R., et al. "A Prospective, Randomized Trial of Unna's Boot versus Duoderm CGF Hydroactive Dressing plus Compression in the Management of Venous Leg Ulcers," *Journal of Vascular Surgery* 15(3):480-86, March 1992.

84. Mayberry, J.C. et al. "Nonoperative Treatment of Venous Stasis Ulcer" in *Venous Disorders.* Edited

by Bergan, J.J., and Yao, J.S.T. Philadelphia: W.B. Saunders Co., 1991.

85. Winter, G.D. "Formation of a Scab and the Rate of Epithelialization of Superficial Wounds in the Skin of a Pig," *Nature* 193:293-94, 1962.

86. Loiterman, D.A., and Byers, P.H. "Effect of a Hydrocellular Polyurethane Dressing on Chronic Venous Ulcer Healing," *Wounds* 3(5):178-81, September-October 1991.

87. Noyes, L.D., et al. "Hemodynamic Assessment of High Compression Hosiery in Chronic Venous Disease," *Surgery* 102(5):813-15, November 1987.

88. Pekanmaki, K., et al. "Intermittent Pneumatic Compression Treatment for Postthrombotic Leg Ulcers," *Clinical & Experimental Dermatology* 12(5):350-53, September 1987.

89. Scurr, J.H., et al. "Regimen for Improved Effectiveness of Intermittent Pneumatic Compression in Deep Venous Thrombosis Prophylaxis," *Surgery* 102(5):816-20, November 1987.

90. Mulder, G., et al. "Study of Sequential Compression Therapy in the Treatment of Nonhealing Chronic Venous Ulcers," *Wounds* 2:111-15, 1990.

91. Allsup, D.J. "Use of the Intermittent Pneumatic Compression Device in Venous Ulcer Disease," *Journal of Vascular Nursing* 12(4):106-11, December 1994.

92. Smith, P.C., et al. "Sequential Gradient Pneumatic Compression Enhances Venous Ulcer Healing: A Randomized Trial," *Surgery* 108(5):871-75, November 1990.

93. Mirand, F., Perez, M., Castigloni, M., et al. "Effect of Sequential Intermittent Pneumatic Compression on Both Leg Lymphedema Volume and on Lymph Transport as Semi-quantitatively Evaluated by Lymphoscintigraphy," *Lymphology* 34:135-141, 2001.

94. Szuba, A., Cooke, J., Yousuf, S., Rockson, S. "Decongestive Lymphatic Therapy for Patients with Cancer-Related or Primary Lymphedema," *The American Journal of Medicine* 109(4):296-300, September 2000.

95. Lund, E. "Exploring the Use of CircAid Legging in the Management of Lymphoedema," *International Journal of Palliative Nursing* 6(8):383-391, September 2000.

96. Ko, D., Lerner, R., Klose, G., Cosimi, A. "Effective Treatment of Lymphedema of the Extremities," *Arch Surg* 133(April):452-458, April 1998.

97. Pagberg, F.T., Johnston, M.V., Sisto, S.A. "Structured exercise improves calf muscle pump function in chronic venous insufficiency: a randomized trial," *J Vasc Surg* 39:79-87, 2004.

98. McCulloch, J.M., et al. "Intermittent Pneumatic Compression Improves Venous Ulcer Healing," *Advances in Wound Care* 7(4):22-26, July 1994.

99. Raju, S. "Axillary Vein Transfer for Postphlebitic Syndrome," in *Atlas of Venous Surgery*. Edited by Bergan, J.J., and Kistner, R.L. Philadelphia: W.B. Saunders Co., 1992.

100. Kistner, R.L. "Transposition Techniques," in *Atlas of Venous Surgery*. Edited by Bergan, J.J., and Kistner, R.L. Philadelphia: W.B. Saunders Co., 1992.

101. Kistner, R.L. "Valve Reconstruction for Primary Valve Insufficiency," in *Atlas of Venous Surgery*. Edited by Bergan, J.J., and Kistner, R.L. Philadelphia: W.B. Saunders Co., 1992.

102. Breu, F.X., Guggenbichler, S. European consensus meeting on foam sclerotherapy. April 4-6, 2003. Tegernsee, Germany.

103. Scurr, J.H. "Alternative Procedures in Deep Venous Insufficiency," in *Atlas of Venous Surgery*. Edited by Bergan, J.J., and Kistner, R.L. Philadelphia: W.B. Saunders Co., 1992.

CHAPTER 15

Arterial ulcers

Mary Y. Sieggreen, MSN, APRN, CS, CVN, APN
Ronald A. Kline, MD, FACS, FAHA
R. Gary Sibbald, BSc, MD, FRCPC (Med)(Derm), FAPWCA, MEd

OBJECTIVES

After completing this chapter, you'll be able to:

- identify the structure and function of the lower extremity arterial system

- assess the signs and symptoms of lower extremity arterial disease and ulcers

- select appropriate vascular laboratory diagnostic testing for lower extremity arterial disease

- evaluate medical and surgical treatment options for lower extremity arterial disease

- design appropriate patient education for prevention and appropriate lifestyle change.

Scope of the problem

Peripheral vascular disease is commonly used to refer to arterial problems in the legs. Some authors also include diseases of the venous and lymphatic systems in their definition of peripheral vascular disease so the reader should be aware that there may be discrepancies in how this condition is discussed.

Patients with leg and foot ulcers may have several different etiologies including arterial, venous, and lymphatic disease along with trauma, infections, inflammatory diseases, and malignancy. This chapter describes the arterial component including anatomy and physiology, as well as examining the treatment of lower extremity arterial ulcers.

Approximately 8% to 10% of patients with leg and foot ulcers have pure arterial insufficiency.[1] It's estimated that between 1% and 22% of the population over age 60 suffers from lower extremity skin ulcers.[2-5] One study found the problem to be underestimated when a self-report survey indicated high numbers of patients cared for their own ulcers without consulting a health care provider.[6] The principal etiology of leg ulcers is chronic venous ulcers and of foot ulcers, arterial disease is much more common.[1,7-9] Although it's understood that chronic wounds have physical, financial, and psychological affects, it's difficult to measure their effects on a patient's quality of life.[10] It's also difficult to obtain accurate etiological information about leg ulcers, because, in about one-third of medical records, no ulcer etiology documentation exists.

Vascular anatomy and physiology

Vascular anatomy includes the arterial, venous, and lymphatic systems. Vascular ulcers may develop in any of these systems from a variety of causes. For the purposes of this chapter, we will confine our discussion to the arterial system.

Arterial system

Lower extremity arterial perfusion begins with adequate cardiac performance. As blood exits the left ventricle, it begins its downward course through the descending thoracic aorta. The intercostal arteries, which arise from the descending thoracic aorta, are the first important collaterals to perfusion in the legs. These become important when they are the sole collaterals in distal aortic occlusive disease. As the aorta exits the thorax and enters the true abdominal cavity, its caliber begins to decrease after every major arterial branch. Its greatest reduction in size occurs distal to the renal arteries.

Lumbar arteries usually arise as paired vessels at each vertebral level in the abdomen. The lumbar arteries become important collateral pathways to the lower extremities in distal aortic occlusions or severe aortoiliac occlusive disease. At the level of the umbilicus, the abdominal aorta bifurcates into the common iliac arteries that in turn branch into internal and external iliac arteries. The internal iliac arteries perfuse the lower sigmoid colon and rectum. They also, by way of the gluteal and pudendal branches, provide another collateral pathway to perfusion of the legs. The external iliac artery becomes the common femoral artery at the level of the inguinal ligament. It's at this level that one can first appreciate the quality of the pulse wave by palpating the femoral artery.

Aspects of the femoral artery

The common femoral artery bifurcates into the superficial femoral artery and the deep femoral artery. The deep femoral artery is the single most important collateral pathway for perfusion of the lower portion of the leg. Its muscular perforators allow reconstitution of the popliteal artery in superficial femoral artery occlusions. The superficial femoral artery becomes the popliteal artery after it exits the adductor hiatus, also known as *Hunter's canal.* (See *Arterial system.*)

The superficial femoral artery is the most commonly occluded artery in the legs of patients with peripheral vascular occlusive disease. Its occlusion infrequently results in significant ischemia to the lower leg. Below the knee, the popliteal artery bifurcates into the tibioperoneal trunk and the anterior tibial artery. The anterior tibial artery proceeds from the popliteal fossa through the interosseous membrane, which connects the tibia and fibula; it then courses down the anterior muscle compartment into the foot. The tibioperoneal trunk at a variable distance then bifurcates into the peroneal artery and the posterior tibial artery.

The peroneal artery courses down toward the ankle in the deep muscular compartment whereas the posterior tibial artery descends into the foot in a more superficial fashion. The peroneal artery provides important muscular profusion branches. It's commonly patent even in the presence of severe lower-extremity peripheral vascular occlusive disease.

Aspects of the tibial arteries

The anterior and posterior tibial arteries proceed into the foot with the anterior tibial artery becoming palpable as it becomes the dorsalis pedis artery. The posterior tibial artery then courses behind the medial malleolus and at this level also becomes palpable. The posterior tibial artery provides both deep and superficial components to the plantar arch. Perforators from the plantar arch provide arterial perfusion to the heel, sole, and branches to the digits.

The anterior tibial artery eventually communicates with the plantar arch forming a

Arterial system

This illustration shows the major arteries of the lower extremities.

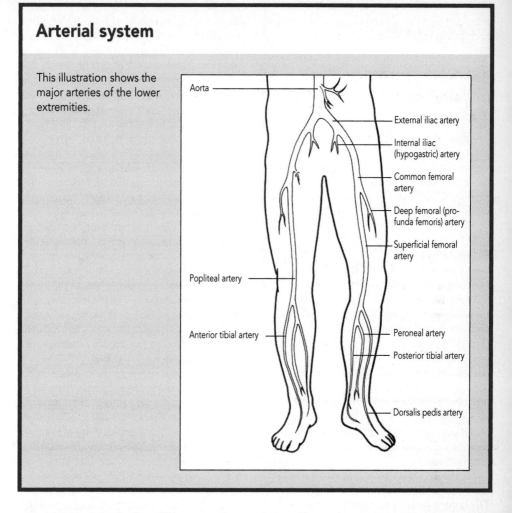

complete circuit in the foot. The peroneal artery, although it stops above the level of the ankle joint, does provide medial and lateral tarsal branches that communicate with the distal most portions of the anterior tibial and posterior tibial arteries. This is another important collateral pathway for revascularization of the plantar arch in patients with occlusive disease. Vascular surgeons can perform bypass operations to any of these named vessels with modern procedures successfully bypassing more distal vessels.

Arterial wall architecture
The arterial wall typically consists of three lamina. The outer lamina, the adventitia, is a layer of loose connective tissue that provides moderate strength to the arterial wall. The media, or middle layer, contains both elastic and muscular fibers and is responsible for arterial strength, elasticity, and contractility. The intima, the innermost layer, is the endothelial lining of an artery and a few cell layers thick. As the arterial tree descends from the center to the periphery, muscular functions become more evident. Vessels below the common femoral artery have a greater propensity for rapid size adjustments in direct relationship to perfusion. The tibioperoneal vessels can quickly accommodate changes in perfusion by relaxation or dilatation.

Arterial wall

In the layers of the arterial wall shown here, the plaque formation and thrombus significantly reduce blood flow through the vessel.

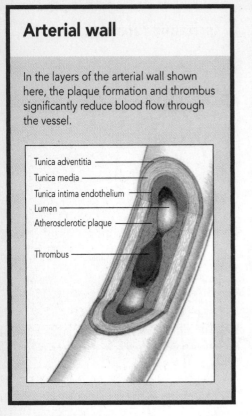

Tunica adventitia
Tunica media
Tunica intima endothelium
Lumen
Atherosclerotic plaque
Thrombus

Arteries are capable of increasing in size to maintain constant shear stress when atherosclerotic accumulation decreases luminal surface area. However, once a stenosis reaches 50% of the vessel diameter, the artery loses its ability to relax any further and any increase in atherosclerotic accumulation impedes arterial perfusion. Further restriction in flow through this stenotic area results in a decrease in the diameter of the artery distal to the stenosis in order to accommodate diminished blood flow. Compliance of an artery decreases as the arterial wall becomes more rigid as seen in calcific atherosclerosis. (See *Arterial wall.*)

Arterial perfusion

As blood descends through successively smaller arterial conduits, it eventually reaches the arteriolar level. Blood flow (rheologic factors) in this precapillary bed play an important role in perfusion. Blood is a non-Newtonian thixotropic fluid; that is, its viscosity is inversely proportional to its shear rate. Shear rate can be equated to the velocity of blood flow. The slower blood is propulsed the more viscous it becomes. The primary determinant of whole blood viscosity at any given shear rate is the hematocrit. As red cell mass increases, blood viscosity markedly increases and the flow decreases.

Dehydration or polycythemia, two of many disease states that increase whole blood viscosity, can result in a sludging of blood in the precapillary bed and decrease arterial tissue perfusion. In many elderly patients with arterial occlusive disease, even mild dehydration can result in poor extremity perfusion. Simple rehydration can reduce the red cell mass and allow for better perfusion. In other cases of increased blood viscosity, such as multiple myeloma, plasmapheresis may be necessary to remove the abnormal concentrations of proteins. Nonetheless, in the "normal" atherosclerotic patient, it's the red cell mass, measured by hematocrit, which is the primary determinant of viscosity.

As blood proceeds into the capillary bed, the diameter of the vessel approaches that of the red cell—approximately 8 microns in diameter. Red cells pass through capillaries sequentially. Red cell deformability plays a role in perfusion at this level. In conditions in which the red cell membrane is relatively rigid, tissue perfusion decreases because of increased transit time for a red cell to pass from the precapillary to postcapillary level. Although nutrient and oxygen extraction are increased by this increase in transit time, the per unit perfusion of the tissues is overall decreased. Medications such as pentoxifylline reportedly facilitate red cell deformability, thereby increasing the per unit perfusion of tissues.[7,8]

In normal states, arterial tissue perfusion is well above minimal requirements. Certain tissues, such as muscle, can change their metabolic requirements. Muscle becomes more efficient under anaerobic conditions—for example, in a trained person who engages in long-distance running. The process is gradual, but it's useful in patients with claudication. A regular exercise program can increase the distance walked before claudication occurs. The skin does not have the same kind of compensatory mechanism where exercise can gradually increase blood flow.

Arterial ulcer pathophysiology

The pathophysiology of vascular ulcers varies according to the type of ulcer. Arterial ulcers are wounds that will not heal due to compromised or inadequate arterial blood flow. Precipitating events for arterial ulcers vary. Limbs with arterial compromise may have minimal but adequate blood flow to maintain tissue viability. Ischemic lower extremity ulcers are often precipitated by trauma or infection.

The location of traumatic ulcers varies depending on the cause, but these wounds are commonly found on the foot or on the anterior tibial area of the lower leg. Traumatic ulcers may be caused by an acute physical injury, such as blunt trauma (for example, bumping into a piece of furniture or dropping a heavy object on the foot), or by acute or chronic pressure (such as the continual pressure from ill-fitting footwear). Several other conditions may be responsible for tissue breakdown, including thermal extremes, chemicals, or a localized clot or embolus, which can also lead to decreased cellular nutrition from impaired arterial flow. Regardless of the cause, when ischemia is present, wound healing is inhibited. Although some wounds heal in the presence of ischemia, arterial inflow must usually be improved for healing to occur. Injury repair requires more than baseline oxygen consumption and increased tissue nutritional need because diminished arterial flow causes tissue hypoxia in arterial insufficiency and can eventually lead to gangrene or tissue necrosis. (See *Ischemic forefoot*.)

Diagnosing vascular ulcers

Vascular disease and ulcer etiology can be determined by obtaining a thorough patient history and performing a physical examination.

Ischemic forefoot

This photograph shows an ischemic forefoot.

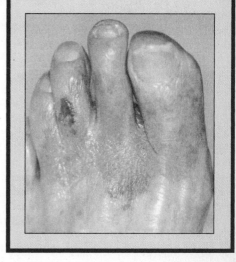

A focused vascular history includes a clear description of the presenting complaint, past medical history for vascular and related conditions, current and previous medications, and risk factors. Signs and symptoms of lower extremity vascular disease may include pain, tissue loss, or change in appearance or sensation. Noninvasive vascular laboratory testing is required to identify the location of vascular pathology.

The first question to ask every patient about his history is allergies. This question is important if there is a known sensitivity to medications that may be ordered or to dyes used for angiography. The next question should be about the patient's medications and then about his occupation.[11]

The important points to remember about a patient's history include remembering the mnemonic ABCDEs,[11] all of which are increased risk factors for arterial disease. They are:

• A_{1C}: Hgb A_{1C} refers to the personal or family history of diabetes or arterial disease. Arterial disease is often manifest at an earlier age in males and individuals that smoke or have other risk factors.

- Blood pressure: Find out if it is elevated and if they are on medications.
- Cholesterol: Elevated cholesterol is a risk factor and the use of statin cholesterol lowering agents may reduce this risk.
- Diet and obesity: Increased weight especially a body mass index above 25 indicates an increased risk for heart and peripheral vascular disease as well as diabetes.
- Exercise: Individuals that exercise regularly have a lower risk of peripheral vascular disease and can build up a greater tolerance to overcome compromised circulation. In general, individuals with leg pain at rest or when in bed have severe ischemia, those that have pain or claudication (aching and throbbing calf muscles) with walking up a few stairs or less than 50 yards have moderate disease, and individuals with symptoms after walking one or two blocks have mild disease.
- Smoking: One cigarette decreases circulation 30% for 1 hour and the more pack-years of accumulated smoking history the greater the risk. Ask patients how many cigarettes they smoke a day and how many years they have been smoking. (Example: 30 years of smoking and half a pack a day is 15 pack years [$30 \times 0.5 = 15$.])

Other risk factors include increased levels of homocysteine and hypothyroidism.[12] If peripheral vascular disease is present, it is also more common to have a history of coronary artery disease and previous stroke.[12]

Physical examination

Skin inspection is an important part of the physical examination. It includes examining the distal extremities for taut or shiny, atrophic skin that's present with arterial disease. Because skin color may indicate arterial perfusion, each toe should be noted and compared with the other foot and toes. Arterial insufficiency causes ischemic tissue to first become pale, progressing to a mottled netlike appearance (livedo reticularis) and subsequently to a dark purple hue, and finally black. Elevating the foot at a 45-degree angle causes the ischemic limb to become pale. Immediately after positioning the ischemic foot in a dependent position, it becomes dark red or ruddy. This finding is the reactive hyperemia of ischemic tissue. There may be a loss of hair distally and the nails may lose their luster and become thickened. Make sure to distinguish nail changes from changes that occur with a fungus infection or psoriasis.

Palpate the skin for temperature changes. The skin of an ischemic limb feels cool or cold, with temperature demarcation that correlates to the diseased artery. Capillary refill time, determined by compressing the skin (dorsum of the foot or toe pad) with the thumb to remove the local profusion leading to a local blanching of color, and releasing the thumb and observing the capillary refill and return of color is a good indicator of arterial skin perfusion. Perform this test with the foot slightly elevated. Normal capillary refill time takes less than 3 seconds to return from pallor to normal skin color.

Palpate pulses for presence, rate, regularity, strength, and equality. The most common objective physical finding is the presence or absence of pulses. Care must be taken when palpating pedal pulses. It's common to mistake a contracting tendon for the presence of a pulse. No universal consensus exists regarding a pulse grading system; conversely, a high degree of observer variability exists in determining the presence or absence of pulses. It can be confusing if clinicians report 2+ or 3+ pulse examinations. Documentation is better facilitated if pulses are recorded as present or absent. However, even this seemingly obvious assessment parameter may not always be accurate. One study found only a 50% chance that two observers would agree with a third observer about the presence or absence of dorsalis pedis or posterior tibial pulses. This same study found the dorsalis pedis congenitally absent in 4% to 12% and the posterior tibial absent in 0.24% to 12.8% of subjects.[13] Additional descriptors of pulse, such as "weak," or "bounding," can be added to clarify your findings.

PRACTICE POINT

The best way to document pulses is to use descriptor terms, such as present or absent, rather than numerical ratings, such as 2+ or

3+. Use modifier words, such as weak or bounding, to further describe and clarify the pulse findings.

Although pulses in the foot may be present at rest, they may disappear with exercise. A patient who presents with claudication but has clearly discernable pulses should have an exercise test done in the vascular laboratory. Clinicians are often tempted to skip the assessment of the elusive popliteal pulse, particularly when the dorsalis pedis and posterior tibial pulses are strong. While good pedal pulses indicate foot perfusion, finding bounding popliteal pulses may indicate a popliteal aneurysm. Popliteal aneurysms can be a source of emboli to the lower leg with resulting tissue or limb loss.

Test patients with foot or leg ulcers for neuropathy. This is a common finding in persons with diabetes but there are several other causes associated with a loss of protective sensation. For example, neuropathy commonly obscures a traumatic or pressure-induced wound in an ischemic limb. Lack of pain sensation and injury awareness prevents the patient with diabetes from seeking appropriate care early. Evaluate neuropathy by testing light touch with monofilaments for the sensory component, examining for dry skin as part of the autonomic component, and eliciting reflexes for the motor component. You can remember to assess for neuropathy with the mnemonic SAM (Sensory, Autonomic, and Motor). An objective assessment of significant neuropathy is best done by using the 5.07 Semmes-Weinstein monofilament.[14] To perform this assessment, ask the patient to close his eyes and indicate when he feels the monofilament. Test the areas over the plantar aspect of the first third and fifth toe; the first, third, and fifth metatarsal head; both sides of the plantar aspect of the midfoot; the plantar heel; and lastly the dorsum of the foot. Place the monofilament on the test position until it bends slightly and then move it to the next position. Record the number of negative sites the patient reports and if there are 4 or more negative sites, then neuropathy is present that indicates a loss of protective sensation.

PRACTICE POINT

Use the mnemonic SAM to assess for neuropathy:
Sensory
Autonomic
Motor

Arterial signs and symptoms

Arterial insufficiency is commonly associated with complaints of pain[15] resulting from atherosclerotic arterial changes interrupting blood flow to tissues.[16] Arterial pain is characteristically described as claudication or rest pain—that is, pain that occurs with exercise and is relieved by rest; it occurs in the muscle group distal to the stenosed or occluded artery. While the calf is the most common location for claudication, it can also occur in the buttocks, thighs, or feet and is predictable and reproducible. Claudication is described by patients as cramping, aching, or muscle weakness.

PRACTICE POINT

When taking a history it's important to find out exactly how far the patient can walk before he needs to stop; a shorter distance indicates more severe atherosclerosis. Reported changes in ambulatory distance may indicate progressive atherosclerotic disease.

The patient with leg ulcers and poorly perfused tissue commonly seeks care because of sharp, severe, and possibly, constant pain at the ulcer site and the distal extremity. Pain that occurs at rest represents inadequate perfusion and is a sign of threatened limb viability. The patient may describe waking up at night with pain across the distal metatarsal area of the foot. In an attempt to relieve the pain, the patient will get out of bed and lower the foot, which has an increased blood flow due to increased hydrostatic pressure, to

Blue toe syndrome

This photograph shows "blue toe syndrome" in the second toe caused by tissue ischemia from arteriosclerosis.

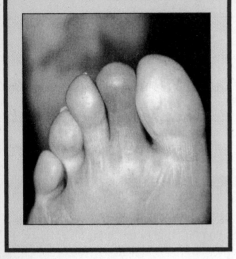

improve tissue perfusion. The patient may even ambulate. The ischemic pain is also relieved by the small contribution of blood flow from collateral vessels. The patient with pain at rest may begin sleeping with his legs dependent and leg edema may develop due to the chronic dependent position.

PRACTICE POINT

Rest pain represents end-stage arterial insufficiency and commonly requires surgical intervention.[17,18]

Patients with extensive sensory neuropathy—for example, those with diabetes—may not experience pain even with severely ischemic ulcers. On the other hand, these patients may experience such intense hyperesthesia associated with the neuropathy that they cannot bear the light touch of stockings. Ulcers in patients with neuropathy are typically found on the plantar side of the foot and are surrounded by calluses from long-term local pressure. These patients may describe the sensations of burning, stinging,

shooting, and stabbing pain rather than the more characteristic gnawing, aching, throbbing, and tender pain associated with an acute injury of peripheral vascular disease.

When obtaining a history, note previous arterial surgery for vascular disease, including coronary artery disease and cerebral vascular disease. Vascular disease isn't limited to any one organ but can occur in all body systems. Document all medications, especially vasoconstrictor drugs. Ischemic symptoms are exacerbated by nicotine. Patients with symptomatic vascular disease may aggravate their symptoms by using tobacco, nicotine gum, or nicotine patches for smoking cessation.

Another arterial finding upon examination is gangrene. In ischemic tissue, gangrene initially appears pale, then blue-gray, followed by purple and, finally, black. Gangrenous tissue eventually becomes black, hard, and mummified. The hardened tissue isn't painful, but significant pain may be present at the line of demarcation between the gangrene and the live but ischemic tissue. Gangrene may be a small skin lesion or extend to an entire limb depending on the location of the arterial lesion. If a small patch of skin is affected, the skin will dry and fall off, producing a skin ulcer. Large areas of gangrene may require debridement, skin graft, or potential amputation.

Other findings upon examination are ulcers that may appear as small black or dark purple dots, circular areas found on the distal toes, or localized infarcts around the toe nail beds. (See *Blue toe syndrome*.) Ulcers found in these areas are caused by tissue ischemia from arteriosclerosis or by atheromatous debris embolizing from a proximal artery. Arterial ulcers may also be found between the toes, starting as a small moist macerated spot on the skin surface extending deep into the bony structure of the foot.

Arterial ulcers typically have distinct borders with a pale-gray or yellow-dry base. They may contain exposed tendons, fascia, fat, muscle, bone, or joint structures in their base. The surrounding tissue may appear pale compared to skin elsewhere on the body or it may be reddened if the leg is dependent. Chronic ischemic skin may appear thin and shiny. Foot elevation will produce skin pallor. The red or ruddy color of a dependent ischemic limb is called *dependent rubor* or *reactive hyperemia*. (See *Dependent rubor*.) Even in a person of color, the difference in hue is discernible when the ischemic limb is compared to the contralateral well-perfused limb.

Arterial pressure is one of the most reliable physical findings in peripheral arterial disease.[19] However, lower extremity blood pressures aren't obtained as a part of the routine physical examination. Bilateral brachial pressures should always be obtained on the initial examination to identify whether a discrepancy exists between them. The correct pressure is always the higher of the two pressures. This pressure is used to determine the ankle-brachial index when assessing lower extremity perfusion.

Vascular testing

Although an experienced vascular clinician can make a vascular diagnosis on history and physical examination alone, vascular laboratory studies help pinpoint the diagnosis. The presence, location, and severity of arterial disease is confirmed by vascular laboratory procedures. Information obtained by vascular studies can predict potential ulcer healing (healable ulcer) when the cause is arterial insufficiency.[7] Laboratory tests differentiate among conditions contributing to a nonhealing ulcer.

Noninvasive vascular testing is divided into direct tests that image the vessel itself and indirect tests that demonstrate changes distal to the diseased vessel. These tests include segmental arterial Doppler ultrasound with pressures, arteriogram, ankle-brachial index (ABI), transcutaneous pressure of oxygen ($tcPO_2$), and toe pressures.

Handheld Doppler ultrasound

A Doppler ultrasound transmitting probe sends a signal, which is reflected from an object to the receiving probe. If the signal strikes a moving object such as blood cells, a frequency shift is detected and reflected as

Dependent rubor

Foot elevation produces skin pallor in patients with ischemic skin. When dependent, the ischemic limb will have a red or ruddy color, as shown here in the patient's right leg. This is called dependent rubor or reactive hyperemia.

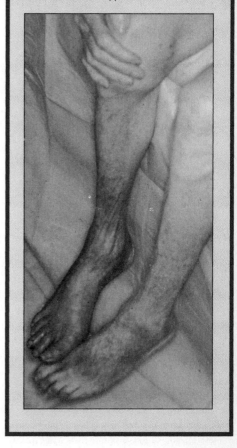

sound. The audible signals of arterial flow patterns can then be determined. The handheld Doppler is used to detect an audible signal on the dorsum of the foot or ankle (dorsalis pedis or posterior tibial artery). A blood pressure cuff is then placed around the lower calf and inflated until the audible signal disappears. The cuff is then slowly deflated and when the signal returns the systolic pressure is determined from the reading on the cuff

Arteriogram

The arteriogram below shows iliac stenosis.

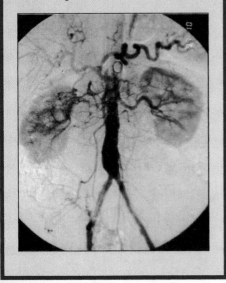

strates the normal triphasic signal representing the three phases of the pulsation in a normal peripheral artery. The first wave represents forward flow of blood and arterial distention. The second phase represents the arterial relaxation and subsequent retrograde flow of blood. The third phase or portion of the triphasic Doppler signal is believed to represent the bulging of the aortic valve, which occurs during diastole.

The third phase of the triphasic arterial signal is first lost as an artery becomes less compliant and is followed by loss of the second phase of the triphasic Doppler signal. With worsening occlusive disease proximal to the area of auscultation, the normally sharp first wave becomes flattened and broader. In severely diseased arteries, the Doppler signal can be a monophasic, low-amplitude wave. The minimum systolic pressure that can result in forward Doppler flow is used in the calculation of the ABI, a measurement of arterial perfusion in the leg. (See *Arterial waveform changes.*)

gauge. The procedure is then repeated on the arm for the brachial artery. If the leg pressure is 80 mm Hg and the arm pressure 100 mm Hg then the ankle brachial pressure ratio is 80/100 mm Hg or 0.80.

Arteriogram

An arteriogram is an invasive test used to identify an operative lesion in the arterial system by outlining the patent arterial lumen. (See *Arteriogram.*) Indications for a surgical procedure include incapacitating claudication, rest pain, nonhealing ulcers, and gangrene. An arteriogram is not indicated unless a bypass or dilation procedure can be performed. It's also not indicated when the patient is too ill for surgery or is refusing surgical intervention.

Arterial testing

Propagation of a pulse wave originating in the heart is easily measured by auscultation of a peripheral artery with Doppler ultrasound. Recording the Doppler shift demon-

Ankle-brachial index

Additional tests for arterial disease include ankle-brachial index (ABI), segmental pressures and waveforms, duplex ultrasound, and exercise treadmill for claudication. Perfusion is indirectly measured in a vascular laboratory by the ABI—the Doppler systolic pressure of the brachial artery divided into the ankle systolic pressure. ABI ratios reflect the degree of perfusion loss in the lower extremity.

In most individuals, the resting ankle pressure in a supine position is equal to the brachial pressure, with an ABI value of one. An individual with claudication may have a normal ABI in this position and have it drop during exercise. Patients with pain even in the resting state will have an abnormally low ABI. With exercise, the ABI in the patient with resting pain usually doesn't fall because the arteries are already maximally dilated. Inadequate perfusion creates local tissue factors that result in vasodilatation. Collateral pathways can't provide the additional tissue perfusion required resulting in rest pain. A patient with ischemic tissue loss usually has a perfusion picture more consistent with rest

Arterial waveform changes

The arterial changes corresponding to occluded arteries are illustrated here.

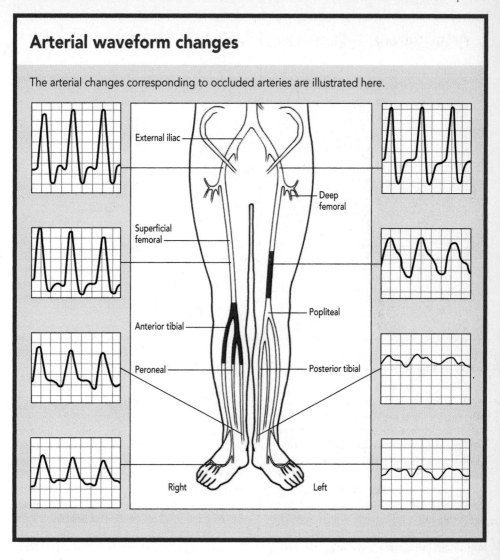

pain than claudication.[7] (See *Obtaining an ankle-brachial index*, page 328.)

Segmental pressures

Segmental pressures have been used since the 1950s to determine the location of arterial vascular lesions.[20] Pressures obtained at the level of the thigh, above the knee, calf, and ankle are compared with each other and pressures in the other leg. An arterial lesion can be isolated with a 20 mm Hg gradient between cuff pressures. If no pressure gradient exists on a limb that claudicates, the pa-

tient is asked to exercise and repeat pressures are obtained.

A palpable pulse indicates an arterial flow pressure of approximately 80 mm Hg or more in the foot. With calcification of the intima, the arterial pressures derived in the larger vessels of the leg can be falsely elevated. If an ABI is over 1.2 the results are not reliable. The vascular laboratory will then have to rely on accessory tests, such as the toe pressure procedure or transcutaneous oxygen saturation level test ($TCPO_2$).

Obtaining an ankle-brachial index

To obtain an ankle-brachial index (ABI), you'll need a sphygmomanometer and a Doppler device. The procedure is performed as follows:

- Take the bilateral brachial blood pressure while the patient is supine. The higher of the two systolic pressures is used as the brachial pressure in the ratio.
- Place the blood pressure cuff on the leg just above the malleoli. Place the Doppler probe at a 45-degree angle to the dorsalis pedis or posterior tibial artery.
- Inflate the cuff until the Doppler signal is obliterated. With the Doppler probe over the artery, slowly deflate the cuff until the Doppler signal returns. Record the number as the ankle systolic pressure.
- Divide the ankle pressure by the higher of the two systolic pressures. The ratio obtained is the ABI.

ABI Interpretation

ABI	Interpretation
1.0	Normal
0.75 to 0.90	Moderate disease
0.50 to 0.75	Severe disease
Less than 0.5	Rest pain or gangrene
Unreliable	Diabetes

Toe pressures

Toe pressure tests measure the flow through the large toe where the vessel is small enough that calcium deposits don't circle the entire vessel and compressibility is usually always present. A toe pressure of 50 mm Hg or higher even in a person with diabetes is usually adequate for healing. Toe pressures of 20 to 30 mm Hg usually indicate some vascular compromise and the wound healing will be more difficult. Pressures below 30 mm Hg may be adequate if the skin is intact but as soon as injury results and disrupts the cutaneous barrier, the vascular supply is often inadequate for the repair process.

EVIDENCE-BASED PRACTICE

A falsely-high pressure reading is commonly seen in patients with diabetes due to incompressible artery walls caused by medial sclerosis of the arteries.[18] When the vessels are incompressible, toe pressures are obtained because they're reported to be more accurate.

Treating vascular ulcers

"When treating vascular ulcers, follow the preparing the wound bed paradigm."[21,22]

- Treat the cause: bypass, stents, or dilation with a consult to a vascular specialist
- Patient-centered concerns: pain, quality-of-life, and activities of daily living
- Local wound care:
  – Healable wound—debridement, moisture balance, and bacterial balance
  – Maintenance wound—procedures may be more conservative because of patient or system factors causing the wound to not heal
  – Nonhealable wound—requires conservative debridement, moisture reduction, and bacterial reduction.

With a healable wound you should actively promote debridement of slough or nonviable tissue to create a clean wound. This may including bleeding postdebridement or the use of mechanical, enzymatic, or autolytic debridement methods with dressings (usually alginates, hydrogels, or hydrocolloids).

A maintenance wound—one that could heal but patient factors, such as smoking or inconsistent treatment, excessive obesity, or uncontrolled diabetes, can make sustained healing of the wound less likely—requires conservative debridement accompanied by local wound care for bacterial and moisture balance. If a wound doesn't have enough blood supply to heal, gangrene should be allowed to dry and demarcate. This can be done by removing the soft slough often around the proximal intersection of the necrotic and viable tissue but leaving the necrotic cap intact. Moisture and bacterial reduction may be best served with antiseptic agents, such as povidone-iodine and chlorhexidine, that can reduce bacterial counts with acceptable tissue toxicity.[22] Both of these agents have a broad spectrum of action, a sustained residual effect, and acceptable tissue toxicity for this indication. Agents such as sodium hypochlorite, quaternary ammonium agents, and various aniline dyes (crystal violet) have higher cellular toxicities and more limited antibacterial effects.[22]

Wound infection

It's important to remember that all chronic ulcers contain bacteria (contamination). When the bacteria is attached to tissue and multiplies, it becomes colonized and can lead to damage that will delay healing (such as with critical colonization, increased bacterial burden, covert infection, and superficial infection). Patients with critical colonization don't have all the classic signs and symptoms of a deep tissue infection. Infection can be diagnosed with a bacterial swab that helps identify resistant organisms or serves as a guide to antimicrobial therapy. You should examine the superficial compartment of the wound bed for more than one sign of bacterial damage. The key features of a wound bed can be remembered as NERDS.©[23] (See NERDS© and STONES© in chapter 7, Wound bioburden, and in the color section, pages C7 to C9.)

Topical treatment for critically colonized wounds could include the various new silver dressings or cadexomer iodine in healable wounds, and povidone-iodine or chlorhexidine in wounds with inadequate blood supply to support healing.

Deep tissue infection requires systemic antimicrobial agents. The classical signs of warmth, tenderness, swelling, and erythema can be supplemented for persons with chronic wounds by the mnemonic STONES.©[23] (See NERDS© and STONES© in chapter 7 and in the color section, pages C7 to C9.)

Obviously, if exudate and smell are present, you need to use other criteria to determine if the ulcer has superficial or deep tissue infection.

PRACTICE POINT

- The diagnosis of superficial or deep tissue infection should be made clinically with a bacterial swab to help with treatment decisions.
- Persons with diabetes, neuropathy, and foot ulcers often have a falsely-negative X-ray of the foot for osteomyelitis and other criteria should be used such as probing bone to make a diagnosis.[24]
- The use of bone scans is limited because they're expensive and may give false-positives in the presence of inflammation. (Magnetic resonance imaging may be more helpful diagnostically.)

Wound cleaning

A clean wound, free from dead tissue and wound debris, is necessary for healing to occur. Many commercial wound cleaners have some cytotoxicity but they have surfactant properties that are often useful. Povidone-iodine, chlorhexidine, hydrogen peroxide, and 0.25% acetic acid have been shown to interfere with fibroblast formation and epithelial growth.[25-28] The selected use of these agents, particularly povidone-iodine and chlorhexidine, should be reserved for wounds that don't have the ability to heal or for time-limited use in wounds where bacterial burden is more important than cellular toxicity.

EVIDENCE-BASED PRACTICE

The advantage of wound cleaning should be weighed against damaging new tissue growth.[29]

The safest wound cleaner is 0.9% saline solution or water. Wounds should be cleaned with a force strong enough to dislodge debris but gentle enough to prevent damage to newly growing tissue. The pressure to accomplish this goal ranges from 4 to 15 psi.[30] A 19G needle or 19G angiocatheter distributes approximately 8 psi when used with a 35-cc syringe. A Baxter cap on a saline irrigation bottle is a less expensive method to distribute an adequate amount of pressure. Hydrotherapy or whirlpool debridement has been used to aid in cleaning and debridement of arterial ulcers.[31] This may suggest that vigorous irrigation is the significant factor in cleaning the wound. (For more information about wound cleaning, see chapter 7, Wound bioburden.)

Dressings chosen for specific wounds depend on the wound bed condition and the goal for the wound. Many new dressings are designed to support moist wound healing (see chapter 9, Wound treatment options). Because the skin is fragile in patients with either arterial or venous disease and can be easily injured, tape and adhesive products should be used with extreme caution. We recommend the use of other methods of securing dressings that won't injury the skin. Of the available adhesive products, soft silicones are less likely to cause local trauma during dressing changes.

PRACTICE POINT

The preferred attachment device for dressings on vascular leg ulcers is a gauze roll, or commercial devices (such as netting or tube gauze) that hold dressings in place without adhesive, which can damage fragile skin.

Arterial ulcer treatment

Treatment of arterial ulcers must include increasing the blood supply to the area. Positioning the extremity in a dependent position may facilitate blood flow by gravity through collateral vessels. Use caution if devices such as a foot cradle are used for protection because an insensate foot is subject to trauma from the cradle's hard wood or met-

al. Debridement of gangrene should not be performed in the presence of ischemia because the blood flow is insufficient to heal the new surgical wound. Ulcers without adequate arterial inflow must be kept dry—in contrast to the principle of moist-wound healing for ulcers with adequate blood supply. Moisture provides a bed for bacterial growth if eschar or gangrenous tissue are present. This tissue, if kept dry, can be left in place until demarcation or debridement is indicated.

Ulcers with adequate blood supply that are expected to heal should be dressed with products that support moist wound healing principles. These dressings include moist saline gauze, hydrocolloids, thin films, and foams. The surrounding intact tissue should be protected from fluid accumulation, which can macerate the healthy skin at the ulcer border.

Arterial reconstruction is the treatment of choice to improve the circulation for most patients.[32] Percutaneous intraluminal balloon angioplasty is a consideration for discreet short lesions in the proximal arteries. Treatment for arterial leg ulcers requires reinstating arterial inflow before any other treatment is established. This is usually preceded by a noninvasive vascular test, an arteriogram followed by an angioplasty or surgery. Simultaneously, local ulcer treatment can be determined. Usually the arterial ulcer has a dry ulcer bed. The patient may have several punctate ulcers with regular borders, as well as dry eschar or gangrene distal to the most perfused tissue—usually the tips of the toes or an entire toe. This tissue must be kept dry until adequate arterial perfusion occurs. Moistened gangrenous tissue can provide a medium for bacterial growth. (See *Keeping gangrene dry*.)

Surgical treatment for arterial ulcers

Surgical treatment should be considered when patients have incapacitating claudication, rest pain, nonhealing ulcers, or progressive gangrene and infection that can not be controlled. For arterial ulcers, surgical treatment is aimed at restoring tissue perfusion. Bypass grafting may be done using prosthetic grafts or autogenous veins, either reversed or in situ. Percutaneous balloon angioplasty and stent insertions are options, but, other than the common iliac arteries, have poor long-term results, although results of some of these techniques are improving. Ulcers with large skin loss may need skin grafting to close the defect.

The treatment of ulceration due to arterial insufficiency depends on the level that the occlusive disease occurs. Surgeries for arterial insufficiency are generally grouped under three major areas:

- aortoiliac bypass
- femoropopliteal bypass
- distal bypass.

Restoring tissue perfusion

In many patients the occlusive disease is multileveled. The "rule of thumb" is to improve inflow first in these patients and then, if necessary, perform an outflow procedure. Usually inflow involves the aortoiliac segments. The exact surgery is tailored to the individual patient's physiologic status and need. For example, an elderly, frail patient with severe aortoiliac occlusive disease may not be a candidate for an aortobifemoral bypass graft. In this type of patient, an axillobifemoral bypass graft is considered. By avoiding intra-abdominal surgery and clamping of the abdominal aorta, the overall morbidity for these surgeries can be reduced. However, the trade-off for this is that an axillobifemoral bypass graft generally doesn't have the long-term patency rates that an aortobifemoral bypass graft does.

Percutaneous balloon angioplasty

A more recent development in the treatment of aortoiliac occlusive disease has been percutaneous balloon angioplasty with or without stent placement. Isolated short-segment stenoses can be successfully treated with balloon angioplasty. Short-segment stenoses are generally defined as those of less than 10 cm in length, commonly less than 5 cm. With more recent advancement in stent placements, acute occlusions occurring due to atherosclerotic plaque rebound have been decreased. The long-term patency rate for stents approaches that of arterial bypass but only in the aortoiliac segments. Infra-inguinal bal-

Keeping gangrene dry

Gangrenous tissue must be kept dry until adequate arterial perfusion is restored to the area. In the photograph below, the necrotic toes are left open to the air with alcohol wipes placed between them to promote drying.

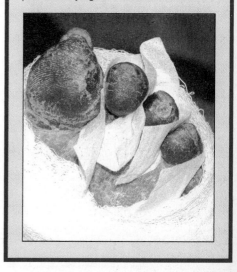

loon angioplasty with or without stent placement is still inferior treatment versus surgical intervention. However, this still holds a place in the treatment of high-risk patients.

Femoropopliteal bypass graft

A femoropopliteal bypass graft is the standard treatment for femoral popliteal disease. In contrast to an aortoiliac bypass, where the bypass conduit is that of a synthetic material, the femoropopliteal segment may have either a prosthetic conduit or an autogenous venous conduit. The patency rate for a bypass of the femoral popliteal segment depends upon the choice of conduit and the distal level of the bypass. In an above-knee femoropopliteal surgery, the patency rate between autogenous vein and prosthetic material has no significant difference, although long-term patency rates are better when an autogenous venous conduit is used. In a below-knee femoropopliteal bypass, prosthetic material is far inferi-

Graft patency rates

This chart shows the percentage of grafts that remain patent after 1, 2, 3, and 4 years.

Type of graft	1 year	2 years	3 years	4 years
ABOVE-KNEE FEMOROPOPLITEAL GRAFTS				
Reverse saphenous vein	84%	82%	73%	69%
Polytetrafluoroethylene (PTFE)	79%	74%	66%	60%
BELOW-KNEE FEMOROPOPLITEAL GRAFTS				
Reverse saphenous vein	84%	79%	78%	77%
PTFE	68%	61%	44%	40%
Limb salvage				
Reverse saphenous vein	90%	88%	86%	75%
In-situ vein bypass	94%	84%	83%	
INFRAPOPLITEAL GRAFTS				
Reverse saphenous vein	84%	80%	78%	76%
PTFE	46%	32%	21%	
Limb salvage				
Reverse saphenous vein	85%	83%	82%	82%
PTFE	68%	60%	56%	48%
AT OR BELOW-ANKLE GRAFTS				
Reverse saphenous vein	85%	81%	76%	
In-situ vein bypass	92%	82%	72%	
Foot salvage	93%	87%	84%	

or to that of autogenous venous conduits.[33] An autogenous venous conduit should be used in the below-knee position whenever possible. (See *Graft patency rates*.)

Below-knee femoropopliteal bypasses using veins have a higher patency rate than above-knee femoropopliteal bypasses because a certain amount of atherosclerotic disease at the level of the knee joint can be missed if only anterior-posterior arteriography views are obtained. For this reason, many vascular surgeons require oblique views of the popliteal artery so as to preclude this as a source of decreased long-term patency rates.

Distal bypass

A distal bypass, below the tibial perioneal trunk, requires an autogenous venous conduit. It's reserved for patients with tissue loss when pulsatile arterial perfusion to an ischemic area is desired. Although somewhat controversial, either a reversed venous bypass or an in situ bypass can be performed. Patency rates in large series regarding these two techniques is equivalent. The in situ technique is generally reserved for patients with considerable size disparity between the proximal and distal venous conduit, such as the greater saphenous vein. An in situ bypass is technically more demanding and requires more operative time than a reversed venous bypass. Nonetheless, the overall patency between the two techniques is equivalent. Some vascular surgeons advocate the use of prosthetic material for distal bypasses with the creation of a controlled arterial venous fistula in order to promote long-term patency rates of the prosthetic conduit.

A patient who has calf claudication requires improved perfusion to the posterior calf muscles. Claudication can occur in the buttocks, thighs, or to isolated compartments of the lower legs. The perfusion of the respective symptomatic musculature is what determines the level of the outflow portion of the bypass. In patients with combined aortoiliac superficial femoral popliteal disease, 90% of the claudication can be cured by merely improving the inflow to the profundal system by some form of aortoiliac bypass. It's for this reason that routine combined aorto-femoral and femoropopliteal bypasses should be avoided. In patients with lifestyle-limiting claudication with isolated superficial femoral artery disease, a femoropopliteal bypass is usually all that's required.

Patients with ischemic tissue loss commonly require pulsatile arterial flow to heal their lesions. If these lesions occur in the foot, then whatever bypass is necessary to restore pulsatile arterial flow to the affected area should be performed. If this requires a femoral distal bypass then this is usually the surgery chosen. Combined with the appropriate vascular bypass procedure, an area of ischemic tissue loss with gangrenous edges should be debrided to create viable tissue. However, in some patients, if the area of loss is that of dry gangrene, autoamputation can be anticipated once adequate perfusion is restored. Some clinicians allow the gangrenous eschar to autoamputate to enable normal epithelial coverage of the underlying eschar before eschar separation. If, however, the area of tissue loss involves a digit, amputation with primary closure may be recommended if no infection is present. This can be done in conjunction with the vascular bypass procedure, or the procedures can be separated by several days if deemed appropriate.

Arterial reconstruction with an in situ graft may be used to revascularize the lower extremity well below the knee. An in situ graft is a vein left in its natural location, anastomosed to the arterial system above and below the arterial stenoses, after the valves are lysed. This procedure allows the surgeon to reconstruct the smaller distal arteries in the lower extremity near the foot. These reconstructed vessels are close to the skin surface. The surgeon must use extreme care to not cause injury to underlying vessels when using sharp debridement for these necrotic ulcers. Autolytic debridement is a safer debriding alternative.

Medical treatment

The medical treatment of arterial disease may include the use of antiplatelet drugs, such as aspirin or clopidogrel, that inhibit the binding of adenosine triphosphate (ATP). Clopidogrel has been shown to be slightly better than aspirin in a comparative study.[34] In addition, cilostazol[35-37] has been used not only to decrease platelet aggregation, but also to act as a vasodilator that may facilitate an increase in exercise capacity. However, it can not be used in patients with heart failure. In addition, building up exercise tolerance with a conditioning program may also be important.

Measuring healing

Calculating healing rates is problematic when no standard measurement for wound healing parameters exists. Following wounds to complete healing is one method, but this method is not satisfactory if changes in therapy are needed. Healing rates can be expressed as percent of ulcer area, measurement of change in ulcer perimeter, or percent of ulcer area healed. However, the perimeter and surface area is much greater in large ulcers. Using these measurements will give erroneously high healing rates for larger ulcers compared with smaller ulcers. For example, if the percent of ulcer healed is used as a measurement, smaller ulcers will appear to heal faster than large ulcers by comparison.

In another method, ulcers are traced on a celluloid screen, then measured. The area and

---

PATIENT TEACHING

Teaching about arterial ulcers

Teach the patient with an arterial ulcer to:
- monitor arterial or graft patency by palpating pulses
- recognize signs and symptoms of graft failure and what to report
- avoid nicotine in any form
- begin or maintain a regular exercise program
- manage blood glucose, if diabetes is present
- control hyperlipidemia
- manage hypertension
- reduce weight, if indicated
- perform meticulous foot care
- manage ulcer care.

---

circumference of the tracing are calculated by a computer program. In general, a healing trajectory will be established if a wound is 20% to 40% smaller by week 4 and that wound should heal by week 12 provided that the same healing rate is maintained.[38-40]

However, there are some patients that do not heal at the expected rate. If tissue damage has progressed beyond salvage, surgery is too risky or the limitations of the ischemic limb are interfering with quality of life; amputation then must be considered.

Patient education

The patient may inadvertently neglect his ulcer or fail to use prevention measures if he doesn't understand the nature of the condition. Be sure to educate your patient about the reason the ulcer developed and the treatment rationale. Patient-centered concerns should be central to the treatment process and active involvement by the patient includes the recognition and reporting of changes that indicate problems with healing. Patient and family education should also include assessment of patient and family needs and level of comprehension about the arterial ulcer and its etiology. Teaching methods vary and should be chosen to facilitate the most appropriate method for the patient and his family.

Risk factors

Factors that increase risk for arteriosclerosis include smoking, diabetes, hyperlipemia, and hypertension.[41] Smoking is a risk factor in 73% to 90% of patients with atherosclerotic arterial disease. Up to 30% of patients with arterial disease are reported to have diabetes,[42] and of those patients with diabetes, 16% to 58% have arterial disease.[43-45] Hypertension is present in 29% to 39% of patients with atherosclerosis, and 31% to 57% of patients with atherosclerosis have hyperlipidemia.[42] Risk factor modification is part of the treatment for vascular ulcers to reduce the possibility of further breakdown.

Patients can help themselves by positioning and reducing activities that impair blood flow. After a surgical or percutaneous intervention to restore arterial flow, the patient should continue behaviors that promote vascular health and reduce risk factors. (See *Teaching about arterial ulcers*.)

Smoking cessation

Smoking cessation is critical for patients with arterial insufficiency. The direct relationship between tobacco use and ischemia is well-known. Smokers are nine times more likely to develop claudication than nonsmokers.[46] However, the link between smoking and vascular disease isn't well recognized by many patients; in one study, only 37% of smokers with peripheral vascular disease understood the strong association between smoking and vascular disease.[47] Patients must be informed of the negative effects of smoking on the vascular system and be referred to smoking cessation specialists if needed. Teach the patient the ABCDEs mnemonic to remember the risk factors of arterial disease.[11]

Summary

Success in managing arterial ulcers requires a total patient commitment. Risk factors and ulcer management are so dependent upon the patient's activities that the patient must have as much information as possible to participate in the treatment process. An understanding of the peripheral vascular blood supply and the need for adequate tissue oxygenation is critical to the management of arterial ulcers in the legs and feet.

Arterial reconstruction is the hallmark of treatment for arterial disease. In general, dry arterial ulcers or those with fixed, stable, dry eschar should be kept dry until the tissue is revascularized.. Economic concerns make it imperative to choose the appropriate dressings and treatment. Research demonstrates little increased benefit of the newer treatments over the old in healing rates; however, some modern wound dressings often improve quality-of-life and pain issues.

Show what you know

1. Risk factors for the development of arterial ulcers include all of the following except:

A. smoking.
B. hypercholesterolemia.
C. diabetes mellitus.
D. varicose veins.
E. hypertension.

ANSWER: D. Varicose veins of the lower legs are an early sign of venous insufficiency and the presence of venous disease is not a known risk factor for the development of arterial disease. Smoking, hypercholesterolemia, diabetes mellitus, and hypertension are risk factors for arterial disease.

2. Patients with arterial ulcers that do not have adequate blood supply to heal should have local wound care that includes:

A. aggressive local debridement to bleeding tissue.
B. silver dressings that promote moisture balance.
C. local antiseptics such as povidone-iodine and chlorhexidine.
D. moisture balance dressings such as a hydrogel.

ANSWER: C. In patients without the ability to heal, antimicrobials that will work with moisture reduction, such as povidone-iodine or chlorhexidine, are a necessary treatment. Other treatments include conservative debridement of the slough, moisture reduction, and antibacterials that work in a dry environment. For silver to be effective in a wound bed, it requires moisture to be converted to the ionized form and this is contraindicated in ulcers without the ability to heal.

3. Which of the following is most likely to be associated with an arterial ulcer?

A. Lipodermatosclerosis
B. Reduced blood flow
C. Edema
D. Systemic hypertension
E. Diabetes mellitus

ANSWER: B. An arterial ulcer by definition is always associated with arterial insufficiency or reduced blood flow (100%). Lipodermatosclerosis and edema are associated with venous ulcers. There is a less common but significant association of arterial ulcers with diabetes (30%) and hypertension in 29% to 39% of patients.

4. The ankle-brachial index (ABI) is an indicator of loss of perfusion in the lower extremity.

A. True
B. False

ANSWER: A. Perfusion of the lower extremity is indirectly measured by the ABI.

5. Surgical treatment for arterial ulcers most commonly includes:

A. a graft.
B. valvoplasty.
C. a bypass graft.
D. phlebectomy.

ANSWER: C. Arterial ulcers are associated with arterial insufficiency and a bypass graft is meant to restore the arterial circulation to the ischemic tissues. The other options are incorrect.

References

1. Young, J.R. "Differential Diagnosis of Leg Ulcers," *Cardiovascular Clinics* 13(2):171-93, 1983.
2. Cornwall, J.V., et al. "Leg Ulcers: Epidemiology and Aetiology," *British Journal of Surgery* 73(9):693, September 1986.
3. Coon, W.W., et al. "Venous Thromboembolism and Other Venous Disease in the Tecumseh Community Health Study," *Circulation* 48(4): 839-46, October 1973.
4. Dewolfe, V.G. "The Prevention and Management of Chronic Venous Insufficiency," *Practical Cardiology* 6:197-202, 1980.
5. Callam, M.J., et al. "Chronic Ulcers of the Leg: Clinical History," *British Medical Journal* (Clinical Research Edition) 294(6584):1389-91, May 30, 1987.

6. Nelzen, O., et al. "The Prevalence of Chronic Lower-limb Ulceration has been Underestimated: Results of a Validated Population Questionnaire," *British Journal of Surgery* 83(2):255-58, February 1996.

7. Rutherford, R.B. "The Vascular Consultation" in *Vascular Surgery,* Vol. 1, 4th ed. Philadelphia: W.B. Saunders Co., 1995.

8. Moore, W.S. (ed.) *Vascular Surgery: A Comprehensive Review,* Philadelphia: W.B. Saunders Co., 1991.

9. Browse, N.L., et al. *Diseases of the Veins: Pathology, Diagnosis, and Treatment.* London: Edward Arnold, 1988.

10. Phillips, T.J., and Dover, J.S. "Leg Ulcers," *Journal of the American Academy of Dermatology* 25(6 Pt 1):965-89, December 1991.

11. Sibbald, R.G, and Ayello, E.A. "Assessing Arterial Disease History Using ABCDE'S Mnemonic." E-alert. *Advances in Skin and Wound Care.* (In Press) 2007.

12. Aronow, W.S. "Management of Peripheral Arterial Disease," *Cardiology in Review* 13(2):61-68, March-April 2005.

13. Lubdbrook, J., et al. "Significance of Absent Ankle Pulse," *British Medical Journal* 1:1724, 1962.

14. Mayfield, J.A., Sugarman, J.R. "The Use of the Semmes-Weinstein Monofilament and Other Threshold Tests for Preventing Foot Ulceration and Amputation in Persons with Diabetes," *Journal of Family Practice* 49(11 Suppl):S17-S29, November 2000.

15. Taylor, L.M., and Porter, J.M. "Natural History and Nonoperative Treatment of Chronic Lower Extremity Ischemia" in *Vascular Surgery: A Comprehensive Review.* Edited by Moore, W.S. Philadelphia: W.B. Saunders Co., 1993.

16. Blank, C.A., and Irwin, G.H. "Peripheral Vascular Disorders: Assessment and Intervention," *Nursing Clinics of North America* 25(4):777-94, December 1990.

17. Fahey, V.A., and White, S.A. "Physical Assessment of the Vascular System" in *Vascular Nursing.* Edited by Fahey, V.A. Philadelphia: W.B. Saunders Co., 1994.

18. Baker, J.D. "Assessment of Peripheral Arterial Occlusive Disease," *Critical Care Nursing Clinics of North America* 3(3):493-98, September 1991.

19. Brantigan, C.O. "Peripheral Vascular Disease: A Comparison between the Vascular Laboratory and the Arteriogram in Diagnosis and Management," *Colorado Medicine* 77(9):320-27, September 1980.

20. Winsor, T. "Influence of Arterial Disease on the Systolic Blood Pressure Gradients of the Extremity," *American Journal of Medical Science* 220, 1950.

21. Sibbald, R.G, et al. "Preparing the Wound Bed 2003: Focus on Infection and Inflammation," *Ostomy/Wound Management* 49(11):24-51, November 2003.

22. Sibbald, R.G, et al. "Best Practice Recommendations for Preparing the Wound Bed: Update 2006," *Wound Care Canada* 4(1):R6-R18, 2006.

23. Sibbald, R.G., et al. "Increased Bacterial Burden and Infection: The Story of NERDS and STONES," *Advances in Skin and Wound Care* 19(8):462-63, October 2006.

24. Grayson, M.L., et al. "Probing to Bone in Infected Pedal Ulcers. A Clinical Sign of Underlying Osteomyelitis in Diabetic Patients," *JAMA* 273(9):721-23, March 1, 1995.

25. Lineaweaver, W., et al. "Topical Antimicrobial Toxicity," *Archives of Surgery* 120(3):267-270, March 1985.

26. Lineaweaver, W., et al. "Cellular and Bacteriologic Toxicities of Topical Antimicrobials," *Plastic & Reconstructive Surgery* 75(3):94-96, March 1985.

27. Cooper, M., et al. "The Cytotoxic Effects of Commonly Used Topical Antimicrobial Agents on Human Fibroblasts and Keratinocytes," *Journal of Trauma* 31(6):775-84, June 1991.

28. McCauley, R.L., et al. "In Vitro Toxicity of Topical Antimicrobial Agents to Human Fibroblasts," *Journal of Surgical Research* 46(3):267-74, March 1989.

29. Maklebust, J. "Using Wound Care Products to Promote a Healing Environment," *Critical Care Nursing Clinics of North America* 8(2):141-58, June 1996.

30. Maklebust, J., and Sieggreen, M. *Pressure Ulcers: Guidelines for Prevention and Management,* 3rd ed., Springhouse, Pa.: Springhouse Corp., 2001.

31. Niederhuber, S.S., et al. "Reduction of Skin Bacterial Load with Use of Therapeutic Whirlpool," *Physical Therapy* 55(5):482-86, May 1975.

32. Husni, E.A. "Skin Ulcers Secondary to Arterial and Venous Disease," in *Chronic Ulcers of the Skin.* Edited by Lee, B.Y. New York: McGraw Hill, 1985.

33. Dalman, R.L. "Long-term Results of Bypass Procedures in *Basic Data Underlying Clinical Decision Making in Vascular Surgery.* Edited by Porter, J.M. and Taylor, L.M. *Annals of Vascular Surgery* 141-43, 1995.

34. CAPRIE Steering Committee. "A Randomised, Blinded, Trial of Clopidogrel versus Aspirin in Patients at Risk of Ischaemic Events," *Lancet* 348:1329-39, 1996.

35. Hughson, W.G., et al. "Intermittent Claudication: Prevalence and Risk Factors," *British Medical Journal* 1(6124):1377-79, May 27, 1978.

36. Clyne, CA., et al. "Smoking, Ignorance, and Peripheral Vascular Disease," *Archives of Surgery* 117(8):1062, August 1982.

37. Cavezzi-Marconi, P. "Manual Lymphatic Drainage," in *Phlebolymphoedema: From Diagnosis to Therapy.* Edited by Cavezzi, A., and Michelini, S. Bologna, Italy: Edizioni PR, PR Communications, 1998.

38. Falanga, V., et al. "Initial Rate of Healing Predicts Complete Healing of Venous Ulcers," *Archives of Dermatology* 133(10):1231-34, October 1997.

39. Margolis, D.J., et al. "The Accuracy of Venous Leg Ulcer Prognostic Models in a Wound Care System," *Wound Repair and Regeneration* 12(2):163-68, March-April 2004.

40. Margolis, D.J., and Kantor, J. "A Multicentre Study of Percentage Change in Venous Leg Ulcer Area as a Prognostic Index of Healing at 24 Weeks," *British Journal of Dermatology* 142(5):960-64, May 2000.

41. Barnes, R.W. "The Arterial System" In *Essentials of Surgery.* Edited by Sabiston, D.C. Philadelphia: W.B. Saunders Co., 1987.

42. Coffman, J.D. "Principles of Conservative Treatment of Occlusive Arterial Disease" in *Clinical Vascular Disease.* Edited by Spittell, J.A. Philadelphia: F.A. Davis, 1983.

43. Kilo, C. "Vascular Complications of Diabetes," *Cardiovascular Reviews & Reports* 8(6):18-23, June 1987.

44. Levin, M.E., and Sicard, G.A. "Evaluating and Treating Diabetic Peripheral Vascular Disease: Part 1," *Clinical Diabetes* 62-70, May-June 1987.

45. Dowdell, H.R. "Diabetes and Vascular Disease: A Common Association," *AACN Clinical Issues* 6(4):526-35, November 1995.

46. Hughson, W.G., et al. "Intermittent Claudication: Prevalence and Risk Factors," *British Medical Journal* 1(6124):1377-79, May 27, 1978.

47. Clyne, CA., et al. "Smoking, Ignorance, and Peripheral Vascular Disease," *Archives of Surgery* 117(8):1062, August 1982.

CHAPTER 16

Diabetic foot ulcers

Lawrence A. Lavery, DPM, MPh
James McGuire, DPM, PT, CPed, CWS, FAPWCA
Sharon Baranoski, MSN, RN, CWOCN, APN, DAPWCA, FAAN
Elizabeth A. Ayello, PhD, RN, APRN,BC, CWOCN, FAPWCA, FAAN

OBJECTIVES

After completing this chapter, you'll be able to:

- state the significance of foot ulcers in patients with diabetes as a health care problem

- list strategies for preventing foot ulcers in patients with diabetes mellitus

- describe wound characteristics and assessment parameters for a patient with diabetes mellitus

- list options for reducing pressure for a patient with diabetes mellitus with a foot ulcer

- discuss the rationale for use of diagnostic imaging.

Diabetes: A growing problem

The American Diabetes Association (ADA) defines diabetes as "a disease in which the body doesn't produce or properly use insulin." Diabetes incidence has increased 48% in the last 10 years, with a 70% increase in patients in their 30s. However, of the 20.8 million Americans (7% of the population) who have diabetes, only 14.6 million are diagnosed, leaving over one-third, or 6.2 million, people unaware that they have diabetes. Blacks, Hispanics, Native Americans, and Asian-Americans have the highest prevalence of diabetes mellitus.[2]

Between 5% and 10% of people with diabetes have type 1 diabetes—the autoimmune form of the disorder that causes destruction of pancreatic b-cells and requires insulin therapy to prevent life- threatening complications. Type 1 diabetes is characterized by a sudden onset of clinical signs and symptoms associated with hyperglycemia, with a strong propensity for the development of ketoacidosis. However, although the clinical onset may be abrupt, the pathophysiologic insult is a slow, progressive phenomenon.[2]

Between 90% and 95% (or 19.7 million Americans) have type 2 diabetes, making it the most common form of diabetes mellitus[1]; it's also severely underdiagnosed.[3] Indeed, almost 30% of patients with type 2 diabetes don't know it.[3] This failure to diagnose this patient population results in progressive morbidity and mortality, with severe insulin resistance existing for years before the onset of hyperglycemia. Patients with type 2 diabetes have this relative insulin deficiency because their bodies either fail to make enough insulin or are unable to use insulin properly. Additionally, type 2 diabetes is a heterogeneous disorder for which specific secondary genetic causes of the metabolic syndrome are being rapidly identified. Type 2 diabetes, which is usually seen in older adults, is now being seen in a much younger population.[2]

Diabetes is the single most common underlying cause of lower-extremity amputation in the United States. Foot problems are one of the most common complications in diabetics leading to hospitalization.[4-7] Indeed, admissions for foot complications account for 20% to 25% of all hospital days for patients with diabetes.[4,8,9] In the United States, there are approximately 120,000 nontraumatic lower-extremity amputations performed each year, with 45% to 83% of these amputations involving patients with diabetes.[7,10,11] The risk of lower-extremity amputation in diabetics is 15 to 46 times higher than in nondiabetic patients.[4,5,7,10] After the initial amputation, the risk of reamputation or amputation of the contralateral extremity is also high—9% to 17% of patients will experience a second amputation within the same year[4,12] and 25% to 68% will have an amputation of the contralateral extremity within 3 to 5 years.[4,13,14] The 5-year survival rate after a lower-extremity amputation ranges from 41% to 70%.[10,14]

Diabetes is a contributing factor in 75% to 83% of all amputations among Blacks, Hispanics, and Native Americans.[4,7,15] The incidence of lower-extremity amputation is 1.5 times higher in Hispanics and 2.1 times higher in Blacks compared to non-Hispanic whites. (See *ADA contact information.*)

Etiology and risk factors of foot ulcers

A number of local and systemic risk factors for foot ulceration and amputations should be considered in the prevention and treatment of the diabetic foot. (See *Ulceration and amputation risk factors in diabetic patients,*

ADA contact information

The American Diabetes Association (ADA)[2] offers much information for the diabetic patient and his family, as well as for health care professionals. General information about diabetes is available, along with advice on exercise, nutrition, and daily meal planning. To contact the ADA:

1701 N. Beauregard Street
Alexandria, VA 22311
1-800-DIABETES
www.diabetes.org

page 340.) Perhaps the strongest and easiest risk factor to identify is the presence of a previous ulceration or amputation, which indicates the potential for recurrence due to scar formation or biomechanical abnormalities. The underlying pathology usually isn't reversible, and most disease processes affecting the diabetic foot will continue to worsen over time.

Neuropathy
In patients with neuropathy, pain, the primary natural warning system that alerts the body to take action and seek medical care, is defective. Diabetic neuropathy alters the biomechanics of the foot, which causes increased shear and pressure on the sole, resulting in an increased risk for injury and complications. Usually, patients with diabetes present with sensory, motor, and autonomic neuropathy, all of which have a devastating impact on multiple systems in the foot.

Sensory neuropathy contributes to an inability to perceive injury to the foot due to what's commonly referred to as loss of protective sensation or LOPS.[16] Motor neuropathy contributes to wasting of the intrinsic muscles of the foot; muscle imbalance; structural foot deformity, such as claw toes and subluxated metatarsophalangeal joints; and limited joint mobility. Autonomic neuropathy

Ulceration and amputation risk factors in diabetic patients

Risk factor	Relative risk or odds ratio
LOCAL RISK FACTORS	
History of foot ulcer or amputation	1.6 to 18
Sensory neuropathy	2.2 to 18.4
Structural foot deformity (hallux valgus, claw toes) or limited joint mobility (hallux rigidus, equinus)	3.3 to 3.5
Peripheral vascular disease	2.4 to 3.0
Abnormal foot pressures	2.0 to 5.9
SYSTEMIC RISK FACTORS	
Hypertension	
Hyperlipidemia	1.02 to 2.13
Hyperglycemia	1.02 to 6.4
Male gender	1.3 to 3.2
Duration of diabetes	2.6 to 5.2
Age over 65	1.06 to 3.0
Retinopathy	2.0
Poor vision	1.07 to 3.7
Proteinuria	1.9
Obesity	2.4
	1.2

Adapted with permission from Lavery, L.A., and Gazewood, J.D. "Assessing the Feet of Patients with Diabetes," *Journal of Family Practice* 49(11 Suppl):S9-S16, November 2000.

causes shunting of blood[17] and loss of sweat and oil gland function, which leads to dry, scaly skin that can easily develop cracks and fissures. The combined effect of these neuropathies results in a foot that can't respond to pain and with severe biomechanical impairment, and skin that's poorly nourished and hydrated.

Neuropathy is one of the most prominent risk factors of lower extremity complications[7,16], such as full-thickness ulcerations, with sensory neuropathy as a pivotal component of the critical pathway for the development of ulcers and amputations. Three primary pathways or mechanisms of injury have been identified in the development of foot ulcers. They include wounds that result from ill-fitting shoes (low-pressure injuries that are associated with prolonged or constant pressure), ulcers on weight-bearing areas (repetitive moderate pressure and shear forces on the sole), and penetrating injuries from puncture wounds or other traumatic events (high-pressure injuries with a single exposure of direct pressure).

Several screening methods can be used to identify sensory neuropathy, including vibration testing with a 128 Hz tuning fork (shown top of next page), vibration perception threshold (VPT) testing with a VPT Tester (Xilas Medical San Antonio, Texas), and pressure assessment with Semmes-Weinstein monofilaments (SWM).[16,18,19] Although these methods are noninvasive and

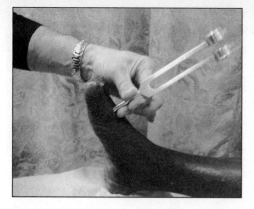

have good sensitivity and specificity to identify patients with loss of protective sensation,[20] the SWM, in particular, may present several problems, which should be considered before using it. SWM should be purchased from a vendor that sells calibrated instruments because considerable variability exists among different brands of monofilament.[21] Booth and Young found that some brands of monofilaments buckle at greater than 8 g of force rather than the 10 g for which they're designated.[21] In addition, the material properties of the monofilament wear out after repetitive testing. Young and colleagues[22] found that after 500 cycles of testing (or the equivalent of testing 10 sites on each foot for 25 patients) there was an average reduction of 1.2 g of testing force. A worn-out monofilament may result in patients being diagnosed as having LOPS when they are not at risk. (See *Assessing protective sensation with a monofilament,* page 342.)

For more consistent testing, a VPT testing instrument or VPT meter is useful. The VPT is a quantitative device that measures large nerve function. It's less prone to inter-operator variation than the monofilaments and it doesn't need to be replaced to continue providing accurate results. The VPT meter (XILAS Medical, San Antonio, Texas) is a hand-held device with a rubber head that's applied to a bony prominence, such as the medial aspect of the first metatarsal head or the tip of the great toe. The unit contains a linear scale that displays the applied voltage, ranging from 0 to 100 volts. The amplitude is then slowly increased until the patient can feel the vibration. The inability to feel greater than

25 volts is indicative of loss of protective sensation and puts the patient at risk of ulceration and amputation.

Wunderlich[20] and Armstrong[16] suggested using a combination of modalities—the SWM, a VPT test, and the University of Texas Subjective Peripheral Neuropathy Verbal Questionnaire, a simple four-question evaluation—to optimize screening for neuropathy. Using a single instrument to diagnose sensory neuropathy with loss of protective sensation will probably miss a subgroup of "at-risk" patients. (See *University of Texas Subjective Peripheral Neuropathy Verbal Questionnaire,* page 343.)

Peripheral vascular disease

Peripheral vascular disease (PVD) in patients with diabetes is characterized by multiple occlusive plaques of small- and medium-sized arteries of the infrapopliteal vessels.[17] PVD puts the patient with diabetes at greater risk for foot ulcers, infections, and amputations.[7,23] Several theories attempt to explain the microvascular changes that occur in diabetes mellitus. One theory proposes that increased microvascular pressure and flow results in injury to the vascular endothelium, which, in turn, causes the release of extravascular matrix proteins. This results in microvascular sclerosis and thickening of the capillary basement membrane. Capillary fragility also leads to micro-hemorrhage, which could be the reason that infection spreads through the tissue planes in patients with diabetes.[17,24] LoGerfo and colleagues[25,26] believe that there is no microcirculatory occlusive process; rather, they suggest that some other physiologic abnormality occurs.

Evaluating vascular status should include a thorough history of symptoms of intermittent claudication, ischemic rest pain, and peripheral vascular surgery; clinical signs of ischemia, such as skin temperature, dependent rubor, pallor, hair loss, and shiny skin; and a clinical assessment of lower-extremity pulses.[27]

If pulses can't be palpated during the assessment, use a Doppler ultrasound to assess for pulsatile flow and to calculate an ankle-

PRACTICE POINT

Assessing protective sensation with a monofilament

A Semmes-Weinstein 10-g (5.07 log) monofilament is commonly used to assess protective sensation in the feet of patients with diabetes. You can order the Semmes-Weinstein monofilament from the following companies:
- Center for Specialized Diabetic Foot Care: 1-800-543-9055
- North Coast Medical, Inc.: 408-283-1900
- Sensory Testing Systems: 1-888-289-9293
- Smith & Nephew Rehabilitation Division: 1-800-558-8633.

Use the 10-g (5.07 log) monofilament wire on each foot at the following 10 sites:
- plantar aspect of the first, third, and fifth digits
- plantar aspect of the first, third, and fifth metatarsal heads
- plantar midfoot medially and laterally
- plantar heel
- dorsal aspect of the midfoot.

Performing the test

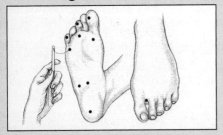

Place the patient in a supine or sitting position. Remove his socks and shoes and provide support for his legs. Touch the monofilament to the patient's arm or hand to demonstrate what it feels like. Then ask him to respond "yes" each time he feels the monofilament on his foot.

Place the patient's foot in a neutral position with his toes pointing straight up, and tell him to close his eyes. Remind him to say "yes" when he feels the monofilament on his foot. Hold the monofilament perpendicular to the patient's foot and press it against the first site, increasing the pressure until the monofilament wire bends into a C shape. Make sure it doesn't slide over the skin. Hold the monofilament in place for about 1 second. Record the patient's response on a foot-screening form. Use a "+" for a positive response and a "-" for a negative response. Then move to the next site.

Test all 10 sites at random and vary the time between applications so that the patient won't be able to guess the correct response. If he has a scar, callus, or necrotic tissue at a test site, apply the monofilament along the perimeter of the abnormality, not directly on it.

Loss of protective sensation is indicated if the patient can't feel the monofilament at any site on his foot. It's essential to teach a patient who has lost protective sensation to inspect and protect his feet.

Adapted with permission from Sloan, H.L., and Abel, R.J. "Getting in Touch with Impaired Foot Sensitivity," *Nursing* 28(11):50-51, November 1998, and from Armstrong, D.G., et al. "Choosing a Practical Screening Instrument to Identify Patients at Risk for Diabetic Foot Ulceration," *Archives of Internal Medicine* 158(3):289-92, February 9, 1998.

brachial index (see *Obtaining an ankle-brachial index* in chapter 15, Arterial ulcers).

Skin and nail examination
Evaluation of the skin and nails is critical to identify the subtle signs of impending injury;

high-pressure areas, cracks, maceration, or fissures in the skin. (See *Skin-care teaching tips*.)

Discoloration of a callus or bleeding under a callus is a sign of a preulcerative lesion. Likewise, deformed and thickened nails are commonly the source of abnormal pressure on the nail bed or ingrown toenails. Common nail disorders seen in patients with diabetes mellitus include onychomycosis (tinea unguium) and onychocryptosis (ingrown toenail).[27] While these are usually minor problems in nondiabetic adults, they can result in cellulitis and osteomyelitis in patients with diabetes, neuropathy, and vascular impairment.

Musculoskeletal examination

In patients with neuropathy, ulcerations typically develop as a result of repetitive pressure and shear on the sole of the foot or from shoe pressure on the top or sides of the foot; however, no clear level of pressure has been

---

University of Texas Subjective Peripheral Neuropathy Verbal Questionnaire

- Do your feet ever feel numb?
- Do your feet ever tingle, as if electricity were traveling into your foot?
- Do your feet ever feel as if insects were crawling on them?
- Do your feet ever burn?[20]

PATIENT TEACHING

Skin-care teaching tips

Teach your diabetic patient the following self-care points:

- Keep your diabetes well controlled. People with high sugar levels tend to have dry skin and less ability to fend off harmful bacteria. Both conditions increase the risk of infection.
- Keep skin clean and dry. Use talcum powder in areas where skin touches skin, such as armpits and groin.
- Avoid very hot baths and showers. If your skin is dry, don't use bubble baths. Moisturizing soaps, such as Dove or Basis, may help. Afterward, use an oil-in-water skin cream, such as Lubriderm or Alpha-Keri. Don't put lotions between your toes—the extra moisture there can encourage fungus to grow.
- Prevent dry skin. Moisturize your skin to prevent chapping.
- Don't scratch dry or itchy skin because doing so can tear the skin, allowing infection to occur.
- Treat cuts right away. Wash minor cuts

with soap and water. Don't use mercurochrome antiseptic, alcohol, or iodine to clean skin because these agents are too harsh. Use an antibiotic cream or ointment only if your doctor says it's okay. Cover minor cuts with sterile gauze. See a doctor right away if you get a major cut, burn, or infection.
- During cold, dry months, keep your home more humid. Bathe less during this weather if possible.
- Use mild shampoos and unscented soaps. Don't use feminine hygiene sprays.
- See a dermatologist about skin problems if you aren't able to solve them yourself.
- Take good care of your feet. Check them every day for sores and cuts. Wear broad, flat shoes that fit well. Check your shoes for foreign objects before putting them on.

Ulcers on digital deformities

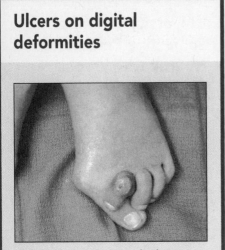

Photograph: J. McGuire. Used with permission.

Metatarsal ulcer

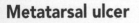

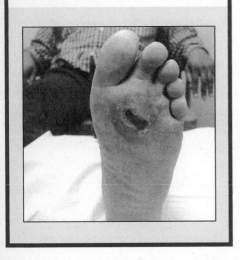

determined to be abnormal or pathologic.[7,28-30] Diabetes alters the biomechanics of patients with preexisting structural and functional foot deformities. Motor neuropathy is thought to contribute to atrophy and weakness of the intrinsic muscles of the foot. This leads to the "intrinsic minus foot" and contributes to the development of high-pressure areas that are predisposed to ulceration.

Ulcers can also occur when digital deformities (cocked-up toes, hammer toes, or claw toes) are irritated by the toe box, or the insole of the shoes. (See *Ulcers on digital deformities.*) The lesser digits contract and sublux dorsally, resulting in a claw toe deformity and a strong plantar flexor force that's produced at the metatarsophalangeal joints.[17,28,31] In many instances, this combination of deformities literally pushes the head of the metatarsal through the bottom of the foot. Limited joint mobility of the ankle and metatarsophalangeal joints, as a result of glycosylation of the gastro-soleus-achilles complex and the peri-articular tissues, further increases pressure on the plantar aspect of the foot. The tips and dorsal aspects of the toes and the area beneath the metatarsophalangeal heads are subjected to increased pressure and friction which, in the presence of loss of protective sensation, can lead to ulceration.[17,28,32] (See *Metatarsal ulcer.*)

Risk stratification

Evaluation of risk factors and risk stratification is important to prioritize the patient's treatment according to their individual needs.[42] Many health care providers either never evaluate the feet or generally consider everyone with diabetes to be "at-risk" for foot problems. This usually leads to no preventive care, but it can also contribute to unnecessary services for low-risk patients. To help evaluate individual risk factors, a risk classification system endorsed by the International Working Group on the Diabetic Foot[42] provides a validated scheme to stratify subjects based on their risk of ulceration and amputation. Key elements of the lower extremity examination should help to risk stratify subjects and identify the frequency and level of preventive care. (See *International consensus on the diabetic foot: Risk categorization.*)

Multidisciplinary strategies

Many strategies are involved in preventing foot complications. Although the specific elements of a multispecialty approach to pre-

EVIDENCE-BASED PRACTICE

International consensus on the diabetic foot: Risk categorization

Category	Risk factors	Ulcer incidence	Amputation incidence	Prevention and treatment
0	No sensory neuropathy	2% to 6%	0	• Reevaluation once a year
1	Sensory neuropathy	6% to 9%	0	• Podiatry every 6 months • Over-the-counter shoes and insoles; evaluate appropriate fit
2	Sensory neuropathy and foot deformity or peripheral vascular disease	8% to 17%	1% to 3%	• Podiatry every 2 to 3 months • Professionally fit therapeutic shoes and insoles • Patient education
3	Previous ulcer or amputations	26% to 78%	10% to 18%	• Podiatry every 1 to 2 months • Professionally fit therapeutic shoes and insoles • Patient education

Adapted with permission from Peters, E.J., and Lavery, L.A. "Effectiveness of the Diabetic Foot Risk Classification System of the International Working Group on the Diabetic Foot," *Diabetes Care* 24(8): 1442-47, August 2001, and from Rith-Najarian, S.J., et al. "Identifying Diabetic Patients at High-Risk for Lower-Extremity Amputation in a Primary Health Care Setting. A Prospective Evaluation of Simple Screening Criteria," *Diabetes Care* 15(10):1386-950, October 1992.

vention haven't been studied, both systemic disease factors and local treatment are believed to be pivotal elements of long-term prevention.

Careful management of systemic disease processes, such as heart failure, renal insufficiency, and diabetes is essential in order to minimize complications. It's critical to control glucose levels to slow the multiple disease processes involved in diabetes-related foot complications. Indeed, hyperglycemia has been associated with higher risk of ulceration and poor healing response in patients with diabetes.[7] Effective glycemic control can be achieved through a comprehensive team effort that addresses dietary management, self-glucose monitoring, proper exercise, ap-

propriate medication, and early recognition and treatment of hyperglycemia.[17]

Several clinical studies have reported a 48% to 78%[33,34] reduction in amputations and a 47% to 49%[35,36] reduction of lower-extremity–related hospitalizations when high-risk diabetic patients are treated in specialty clinics. Indeed, specialty clinics often include multiple specialties that focus on both prevention and care of acute complications. Further, consensus documents for prevention measures related to the "diabetic foot" have been developed by the American Orthopaedic Foot and Ankle Society,[37] the American College of Foot and Ankle Surgery[38], the Registered Nurses' Association of Ontario (www.rnao.org), and the International Working Group on the Diabetic Foot.

Wide-toe shoe with insert

Shoes with a deep toe-box and that are "extra depth" throughout the shoe are the mainstay of diabetic wound preventive care. The shoes typically come with laces, as shown here, or with Velcro closures.

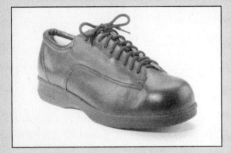

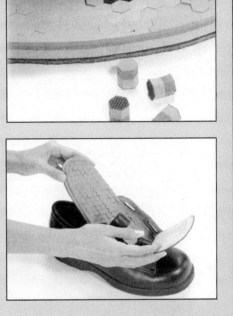

The combination of a correctly sized shoe and an accommodative insole can reduce pressure on the sole, top, and sides of the foot. The insert is customized to relieve pressure, according to the patient's needs, and then placed inside the shoe.

Photographs courtesy of Royce Medical Co.

Frykberg[30] lists the 5 Ps of prevention as meant to provide a mechanism to remind us that preventive care never ends. Diabetes and subsequent foot problems are part of an insidious disease process and require persistent attention and positive reinforcement for the rest of a high-risk patient's life.

 PRACTICE POINT

The 5 Ps of diabetic ulcer prevention:
- podiatry care—persistence
- protective shoes—patience
- pressure reduction—positive reinforcement
- prophylactic surgery—planning
- preventive education—positive attitude.

Podiatric care

Regular foot evaluation is essential to identify new risk factors and prevent impending complications. Podiatric physicians provide for debridement of callus and nails and regular evaluation of shoes and insoles. These routine encounters offer an additional opportunity to reinforce key educational elements, such as the need to avoid going barefoot, hydrate the skin, and inspect the feet daily. Protective footwear and insoles can be prescribed for the patient and then evaluated and monitored for their effectiveness.

Protective footwear and pressure redistribution

The primary role of therapeutic footwear is to protect the foot from repetitive injuries and eliminate the shoe as a source of pathology. Extra depth shoes have a high toe-box with enough depth throughout the shoe to accommodate a total contact molded insole or orthotic. These are often recommended for patients with structural foot deformities, such as claw toes or dislocated metatarsophalangeal joints. These types of shoes usually allow for up to a ⅜"-thick accommodive insole to fit without irritating the top or sides of the foot. (See *Wide-toe shoe with insert.*) The combination of a correctly sized shoe and a protective insole can reduce pressure on the sole, top, and sides of the foot by as much as 20%.[39,40]

Custom-molded shoes are individually made from a mold of the patient's foot. However, because custom-molded shoes can be expensive and can take several weeks or months to make, they're only necessary in a small percentage of high-risk patients with severe foot deformities that can't be accommodated in off-the-shelf shoes.

For patients with less severe deformity, there are a number of more affordable athletic, comfort, and therapeutic shoes with multiple sizes and the extra depth to accommodate a wide variety of foot deformities.

The diabetic shoe bill

Patients with diabetes that are "at risk" for foot disease and who have Medicare Part B are eligible for Medicare's Therapeutic Shoe Bill.[68] In order for a patient to qualify, they must have diabetes and one or more of the following: previous amputation of part or all of either foot; history of a previous foot ulceration; history of preulcerative calluses; peripheral neuropathy, with evidence of callus formation; foot deformity; or poor circulation.

The bill covers one of the following annually: one pair of off-the-shelf depth shoes and three additional pairs of multidensity inserts or custom molded orthoses; one pair of off-the-shelf depth shoes, including a modification and 2 additional pairs of multidensity inserts; or one pair of custom-molded shoes and two additional pairs of multidensity inserts.

PATIENT TEACHING

Always remind your patients to wear properly fitting shoes and insoles to prevent ulceration and recurrence after a foot ulcer has healed.

Prophylactic surgery

Armstrong and colleagues validated a four-tier surgery classification that consists of elective, prophylactic, curative, and emergent surgery. Elective surgery is a planned reconstructive surgery in a patient with foot deformity to eliminate pain or to enhance function. Prophylactic surgery is intended to prevent ulcer recurrence. Curative surgery is intended to facilitate wound healing in a patient with an existing foot wound. Emergent surgery is intended to remove infection or devitalized tissue.[86]

Surgical procedures that fit within the above categories include correcting toe deformities, bunionectomies, achilles tendon lengthening, exostectomy, and amputation. For example, percutaneous lengthening of the Achilles tendon[41] has been shown to reduce foot pressures on the sole in subjects with prior ulceration. This type of surgery has been used as prophylactic and curative.

Lin[84] reported on a cohort of patients with diabetic foot ulcers that had failed to heal after a period of treatment with total contact cast (TCC) immobilization. Using the Achilles lengthening procedure, however, 93% of patients (14/15) healed (on average) in 39 days with no subsequent ulcer recurrence in 17 months.[84] Mueller evaluated the same procedure in a randomized clinical trial and compared neuropathic ulcer healing using TCC immobilization.[85] All of the patients who underwent the surgery healed (n=31) as compared with 88% (n=33) of patients who healed in the TCC group. Further, patients with Achilles lengthening had less than half the incidence of ulcer recurrence (31% vs. 81%) compared to patients in the TCC group.

Preventive education

Many patients receive education during the period when they are initially diagnosed with diabetes. However, continual education and reinforcement is necessary, especially among high-risk patients. In a study of ulcer risk factors, a large proportion of patients both with and without foot ulcers lacked the visual acuity, manual dexterity, or joint flexibility to perform self-examination of their feet. Among ulcer patients, 49% could not position or see their feet, and 15% were legally blind in at least one eye. When patients are obese or have limited joint mobility or impaired vision, education and self-assessment skills should be addressed as well as to the spouse or caregiver.[7] Repetition and positive reinforcement should be practiced by every member of the health care team to help the patient and his family understand the disease process and protection practices.

Temperature monitoring

Home temperature monitoring is a new concept (TempTouch, Xilas Medical, San Antonio, Texas [shown below]) for high-risk pa-

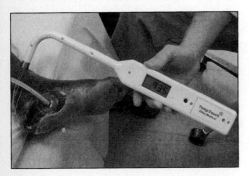

tients to identify early warning signs of tissue injury before a foot ulcer actually develops. Because neuropathy inhibits our natural warning system, local inflammation and pain as a result of tissue trauma go unnoticed. Several studies have used temperature assessment as a surrogate to identify tissue injury in patients "at-risk" for diabetic foot ulcers and pressure ulcers. Indeed, three randomized clinical trials, using temperature assessment, demonstrated a 3- to 10-fold reduction in foot complications among high-risk patients as compared to standard prevention

therapy, consisting of therapeutic shoes and insoles, regular podiatry evaluation, and foot-specific education.[82]

There are two main barriers that contribute to poor results with "standard" prevention practices. First, patients often can't visualize their feet in order to evaluate them.[7] Second, the visual signs of tissue injury are probably too subtle for even the most motivated patient or family member to accurately identify. For instance, in a randomized study by Lavery and colleagues,[83] by the time patients identified "areas of concern," an ulcer had already developed in the majority of patients. Therefore, self-monitoring with an infrared temperature device provides a mechanism to identify the precursor to ulcer and gives the high-risk patient enough time to reduce their activity in order to avoid it.

PRACTICE POINT

Home temperature monitoring can provide objective feedback to warn patients with neuropathy that their feet are injured before an ulcer develops.

Wound characteristics and assessment

Several classification systems can be used to classify diabetic ulcers. The University of Texas ulcer classification system is a validated system that includes a mechanism to document wound depth and the presence of infection and vascular impairment—two pivotal factors in predicting clinical outcomes.[6,43] (See *University of Texas diabetic wound classification system.*) The risk of amputation has been shown to be predictive of amputation as wounds increase in depth (Grade 0 to III) and progress from no infection (Class A), to infection (Class B), to peripheral vascular disease (PVD) (Class C), and to infection and PVD (Class D) using the University of Texas system.

A classification scheme first described by Meggitt[44] and popularized by Wagner[45] has also been used extensively, but has the disad-

University of Texas diabetic wound classification system

	Grade 0	Grade I	Grade II	Grade III
A	Preulcerative or postulcerative lesion, completely epithelialized	Superficial wound, not involving tendon, capsule, or bone	Wound penetrating to tendon or capsule	Wound penetrating to bone or joint
B	Preulcerative or postulcerative lesion, completely epithelialized with infection	Superficial wound, not involving tendon, capsule, or bone with infection	Wound penetrating to tendon or capsule with infection	Wound penetrating to bone or joint with infection
C	Preulcerative or postulcerative lesion, completely epithelialized with ischemia	Superficial wound, not involving tendon, capsule, or bone with ischemia	Wound penetrating to tendon or capsule with ischemia	Wound penetrating to bone or joint with ischemia
D	Preulcerative or postulcerative lesion, completely epithelialized with infection and ischemia	Superficial wound, not involving tendon, capsule, or bone with infection and ischemia	Wound penetrating to tendon or capsule with infection and ischemia	Wound penetrating to bone or joint with infection and ischemia

Reprinted with permission from Armstrong, D.G., et al. "Validation of a Diabetic Wound Classification System: The Contribution of Depth, Infection, and Ischemia to Risk of Amputation," *Diabetes Care* 21(5):855-69, May 1998.

Meggitt-Wagner ulcer classification

Grade	Wound characteristics
0	Preulceration lesions, healed ulcers, presence of bony deformity
1	Superficial ulcer without subcutaneous tissue involvement
2	Penetration through the subcutaneous tissue; may expose bone, tendon, ligament, or joint capsule
3	Osteitis, abscess, or osteomyelitis
4	Gangrene of digit
5	Gangrene of foot

Reprinted with permission from Wagner, F.W. "The Dysvascular Foot: A System for Diagnosis and Treatment," *Foot & Ankle* 2(2):64-122, September 1981, and from Meggitt, B. "Surgical Management of the Diabetic Foot," *British Journal of Hospital Medicine* 227-32, 1976.

vantage of not consistently including depth or infection throughout the system. In addition, osteomyelitis is the only type of infection included and the only vascular parameters are the end-stage disease events of gangrene. Furthermore, the system is difficult to use for more subtle disease processes that are critical for clinical decision-making. (See *Meggitt-Wagner ulcer classification.*)

The ADA Consensus report[1] recommends that a systematic wound assessment include the following questions in the evaluation:
- Has the patient experienced trauma? Is the ulcer a result of penetrating trauma, blunt trauma, or burn?
- What is the duration of the wound? Is the ulcer acute or chronic?
- What is the progression of local or systemic signs and symptoms? Is the wound getting better, is it stable, or is it deteriorating?
- Has the patient had any prior treatment of the wound or previous wounds? What treatments worked? What failed?

In addition, blood glucose control and co-morbidities should be evaluated. Clinical assessment should identify:
- signs of ischemia—adequate blood flow to heal the wound
- signs of soft tissue or bone infection—unpleasant odor, cellulitis, abscess, or osteomyelitis
- wound depth—undermining or exposed tendon, joint capsule, or bone
- appearance—surrounding callus, devitalized tissue, granulation tissue, drainage, eschar, or necrosis.

PRACTICE POINT

Six essentials of the American Diabetes Association's treatment algorithm[48]:
- debridement, early and often
- reducing pressure
- moist-wound healing
- treating infection
- correcting ischemia (below the knee disease)
- preventing amputation.

Debridement

Sharp debridement of the ulcer removes devitalized tissue, reduces the bacterial load of the wound, eliminates proteases from the wound bed, and provides a bleeding wound bed. A diabetic ulcer typically has a thick rim of keratinized tissue surrounding it. Debridement must remove all of the callus and devitalized tissue, so that a clean wound edge is created and all edge pressure from the callus is removed. Enzymatic debridement or autolytic debridement may be an option if

sharp debridement is not possible or if the patient has peripheral vascular disease.[27] Ongoing debridement may be needed throughout the healing process.[17,47] Indeed, higher healing rates have been observed in patients that have had more frequent debridement.[47] In addition, in a post-hoc evaluation from the becaplermin gel pivotal trial, Steed and colleagues reported a higher proportion of healed wounds in both the treatment and placebo study groups when wound debridement was performed more frequently.[46]

Strategies to reduce pressure

Reduction of pressure and shear forces on the foot may be the single most important, yet most neglected aspect of neuropathic ulceration treatment. Off-loading therapy is a key part of the treatment plan for diabetic foot ulcers. The goal is to reduce the pressure at the ulcer site and keep the patient ambulatory.[17,39,49,97] Calhoun and colleagues[17] have defined off-loading as "any measure to eliminate abnormal pressure points to promote healing or prevent recurrence of diabetic foot ulcers." Several methods are available to protect the foot from abnormal pressures. (See *Off-loading modalities and wound healing*.) Off-loading strategies must be tailored to the age, strength, activity, and home environment of the patient. In general, however, more restrictive off-loading approaches will result in less activity and better wound healing. Education is critical to improve compliance with off-loading. The patient must understand that the wound is a result of repetitive pressure, and that every unprotected step is literally tearing the wound apart.

PRACTICE POINT

Methods to off-load the diabetic foot include:
- bed rest
- wheelchair
- ambulatory aids (crutches, walker)
- felted foam padding

Off-loading modalities and wound healing

Off-loading modality	Mean healing time	Percent healed	Source
Total contact cast	• Forefoot ulcers: 30 days • Midfoot and hindfoot ulcers: 63 days	90%	Myerson, M., et al.[50]
Total contact cast	• 38 days	73%	Helm, P.A., et al.[51]
Total contact cast	• 44 days	82%	Sinacore, D.R., et al.[52]
Total contact cast	• Forefoot ulcers: 31 days • Nonforefoot ulcers: 42.1 days	Not reported	Walker, S.C., et al.[53]
Total contact cast	• Midfoot ulcers: 28 days	100%	Lavery, L.A., et al.[54]
Total contact cast Cast boot Half-shoe	• 34 days • 50 days • 61 days	90% 65% 58%	Armstrong, D.G., et al.[55]
Total contact cast Shoe-insole	• 42 days • 65 days	90% 32%	Mueller, M.J., et al. [56]
Scotch cast boot	• 112 days • 181 days	80%	Knowles, E.A., et al.[57]
Half-shoe	• 70 days	96%	Chantelau, E., et al.[58]
Custom splint	• 300 days	Not reported	Boninger, M.L., and Leonard, J.A.[59]

- half-shoes
- therapeutic shoes
- custom shoes
- custom total contact foot orthoses
- custom splints or braces
- prefabricated cast walkers
- total contact casting.

Total contact cast

Total contact casting (TCC) is considered the gold standard for off-loading the foot. Use of TCC reduces pressure at the ulcer site while still allowing the patient to be ambulatory.[17,49] A skilled clinician or technician is required to apply the molded plaster cast to ensure a proper fit. A TCC is a modification of a traditional fracture cast with minimum cast padding and a covering to protect the toes. The cast is molded to the contour of the foot and leg, so that there is no movement within the cast. TCCs are generally changed every 1 to 2 weeks, but in patients with edema or other concerns, the cast may need to be replaced more frequently. (See *Applying a total contact cast,* page 352.)

TCC is one of the most effective ways of treating plantar neuropathic foot ulcers described in the medical literature.[49,53,60] Studies[50,51,52,53,55,56,60-62] have shown that TCC can heal ulcers in six to eight weeks. The proportion of wounds that heal in descriptive and randomized clinical trials with TCC is consistently much higher than those

Applying a total contact cast

The photographs below highlight the major steps in applying a total contact cast.

Foam layer covers toes for protection. Padding is applied over bony prominences before the first layer of casting material is applied.

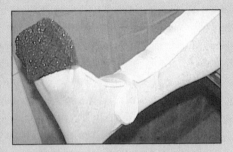

Completed total contact cast.

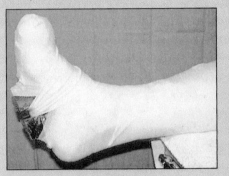

Cast boot covers the total contact cast.

Application of the total contact cast.

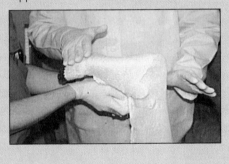

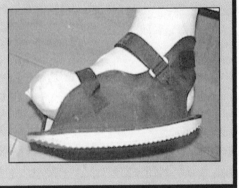

using topical growth factors, bioengineered tissue, or special dressings.[63-66]

One of the main advantages of using a TCC is that it forces patient compliance with off-loading. The ulcer is protected with every step the patient takes. Using TCC to facilitate wound healing is analogous to using a cast to heal a fracture—in both cases, healing is facilitated by rest and immobilization. TCC reduces the patient's activity level,[55] decreases his stride length and cadence, and significantly reduces pressure at the ulcer site.[49,60] The main disadvantages for patients are the same as their complaints with a fracture cast—a cast is heavy and hot, and makes bathing, walking, and sleeping difficult.

PRACTICE POINT

TCC should not be used if wound infection is suspected or present.

Removable cast walkers

In several studies, the removable cast walker has demonstrated that it's comparable to the TCC in pressure reduction.[49,60] Many practitioners consider it their preferred off-loading device because it is less time consuming, easy to apply, and more readily accepted by pa-

tients. In addition, the TCC has several precautions and contraindications that aren't issues with removable walkers. Edema can be
overcome with constant adjustments to the fit
of the device and compression dressings can
be applied in conjunction with the removable
cast boot. Wounds can be inspected regularly
and treated with advanced wound care products such as growth factors, electrical stimulation, and other biologically active dressings. Because the wound and limb can be inspected frequently, the vascular concerns
inherent in the occlusive irremovable TCC
aren't present.

Additional advantages of removable walking boots (as compared to TCCs) are that
they're relatively inexpensive, the protective
inner sole can be easily replaced if it shows
signs of wear, no special training is required
to correctly and safely apply these devices,
and they can be easily removed to assess and
debride the wound, as appropriate.[55-60] It's
also possible to make these walkers into non-
removable devices by securing the walker
with cast material or a non-removable cable
tie. If patients can't remove the walker, the element of forced compliance that makes the
TCC attractive is maintained and the outcomes for healing improve to the levels seen
with the TCC.[88,95,96,97,98]

There are a number of removable walking
boots that have been designed to help protect
and heal foot wounds in diabetics, including
the Royce Active Hex Walker, formerly
known as the DH Pressure Relief Walker; the
Bledsoe Conformer Boot; the DonJoy
Diabetic Walker; and the AirCast Pneumatic
Walker. [95,96] (See *Removable walking boot*.)
In a randomized controlled trial, Armstrong
et al. compared the effectiveness of the TCC,
removable cast walkers, and half-shoes in
their ability to heal neuropathic foot ulcerations in individuals with diabetes. The percentage of healing at 12 weeks was 89.5%
for the TCC, 65.0% for the cast walker, and
58.3% for the half-shoe.[87] When the cast
walker is made non-removable (instant total
contact cast [ITCC]) the difference between
the TCC and cast walker effectively disappears.[89] (See *Irremovable cast walker*.)

Removable walking boot

This photograph shows an example of a
prefabricated, removable walking boot,
which is used as an off-loading device.

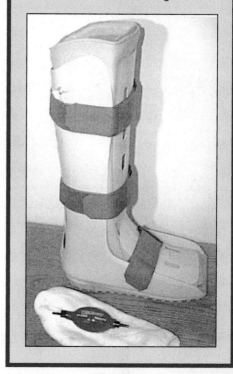

Irremovable cast walker

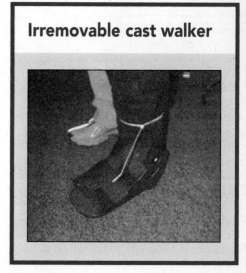

Royce Active Hex Walker

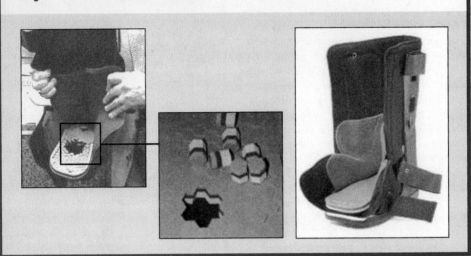

DonJoy High-Tide Diabetic Walker

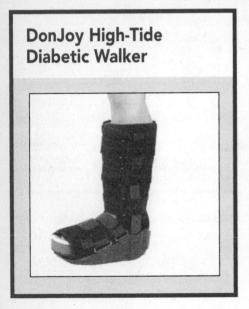

Bledsoe Diabetic Conformer Boot

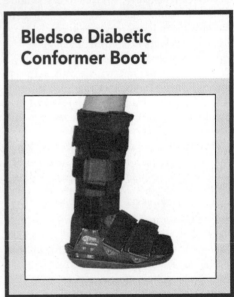

Royce Active Hex Walker

The Royce Active Hex Walker has been shown to be identical to TCCs in pressure reduction at the site of ulcerations on the sole.[60] (See *Royce Active Hex Walker.*) The walker is a low-profile boot with a fixed ankle rocker sole. The interior holds a patented inner sole made up of a series of hexagonal plugs attached to its base by Velcro. The plugs are made of layers of firm density urethane, medium density ethylene vinyl acetate, and soft urethane. The inner sole can absorb shock, conform to the shape of the foot and, because of the independent motion of the hex plugs, reduce shear forces during ambulation. The hex plugs can be removed in areas of high pressure to aid in ulcer healing. Covering the insole with a 2″-thick layer of plastazote secured to the surface with rubber cement, prevents the plugs from loosening with ambulation and reduces edge pressure produced by their removal. In a study by Lavery, the off-loading capacity of the Royce walker was the best of several other cast walkers and comparable to the TCC.[49, 60]

DonJoy Diabetic Walker

A similar system is used in the DonJoy Diabetic Walker, which uses removable diamond-shaped sections, in a plastazote contact layer, thus eliminating the need to cover the removal sections to prevent loosening. (See *DonJoy High-Tide Diabetic Walker.*)

Bledsoe Conformer Diabetic Boot

The Bledsoe Conformer Diabetic Boot also incorporates a fixed ankle-rigid rocker design with a "memory foam" inner sole. In a study by Pollo et al., the Bledsoe walker was shown to be superior to the TCC in off-loading all areas of the foot tested.[89] (See *Bledsoe Diabetic Conformer Boot.*)

AirCast Diabetic Walker

The AirCast Diabetic Walker has a wide-profile rocker sole and a multidensity plastzote inner sole that can be heated or dynamically molded to create a total contact footbed for the walker. (See *Aircast Diabetic Walker.*)

Healing sandals and half-shoes

A number of healing sandals and half-shoes or wedged shoes are available to reduce pressure on the forefoot. (See *Wedged shoe.*) These sandals and shoes are useful for patients who can't tolerate a TCC or for those who need a transitional device after removal of a TCC while they're awaiting therapeutic shoes and insoles. A modification of the Carville healing sandal can be made from a standard surgical shoe with a total contact direct-molded plastazote innersole.[91] (See *Carville healing sandal,* page 356.)

Surgical shoes with a rocker sole design are preferable to the flat design used postoperatively. Royce Medical has a healing sandal utilizing the Active Hex Innersole, described

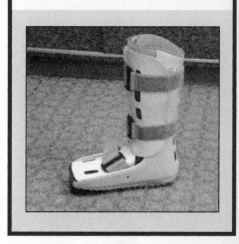

Aircast Diabetic Walker

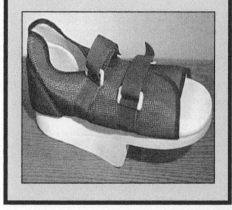

Wedged shoe

This photograph shows an example of a wedged forefront-relief shoe.

above, for the walker that can be used as a transitional device after closing the wound.

The OrthoWedge shoe by Darco products was originally designed to protect the forefoot after elective surgery. The OrthoWedge shoe has a sole that's wedged at a 10-degree dorsiflexion angle, effectively removing from the forefoot area. Studies by Needleman[23] and Lair[67] provide support for its role in

Carville healing sandal

postoperative patients following surgery on the forefoot. However, these types of shoes aren't well accepted by patients because they're difficult to walk in, they typically cause pain of the contralateral extremity, and patients with postural instability can't safely use these devices. Also, most diabetics have equinus and can't tolerate the negative heel position created by the shoe. Further, suspension of the heel during ambulation increases pressure on the forefoot and stresses the midfoot, a common site for collapse in the diabetic Charcot foot. In a randomized clinical trial that compared TCCs to healing sandals and removable cast boots, patients in the healing sandal group were less compliant and used the device during walking significantly less than subjects in the TCC group.[28,54,55]

Ankle-foot orthoses
Custom-made ankle-foot orthoses can be used for lower-extremity pathology, including Charcot fractures, tendon injuries, and neu-

ropathic ulcers. (See *Ankle-foot orthoses*.) The Charcot Restraint Orthotic Walker (CROW), for example, initially was used to treat patients with neuropathic fractures. It provides protection to the neuropathic foot and aids in controlling lower-extremity edema. This device looks like a ski boot; it has a rigid polypropylene shell with a rocker bottom sole.[28] (See *Charcot Restraint Orthotic Walker*, p. 358.)

The primary drawback to custom-made devices is that they typically cost more than $1,000. If the structure of the foot changes or local edema resolves, the device can no longer be used. Since a number of less expensive, off-the-shelf products are now available to treat neuropathic wounds, custom ankle-foot orthoses are used less commonly. Off-the-shelf devices should be replaced at regular intervals since the materials in the insoles will lose their effectiveness over time.[40]

Advanced technologies
Many new treatments have been, and are being developed to improve the outlook for the patient with a diabetic foot wounds. Indeed, several advanced technologies are available for use in treating diabetic foot ulcers that have not responded to standard therapy. In December 1997, the FDA approved the use of becaplermin (Regranex) in patients with diabetic foot ulcers and adequate circulation. This product, a topical gel that contains recombinant human platelet-derived growth factor, promotes wound healing by stimulating cell migration to the wound. Of the patients treated with becaplermin, 50% experienced healing, compared with 35% of patients in the placebo gel control group;[66] mean time to complete healing was also faster in the patients treated with becaplermin. Also, wounds that were debrided and then treated with becaplermin had increased rates of healing when compared to those treated with debridement alone.[47]

Bioengineered skin products are another advanced technology used in wound healing.[75] In 2000, the Food and Drug Administration (FDA) approved the tissue-engineered skin substitute known as Graftskin (Apligraf) for use in noninfected diabetic foot ulcers. This bilayered skin substitute contains cells from human infant foreskins and bovine type I collagen.[63] In a randomized clinical trial by Veves and colleagues[63], patients treated with Apligraf (56%) had more complete wound closure than did patients in the control group receiving standard wound care (38%). The median time to healing was 65 days for Apligraf and 90 days for controls.

A fibroblast-derived, manufactured dermal substitute (Dermagraft) also made from neonatal foreskin was approved by the FDA in September 2001. Results from the randomized clinical trial demonstrated that by week 12, the proportion of wounds that healed in the dermal substitute group was greater as compared to the control group.[65] Ulcers treated with the dermal substitute were 1.7 times more likely to close than those in the control group at any time in the study. Time for wound closure was also significantly faster in the dermal substitute graft group.

Several randomized clinical trials have reported the effectiveness of electrical stimulation to facilitate wound healing in pressure, venous stasis ulcers, and diabetic foot wounds.[76-79] In 2001, Peters[80] reported the results of a randomized clinical trial of 40 subjects with neuropathic ulcers treated with subsensory electrical stimulation compared to a sham device. In the electrical stimulation group, 65% of the patients healed compared with 35% of the patients who had received a placebo. In prospective study of 80 patients, Peters[80] and Baker[81] reported an approximate 60% improvement in healing rates in subjects with electrical stimulation, as compared with controls.

Wounds with inadequate tissue oxygen levels will not heal regardless of the best of care techniques. In 1969, Silver[71] reported on the oxygen gradients in wounds, establishing the need for adequate oxygen in healing tissue. Several authors have suggested hyperbaric oxygen therapy (HBOT) as an adjunct therapy in diabetic patients with adequate arterial circulation and a transcutaneous oxygen level below 40 mm Hg.[72,73] Hyperbaric oxygen therapy is a treatment that requires specialized training and expertise by a physician and a hyperbaric team.

Ankle-foot orthoses

These photographs show examples of custom-made ankle-foot orthoses.

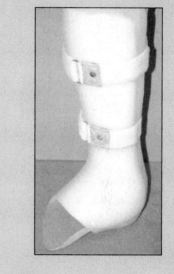

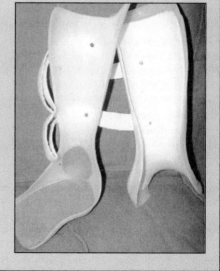

Patients must breathe 100% oxygen while inside a treatment chamber at atmospheric pressure higher than sea. Although *topical* hyperbaric oxygen has been available for decades, there's little scientific evidence to support its effectiveness.[74] Topical treatments

Charcot Restraint Orthotic Walker

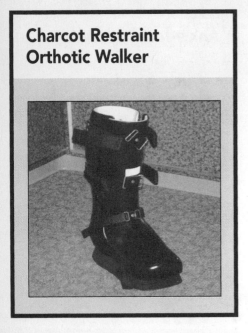

with small chambers over body parts (legs, arms) do not contribute the same effects as HBOT. (See chapter 9, Wound treatment options, for more information on HBOT.)

Small intestinal submucosa of SIS (Oasis) is a freeze-dried extracellular matrix collagen with preservation of several cytokines that remain active. In a study by Niezgoda and colleagues, SIS was compared to becaplermin in 98 patients with diabetic foot ulcers. SIS produced healing in 49% of wounds at 12 weeks; whereas becaplermin produced healing in only 28% of wounds (p-value 0.055). [92,93]

Oxidized regenerated cellulous and collagen ORC (Promgran) has been shown to reduce the concentration of matrixmetalloprotineases in chronic wounds while simultaneously preserving the concentration of growth factors in the wound, thus enhancing wound healing. When combined with ionic silver, Promgran also helped reduce bacterial contamination within the wound bed and facilitated granulation. However, a randomized clinical study of this product didn't show a significant improvement in wound healing compared to standard wound therapy. [64]

Both silver and cadexomer iodine have proved to be safe and effective antiseptics for

use in the treatment of wounds, [94] and numerous silver-impregnated wound dressings have been developed in the past several years. The silver ion is lethal to all bacteria, including MRSA and VRE; few incidences of resistance have been recorded in the literature.

Silver ions kill a broad spectrum of bacteria. By controlling bacterial contamination, topical creams, gels, or dressings using ionic or nanocrystalline silver prevent wounds from progressing to critical colonization and infection. Unfortunately, there are no clinical studies that indicate that these products improve the proportion or rate of healing in diabetic foot wounds, and the recommendations for applications in humans has been based on bench or animal studies.

Diagnostic imaging

Whenever there's an open wound on the foot it's always wise to initially order an X-ray to check for the presence or absence of osteomyelitis. Even if standard X-rays are negative, but the wound has been open for several weeks or if bone can be palpated with a sterile probe, further investigation is warranted. [9]

After X-ray, most clinicians would agree that the magnetic resonance imaging (MRI) is the next diagnostic modality to detect for the presence of osteomyelitis. If X-ray reveals bone destruction and MRI reveals osteomyelitis, a bone biopsy should be obtained prior to considering an ablative procedure such as an amputation.

Technetium bone scans are often ordered in patients with expected infection. These scans show increased uptake in the area of infection but they're nonspecific and also show increased uptake in any area of osseous activity, such as with arthritis or a Charcot fracture. White blood cell labeled bone scans such as an Indium, Technetium bone scan, or Hexamethylpropyleneamine Oxime (HMPAO) can also be compared to standard technetium scan. In the presence of Charcot fracture, the bone will exhibit increased uptake in the technetium scan but not in the labeled scan.

Infection

Identification of foot infections in patients with diabetes mellitus requires vigilance because the normal signs of infection may be blunted or absent.[1] Hyperglycemia impairs leukocyte functioning, including phagocytosis and intracellular killing function.[17] Patients with diabetes may also demonstrate a diminished inflammatory response, even when severe soft tissue and bone infections are present. However, frequent wound culture and use of superficial swab cultures in wounds without clinical signs of infection aren't helpful and should be discouraged. All open wounds have a normal flora of bacteria, and routine swab culture will produce several types of bacteria colonizing the wound.[69,70] Instead, wounds should be thoroughly debrided and cleansed before any cultures are taken. Tissue samples from the base of the wound should be sent for culture. Aerobic and anaerobic cultures should also be ordered when signs and symptoms of infection are present. (See chapter 7, Wound bioburden.)

The ADA[1] recommends that patients with non–limb-threatening infections be treated on an outpatient basis with oral antibiotics to achieve adequate serum levels and address the usual etiologic organisms. *Staphylococcus aureus* and *Streptococcus* are the most common bacteria found in non–limb-threatening infected diabetic foot ulcers.[17,30]

Patients with limb-threatening infections should be hospitalized with administration of parenteral antibiotics and surgical debridement of necrotic and infected tissue. The major pathogens are *S. aureus,* group B streptococci, *Enterococcus,* and facultative Gram-negative bacilli.[1] *Methicillin-resistant S. Aureus* (MRSA) and *Vancomycin-resistant Enterococcus* (VRE) are increasingly common in the population and should be suspected in any wound that has been treated with multiple administrations of antibiotics or in any patient that has been hospitalized in the past.

Care plan for treatment

A comprehensive care plan is vital to treating foot ulcers in persons with neuropathy.[90]

Glycemic control as measured by hemoglobin A1C may influence selection of some advanced therapies. Assessment of vascular supply and adequate circulation is also essential for wound healing.

Summary

Diabetic foot ulcer care is a challenge for both the patient and the health care provider. As our population continues to age, the incidence of diabetes will continue to increase. This increased incidence will lead to more diabetic wounds. A team approach with total involvement of the health care system and the necessary partnership with the patient will be the infrastructure for achieving better outcomes of care.

Early assessment for ulceration in persons with diabetes is essential. A variety of methods must be used to identify at-risk persons. Appropriate skin care and properly fitting shoes is mandatory for any person with diabetes. Clinicians can choose from the many products available to offload the diabetic foot. Infection is an important concern in diabetic ulcers and warrants prompt identification and treatment. Adjuvant therapies coupled with debridement and appropriate dressings can be critical in salvaging the diabetic limb.

Show what you know

1. According to the ADA (2001), how many people are unaware that they have diabetes mellitus?

    A. 50%
    B. 30%
    C. 75%
    D. 25%

ANSWER: B. One-third of people with diabetes are unaware of their condition.

2. The single leading cause of lower-extremity amputation is:

    A. diabetes mellitus.
    B. lymphedema.
    C. arterial occlusion.
    D. venous disease.

ANSWER: A. Diabetes mellitus is the single leading cause of lower-extremity amputation. B, C, D, are not the single leading cause of amputation in diabetic patients. While these conditions can contribute to complications in the diabetic they aren't listed as the leading cause for amputation.

3. According to the ADA, good skin care includes all of the following except:

A. keeping skin clean and dry.
B. applying moisturizers between toes.
C. avoiding very hot showers and tub baths.
D. checking feet daily for cracks or fissures.

ANSWER: B. Moisturizers shouldn't be applied between the toes—fungal infections can occur. All others are ADA recommendations for good skin care.

4. Off-loading strategies must be tailored to the age, strength, activity, and home environment of the patient.

A. True
B. False

ANSWER: A. Off-loading must be tailored to the individual.

5. For which of the following treatment strategies has healing rates for diabetic foot ulcers been found to be comparable to those with Total Contact Casts (TCC)?

A. Wedged shoe
B. Half shoe
C. Wide-toe shoe
D. Walker boot rendered irremovable (ITCC)

ANSWER D. Studies by researchers have found that making walking boots irremovable (nonremovable) that patients had same healing as with the gold standard of off-loading, the total contact cast. The other options are all removable shoes and research has not demonstrated healing rates comparable to TCC.

References

1. "American Diabetes Association: Clinical Practice Recommendations." *Diabetes Care* 21(Suppl 1):1999.
2. American Diabetes Association. www.diabetes. org, cited December 2006.
3. *Centers for Disease Control and Prevention: The Public Health of Diabetes Mellitus in the United States.* Atlanta: Department of Health and Human Services, 1997.
4. Reiber, G.E., et al. "Lower Extremity Foot Ulcers and Amputations in Diabetes," in Mi, H., ed. *Diabetes in America,* 2nd ed. National Institutes of Health 1995.
5. Lavery, L.A., et al. "Increased Foot Pressures After Great Toe Amputation in Diabetes," *Diabetes Care* 18(11):1460-62, November 1995.
6. Lavery, L.A., et al. "Classification of Diabetic Foot Wounds," *Journal of Foot and Ankle Surgery* 35(6):528-31, November-December 1996.
7. Lavery, L.A., et al. "Practical Criteria for Screening Patients at High Risk for Diabetic Foot

Ulceration," *Archives of Internal Medicine* 158(2):157-62, January 26, 1998.
8. Miller, A.D., et al. "Diabetes Related Lower-extremity amputation in New Jersey 1979 to 1981," *Journal of the Medical Society of New Jersey* 82(9):723-26, September 1985.
9. Pecoraro, R.E. "Chronology and Determinants of Tissue Repair in Diabetic Lower Extremity Ulcers," *Diabetes* 40(10):1305-13, October 1991.
10. Lavery, L.A., et al. "In-hospital Mortality and Disposition of Diabetic Amputees in the Netherlands," *Diabetic Medicine* 13(2):192-97, February 1996.
11. van Houtum, W.H., et al. "The Impact of Diabetes-Related Lower-Extremity Amputations in the Netherlands," *Journal of Diabetes and Its Complications* 10(6):325-30, November-December 1996.
12. Lavery, L.A., et al. "Diabetes-related Lower-extremity Amputations Disproportionately Affect Blacks and Mexican Americans," *Southern Medical Journal* 92(6):593-99, June 1999.
13. Edmonds, M.E., et al. "Improved Survival of the Diabetic Foot: The Role of a Specialized Foot Clinic," *Quarterly Journal of Medicine* 60(232):763-71, August 1986.
14. Most, R.S., and Sinnock, P. "The Epidemiology of Lower-Extremity Amputations in Diabetic Individuals," *Diabetes Care* 6(1):87-91, January-February 1983.
15. Lavery, L.A., et al. "Variation in the Incidence and Proportion of Diabetes-Related Amputations in Minorities," *Diabetes Care* 19(1):48-52, January 1996.
16. Armstrong, D.G., et al. "Choosing a Practical Screening Instrument to Identify Patients at Risk for Diabetic Foot Ulceration," *Archives of Internal Medicine* 158(3):289-92, February 1998.
17. Calhoun, J.H., et al. "Diabetic Foot Ulcers and Infections: Current Concepts," *Advances in Skin & Wound Care* 15(1):31-42, January-February 2002.
18. Levin, M. "Diabetic Foot Wounds: Pathogenesis and Management," *Advances in Wound Care* 10(2):24-30, March-April 1997.
19. Rith-Najarian, S.J. et al. "Identifying Diabetic Patients at High-Risk for Lower-Extremity Amputation in a Primary Health Care Setting. A Prospective Evaluation of Simple Screening Criteria," *Diabetes Care* 15(10):1386-95, October 1992.
20. Wunderlich, R.P., et al. "Defining Loss of Protective Sensation in the Diabetic Foot," *Advances in Wound Care* 11(3):123-28, May-June 1998.
21. Booth, J., and Young, M.J. "Differences in the Performance of Commercially Available 10-g Monofilaments," *Diabetes Care* 23(7):984-87, July 2000.
22. Young, R., et al. "The Durability of the Semmes-Weinstein 5.07 Monofilament," *Journal of Foot and Ankle Surgery* 39(1):34-38, January-February 2000.
23. Needleman, R.L. "Successes and Pitfalls in the Healing of Neuropathic Forefoot Ulcerations with the IPOS Postoperative Shoe," *Foot & Ankle International* 18(7):412-17, July 1997.
24. Tooke, J.E., and Brash, P.D. "Microvascular Aspects of Diabetic Foot Disease," *Diabetic Medicine* 13(Suppl 1):S26-S29, 1996.
25. LoGerfo, F.W., and Coffman, J.D. "Current Concepts, Vascular and Microvascular Disease of the Foot in Diabetes. Implications for Foot Care," *NEJM* 311(25): 1615-19, December 20, 1984.

26. LoGerfo, F.W., and Misare, F.D. "Current Management of the Diabetic Foot," *Advances in Surgery* 30:417-26, 1997.

27. Mulder, G.D. "Evaluating and Managing the Diabetic Foot: An Overview," *Advances in Skin & Wound Care* 13(1):33- 36, January-February 2000.

28. Catanzariti, A.R., et al. "Off-loading Techniques in the Treatment of Diabetic Plantar Neuropathic Foot Ulceration," *Advances in Wound Care* 12(9):452-58, November-December 1999.

29. Gibbons, G.W., and Habershaw, G.M. "Diabetic Foot Infections: Anatomy and Surgery," *Infectious Diseases Clinics of North America* 9(1):131-42, March 1995.

30. Frykberg, R.G. "The Team Approach in Diabetic Foot Management," *Advances in Wound Care* 11(2):71-77, March-April 1998.

31. Lavery, L.A., and Gazewood, J.D. "Assessing the Feet of Patients with Diabetes," *Journal of Family Practice* 49(11 Suppl):S9-S16, November 2000.

32. Lavery, L.A., et al. "Ankle Equinus Deformity and Its Relationship to High Plantar Pressure in a Large Population with Diabetes Mellitus," *Journal of the American Podiatric Medical Association* 92(9): 479-82, October 2002.

33. Holstein, P., et al. "Decreasing Incidence of Major Amputations in People with Diabetes," *Diabetologia* 43(7):844-47, July 2000.

34. Larsson, J., et al. "Decreasing Incidence of Major Amputation in Diabetic Patients: A Consequence of a Multidisciplinary Foot Care Team Approach?" *Diabetic Medicine* 12(9):770-76, September 1995.

35. Patout, C.A., et al. "Effectiveness of a Comprehensive Diabetes Lower-Extremity Amputation Prevention Program in a Predominantly Low-Income African-American Population," *Diabetes Care* 23(9):1339-42, September 2000.

36. Runyan, J.W. Jr., et al. "The Memphis Diabetes Continuing Care Program," *Diabetes Care* 3(2):382-86, March-April 1980.

37. Pinzur, M.S., et al. "Guidelines for Diabetic Foot Care," *Foot & Ankle International* 29(11):695-702, November 1999.

38. Frykberg, R.G., et al. "Role of Neuropathy and High Foot Pressures in Diabetic Foot Ulceration," *Diabetes Care* 21(10):1714-19, October 1998.

39. Lavery, L.A., et al. "Reducing Plantar Pressure in the Neuropathic Foot: A Comparison of Footwear," *Diabetes Care* 20(11):1706-10, November 1997.

40. Lavery, L.A., et al. "A Novel Methodology to Obtain Salient Biomechanical Characteristics of Insole Materials," *Journal of the American Podiatric Medical Association* 87(6):260-65, June 1997.

41. Armstrong D.G., et al. "Lengthening of the Achilles Tendon in Diabetic Patients Who Are at High Risk for Ulceration of the Foot," *Journal of Bone & Joint Surgery*, American Volume 81(4):535-38, April 1999.

42. Peters, E.J., and Lavery, L.A. "Effectiveness of the Diabetic Foot Risk Classification System of the International Working Group on the Diabetic Foot," *Diabetes Care* 24(8):1442-47, August 2001.

43. Armstrong, D.G., et al. "Validation of a Diabetic Wound Classification System: The Contribution of Depth, Infection and Ischemia to Risk of Amputation," *Diabetes Care* 21(5):855-59, May 1998.

44. Meggitt, B. "Surgical Management of the Diabetic Foot," *British Journal of Hospital Medicine* 227-32, 1976.

45. Wagner, F.W., Jr. "The Dysvascular Foot: A System for Diagnosis and Treatment," *Foot & Ankle* 2(2):64-122, September 1981.

46. Steed, D.L. "The Wound Healing Society (WHS) Evaluation of the Science to Arrive at Guidelines," *Wounds* 13(5 Suppl. E): 15E-16E, 2001.

47. Steed, D.L., et al. Diabetic Ulcer Study Group. "Effect of Extensive Debridement and Treatment on the Healing of Diabetic Foot Ulcers," *Journal of the American College of Surgery* 183(1):61-64, July 1996.

48. Sheehan, P. "American Diabetes Association (ADA): Presentation of Consensus Development Conference on Diabetic Foot Wound Care," *Wounds* 13(5 Suppl. E):6E-8E, 2001.

49. Lavery, L.A., et al. "Total Contact Casts: Pressure Reduction at Ulcer Sites and the Effected on the Contralateral Foot," *Archives of Physical Medicine & Rehabilitation* 78(11):1268-71, November 1997.

50. Myerson, M., et al. "The Total-Contact Cast for Management of Neuropathic Plantar Ulceration of the Foot," *Journal of Bone & Joint Surgery*, American Volume 74(2):261-69, February 1992.

51. Helm, P.A., et al. "Total Contact Casting in Diabetic Patients with Neuropathic Foot Ulcerations," *Archives of Physical Medicine & Rehabilitation* 65(11):691-93, November 1984.

52. Sinacore, D.R., et al. "Diabetic Plantar Ulcers Treated by Total Contact Casting: A Clinical Report," *Physical Therapy* 67(10):1543-49, October 1987.

53. Walker, S.C., et al. "Total Contact Casting and Chronic Diabetic Neuropathic Foot Ulcerations: Healing Rates by Wound Location," *Archives of Physical Medicine & Rehabilitation* 68(4):217-21, April 1987.

54. Lavery, L.A., et al. "Healing Rates of Diabetic Foot Ulcers Associated with Midfoot Fracture Due to Charcot's Arthropathy," *Diabetic Medicine* 14(1):46-49, January 1997.

55. Armstrong D.G., et al. "Off-loading the Diabetic Foot Wound: A Randomized Clinical Trial," *erratum in Diabetes Care* 24(8):1509, August 2001.

56. Mueller, M.J., et al. "Total Contact Casting in Treatment of Diabetic Plantar Ulcers. Controlled Clinical Trial," *Diabetes Care* 12(6):384-88, June 1989.

57. Knowles, E.A., et al. "Off-loading Diabetic Foot Wounds Using the Scotchcast Boot: A Retrospective Study," *Ostomy/Wound Management* 48(9):50-53, September 2002.

58. Chantelau, E., et al. "Outpatient Treatment of Unilateral Diabetic Foot Ulcers with 'Half Shoes'," *Diabetic Medicine* 10(3):267-70, April 1993.

59. Boninger, M.L., and Leonard, J.A. Jr. "Use of Bivalved Ankle-foot Orthosis in Neuropathic Foot and Ankle Lesions," *Journal of Rehabilitation Research & Development* 33(1):16-22, February 1996.

60. Lavery, L.A., et al. "Reducing Dynamic Foot Pressures in High-Risk Diabetic Subjects with Foot Ulcers: A Comparison of Treatments," *Diabetes Care* 19(8):818-21, August 1996.

61. Sinacore, D.R. "Total Contact Casting for Diabetic Neuropathic Ulcers," *Physical Therapy* 76(3):296-301, March 1996.

62. Caputo, G.M., et al. "The Total Contact Cast: A Method for Treating Neuropathic Diabetic Ulcers," *American Family Physician* 55(2):605-11, February 1, 1997.

63. Veves, A.., et al. "Graftskin, A Human Skin Equivalent, Is Effective in the Management of Noninfected Neuropathic Diabetic Foot Ulcers: A Prospective Randomized Multicenter Clinical

Trial," *Diabetes Care* 24(2):290-95, February 2001.

64. Veves, A., et al. "A Randomized, Controlled Trial of Promogran (A Collagen/Oxidized Regenerated Cellulose Dressing) Versus Standard Treatment in the Management of Diabetic Foot Ulcers," *Archives of Surgery* 137(7):822-27, July 2002.

65. Gentzkow, G.D., et al. "Use of Dermagraft, A Cultured Human Dermis, to Treat Diabetic Foot Ulcers," *Diabetes Care* 19(4):350-54, April 1996.

66. Wieman, T.J., et al. "Efficacy and Safety of a Topical Gel Formulation of Recombinant Human Platelet-Derived Growth Factor-BB (Becaplermin) in Patients with Chronic Neuropathic Diabetic Ulcers. A Phase III Randomized Placebo-Controlled Double-Blind Study," *Diabetes Care* 21(5):822-27, May 1998.

67. Lair, G. *Use of the Ipos Shoe in the Management of Patients with Diabetes Mellitus.* Cleveland: Cleveland Clinic Foundation, 1992.

68. Sugaman, J.R., et al. "Use of the Therapeutic Footwear Benefit among Diabetic Medicare Beneficiaries in Three States," *Diabetes Care* 21(5):777-81, May 1998.

69. Lipsky, B.A., et al. "The Diabetic Foot: Soft Tissue and Bone Infection," *Infectious Diseases Clinics of North America* 4(3):409-32, September 1990.

70. Lipsky, B.A. "Infections of the Foot in Patients with Diabetes," in *The Diabetic Foot*, 6th ed. Pfeifer, M.A., and Bowker, J.H. (eds). St. Louis: Mosby–Year Book, Inc., 2001.

71. Silver, I.A. "The Measurement of Oxygen Tension in Healing Tissue," *Progress in Respiratory Research* 3:124, 1969.

72. Stone, J.A., and Cianci, P. "The Adjunctive Role of Hyperbaric Oxygen Therapy in the Treatment of Lower Extremity Wounds in Patients with Diabetes," *Diabetes Spectrum* 10:1, 1997.

73. Hammarlund, C., and Sundberg, T. "Hyperbaric Oxygen Reduced Size of Chronic Leg Ulcers: A Randomized Double-Blind Study," *Plastic & Reconstructive Surgery* 93(4):829-33, April 1994.

74. Wunderlich, R.P., et al. "Systemic Hyperbaric Oxygen Therapy: Lower-Extremity Wound Healing and the Diabetic Foot," *Diabetes Care* 23(10):1551-55, October 2000.

75. Johnson, P.C. "The Role of Tissue Engineering," *Advances in Skin & Wound Care* 13(2 Suppl 1):12-14, May-June 2000.

76. Kjartansson, J., Lundeberg, T. "Effects of Electrical Nerve Stimulation (ENS) in Ischemic Tissue," *Scandinavian Journal of Plastic & Reconstructive Hand Surgery* 24(2):129-34, 1990.

77. Feedar, J.A., et al. "Chronic Dermal Ulcer Healing Enhanced with Monophasic Pulsed Electrical Stimulation," *Physical Therapy* 71(7):639-49, July 1991.

78. Gault, W.R. "Use of Low Intensity Direct Current in Management of Ischemic Skin Ulcers," *Physical Therapy* 56(3):256-69, March 1976.

79. Lundeberg, T., et al. "Effect of Electrical Nerve Stimulation on Healing of Ischaemic Skin Flaps," *Lancet* 242(8613):712-14, September 1988.

80. Peters, E.J., et al. "Electric Stimulation as an Adjunct to Heal Diabetic Foot Ulcers: A Randomized Clinical Trial," *Archives of Physical Medicine & Rehabilitation* 82:721-25, June 2001.

81. Baker, L.L., et al. "Effects of Electrical Stimulation on Wound Healing in Patients with Diabetic Ulcers," *Diabetes Care* 20(3):405-12, March 1997.

82. Lavery LA, KR Higgins, Lanctot DR, et al. "Preventing Diabetic Foot Ulcer Recurrence in High-Risk Patients: Use of Temperature Monitoring as a Self-Assessment Tool," *Diabetes Care* 30(1):14-20 January 2007.

83. Lin SS, Lee TH, Wapner KL. "Plantar Forefoot Ulceration with Equinus Deformity of the Ankle in Diabetic Patients: the Effect of Tendo-Achilles Lengthening and Total Contact Casting," *Orthopaedics* 5:465-75, May 1996

84. Mueller M, Sinacore D.R. "Effect of Achilles Tendon Lengthening on Neuropathic Plantar Ulcers: a Randomized Clinical Trial," *J Bone Joint Surg* 8:1436-45, August 2003.

85. Armstrong DG, Lavery LA, Frykberg RG. "Validation of a Diabetic Foot Surgery Classification," *Int Wound Journal* 3:240-246, September 2006.

86. Armstrong DG, Nguyen HC, Lavery LA, et al. "Offloading the diabetic foot wound: A randomized clinical trial," *Diabetes Care* 24(6):1019-22, June 2001.

87. Katz IA, Harlan A, Miranda-Palma B, et al. "A Randomized Trial of Two Irremovable Off-loading Devices in the Management of Plantar Neuropathic Diabetic Foot Ulcerations," *Diabetes Care* 28(3):555-59, March 2005.

88. Armstrong DG, Lavery LA, Wu S, et al. "Evaluation of Removable and Irremovable Cast Walkers in the Healing of Diabetic Foot Wounds; a Randomized Controlled Trial," *Diabetes Care* 28(3):551-54, March 2005.

89. Pollo FE, Crenshaw MS, Brodsky MD, Kirksey BS. "Plantar Pressures in Total Contact Casting Verses a Diabetic Walking Boot" Baylor University Medical Center, Dallas, Tex. Accepted for presentation, Annual Meeting of the Orthopedic Research Society, San Francisco, Feb 25-28, 2001

90. Brand P.W. "The Insensitive Foot (including leprosy)," In: Jahass MH (ed). *Disorders of the Foot*, vol 2., Philadelphia: WB Saunders Co., 1266-86, 1982.

91. Mostow E.N., Haraway G.D., Dalsing M., et al. OASIS Venus Ulcer Study Group. Effectiveness of an extracellular matrix graft (OASIS Wound Matrix) in the treatment of chronic leg ulcers: a randomized clinical trial. *J Vasc Surg* 41(5):837-43, May 2005.

92. Niezgoda, J.A., et al. "OASIS Diabetic Ulcer Study Group. "Randomized Clinical Trial Comparing OASIS Wound Matrix to Regranex Gel for Diabetic Ulcers," *Advances in Skin and Wound Care* 18(5):258-66, June 2005.

93. Drosou, Falabella, Kirsner. "Antiseptics on Wounds: An Area of Controversy (Parts I and II)," *Wounds* 15(5), May 2003.

94. McQuire, J.B. "Pressure Redistribution Strategies for the Diabetic or At-risk Foot: Part I," *Advances in Skin and Wound Care* 19(4):213:21 May 2006.

95. McQuire, J.B. "Pressure Redistribution Strategies for the Diabetic or At-risk Foot: Part iI," *Advances in Skin and Wound Care* 19(5):270-77, June 2006.

96. Frykberg, R.G. "Diabetic Foot Ulcers: Pathogenesis and Management," *Am Fam Physician* 66:1655-62, November 2002.

97. Frykberg, R.G. "A Summary of Guidelines for Managing the Diabetic Foot," *Advances in Skin and Wound Care* 18(4):209-14, May 2005.

98. Sibbald, RG, Woo, K, Ayello, EA. "Increased Bacterial Burden and Infection: the story of NERDS and STONES," *Advances in skin and Wound Care* 19(8):447-61 October 2006.

CHAPTER 17

Sickle cell ulcers

Terry Allen Treadwell, MD, FACS
Angela Colette Willis, RN, CWS, CDE
Harold Brem, MD, FACS

The contributions of Marc Gibber, Wound Care Center, The Mount Sinai Medical Center, New York, New York; and Sharon Weinberger, The Mount Sinai Medical Center, New York, New York, to the first edition of this chapter are greatly acknowledged.

OBJECTIVES

After completing this chapter, you'll be able to:

- understand the pathogenesis of sickle cell anemia (or sickle cell disease)

- discuss the pathogenesis of sickle cell ulcers

- differentiate sickle cell ulcers from arterial and venous ulcers

- implement protocols for prevention and treatment of complications of sickle cell ulcers (such as infection).

Sickle cell anemia

Sickle cell ulcers are a complication of sickle cell anemia, an inherited, genetic disorder of the oxygen carrying hemoglobin in red blood cells. Sickle cell anemia (or sickle cell disease) was first reported in 1910 by Dr. J.B. Herrick.[1] It is a disease primarily seen in black individuals and is more prevalent in the United States and Africa. The disease is seen in two main forms: when the individual receives a gene for the abnormal hemoglobin (hemoglobin S) from both the mother and the father, the person has homozygous sickle cell disease, which is the most severe form; when the individual receives only one gene for the abnormal hemoglobin from either the mother or father and the other gene is for normal hemoglobin, the person has heterozygous sickle cell disease, which is the less severe form.

Prevalence and incidence

The patient with homozygous form of sickle cell disease is most likely to develop the sickle cell ulcer. Studies have shown that males are more likely to develop leg ulcers due to sickle cell disease than females.[2] The same study found that 5% of males with sickle cell disease who were over age ten had sickle cell ulcers [2], and 75% of patients over age thirty had a sickle cell ulcer at some time during the

Sickled cells

The diagrams below show a normal red blood cell and a sickled cell.

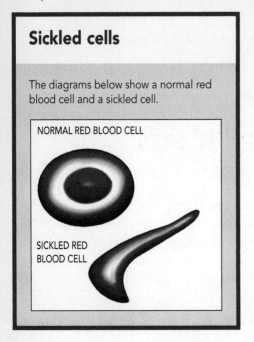

NORMAL RED BLOOD CELL

SICKLED RED BLOOD CELL

course of their disease.[3] With over 80,000 patients in the United States with sickle cell disease[4], this makes the number of patients with sickle cell ulcers significant.

PRACTICE POINT

Lower extremity ulcers in young black patients, especially males, could be due to undiagnosed sickle cell disease.

Ulcer pathogenesis

The abnormal hemoglobin molecule in the red blood cell in the patient with sickle cell disease does not affect the amount of oxygen the red blood cell can carry. After the red blood cell and its hemoglobin give up the oxygen to the tissues, the abnormal hemoglobin causes the red blood cell to distort and become rigid. This results in the cell becoming deformed into a sickle shape (See *Sickled cells*.)

When the red blood cell is reoxygenated, the cell resumes its normal shape. Unfortunately, while the cells are in the sickled shape, they tend to increase blood viscosity and become

"sticky." This causes slowing of the blood flow in small vessels and subsequently clotting of the vessels, which results in ischemia of tissues and organs. Over time the patient suffers repeated episodes of pain, tissue damage, and, eventually, organ failure. Many times the cells become damaged while they are in the sickled shape and have a shortened life-span. Because these cells are removed from the circulation faster than normal, anemia results. (See *Conditions associated with sickle cell anemia.*)

Although the exact cause of sickle cell ulcers is not clear, they have been associated with trauma, infection, severe anemia, and warm temperatures[6] and are most likely to occur in the malleolar area of the lower extremities. Laboratory evaluation has shown that sickle cell ulcer patients have lower hemoglobin levels and higher levels of lactate dehydrogenase (LDH), bilirubin, aspartate transaminase (AST), and reticulocytes than do patients with sickle cell disease with no ulcers.[7] It has been suggested that the sickle cells cause chronic damage to the microcirculation in the skin at the ankle. This damage includes injury to the capillary walls, thickening of the intima lining of the capillary, and increase in permeability of the vessel wall, allowing macromolecules to escape into the tissues.[8] These changes result in the skin having a reduced blood supply, being more susceptible to minor trauma, and being less able to heal.[9] As a result, these areas of involvement are more likely to be the sites of skin breakdown and ulceration. It has also been suggested that a reduction in the amount of the smooth muscle relaxant (nitric oxide) in the microcirculation can result in unrestrained vasoconstriction of the small vessels, ischemia of the skin, and skin necrosis.[9]

Diagnosis
Medical history

Evaluation of the patient with a suspected sickle cell ulcer is of utmost importance so that the correct diagnosis can be made and appropriate treatment planned. The patient's medical history should be recorded, and the events surrounding the ulcer development

Conditions associated with sickle cell anemia

Complication	Cause
"Crisis" with fever and pain	Sickling of cells due to abnormal hemoglobin
Pain in bones, joints, and back	Sickling of cells and ischemia of tissues
Severe abdominal pain	Sickling of cells and ischemia of tissues
Pregnancy problems Fertility problems	Uncontrolled sickling of cells

Increased infections
   Pneumonia
   Urinary tract
	Deficient immune response

Salmonella osteomyelitis	Ischemia of bones, bone infarcts, sepsis
Chronic leg ulcers	Sickling of cells and ischemia of tissues
"Hand-foot" syndrome	Sickling of cells and ischemia of bones
Avascular necrosis of femoral or humeral head	Ischemic necrosis of bones due to sickling
Visual problems	Ischemia of retina due to sickling
Pulmonary infarction	Ischemia of lung due to sickle cell emboli

Congestive heart failure
   Cardiac murmurs
   EKG abnormalities
	Myocardial ischemia

Jaundice	Hemolytic anemia Gallstone production and obstructive jaundice
Cirrhosis of liver	Ischemia of liver and cell necrosis
Hepatitis	Multiple blood transfusions
Enlarged spleen (infancy only)	Increased blood production
Splenic infarction (late teens, adult)	Ischemia of tissue due to sickling of cells

Renal dysfunction
   Hematuria
   Infections
	Ischemia of kidney with infarction of tissue

Renal vein thrombosis	Sickling of cells
Priapism (especially in children)	Sickling of cells

(continued)

Conditions associated with sickle cell anemia (continued)

Complication	Cause
Impotence	Damage of penis by priapism and ischemia
Anemia	Hemolysis of abnormal cells
"Aplastic crisis"	Failure of bone marrow to produce cells due to infarction of marrow
Folate deficiency	High folate requirement of hemolytic anemia

Adapted from Conley, C. Lockard, "The Hemoglobinopathies and Thalassemias" in *Textbook of Medicine*, eds. Beeson, PB, McDermott, W, 13th Edition, W.B. Saunders Co., Philadelphia, pp.1501-1503, 1971.

should be investigated. Is this the first ulcer the patient has had? How long has the ulcer been present? How did the ulcer first develop? Was there trauma to the area? How did the area first look? Any history of lower extremity edema, unexplained swelling of the hands, feet, or knees, osteomyelitis, episodes of abdominal or joint pain, episodes of severe unexplained pain, recurrent urinary tract infections or pneumonia, or anemia should be noted. Sickle cell patients are prone to develop unexplained episodes of fever which tend to resolve without therapy. These patients may carry a diagnosis of FUO (fever of unknown origin).

Physical examination

A complete physical examination should be part of the evaluation of the patient. Vital signs, especially temperature, should be taken because, as mentioned above, unexplained fever may be a sign of sickle cell disease. Abdominal examination can detect enlargement of the liver and spleen. Examination of the extremities is also important to evaluate the ulcer and for the presence and degree of edema.

The presence of scars or other skin problems of the extremities may indicate previous ulcer incidence. The location of the ulcer or ulcers is important as most sickle cell ulcers are found on the lower one third of the leg and usually over the medial or lateral malleoli (or both) of the ankle[6]. The size of each ulcer should be measured by determining the length and width or by using one of the more advanced measuring modalities described elsewhere in the book. (See chapter 6, Wound assessment.)

The presence of an ulcer in a patient with varicose veins, venous insufficiency, and sickle cell disease can be especially troublesome as it may lead to misdiagnosis. (See *Undiagnosed sickle cell ulcer treated initially as a "venous ulcer."*) In addition, venous incompetence in the patient with sickle cell disease may predispose him for ulcer development and is highly correlated with the development of a recurrent sickle cell ulcer.[10] Noninvasive venous studies can be helpful in establishing the correct therapeutic approach in these patients.

 PRACTICE POINT

Misdiagnosis—and thus, mistreatment—of sickle cell ulcer as a venous "stasis" ulcer makes it imperative to get the differential diagnosis correct.

Ulcer assessment

Examination of the wound bed is essential to determine the presence of granulation tissue or fibrinous material ("slough"). (See photographs in the color section, pages C10 and

C11.) In addition, the presence of cellulitis or peri-ulcer erythema should also be documented and the presence and character of any drainage noted. Tenderness of the lower extremity to palpation or the presence of pain in the ulcer or surrounding area should be also recorded. A brief vascular examination should always be performed to be sure the patient has adequate blood flow to the area. The presence of dorsalis pedis and posterior tibial pulses should be noted. If there is a question about the adequacy of the circulation, the patient will need to be referred for noninvasive vascular studies or arteriography. The microcirculation in the periwound area can be evaluated with the laser Doppler and TcPO$_2$ measurements, if available.

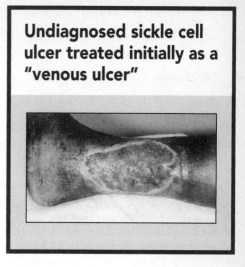

Undiagnosed sickle cell ulcer treated initially as a "venous ulcer"

PRACTICE POINT

A complete history and physical examination are vital when evaluating a patient with a sickle cell ulcer.

Laboratory assessment

Laboratory evaluation depends on the condition of the patient. If the patient does not have a diagnosis of sickle cell disease, but it's suspected the clinician should order blood tests that check for anemia, sickle cells, and abnormal hemoglobin. This usually involves a complete blood count (CBC), sickle "prep," and a hemoglobin electrophoresis. However, although hemoglobin electrophoresis is considered the diagnostic tool of choice, it has its limitations especially if the patient has had recent blood transfusions.[5] In such a case, referral to a hematologist may be necessary. If the patient with known sickle cell disease has an ulcer, the laboratory workup should consist of a CBC with differential white blood cell count and reticulocyte count.

Patients with sickle cell disease are especially prone to developing infections; therefore, it is important to obtain a wound culture using appropriate technique if the wound appears infected or is covered by a biofilm. We have found that a significant number of patients with sickle cell ulcers

have wounds covered by biofilm, which must be removed before the ulcer can heal. (See photographs in the color section, page C23.) The most frequent way to remove a biofilm is with sharp debridement, but recently we have turned to ultrasonic debridement techniques, which are less painful for the patient. (See photographs in the color section, page C23.) Currently, although other methods for removing biofilms are still considered experimental, it's hoped that they will be available in the near future. (See chapter 7, Wound bioburden.)

Infection and osteomyelitis

Patients with sickle cell disease and a deep, painful ulcer should be evaluated radiologically for the presence of osteomyelitis especially if the patient has fever or leukocytosis. In particular, patients with sickle cell disease are prone to developing salmonella osteomyelitis.[5] Radiologic evaluation can be done by several methods. Plain film X-rays are the least sensitive method and usually don't any evidence of osteomyelitis until late in the course of the infection. In addition, they can be especially confusing in the patient with sickle cell disease as the disease can result in periosteal elevation and other bone changes mimicking osteomyelitis.[5] Nuclear medicine bone scans are slightly more helpful, but it must be remembered that routine bone scans only detect areas of inflammation.

Also, if the patient has an ulcer overlying the bone in question, the bone scan is virtually useless. Magnetic resonance imaging appears to be the imaging modality of choice in terms of sensitivity and specificity. It has been suggested that bone biopsy and culture may be the only definitive way to determine if osteomyelitis is present[6], but it should be done with great care so as not to cause an infection in the bone. Biopsy of the wound bed and wound margin may be advisable if the ulcer has been present for over three months, does not respond to therapy, or just doesn't "look right." This should be done to rule out the possibility of malignancy and can help with the diagnosis.[12]

Pain

Because of the painful nature of sickle cell ulcers and the need to do biopsy cultures, the practitioner must be aware of recent studies about the use of topical and local anesthetics. Berg, et.al. have shown that EMLA cream, a topical anesthetic agent commonly used before doing wound biopsies, is highly antibacterial.[11] Within one hour of exposure to EMLA cream, most common bacteria were killed. This included strains of *Staphylococcus aureus* (both methicillin-resistant and methicillin-sensitive strains), Streptococcus pyogenes, *Escherichia coli,* and *Pseudomonas aeruginosa.* Injected solutions of 1% lidocaine were also found to be antibacterial for the same organisms but at greater than two hours after local injection. It is the recommendation of the authors that EMLA cream not be used for anesthesia when biopsy cultures are being done. Local injection of preservative-free 1% lidocaine would be satisfactory to use if the biopsy culture is done within two hours of the injection.[11]

Although sickle cell ulcers tend to be extremely painful, pain assessment is an area that can be easily overlooked as, often times, the patient is fearful of experiencing even more pain and may not want you to look at the ulcer much less touch it. This makes debridement and treatment of these ulcers very difficult. (A useful pain assessment tool for evaluating a patient's pain is outlined elsewhere in this book [see chapter 12, Pain management and wounds]). It has been the author's experience that if the provider does not address the pain problem many of the patients will not return for follow-up care. Indeed, most patients would rather keep their ulcer than deal with potentially being in more pain than they already are. For this reason, significant debridements must by done with some type of anesthesia, either topical anesthesia (xylocaine ointment), injectable local anesthesia, regional anesthesia, or general anesthesia. Some of these techniques will require hospitalization of the patient.

Pain control can be managed with topical anesthetic agents. Topical xylocaine ointment or EMLA cream can be used on a regular basis for pain control. Applied every four to six hours, these agents can make the patient's daily activities much more manageable. It also makes dressing changes more comfortable. Other therapies, including opioid analgesics and regional medications (xylocaine patches), are useful but many times have to be managed by a pain specialist. (See chapter 12, Pain management and wounds.)

PRACTICE POINT

Sickle cell ulcers are extremely painful. Evaluation and treatment of the patient's pain should be a top priority and should be the first steps in instituting therapy for the ulcer.

Treatment

Treatment of sickle cell ulcers can be challenging and frustrating. Even in this day of evidence-based therapies, it is noteworthy that there are no published trials of treatments of sickle cell ulcers.[6] One of the more interesting findings about the treatment of sickle cell ulcers is that most ulcers will heal with prolonged bed rest[6] Obviously, this is not a practical therapy as hospitalization is no longer possible and complete bed rest at home is not realistic. However, any therapy that results in a long period of immobilization, such as from operative intervention, must take into account that the bed rest is healing the ulcer, not the treatment. With this in mind one must begin with the basics of what we know constitutes good wound care.

The basics of good wound care include debridement of devitalized tissue, control of infection, assurance of adequate circulation, and maintenance of a moist wound environment. The major addition in the treatment of sickle cell ulcers is control of wound pain. Many times the ulcers are so painful that manipulation of the wound is impossible. Treatment of the wound with topical anesthetics has been previously addressed and must not be overlooked. If the therapy for the wound is painful, most people will forgo your advice and treat the ulcers themselves in ways that do not cause more pain. It is unfortunate that many of these patients are labeled as "noncompliant" when it is a poor choice of therapy by the clinician and not the compliance of the patient that should be in question. Once the pain is controlled, the wound can be debrided and treated, as indicated.

The evaluation of sickle cell ulcers for infection and the evaluation of the patient for circulation problems have been covered previously. The importance of moist wound care has been known since Winter's publication in 1963.[13] It is now known that wounds treated with wet-to-dry dressings do not heal well and removing a dry dressing that adheres to the wound causes pain and wound reinjury.[14] Wounds treated with moist wound healing heal faster, are less painful, and have less scarring. There are numerous wound dressings currently available which will maintain a moist wound environment. (See chapter 9, Wound treatment options.)

If the wound is felt to be infected, topical antimicrobials should be considered. Oral or I.V. antibiotics are only indicated if the patient has a leukocytosis, cellulitis, or fever. Silver dressings have become popular in the treatment of the wound with a clinically significant bacterial burden (critical colonization) or with frank infection. There are numerous silver dressings available for use on these wounds. It is these authors opinion that, at this time, one should pick the silver dressing that best meets the patient's needs instead of debating the amount of silver in the dressing. It there is excess drainage pre-

sent, a silver alginate, hydrocolloid, or foam might be indicated. If there is significant odor, then a silver dressing with odor control properties might be most beneficial. If only a bandage delivering silver ions is needed, those are also available. It is suggested that once the bacterial burden is under control, the silver dressing should be discontinued and other moisture control dressings used. This is because of the potential for toxicity of the silver to the growing tissues.[15,16] Dressings containing Cadexomer iodine are useful in treating wounds critically colonized with bacteria or wounds which are infected.[17, 18]

Other therapies that may be helpful include oral zinc sulfate (200 mg three times/day)[19] and zinc oxide impregnated Unna boots. An Unna boot applied to the lower extremity and covered with an ace wrap has been especially beneficial for patients with edema. The bandages are changed weekly until the ulcer has healed.[6] A recent series of patients treated with the topical growth factor, molgramostim (GM-CSF), reported some degree of success in the treatment of these very difficult wounds. [20]

The revival of the use of natural honey, a therapeutic product as old as Egyptian medicine, for treatment of sickle cell ulcers has been tried and has met with mixed results.[21] Because natural honey is unsterile, some important implications must be considered for treatment of wounds, the most serious of which is the presence of clostridial spores which could cause wound botulism. However, the introduction of the sterilized honey product, Manuka honey from New Zealand, opens new opportunities for the treatment of sickle cell ulcers.[22]

The use of the human tissue-engineered skin in the treatment of sickle cell ulcers has met with some degree of success. [23] Prior to applying any advanced therapy product the wound bed must be well prepared, which means assuring that the wound bed has been debrided to remove all necrotic tissue, that infection has been controlled, and that the wound environment has been optimized.[24] To achieve the goal of wound environment optimization, one author recommends pretreating the wound with a protease modulating agent for two to three weeks to reduce the abnormal protease levels.[27] These agents include oral or topical Doxycycline or an oxidized, regenerated cellulose (ORC) collagen product.[25,26] His early data show that pretreatment of any chronic wound with these protease modulating agents prior to application of human skin equivalent improves the healing rate.[27] Once treated with the tissue-engineered skin product, the patients experience significant relief of their pain as well as healing of their ulcer. (See photographs in the color section, page C24.) One patient's ulcer healed within 8 weeks of one application of the human tissue-engineered skin. Over eighty percent of our patients treated with human skin equivalent will heal with only one application.[27] It is also of note that sickle cell ulcers treated with tissue engineered skin seem to have a more "normal" appearing and stable scar. (See photographs in the color section.)

One of the treatments of sickle cell disease is hydroxyurea, which is known to improve symptoms associated with sickle cell disease. Unfortunately, hydroxyurea is known to cause leg ulcers in patients taking this medication.[29,30] The medication must be stopped before the ulcer will heal.[31] Fortunately, it has been found that ulcers related to hydroxyurea therapy respond promptly to treatment with tissue engineered skin.[31]

The use of the split-thickness skin graft to treat patients with sickle cell ulcers may be a reasonable therapeutic alternative. However, the procedure requires hospitalization and anesthesia, thus making it less cost-effective. It has also been reported that split-thickness skin grafting has a very low success rate in healing sickle cell ulcers and in those that do heal, the recurrence rate is very high.[28] Success has been noted with the use of muscle flaps, myocutaneous flaps, and free flaps to cover large lower extremity sickle cell ulcers[32,33] but not uniformly.[34]

Transfusion therapy has been tried in the treatment of patients with sickle cell ulcers who have been resistant to all other therapies. The goal of the therapy is to keep the hematocrit between 30-35 volume percent and the percentage of normal hemoglobin (hemoglobin A) greater than 70% of the total.[28]

Another interesting approach to treating sickle cell ulcers has been the use of I.V. arginine butyrate. The concept is that the arginine butyrate will change the concentration of abnormal hemoglobin, thus allowing the wounds to heal. Two studies have shown reasonable success with this method[35, 36], but no randomized controlled trials have been done as of this time.

Other therapies for sickle cell ulcers include medications, such as pentoxifylline (Trental); negative pressure wound therapy; hyperbaric oxygen therapy; electromagnetic stimulation; and nitric oxide stimulation. Others therapies are still considered experimental, and their utility in treating these patients with difficult wound problems will be determined by future studies.

It is our impression that sickle cell ulcers will respond better to any therapy if the sickle cell disease is under control. If the patient's anemia is profound (below 5 grams Hg/ 100 cc) or if the abnormal hemoglobin-containing cells represent greater than 50% of the total volume of red blood cells, the chance of any therapy working is problematic. This has recently been supported by work reported by Eckman and Platt.[28]

Preventing ulcers

Prevention of sickle cell ulcers is of utmost important. The patient with sickle cell disease must be instructed in the importance of good skin care and methods to keep the skin moisturized and to avoid trauma to the lower legs and ankles. For example, the patient should use insect repellants to avoid insect bites. It has been noted that edema is the single most common occurrence prior to recurrence of an ulcer.[28] For this reason, the importance of treating lower limb swelling should be emphasized including the use of support hose or elastic wraps. The patient should also be instructed to treat any minor injury to the lower extremities aggressively and seek medical care promptly. The clinician should inspect the lower extremities of sickle cell patients at each visit and review the preventative measures with them routinely.

PRACTICE POINT

Always look for edema on the lower extremities of patients with sickle cell disease as it is a critical indicator prior to ulceration.

Summary

Sickle cell ulcers are a potential reality for any person with the inherited disease—sickle cell anemia. The success of therapy is multifactorial, which involves optimizing the patient's sickle cell disease and using several therapeutic modalities to treat the ulcer. It is the hope that in the near future, research will provide more satisfactory therapies to treat these difficult wounds.

Show what you know

1. *Which of the following is NOT correct?*

   A. Sickle cell disease is an inherited disease of the blood's hemoglobin molecule.
   B. Sickle cell disease is seen primarily in black individuals.
   C. Higher risk of developing an ulcer is seen in individuals with heterozygous sickle cell disease.
   D. The most severe form of sickle cell disease is seen when an individual inherits an abnormal hemoglobin gene from both parents.

ANSWER: C. Persons with heterozygous sickle cell disease receive only one gene for abnormal hemoglobin from one of their parents and are at less risk of ulceration than persons who have abnormal hemoglobin genes from both parents (homozygous). A, B, and C are true statements.

2. *Sickle cell ulcers are more likely to develop in males with sickle cell disease than females.*

   A. True
   B. False

ANSWER: A

3. *Which one of the following can signal that a patient with sickle cell disease might ulcerate?*

   A. Edema
   B. Hemoglobin A1C of 7
   C. Absence of fever
   D. Resolution of pain in the leg

ANSWER: A. Edema is a key indicator that a person with sickle cell disease may get an ulcer. B is incorrect as hemoglobin A1C is not related to sickle cell disease but to diabetes mellitus. C is incorrect as patients with sickle cell often have fever of unknown origin. D. Pain is frequently part of sickle cell ulcers.

4. *Which one of the following is not part of the evaluation of the patient with a sickle cell ulcer?*

   A. History including a family history
   B. General physical examination
   C. Assessment of wound bed and pulses
   D. A bone scan

ANSWER: D. A bone scan is virtually useless in diagnosing osteomyelitis while MRI is preferred. A, B, and C, are all correct and should be part of the assessment of a patient with a sickle cell ulcer.

5. *Comprehensive treatment of the patient with sickle cell ulcer could include all of the following* except:

   A. Restrict dietary iron intake
   B. Debridement of the ulcer
   C. Wound pain management
   D. Compression modalities

ANSWER: A. There is no reason to restrict iron in the diet of persons with sickle cell disease. B, C, and D are all important parts of the holistic plan of care of patients with a sickle cell ulcer.

References

1. Herrick JB. "Peculiarly Elongated and Sickle-Shaped Red Blood Corpuscles In a Case of Severe Anemia," *Trans Assoc Am Physicians* 25:553, 1910.
2. Powars DR, Chan LS, Hiti A, Ramicone E, Johnson C. "Outcome of sickle cell anemia: a 4-decade observational study of 1056 patients," *Medicine (Baltimore)* 84:363-76, 2005.
3. Charache S. "One view of the pathogenesis of sickle cell diseases," *Bull Eur Physiopathol Respir* 19: 361-66, 1983.
4. Sickle-cell Anaemia Fifty-Ninth World Health Assembly: World Health Organization, 2006.
5. Conley, C. Lockard, "The Hemoglobinopathies and Thalassemias" in *Textbook of Medicine*, eds. Beeson, PB, McDermott, W, 13th Edition, W.B. Saunders Co., Philadelphia, pp.1501-1503, 1971.
6. Management of Sickle Cell Disease, the Sickle Cell Information Center; at www.scinfo.org/nihnew-chap22.htm; accessed 12/27/06.
7. Nolan VG, Adewoye A, Baldwin C, et.al. "Sickle cell ulcers: association with haemolysis and SNPs in Klotho, TEK and genes of the TGF-Beta/BMP pathway," *Br J Haematol.* 133(5):570-578, 2006.
8. Morris CR, Kuypers FA, Larkin S, Sweeters N, Simon J, Vichinsky EP, Styles LA. "Arginine therapy: a novel strategy to induce nitric oxide production in sickle cell disease," *Br J Haematol* 111:498-500, 2000.
9. Aslan M, Freeman BA. "Oxidant-mediated impairment of nitric oxide signaling in sickle cell dis-

ease—mechanisms and consequences," *Cell Mol Biol (Noisy-le-grand)* 50:95-105, 2004.

10. Clare A, FitzHenley M, Harris J, Hambleton I, Serjeant GR. "Chronic leg ulceration in homozygous sickle cell disease: the role of venous incompetence," *Br J Haematol.* 2002; 119(2):567-571

11. Berg JO, Mossner BK, Skov MN, et.al. "Antibacterial Properties of EMLA and Lidocaine in Wound Tissue Biopsies for Culturing," *Wound Rep Reg* 14:581-585 , 2006

12. Ackroyd JS, Young AE. "Leg ulcers that do not heal," *Br Med J* 286:207-208. 1983

13. Winter, G.D. "Formation of the Scab and the Rate of Epithelialization of Superficial Wounds in the Skin of Young Domestic Pigs," Nature 193:293-94, 1962.

14. Ovington LG. "Hanging wet-to-dry dressings out to dry," *Home Healthc Nurse* 19:477-83, 2001.

15. Leaper DJ. "Silver dressings: their role in wound management," *Int Wound J* 3:282-294, 2006.

16. Alvarez OM, Mertz PM, Eaglstein WH. "The effect of occlusive dressings on collagen synthesis and re-epithelialization in superficial wounds," *J Surg Res* 35:142-8, 1983.

17. Lamme EN, Gustafsson TO, Middelkoop E. "Cadexomer-iodine ointment shows stimulation of epidermal regeneration in experimental full-thickness wounds," *Arch Dermatol Res* 290:18-24, 1998.

18. Holloway GA, Jr., Johansen KH, Barnes RW, Pierce GE. "Multicenter trial of cadexomer iodine to treat venous stasis ulcer," *West J Med* 1989;151:35-38, 1989.

19. Serjeant GR, Gallaway RE, Gueri MC. "Oral zinc sulphate in sickle cell ulcers," *Lancet* 2:891-892, 1970

20. Mery L, Girot R, Aractingi S. "Topical effectiveness of molgramostim (GM-CSF) in sickle cell leg ulcers," *Dermatology* 208:135-37, 2004.

21. Okany CC, Atimomo CE, Akinyanju OO. "Efficacy of natural honey in the healing of leg ulcers in sickle cell anemia," *Niger Postgrad Med J* 11(3): 179-181, 2004.

22. *Honey: A Modern Wound Management Product.* Ed. White Richard, Cooper Rose, Molan Peter. Wounds UK Publishing, 2005

23. Gordon S, Bui A. "Human skin equivalent in the treatment of chronic leg ulcers in sickle cell disease patients," *J Am Podiatr Med Assoc.* 93(3):240-241, May-June 20

24. Schultz GS, Falanga V, et. al. "Wound bed preparation: A systematic approach to wound management," *Wound Rep Reg* 11(Supp):1-28, 2003.

25. Chin GA, Schultz GS. "Treatment of chronic ulcer in diabetic patients with a topical metalloproteinase inhibitor, doxycycline," *Wounds* 15(10):315-323, 2003.

26. Cullen, B., et.al. "Mechanism of action of Promogran, a protease-modulating matrix, for the treatment of diabetic foot ulcers," *Wound Rep Reg* 10:16-25, 2002.

27. Treadwell TA. Unreported data, Institute for Advanced Wound Care, 2006.

28. Eckman J, Platt A. Leg Ulcers. Sickle Cell Information Center Guidelines at www.scinfo.org/legulcr.htm accessed 12/3/06

29. Best JP, Daoud MS, Pittelkow MR, Petit RM. "Hydroxyurea-induced leg ulceration in 14 patients," *Ann Int Med.* 128: 29-32, 1998.

30. Weinlich G, Schuler G, Greil R, Kofler H, Fritsch P. "Leg ulcers associated with long-term hydroxyurea therapy," *J Am Acad Dermatol.* 39: 372-374, 1998.

31. Flores F, Eaglstein WA, Kirsner RS. "Hydroxyurea-induced leg ulcers treated with Apligraf," *Ann Intern Med* 132(5): 417-418, March 2000.

32. Heckler FR, Dibbell DG, McCraw JB. "Successful use of muscle flaps or myocutaneous flaps in patients with sickle cell disease," *Plast Reconst Surg* 59:902-908, 1997.

33. Khouri RK, Upton J. "Bilateral lower limb salvage with free flaps in a patient with sickle cell ulcers," *Ann Plast Surg* 1991;27:574-6.

34. Richards RS, Bowen CVA, Glynn MFX. "Microsurgical free flap transfer in sickle cell disease," *Ann Plastic Surg* 29:278-281, 1992.

35. Sher GD, Olivieri NF. "Rapid healing of chronic leg ulcers during arginine butyrate therapy in patients with sickle cell disease and thalassemia," *Blood* 84:2378-2380, 1994.

36. Atweh GF, Sutton M, Nassif I, Boosalis V, Dover GJ, Wallenstein S, Wright E, McMahon L, Stamatoyannopoulos G, Faller DV, Perrine SP. "Sustained induction of fetal hemoglobin by pulse butyrate therapy in sickle cell disease," *Blood* 93:1790-97, 1999.

CHAPTER 18

Surgical wounds, tubes, and drains

Joyce M. Black, PhD, RN, CPSN, CWCN, FAPWCA
Steven B. Black, MD, FACS

OBJECTIVES

After completing this chapter, you'll be able to:

- explain the intrinsic and extrinsic causes of surgical wounds that have failed to heal

- describe the reconstructive ladder and how it's used to plan reconstruction

- manage the patient with fistulas

- describe the principles that guide care of patients who require tissue or bone transplantation for wound closure

- describe strategies to manage tubes and drains.

Surgical wounds are common in hospitalized patients; however, due to the body's amazing ability to heal acute wounds, they're seldom seen by wound care specialists, unless they have failed to heal. This chapter will address common surgical wounds, complex wounds healed via surgical procedures, and surgical wounds that have failed to heal in a timely manner.

Assessment

When examining a patient with a nonhealing surgical wound, it's imperative that the initial reason for surgery and the operation performed be fully understood. The answers to these questions must be clear in the examiner's mind: What was the preoperative condi-

tion that required surgery? For example, did the patient have gastric bypass or repair of abdominal lacerations? What was the patient's condition before surgery? Was the patient healthy or was the patient chronically ill due to diabetes or cancer? What was the intended operation? Were organs or tissues removed? Were foreign materials implanted? Was the operation carried out as planned? For example, has the wound been closed with permanent sutures or mesh? Has healing been occurring along a normal trajectory until now? If so, what has happened to alter the course of healing? What medications is the patient taking that might impact healing? Has the nutritional status of the patient been normal since surgery? Was it normal prior to surgery?

From this initial assessment, a comprehensive understanding of the patient who has the wound, not just the wound itself, will be obtained. And, although treating the wound is of utmost importance, also treating the patient, whose body will heal the wound, is equally imperative.

Extrinsic and intrinsic causes of nonhealing wounds

Causes of nonhealing wounds can be grouped into two large categories: extrinsic and intrinsic. Extrinsic causes are those factors that exist outside of the wound, such as pressure, smoking, and malnutrition. Intrinsic factors exist within the wound, such as infection, tension, and arterial insufficiency. Determining which of these factors is present in a wound is an important initial step in wound care as well as removing any obstacles to healing; local treatments won't be effective in maintaining the wound if the underlying cause of the disruption in healing is not addressed.

Early wound care focuses on removing the obstacles to healing. Although it seems that wound care has seen technological advances, the great 16th century surgeon, Ambrose Pare, is still correct in that we, as health care providers, don't heal wounds, we create them and nature heals them.[1] Indeed, our role is to support the body so that the wound can heal. Wound care practitioners must exercise caution when moving too quickly into treatments for wounds until the underlying causes of the delay in wound healing is fully understood.

Goals of care

For acute wounds, wound closure with the return of form and function are the usual goals of care. Left alone to close via contraction and scar formation, wounds seldom have either form or function and will often recur and look unpleasant. The ability to reach ideal and complete healing without unsightly scarring, such as seen in fetal wounds is impossible. Therefore, the return of acceptable healing with sustained function and anatomic continuity becomes the ideal end point.

Reconstructive ladder and planning reconstruction

A decision-making process in choosing the method to achieve wound closure is based on the following information and the "rungs" of the reconstructive ladder. (See *Reconstructive ladder.*)

Is the wound missing tissue?

If the wound hasn't lost any tissue, it may be possible to close it primarily. Wounds are capable of healing by primary intention, which occurs when the wound edges are approximated (pulled together), and retained by sutures, staples, or glue. The dynamics of healing begin, and new tissue synthesis begins to occur. A healing ridge (an induration beneath the skin, extending to approximately 1 cm) forms directly under the suture line between days 5 and 9 after surgery.

What kind of tissue, if any, is missing?

Wounds that only lack portions of skin may be allowed to granulate closed if they're small, or skin may be grafted to speed the healing process. Wounds that lack tendon, muscle, or bone may require transplantation of these tissues to provide form and function. Such operations require flaps of skin, muscle, fascia, or bone. Such flaps are named for their composition, such as an osteocutaneous flap, which is a bone and skin flap. Another type of flap is the free flap, which employs the surgical technique of freely removing tissue from one area with the nutrient artery and vein intact and moving the tissue to the recipient site. The vessels are reanastomosed using a microscope. A radial free-arm flap contains radius bone, overlying muscle, and skin. It is commonly used to reconstruct the face after wide excision of cancer of the mandible and floor of the mouth.

What donor-site morbidity may occur?

Donor sites have some form of scarring and may exhibit some loss of function, depending on the tissues removed. Once skin is removed for a skin graft, moist wound-healing techniques should usually be implemented at the donor site to minimize scarring and postoperative pain. For example, when the breast is reconstructed using the latissimus muscle from the back, the woman may lose some function of the shoulder. Although some patients perceive the loss of function as tolerable, other patients—for example, a tennis player—may undoubtedly perceive it differently. If a thumb is lost, a patient may opt to transplant the great toe to provide opposition for hand function; however, most people wouldn't want to sacrifice a thumb to replace the great toe. In other words, the degree of loss a patient is willing to experience is proportional to his need for the sacrificed tissue.

What's the simplest method to achieve wound closure?

The easiest method available to close the wound is often used first. Wounds that can heal on their own via granulation and epithelialization are allowed to do so. Skin grafting is the next simplest method and is used to treat wounds that are missing only skin. Skin grafting can be full- or partial-thickness, depending on the kinds of tissue missing in the recipient site and the condition of the recipient site. Wounds that could close on their own, but with accompanying contracture and loss of function, may also be grafted. If muscle is missing, muscle flaps may be used to fill the wound defect or cavity, but the muscle isn't made functional (that is, an insertion, origin, and nerve aren't restored to create a functional muscle). The blood supply to the muscle is restored so that it remains viable. The ample blood flow into muscle is commonly used to treat complex wound problems such as osteomyelitis; restored blood flow may also transport antibiotics and immune cells to the wound.

Muscle has been shown to supply overlying islands of skin through a series of vessels that perforate the muscle body. Surgeons can

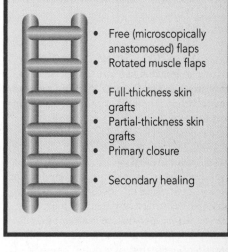

Reconstructive ladder

The reconstructive ladder is used to determine the method to replace missing tissue from a wound bed. The ladder shows the simplest method—simply allowing the wound to heal on its own—at the bottom of the ladder.

- Free (microscopically anastomosed) flaps
- Rotated muscle flaps

- Full-thickness skin grafts
- Partial-thickness skin grafts
- Primary closure

- Secondary healing

simultaneously transplant a muscle and the island of skin to both fill a wound cavity and provide skin coverage. Such a flap is called a musculocutaneous flap. Often the specific muscle is noted, as in the case of the tensor fascia lata flap, which is used to close a trochanteric pressure ulcer. If a large amount of skin is missing, the muscle may be transplanted and then covered with skin grafting to achieve the same effect. Such an operation is called a muscle-flap and split-thickness skin graft, with the specific muscle being grafted added to the name.

Muscle is brought to the recipient site in one of two ways:
- it's rotated along an arc with its original blood supply left intact
- it's freed from its blood supply and the artery and vein are reattached via the microscope at the recipient site.

Freeing the muscle, skin, and other parts of a flap allows the flap to be used for reconstruction in areas that the muscle normally couldn't reach, such as the lower third of the leg.

It's important to note that, as often as possible, tissue should be replaced with similar tissue. Similar hair bearing, appearance, and thickness improve aesthetic appearance on the reconstructed wound. This process of choosing a method to close a wound has been called a reconstructive ladder. (See *Reconstructive ladder.*) The easiest method, secondary healing, is at the bottom of the ladder.

Wounds without missing tissues

Some wounds don't require grafts because they aren't missing tissue, or local tissues can be undermined and lifted to close the original wound.

Simple lacerations

Traumatic wounds are often missing little or no tissues and can be closed primarily; however, the full extent of the injury must be known before any closure is attempted. Laceration of arteries and veins is usually obvious by the amount of bleeding present. Facial lacerations are especially bloody due to the robust blood supply in the face. The patient with a facial laceration is assessed for function of motor and sensory nerves, muscle, parotid and salivary glands in the area prior to injection with lidocaine, which would obscure the findings. Repair of these tissues (vessels, tendons, ligaments, and nerves) is commonly completed in the operating room for its sterile environment sometimes with the benefit of the operating microscope. Wounds are copiously irrigated to remove any debris. Skin closure is accomplished by undermining surrounding tissues to facilitate their movement and suturing layers of tissue with minimal tension. Drains may be placed in wounds with contamination or large amounts of dead space. The appearance of the wound should ideally mimic the ipsilateral appearance. However, traumatic amputation or extensive debridement may leave less than acceptable appearance.

Removing all forms of tension on the wound reduces the scar. Wounds that must be mobilized to gain function, such as incisions over joints, heal with wider scars and this may be disturbing to the patient's self-image. Stinted dressings, immobility (for example, limited chewing or talking with facial lacerations), and thin applications of topical antibiotics may help to minimize scars. Moist wound-healing techniques, used throughout the healing process, will minimize healing time and, potentially, the amount of scarring. However, it's important for the patient, the patient's family, and members of the healthcare team to realize that scarring is inevitable and only after the scar has matured, which can take more than 1 year, will scar revision be attempted. Silicone-based dressings may be used over some healed wounds to help minimize scar build-up during the maturation phase.

Extensive lacerations

Extensive lacerations, even though unsightly, are seldom life-threatening. Lifesaving care of the heart, lungs, and brain precedes definitive wound care. Initial wound care includes debridement of obvious dirt, glass, grass, or other foreign bodies. Massive lacerations are packed with moist dressings to prevent tissue desiccation and, when the patient is stable, the wounds are debrided and surgically closed, if possible. Extensive wounds may require multiple debridements until viable tissue is present; these wounds may also require more complex forms of delayed closure, such as flaps.

Wounds that are not closed within the first 6 hours after injury are considered contaminated and cannot be primarily closed after that time. Some clean facial wounds are an exception to this rule, and their closure may be delayed longer in healthy patients who are on antibiotics.

Penetrating abdominal wounds

Penetrating abdominal wounds include stab wounds, impalements, gun shots and so forth. These are serious wounds due to direct tissue injury, risk of contamination and sepsis, and the potential for excessive bleeding. Depending on the degree of contamination from environmental agents (e.g., dirt) or penetration of the bowel or bladder, the wound may not be completely closed. Frequently in traumatic injuries, these wounds are not closed external to the fascia. If the fascia cannot be closed, leaving the abdomen open is also a challenge. These patients require multiple re-explorations while simultaneously reducing or controlling abdominal fluid secretion and preserving the fascia for closure. Currently, no protocols exist for the management of the open abdomen and care is based on clinical judgment.

Abdominal compartment syndrome

Abdominal compartment syndrome (ACS) is similar to compartment syndrome of the extremity. Normal intra-abdominal pressure ranges from 0 to 5 cm water (H_2O); determining intra-abdominal pressure can be done by using simple water-column manometry with a bladder catheter. However, when it is mildly increased to 10 to 15 cm H_2O cardiac index rises due to compression of the vena cava. With further elevations, there is progressive organ dysfunction due to intra-abdominal hypertension on the abdominal organs. Direct compression on the hollow intestine and portal-caval system causes them to collapse. When the bowel is compressed it becomes ischemic, allowing bacteria to thrive. Vasoactive substances, such as histamine and serotonin increase endothelial permeability, further capillary leakage impairs red cell transport, and ischemia worsens. As pressure rises, ACS not only impairs visceral organs, but also damages the cardiovascular and the pulmonary systems; it may also cause a decrease in cerebral perfusion pressure. Therefore, ACS should be recognized as a possible cause of decompensation in any critically injured patient.[2]

Why include ACS in a wound healing chapter? Because the treatment of ACS is not closure of the abdomen. If the abdomen is at all difficult to close, this procedure should be abandoned and alternative techniques applied. A good rule of thumb is that if, when looking at the abdomen horizontally, the gut can be seen above the level of the wound,

consider leaving the abdomen open and use temporary closure.

The easiest method of controlling the open abdomen is to use a silo-bag closure.[3] This short term therapy has increasingly been replaced by negative wound pressure therapy (NPWT). The use of NPWT has been shown to allow successful fascial closure in patients who in the past would have required mesh grafting for closure. While NPWT increases the use of primary closure, it also shortens time to recovery.[4]

Fistula

Fistula are defined as abnormal openings between two epithelial surfaces. Fistulas can be therapeutic (colostomy, tracheostomy) or pathologic (enterocutaneous, rectovaginal). Fistula between the small and large bowel represent significant problems and require specialized management. The incidence of fistulas is on the rise due in part, to the use of open abdominal procedures in the treatment of sepsis and trauma. In addition, the growing use of mesh to repair abdominal wounds is also contributing to the number of cases.

Fistulas are classified by the tissue involved, if they are external or internal, simple or complex, and by the amount of effluent (output) from them. The name given to the fistula provides information on which two body areas are connected. For example, a enterocutaneous fistula is an external fistula from the small intestines to the skin. External fistula empty to the environment while internal fistula empty into other organs. A simple fistula is one with a direct and often short tract. A complex fistula is often associated with abscess and involves organs or open wounds. High output fistula produce more than 500 ml/day; low output fistula produce less than 200 ml/day. All of these characteristics are important to identify in order to facilitate closure. Although there hasn't been definitive research on the most efficacious methods for treating fistulas, overall, 30% to 70% of fistulas close. However, those fistulas that open into granulating wounds have only a 6% to 10% chance of closure.[5]

Management of the patient with an entero-cutaneous fistula has 3 phases: stabilization, investigation, and treatment. Stabilization includes replacement of fluids lost through the fistula (high output fistulas can lead to hypovolemia) or immediate surgery if uncontrolled sepsis, hemorrhage, or evisceration is present. Investigation of the anatomical nature of the fistula and for the presence of abscesses assists in determining the final care plan. Instillation of dye through a postoperative fistula or a CT scan helps determine the anatomy of the fistula tract.

The patient is NPO to reduce the output from the GI tract. However, returning the patient to a positive nitrogen balance is essential. Therefore, hyperalimentation (TPN) with lipids may be given, although oral feeding may be used if the patient can absorb the nutrients. Patients who have increased effluent after feeding will likely need to be fed parenterally. Patients with high output proximal small bowel fistulas will almost always need parenteral feeding and may benefit from GI decompression. Recently, somatostatin and octreotide have been added to support metabolism for these patients.[5]

If the fistula includes an abscess, the abscess must be drained and antibiotics given. Gram negative and anaerobic organisms are the most common culprits.

Spontaneous closure of fistulas may occur, but only after sepsis is controlled and nutrition is adequate. Colonic fistula can require 30 to 45 days to heal, whereas ileal fistula can take 45 to 60 days to heal. Of fistulas that close, 90% do so within 5 weeks.[6] If surgical repair is desired, it should not be done prematurely. Indeed, premature attempts to operate on inflamed, ischemic, or necrotic tissue increases the risk of peritonitis and leads to the formation of dense adhesions and recurrent fistulas. Definitive therapy will likely require resection of the fistula or diversion of the fecal stream proximal to the fistula.

Initially, the use of NPWT was contraindicated in fistulas. However, NPWT has produced good results (closure) in patients with low output fistula. It also appears that NPWT may be helpful when used to occlude the fistula.[4]

Containment of effluent

A major issue for treating fistula (and all of wound care) is containment of effluent, control of odor, and protection of the surrounding tissues. The goal is to design a containment system that collects effluent, protects perifistular tissues, allows measurement of volume, and controls odor. Many systems have to be designed specific to the patient and require considerable clinical experience and judgment. There are four major concerns: odor, access, effluent and fistula opening.

Is odor a problem?

If so, the drainage should be deodorized by placing liquid deodorants, charcoal, or ground Flagyl in the collection bag. Changing the dressings often or deodorizing the room can also be done. If dressings are changed often, be certain that perifistular skin is well protected. Some of the commercial deodorizers can be quite potent, so it is important to ask the patient how he's tolerating it.

Is access to the fistula or drainage needed?

If yes, two-piece systems or wound management systems are required. If not, one-piece pouches, or catheters placed into the fistula and placed to gravity or suction can be used.

Is the effluent greater than 100 ml in 24 hours?

If not, the fistula can be covered with gauze, foam, alginate or other dressings to absorb the drainage. If yes, individualized plans and approaches are warranted. Many of the same products used for traditional GI or GU stomas can be used with varying degrees of success to pouch a high-output fistula.

An esophageal fistula can be difficult to manage due to the salivary amylase in the drainage and the usual curves of the neck. A retracted penis pouch, pediatric ostomy pouches, and fecal incontinence bags can provide containment for neck fistulas.[7]

Is the fistula opening greater than 3 inches?

Fistulas that have openings that are larger than 3 inches are treated with many containment systems. These include one-piece or two-piece ostomy systems (depending on the need for access), wound management systems, red, rubber catheters-to-wall suction systems, and incontinent collection systems.[8]

Wounds requiring tissue transplantation for closure

Tissue transplantation is a phrase used to describe closure techniques for a group of wounds that have missing tissue. In order to achieve closure, various tissues (skin, muscle, fascia, bone) can be grafted or flapped into the wound. These wounds can be quite complex to manage.

Nonhealing surgical wounds

Nonhealing surgical wounds are slow to heal because of underlying disease states, such as poorly controlled diabetes, protein-calorie malnutrition, compromised immunity, and infection. By convention, any surgical wound of 3 to 4 weeks duration that is not responding to conventional therapy is considered nonhealing.

Infection, including the development of biofilms is a common culprit. Common bacterial causes include *Staphylococcus, Pseudomonas,* and *Enterobacter*. Debridement and low-frequency ultrasound debridement destroys the biofilm and is an important component of wound care. [9]

Abdominal wound dehiscence and evisceration

Wound dehiscence is the separation of the edges of a surgical wound. The strength of a wound lies in the musculoaponeurotic layer of the abdomen. In the early postoperative period, wounds stay closed due to the strength of the sutures used or through normal healing processes as muscles regain their strength. However, some wounds are susceptible to dehiscence, thus requiring tissue transplantation.

Risk factors for wound dehiscence may be technical or related to the patient factors. Technical factors are due to the type of closure used. Indeed, wound dehiscence may occur because sutures break, sutures stretch or cut through the tissues, knots slip, the suture was too thin, or an insufficient number of sutures were used. Closure is best achieved when long-lasting, absorbable or permanent sutures are used, with secure knots that do not slip nor invite bacteria to harbor in them. Sutures should be placed about 1 cm from the abdominal wound and 1 cm apart. This closure places the suture in healthy fascia that will not be cut by suture material. In wounds that are healing securely, a healing ridge of palpable thick tissue about 0.5 cm appears along the incision. This ridge is almost always absent in wounds that rupture.

Patient factors that precipitated wound dehiscence have been reported in a large retrospective study. The most significant factors for dehiscence were being over age 65, emergency operation, cancer, hemodynamic instability, intra-abdominal sepsis, wound infection, hypoalbuminemia, obesity, and use of steroids. Factors that were not significant included gender, anemia, and the presence of diabetes mellitus and pulmonary disease. Overall morbidity and mortality were 30% and 16%, respectively, correlating directly with the number of risk factors.[10]

Obesity, heavy coughing or retching and ascites, all which strain the wound during healing, predispose to dehiscence. However, many surgeons believe that if the wound is closed securely, these complications will not occur. Usually the first sign of an impending problem is the discharge of serosanguineous fluid from the wound, but some patients present with sudden evisceration following an episode of coughing or retching. When the edges of the wound separate and internal organs such as the gut are protruding from the wound, this is known as evisceration.

Evisceration is a frightening experience for the patient. Immediate treatment includes remaining calm, medicating for pain, and keeping the viscera moist with a sterile moist towel to hold the abdominal contents into the abdomen. Exposed intestines should not be forced back into the abdomen. The patient should be kept NPO and prepared for immediate surgery. Lower the head of the bed so it is flat or no more than 20 degrees.[10] Monitor the patient's vital signs and assess for signs and symptoms of shock.[10] The wound is explored urgently in surgery, devitalized tissue is excised, and the abdomen is closed with nonabsorbable suture interrupted suture taking secure bites into healthy tissue. Hernia formation is relatively common, reaching 30% in wounds that eviscerated and re-closed. If the wound has dehisced and that patient cannot tolerate another anesthetic, the wound can be packed with dressings, an abdominal binder used or a vacuum- assisted closure applied to obtain secondary healing. These wounds will inevitably develop hernia.

Median sternotomy

Median sternotomy incisions are extremely complex wounds to close following surgery. Bone is usually repaired with rigid fixation and immobilization but the sternum is often closed with wire and subjected to constant movement with respiration. Further, the operations through sternotomy are often long and bloody, so the fact that some sternotomy incisions become infected and dehisce should not be surprising.

Indeed, infected medial sternotomy[12] wounds following cardiac surgery are a dreaded complication. High-risk patients include obesity (BMI over 30), diabetes, heart failure, previous myocardial infarction, urgent operative status, and hypertension. Perfusion time over 200 minutes, use of an intra-aortic balloon pump, and three or more distal anastomoses are risk factors for very serious infections but these conditions rarely occur. Control of blood glucose and improvement of heart failure prior to surgery are helpful interventions. Sternal incision contamination from intranasal organisms can be reduced by using intranasal Bactroban (mupirocin) ointment.[11] Additionally, the use of transparent adhesive dressings is also helpful to prevent environmental exposure while the wound closes.[13,14]

Early wound infection, such as the aforementioned suppurative mediastinitis, appears as cellulitis, purulent wound drainage, and obvious tracking between the skin, sternum, and mediastinum. Left untreated, these infections smolder down into the mediastinum and may even extend into aortic suture lines, prosthetic grafts, and intracardiac prosthesis.

Local wound care is based on the needs of the wound and the condition of the patient. Wound-bed preparation may include packing, debridement, or the use of NPWT, which may be used as a first line of treatment to drain the superficial infection down to the sternum because it splints the chest wall. NPWT can be used as a bridge to allow the patient to recover or stabilize. Preliminary data show improved survival rates of patients with mediastinitis who were treated with NPWT.[4]

For wounds that are packed, caution is required when treating deep wounds. One continuous piece of rolled gauze is the preferred method to avoid losing single dressings in the cavities. Further, if wounds require topical application of solutions, the large amount of open tissue will quickly absorb the fluids. Use of such products as povidone-iodine solution in these large wounds has resulted in iodine toxicity due to the large absorptive surface. Wounds that extend to the myocardium or around the myocardium should be gently packed between heartbeats. Packing the wound tightly can constrict myocardial filling during relaxation; therefore, the wound must be tucked loosely with gauze.

Chest wall reconstruction

Stabilization of the patient prior to surgery includes maximizing heart and pulmonary function, improving nutrition, and preparing the wound bed. Defects following excision of a tumor, tissue loss from infection of the pleural space, or dehiscence of sternal wounds after coronary bypass grafting are chest wall wounds that usually require reconstruction.

Failure to stabilize the chest wall can lead to paradoxical chest motion with breathing, leading to compromised respiratory function.

Loss of the sternum is especially complex, because without the sternum, ribs are pulled inward with inspiration (e.g., flail chest). Patients can usually tolerate the loss of 4 ribs, if the wound is closed with muscle flaps, like the latissimus dorsi flap. Massive chest injuries or defects will require bony reconstruction; if bone is not used, acrylics or synthetic mesh can be used. However, the risk of infection and rejection are ever-present when synthetic materials are used. [14-16]

When a defect is limited to skin and subcutaneous tissue, local skin flaps can frequently be used to close the wound. A skin flap can be rotated or advanced to cover the wound. The deltopectoral skin flap can also be used to cover chest wounds, although its blood supply is stretched to do so. The principle blood supply to the flap is from two large perforating arteries arising from the second or third intercostal space lateral to the sternal border. Therefore, any tension of the flap or chest can interfere with blood supply to the flap. The weight and torsion of the breast tissue or an obese chest can place tension on the flap, so a loose fitting bra or binder should be used to support the tissue.

PRACTICE POINT

Immediately report to the surgeon any signs of flap ischemia, such as pale, dusky, mottled, or cool tissue.

When the defect is greater, several muscles may be needed for reconstruction, depending on the location of the wound. The latissimus dorsi, pectoralis major, rectus abdominus, and trapezius are the most common muscles used for chest wall reconstruction. [15] The pectoralis muscle is commonly used because it is near the defect. Its blood supply is through the thoracoacromial artery, located in the axilla. The muscle is also supplied with perforating arteries from the internal mammary artery. If the pectoralis muscle is used, the patient will lose some of the ability to adduct and rotate the arm and may have some weakness with lifting. Due to severity of the defect, this donor site mobility is usually justified.

Following surgery, vascular inflow and outflow must be closely monitored. Arterial insufficiency in the flap is a major hazard and problems occur from too much tension on the artery, hematoma in the underlying tissue, extravasated blood, increased blood viscosity, spasm of the artery, or injury or disease of the arterial vessels. Venous outflow problems occur from edema in the flap or compression of the veins. A flap with arterial inflow problems will appear pale and feel cool. Flaps with venous congestion will look engorged, purple and feel tense or full. [16]

Pressure ulcer repair

Repairing a pressure ulcer site is a process containing multiple steps that begin well before surgery. After the pressure ulcer bed is clean, it can be surgically closed. However, before any decisions are made for surgery, such plans must be considered in light of the patient's situation, condition and goals. While various surgical options may be technically possible, doing these operations for the right reasons is an essential first step. Surgery shouldn't be entered into lightly. For some patients, not closing the wound surgically may be the final decision. With proper nutrition, pressure relief, and local wound care, deep pressure ulcers may remain stable for the duration of the patient's life. Adjunctive therapies, such as NPWT, electrical stimulation, and the use of bioengineered tissue products, may be considered to help with closure of these chronic wounds.

Preparing the patient for surgery

Prior to any surgery, the patient's nutritional status and comorbidities must be controlled. Although operative blood loss is usually modest with this type of surgery, general anesthesia is commonly used and the patient must be able to tolerate the stress.

If the pressure ulcer is, in large part, due to malnutrition, surgery should be delayed until the patient has achieved positive nitrogen balance. Calorie counts provide clear data on actual intake of protein and calories, and adjustments can be made to reach ideal levels of intake of 25 to 35 cal/kg of calories and 1.5 to 3.0 g/kg of protein. Monitoring albumin is a reasonable marker, although the half-life of albumin is 20 to 21 days, which seldom reflects current nutritional status. Further, albumin is also lowered by inflammatory processes. With a half-life of 3 days, serum prealbumin is now accepted as a better marker for assessing visceral protein status. In patients with impaired renal function, prealbumin is artificially high because it is not removed with dialysis. Therefore, patients on dialysis should be classified as malnourished if prealbumin is less than 30 mg/dl, whereas the usual normal range is 16 to 35 mg/dl. More accurate nutritional information on protein status can benefit the healing potential for the patient. It's important to recognize that patients who are malnourished are usually deficient in vitamins (especially vitamin C) and minerals (especially zinc and iron); these supplements should be given throughout the course of care.

If the ulcer is due primarily to pressure (such as ischial ulcers in a paraplegic patient), pressure must be redistributed both before and after surgery. Long-term plans for continued pressure redistribution must be included in the operative plan, such as fitting the patient for a wheelchair and appropriate off-loading device, and teaching him pressure-relief techniques to avoid high rates of recidivism. If the ulcer is due to a combination of erosion, shear, and pressure (such as ulcers on the sacrum in a patient with dyspnea and incontinence), all contributing factors need to be addressed. Similarly, long-term pressure reduction and proper skin care management must be included in the care plan. There is a finite number of available flaps; therefore, all efforts must be directed to prevent recurrent ulcers, especially through education of the patient.

Wound infection may not be evident from the surface appearance of the wound. The presence of osteomyelitis should be considered and ruled out in all stage III and IV ulcers. The work-up for suspected osteomyelitis includes a complete blood count, erythrocyte sedimentation rate, and X-rays. This combination of studies has a sensitivity of 73% and specificity of 96%.[17] CT bone scans can be used to diagnose, as needed. Biopsy after adequate debridement can also be used if osteomyelitis is still suspected and the above studies are negative.

Other infections must also be controlled prior to surgery. Urinary tract infections (UTIs) are common in people with diabetes, elderly women, patients with catheters, and those with sacral wounds. Urosepsis is a serious complication and should be considered as the cause of changes in mental status, mal-

nutrition, or changes in vital signs. Chronic urinary antibiotics may be needed for persistent UTIs. Wound infection can also lead to sepsis. (See chapter 7, Wound bioburden.)

Spasms are often a contributing factor to both shear and friction injuries and may also complicate a postoperative course by putting undo tension on wound closure sites. Spasms are common after spinal cord injury due to loss of supraspinal inhibitory pathways. The higher the level of spinal cord injury, the more likely spasms will occur. People with cervical injury have almost a 100% chance of spasm compared to those with injury in the lower thoracic or lumbar spine, who have a 50% chance of spasm. Spasm must be controlled prior to surgery with medications such as baclofen (Lioresal) or dantrolene (Dantrium). Botulism toxin (Botox) can also be injected into the muscle to attempt to reduce spasm; however, the efficacy of this treatment is unrecorded. Spastic limbs may lead to wound dehiscence and postoperative wound complications, and therefore must also be controlled.

Contracture develops in patients with longstanding denervation due to tightening of the muscle and joint capsules. Because hip flexors are so strong, hip contraction is common and can make positioning difficult, with bony prominences resting upon each other and leading to ulcers. Contractures can be minimized and even prevented with proper, persistent positioning, splinting, and a program of aggressive (often passive) range-of-motion exercises. Patients with significant contracture can't be placed in a supine position; if surgery is performed on one hip, only one side will be available as a turning surface, which will require a sophisticated pressure redistribution system to prevent complications or undue pressure at the other hip. A defined turning schedule is essential in these cases. If contractures can be released via tenotomy, the wound may heal. However, leaving a limb flaccid after tenotomy may leave the patient more immobile.

Preparing the wound for surgery

Debridement of nonviable tissue is an important first step in the treatment of full-thickness necrotic pressure ulcers or infected, dehisced surgical wounds. Debridement of adherent eschar in pressure ulcers is advised to reduce the wound bioburden and risk of sepsis. The true stage of a pressure ulcer can't be determined until adequate debridement has been performed because the true depth of the wound is obscured. Debridement can create extensive wounds. For example, pelvic pressure ulcers can extend to the scapula and to the vagina or trochanters. Removal of necrotic tissue may enhance the wound healing cascade and diminishes the risk of infection. (See chapter 8, Wound debridement.) Dry and stable gangrene should not be removed from foot ulcers in patients with impaired arterial supply. Changing a closed and stable wound to an open and ischemic wound creates a greater problem.

Wound debridement is most thoroughly completed in the operating room. Bedside debridement may be used to unroof hard eschar, but can seldom be completed to the level of a clean wound bed. Enzymatic debridement will often provide reasonable wound debridement, but may take many weeks. However, in the patient who is a poor surgical risk, enzymatic agents are a good alternative.

Determining which wounds would benefit from debridement is the first step. Generally necrotic tissue is understood to be a healing deterrent because it allows infection. Necrotic tissue has no blood supply so antibiotics and antibodies are not present in it. The wound and surrounding tissues should be examined fully to assess for fluid collection, abscess formation, and extensions into surrounding tissues.

Whether or not heels should be debrided remains controversial. Most clinicians feel that stable, dry, adherent eschar on the heels shouldn't be debrided. The foot, especially the posterior heel, has very limited blood flow and only subcutaneous fat. Once the underlying fatty tissue is exposed to the environment, it may quickly become infected due to desiccation and its limited blood flow. If bone is exposed during debridement, osteomyelitis may be an inevitable occurrence.[17] Stable, dry eschar that has no openings should be left intact, assessed often, and off-loaded completely with pillows under the calves or floating the heel in orthotic splints/boots. The phrase "float the heels" is an appropriate order to convey the idea that no pressure is to be applied to the heels. If the eschar softens or breaks or the tissue around the ulcer becomes fluctuant or inflamed, the tissue should be excised to prevent deeper bacterial invasion and sepsis. Chemical debridement may be needed to continue the process of wound bed preparation. Moist wound-healing techniques should be instituted at this time. Off-loading should continue throughout the course of treatment.

Flaps for pressure ulcer repair

Large areas of skin or skin and muscle may be missing from a pressure ulcer. Surgical repair options depend on what kind of tissue needs replacement. If skin is missing on a sacral wound, for example, rotational flaps of skin or skin and fascia can be rotated to close the wound. If muscle is missing, such as in a deep stage IV ulcer, the gluteus may be used to provide padding and protection of the bony structures. The muscle moved into the wound doesn't function as muscle; it atrophies over time due to denervation. Muscle tissue provides padding and robust blood supply to combat osteomyelitis. Muscle also carries more skin with its named blood vessels, so more skin can be moved without ischemia developing. (See *Flaps for pressure ulcer repair,* page 384.)

Postoperative care

The transplanted muscle flap requires adequate perfusion of arterial blood and drainage of venous blood to survive. Because a limited number of flaps are available to reconstruct any wound, the threat of flap failure is great. Early flap failure is most commonly due to arterial spasm or clots in the venous drainage. Flaps that have impaired arterial flow appear pale, have poor to absent capillary refill, and show sluggish bleeding when lanced. These wounds require quick restoration of their arterial supply by opening the wound and examining the arterial anastomosis site. Occasionally, arterial spasm is the culprit. Spasm can be treated by posi-

Flaps for pressure ulcer repair

This chart presents closure options for pressure ulcers at common sites.

Pressure ulcer site	Muscle flap options	Skin or fasciocutaneous flap options
Sacral ulcer	• Gluteus maximus (superiorly or inferiorly based)	• Transverse or vertical lumbosacral
Ischial ulcer	• Gluteus maximus (superiorly based) • Biceps femoris • Semimembranosus • Semitendinosus • Tensor fascia lata (may retain sensation)	• Posterior thigh advancement flap with skin graft of donor site • Posterior V-Y advancement flap • Medial thigh rotation flap
Trochanteric ulcer	• Tensor fascia lata (may retain sensation)	

tioning the flap dependently and warming the area.

PRACTICE POINT

Early signs of arterial flap failure are:

• pale color
• capillary refill poor or absent
• bleeding sluggish when lanced
• loss of audible pulses by Doppler.

Flaps that have impaired venous drainage appear dark blue and swollen. The problem is seldom a faulty anastomosis site; usually, it results from the sluggish exit of venous blood. Venous congestion can be treated by elevation and application of leeches to drain excess blood from the flap. NPWT may also be recommended to decrease fluid collection. Drains are commonly used to empty fluid accumulation in dead space, and can be left in place for a week or longer until drainage has subsided.

Tension on the incision line can lead to dehiscence. Bolster dressings are typically used to close the wound with little tension. Suture lines are slow to heal, especially in the denervated patient, and sutures are left in place for at least 3 weeks. Due to poor approximation and tensile strength, great caution must be used when moving the patient to avoid pulling on the suture line. It's possible to tear open a late-stage surgical repair, which commonly leads to complete flap failure.

Pressure relief is crucial following flap repair. Surgeons usually prescribe air-fluidized beds or low-air-loss beds for 2 to 6 weeks. Large skin flaps are especially prone to failure because of tension on the distal edges of the flap. If fecal incontinence is likely, the patient may be placed on a low residue diet and constipating medications. Diverting colostomy may be required prior to flap closure in extreme cases to prevent contamination of the surgical site with stool.

The patient must be compliant with off-loading strategies after a surgical flap for wound closure to prevent breakdown of the surgical repair. This involves not only immediate postoperative pressure redistribution, but continued interventions of pressure relief and reduction after complete healing has occurred, especially in patients confined to wheelchairs. Proper chair cushions and weight shifts are essential.

Leg reconstruction

Tissue defects of the leg can be reconstructed with muscle flap covered with skin grafts, myocutaneous flaps, or free flaps, depending on the location of the wound and available tissue. Attempts are made to salvage the leg unless there is irretrievable nerve or vessel damage. Major soft tissue injuries with or without bone involvement provide an environment favorable for infection. Wound care is commonly completed in the operating room, where debridement can be performed in a sterile atmosphere. Definitive wound coverage often includes rectus abdominus, gluteus, rectus femoris, gastrocnemius, and soleus muscle.

Following surgery, it's imperative to monitor the flap for signs of vascular compromise. These situations are emergent, and without immediate intervention, the limb may be lost due to ischemia. Prompt and accurate reporting of unusual findings must be made to the attending surgeon.

PRACTICE POINT

Monitor for the following signs of vascular compromise:
- pallor and coolness
- lack of pulses
- pain with movement
- slow or absent capillary refill
- Inability to move extremity

Necrotizing fasciitis

Necrotizing fasciitis, formerly called streptococcal gangrene, is a rapidly progressive skin infection. Although beta-hemolytic *Streptococcus pyrogenes* is the most common organism, no single organism is responsible for the infection. Frequently, necrotizing fasciitis is caused by two organisms acting in concert, called synergistic gangrene. Gram-positive bacteria (including staphylococcus), gram-negative bacteria, anaerobic (including gas gangrene caused by *Clostridium perfringens*), marine vibrio, and fungi have been identified. Necrotizing fasciitis due to beta-hemolytic streptococcal organisms is highly sensitive to

---

Conditions leading to necrotizing fasciitis

The conditions listed below place patients at risk for necrotizing fasciitis.
- Age 50 and older
- Alcoholism
- Anal fissure
- Atherosclerosis
- Diabetes mellitus
- Diverticulum
- Hemorrhoids
- Hypertension
- Immunosuppression
- Intravenous drug use
- Malignancy
- Malnutrition
- Obesity
- Renal failure
- Surgery
- Trauma
- Urethral tear

Adapted with permission from Ault, M.J., et al. "Rapid Identification of Group A Streptococcus as a Cause of Necrotizing Fasciitis," *Annals of Emergency Medicine* 28(2):227-30, August 1996.

---

antibiotics. However, antibiotics don't penetrate necrotic tissue so delays in treatment can lead to a 75% mortality.[18] Necrotizing fasciitis is known to the public as "flesh-eating bacteria."

Many conditions increase risk of necrotizing fasciitis. (See *Conditions leading to necrotizing fasciitis.*) Necrotizing fasciitis appears to develop following a breach in the integrity of a mucous membrane barrier, especially in the abdomen and perineum. The extremities are also commonly involved. A malignancy may also give rise to a portal of entry. In males, leakage into the perineal region can result in a syndrome called Fournier's gangrene, characterized by massive swelling and tissue loss of the scrotum and penis with extension into the perineum, the abdominal wall, and legs.

A reddened, painful, swollen area of cellulitis accompanied by severe local pain and fever are the most common early signs. More generalized swelling develops and is followed by brawny edema. With progression, dark red induration of the epidermis appears, along with bullae (filled with blue or purple fluid). Later, the skin becomes friable and takes on a bluish, maroon, or black color. By this stage, thrombosis of blood vessels in the dermal papillae is extensive. Extension of infection to the level of the deep fascia causes this tissue to take on a brownish-gray appearance of frank gangrene. Skin is a very effective barrier preventing bacteria from invading the body, and likewise, skin is also able to trap organisms within the body leading to rapid spread along fascial planes and through venous channels and lymphatics. Patients in the later stages are toxic and frequently manifest septic shock and multiorgan failure. Skin inflammation is rapidly followed by necrosis of superficial fascia, subcutaneous fat, and in some cases, muscle. Necrotizing fasciitis is commonly seen in conjunction with severe systemic toxicities

PRACTICE POINT

The hallmark of necrotizing fasciitis is pain out of proportion to physical findings.

Diagnosis and treatment

Aspiration cultures from the wound edge or punch biopsy with frozen section may be helpful if the results are positive, but false-negative results occur in approximately 80% of cases. There is some evidence that aspiration alone may be superior to injection and aspiration using normal saline solution. However, deep biopsy and frozen section histopathology may confirm diagnosis. Frozen sections are especially useful in distinguishing necrotizing fasciitis from other skin infections such as toxic epidermal necrolysis.

PRACTICE POINT

In cases of suspected necrotizing fasciitis, myositis, or gangrene, early, aggressive surgical exploration is necessary to:
- visualize deep structures
- remove necrotic tissue
- open compartments to decrease pressure
- obtain tissue for Gram stain for aerobic and anaerobic organisms
- repeat debridements.

Repeated debridements are usually necessary until all devitalized tissue is removed. Broad-spectrum antibiotics are started I.V. pending more specific culture results.

Appropriate empirical antibiotic treatment for necrotizing fasciitis from group-A streptococcal organisms is commonly clindamycin plus penicillin G and cephalosporin (first- or second-generation). Mixed aerobic-anaerobic infections can be treated with ampicillin and sulbactam, cefoxitin, or combinations of clindamycin, metronidazole, ampicillin, or ampicillin, sulbactam, and gentamicin. Group A streptococcal and clostridial infection of the fascia or muscle carries a mortality rate of 20% to 50% even with penicillin treatment. Hyperbaric oxygen treatment may also be useful as many of these infections have an anaerobic or micro-aerophilic component. Antibiotic treatment should be continued until all signs of systemic toxicity have resolved, all devitalized tissue has been removed, and granulation tissue has developed. Multiorgan system failure is not uncommon.

Following debridement, the wounds are packed open. The packing can be extensive and may be completed in the operating room with daily debridement. Definitive treatment may include amputation or extensive skin grafting after the infection is under control and the wounds show evidence of granulation. It's essential that the dressings stay moist to prevent desiccation of tissue. It may be helpful to use products with a higher absorptive capacity than gauze to manage fluid from draining wounds.

Tubes and drains

Traditionally, surgeons have utilized tubes and drains based on surgical teaching and tradition However, with the development of evidence-based medicine, these approaches are being evaluated and challenged. As a result, this aspect of surgical wound care is evolving.

Nasogastric tubes

In the past decade, the routine use of nasogastric (NG) tubes for all patients undergoing GI surgery has become increasingly rare. A meta-analysis of 26 trials (N – 3,964) concluded that NG tubes are unnecessary in elective surgical patients and may even cause pneumonia, atelectasis, fever, and prolongation of time to oral feeding. [19] Today, NG decompression is usually limited to those patients undergoing esophageal or gastric operations for upper intestinal decompression and to decrease tension on alimentary anastomosis. The other group of patients who are managed with NG tubes are those with intestinal obstruction or with severe prolonged ileus, usually related to intra-abdominal sepsis. However, NG decompression is appropriate on a selective basis for any patient in whom severe nausea, vomiting, or gastric distention develops.

Patients with NG tubes need to have frequent oral care (every 2 to 4 hrs), confirmation of the placement of the tube, and assessment of the consistency and amount of the drainage from the tube. Despite being anchored with tape or other devices, NG tubes can coil in the esophagus or the back of the throat and hamper breathing. Patients report considerable discomfort from NG tubes; however, sucking on ice helps to alleviate the sensation. Be certain to include the fluid consumed from ice as intake (1 cup of ice = 80 ml of water). Finally, in unconscious patients, an NG tube can cause a pressure ulcer on the nares. The condition of the skin around the tube is an important aspect of daily nursing assessment.

Feeding tubes

Enteral tube feeding is an important adjunct in the treatment of both acute and chronically ill patients who cannot consume adequate calories and protein. Tubes can be placed to deliver nutrient into the stomach, duodenum or jejunum. NG tubes are easily placed, whereas postpyloric tube placement is more difficult. Patients at high risk of aspiration, such as those with gastric atony or gastroparesis, and patients with pancreatitis, where it is considered desirable to feed beyond the ampulla, should be considered for a postpyloric tube. However, aspiration remains a risk in any patient who is fed artificially. Soft and pliable feeding tubes can pass easily into the trachea even in intubated patients and can cause a pneumothorax or a pneumonia if feedings are given without confirmation that the location of the tip is correct.

For those patients who will require long-term feeding, enterostomies—permanent or temporary—can be placed into the stomach or jejunum. Skin infections are usually minor and can be managed with local wound care (dressing changes) and antibiotics. Major infections are extremely rare (<1.6% of cases).[20] with peritonitis occurring infrequently. The more common complications involving gastrostomy tubes are excessive leakage of gastric intestinal fluids onto the skin. The balloon in the stomach can create too much tension on the gastric mucosa and lead to ulceration or erosion; both of which require correct application of tension, optimal fixation of the tube, and local wound care.

Skin care around the tube

Skin around the tube insertion site should be assessed daily for signs of breakdown, infection or excoriation. Leakage of gastric content onto the skin is not uncommon and the tube will need to be examined for leaks and stabilized to prevent movement in and out of the abdomen. For the first week following placement, the insertion site and external retention device should be cleansed with normal saline. Half-strength hydrogen peroxide can be used to remove crusts. After the first week, the stoma site should be cleaned with soap and water, including beneath the external retention device.

A gastrostomy tube should be rotated 360 degrees daily, according to the manufacturers' recommendations. The tube should be checked for its ability to be moved in and out of the abdominal wall; ¼ inch (0.5. cm) is normal. If the tube cannot be moved even slightly, notify the physician as this may indicate that it has become imbedded in the tissues, and thus eroded into the stomach wall. This problem is called "buried bumper syndrome."

Tube blockage is common with crushed medication, inadequate flushing (particularly with nasojejunal tubes, which tend to be longer and of finer bore), or precipitation of protein in the feeding. Ideally, tubes should be regularly flushed with water, every 6 hours in the case of nasojejunal tubes, and flushed before and after use. To avoid a clogged feeding tube, thoroughly flush enteral feeding devices every 4 to 6 hours during continuous feedings and whenever feedings are on hold, before and after administration of feedings and medications, and after checking residuals. Always use a large syringe (30 to 60 ml) for flushing to prevent rupturing the tube. Irrigate the tube with 20 to 30 ml of tepid water—no fluid has been found to be superior to water for maintaining patency. If the feeding tube has a Y port connector, flush through the side port. Otherwise, disconnect the feeding infusion and flush directly into the tube.

Long intestinal tubes

Long intestinal tubes (e.g., the Cantor tube and the Miller-Abbott tube) are occasionally used in patients with partial small-bowel obstruction early after operation, although mechanical bowel obstruction usually necessitates early operation. Because continued movement of the tube distally is dependent on peristalsis, these tubes are of little value in patients with paralytic ileus. The Cantor tube is made of silicone-coated polyvinyl chloride and has a small balloon tip. The tip is filled with mercury, passed through the nose, and allowed to advance into the small intestine either passively or under fluoroscopic guidance. The tube is not secured to the nose or face so that it can move distally. Changing the position of the patient (right side initially, then left) can help advance the tube. Removal of the tube is accomplished by pulling approximately 30 cm of tube out of the nose every 1 or 2 hours and either taping or clamping it to prevent slippage.

Biliary drainage catheters

Biliary tract drains include cholecystostomy tubes, percutaneous drains, endoscopically placed nasobiliary tubes, and T tubes. Cholecystostomy tubes can be placed under local anesthesia and are used in patients who cannot tolerate cholecystectomy. Percutaneous cholecystostomy tubes can also be inserted with fluoroscopy guidance. Nasobiliary tubes are placed during endoscopy to alleviate common bile duct (CBD) obstruction.

T tubes are placed in the CBD following surgery to explore or repair it. The T-shaped end of the tube is used to stent the duct. The long end of the T tube is then brought out of an incision, sutured to the skin, and attached to a drainage bag. A T tube usually drains most of the bile produced (600 to 700 ml daily) initially. A decrease in the volume of bile drained indicates patency of the distal duct and free flow into the duodenum. The tube can be removed by gentle withdrawal; alternatively, the tube is clamped, and if the patient continues to do well, it is removed on an outpatient basis after 1 to 2 weeks. Bile is caustic, so caution must be used when emptying biliary drains to avoid contact with the patient's skin.

Drains

Various tubes and associated devices have been used to drain purulent materials, blood, or serum from body cavities or dead space created during surgery. These include Penrose drains (very soft rubber tubes), closed-suction drains (e.g., Jackson-Pratt or Hemovac drains), and sump drains (multiple-lumen tubes that draw air into one interior lumen and fluid from a companion tube). Controlled clinical trials in elective surgical patients indicate that routine use of drains does not improve outcomes for patients undergoing cholecystectomy, colon surgery[21,22] thyroid surgery,[23] or hip and knee replacement.[24] Postoperative drainage does, however, reduce serum formation and other wound problems after mastectomy.[25] Postmastectomy wound drainage can be managed on an outpatient basis, thus won't hinder or delay discharge.

Drainage tubes are indicated in esophageal, pancreatic, duodenal, hepatic, or pelvic surgery when there is a significant chance for leakage of bile, enteric contents, lymphatic, or pancreatic fluid. Drains can also be used to collapse a large dead space and to prevent seroma formation. When prophylactic or therapeutic drainage is instituted, many options of drainage exist, including closed-suction drains, sump drains, and percutaneous catheter drains. Drain removal is directly related to the reason for drain placement. For example, a drain placed at the time of a distal pancreatic resection will not be removed until the patient is tolerating a full diet by mouth, thereby maximally stimulating the pancreas and allowing assessment for a pancreatic leak.

Errors in tubes

Patients in the intensive care unit (ICU) often have many tubes, including I.V. lines, feeding tubes, chest drainage tubes, central venous catheters, and wound drains. The number of tubes can be confusing, especially if the drain is not labeled, and this can lead to errors related to invasive line, tube, and drain (LTD) placement, maintenance, or removal. A study was done through an anonymous web-based ICU Safety Reporting System to report unsafe conditions and events in ICUs that could or did lead to patient harm. Researchers identified 114 LTD incidents (including one patient death directly related to an LTD incident) at 18 ICUs in the United States and over 60% were considered preventable. Of patients who suffered LTD incidents, 56% sustained physical injury and 23% had either an actual or anticipated longer hospital stay. LTD incidents were 3 to 4 times more likely to occur in the operating room, on a holiday, or in patients with medically complex conditions. They were nearly 8 times more likely to occur in patients ages 1 to 9 years than in older patients.[26] The study concluded that the clinicians' knowledge and skills helped prevent LTD incidents, whereas team communication was less likely to prevent them (probably because LTD procedures usually depend on a single individual).

Summary

Understanding the etiology of complex wounds is a critical first step in developing an effective treatment plan. Recognition of unique characteristics of each of these wound categories will enable the clinician to correctly identify the wound. The goal of care for acute wounds is wound closure with the return of form and function. Use of the reconstructive ladder can assist clinicians in the decision-making process. Surgical management may be part of the care plan for complex acute and chronic wounds. Maintaining the patency of drains and tubes as well as assessing and protecting the skin around drains and tubes is imperative.

Show what you know

1. Which of the following situations depicts the use of the simplest method for closure of the wound described?

    A. A skin graft of a venous stasis ulcer
    B. Secondary healing of a calcium extravasation
    C. Primary closure for a sternal incisional dehiscence
    D. A free fasciocutaneous flap for a stage III pressure ulcer

ANSWER: B. Secondary healing is the simplest method for any wound, but in many deep wounds secondary healing will require excessive scar and time. Venous stasis ulcers and sternal dehiscence can sometimes heal secondarily, so skin grafting would be more complex. A stage III ulcer should be able to heal with other methods than free flaps, which are the "top of the line" surgical options.

2. Which of the following wounds might require a musculocutaneous flap for closure?

    A. A large burn on the face
    B. Calciphylaxis of the lower legs
    C. Radiation necrosis of the chest wall
    D. A stage II pressure ulcer on the trochanter

ANSWER: C. Only the radiation of the chest wall is a wound with muscle involvement. In addition, the additional blood supply brought into the area by the muscle will often be used to treat any osteomyelitis.

3. Which of the following signs might indicate arterial impairment in a flap?

    A. Pain and coolness
    B. Pallor and warmth
    C. Slow capillary refill and pain
    D. Slow capillary refill and pallor

ANSWER: D. The loss of arterial inflow will render a flap pulseless (often only by Doppler), so delays in capillary refill are seen first, and pallor. If the early signs are not recognized, the flap can become cyanotic and eventually lose tissue.

4. You discharged a patient with ischial ulcers from the hospital after 6 weeks of local wound care. Upon return to the clinic, the wounds have recurred and are necrotic. Which of these causes of recurrence should be investigated first?

A. Presence of urinary incontinence
B. Inadequate pressure relief in seating
C. Deterioration of nutritional status
D. Development of ischial osteomyelitis

ANSWER: B. A hospitalized patient often has pressure reduction via beds and chair cushions. In addition, the nurses remind the patient to off-load. Once discharged, the lack of these devices and cues can quickly lead to deterioration. The other factors can contribute and should be considered too.

5. Which statement about fistula care is true?

A. NPWT is contraindicated for treating fistulas.
B. External fistula empty into an organ.
C. Low output fistula produce less than 200 ml per day.
D. Fistulas that open into granulating wounds have the best chance of healing.

ANSWER: C. Exudate from low output fistula is les than 200 ml per day while high output fistulas produce more than 500 ml per day. B is incorrect as external fistulas empty to the environment while internal fistula empty into an organ. A is incorrect as NPWT can now be used to treat patients with a fistula. D is incorrect . While 30-70% of fistulas do close, fistulas that open into granulating wounds have the poorest chance of closure at only 6-10%.

References

1. Levine, J. "Historical Notes on Pressure Ulcers: The Cure of Ambrose Pare," *Decubitus* 5(2):23-24, 26, 1992.
2. Paylidis, T.E., et al. "Complete Dehiscence of the Abdominal Wound and Incriminating Factors," *European Journal of Surgery* 167(5):351-55, 2001.
3. Doughty, D. "Preventing and Managing Surgical Wound Dehiscence," *Home Health Nurse* 22:364-67, 2005
4. Argenta, L., et al. "Vacuum-assisted Closure: State of the Clinical Art," *Plastic and Reconstructive Surgery* 117(7S):127S-142S, 2006.
5. Dudrick, S., Mahaaraj, A.R., and McKelvey, A. "Artificial Nutritional Support in Patients with Gastrointestinal Fistulas," *World Journal of Surgery* 23:570-76, 1999.
6. Maykel, J.A. and Fischer, J.E. "Current Management of Intestinal Fistulas," in *Advances in Surgery*. Edited by Cameron, J.L., St. Louis: CV Mosby, 2003.
7. Zimmnicki, K. "Products for Managing Neck Fistulas," *ORL-Head and Neck Nursing* 24(3):26, 2006
8. Kozell, K. and Martins, L. "Managing the Challenges of Enterocutaneous Fistula," *Wound Care Canada* 1(1):10-14, 2002.

9. Breuing, K.H., et al. "Early Experience Using Low-frequency Ultrasound in Chronic Wounds," *Annals of Plastic Surgery* 55(2):183-87, 2002.
10. Moz, T. "Wound Dehiscence and Evisceration," *Nursing* 34(5):88, 2004.
11. Maciver, R.H., et al. "Topical Application of Bacitracin Ointment is Associated with Decreased Risk of Mediastinitis After Median Sternotomy," *Heart Surgery Forum* 9(5):E750-33, 2006.
12. Finkelstein, R., et al. "Surgical Site Infection Rates Following Cardiac Surgery: The Impact of a 6-year Infection Control Program," *American Journal of Infection Control* 33(8):450-54, 2005.
13. Fowler, V., et al. "Clinical Predictors of Major Infections After Cardiac Surgery," *Circulation* 112(9) Suppl.:I358-65, 2005.
14. Ahumada, L.A., et al. "Comorbidity Trends in Patients Requiring Sternotomy and Reconstruction," *Annals of Plastic Surgery* 54(3):264-68, 2005.
15. Seyfer, A. "Chest Wall Reconstruction," in *Plastic Surgery: Indications, Operations and Outcomes.* Edited by Achauer, B. St. Louis: Mosby-Year Book, Inc., 2001.
16. Black, S.B. and Eastman, S. "Repair and Care of Chest Wall Defects," *Plastic Surgical Nursing* 21(1):13-19, 2001.
17. Lewis, V.L., et al. "The Diagnosis of Osteomyelitis in Patients with Pressure Sores," *Plastic and Reconstructive Surgery* 81(2):229-32, February 1988.
18. Chapnick, E.K. and Albert, E.I. "Necrotizing Soft Tissue Infections," *Infectious Disease Clinics of North America* 10:838-43, 1996.
19. Cheatham, M.L., et al. "A Meta-analysis of Selective Versus Routine Nasogastric Decompression After Elective Laparotomy," *Annals of Surgery* 221(5): 469-78, 2005.
20. Marik, P.E. and Zaloga, G.P. "Meta-analysis of Parenteral Nutrition Versus Enteral Nutrition in Patients with Acute Pancreatitis," *BMJ* 328:1407-11, 2004.
21. Urbach, D.R., et al. "Colon and Rectal Anastomoses Do Not Require Routine Drainage: A Systematic Review and Meta-analysis," *Annals of Surgery* 229(2):174-80, 1999.
22. Karliczek, A., et al. "Drainage or Nondrainage in Elective Colorectal Anatomosis: A Systematic Review and Meta-analysis," *Colorectal Disease* 8(4):259-63, May 2006.
23. Pothier, D.D. "The Use of Drains Following Thyroid and Parathyroid Surgery: A Meta-analysis," *Journal of Laryngology and Otology* 119(9):669-71, 2005.
24. Parker, M.J., et al. "Closed Suction Drainage for Hip and Knee Arthroplasty: A Meta-analysis," *Journal of Bone and Joint Surgery American* 86-A(6):1146-62, 2004.
25. Katsumasa, et al. "Evidence-based Risk Factors for Seroma Formation in Breast Surgery," *Japanese Journal of Clinical Oncology* 36(4):197-206, 2006.
26. Needham, D.M., et al. "A System Factors Analysis of 'Line, Tube, and Drain' Incidents in the Intensive Care Unit," *Critical Care Medicine* 33(8):1701-707, 2005.

CHAPTER 19

Atypical wounds

Tami de Araujo, MD
Robert S. Kirsner, MD, PhD

OBJECTIVES

After completing this chapter, you'll be able to:

- recognize the importance of identifying atypical wounds

- state the need for wound biopsies in determining the etiology of an atypical wound

- describe the various clinical manifestations of atypical wounds.

Types of atypical wounds

Prolonged pressure (pressure ulcers), venous insufficiency (venous leg ulcers), complications of longstanding diabetes mellitus (diabetic foot ulcers), or poor vascular supply (arterial ulcers) are the most common causes of chronic wounds. Wounds due to uncommon etiologies, called *atypical wounds,* are less frequently encountered and less well-understood. Their prevalence hasn't been studied extensively, but it's estimated that, of the more than 500,000 leg ulcers in the United States, 10% may be due to unusual causes.[1] A variety of etiologies may cause atypical wounds,[2] such as infections, external or traumatic causes, metabolic disorders, genetic diseases, neoplasms, or inflammatory processes.

It's critical to recognize when a wound is caused by an etiology other than prolonged pressure, neuropathy, or abnormal vascular supply so that a correct diagnosis can be made and the appropriate therapy provided. A wound should be evaluated for an atypical etiology if:

- it's present in a location different from that of a common chronic wound

- its appearance varies from that of a common chronic wound

- it doesn't respond to conventional therapy.

For example, the thigh is an atypical location for a pressure, venous, arterial, or diabetic ulcer, and should raise the suspicion of an atypical cause. A wound on the medial aspect of the leg but extending deep to the tendon would be considered atypical despite being a common location, because the depth of this wound is atypical for venous ulcers. Finally,

Potential etiologies of atypical wounds

Although not all-inclusive, this list presents some of the most commonly encountered etiologies for an atypical wound.

Inflammatory causes
- Vasculitis
- Pyoderma gangrenosum

Infections
- Atypical mycobacteria
- Deep fungal infections

Vasculopathies
- Cryoglobulinemia
- Cryofibrinogenaemia
- Antiphospholipid antibody syndrome

Metabolic and genetic causes
- Calciphylaxis
- Sickle cell anemia

Malignancies
- Squamous cell carcinoma
- Basal cell carcinoma
- Lymphoma
- Kaposi's sarcoma

External causes
- Burns
- Bites
- Stings
- Radiation

any wound that isn't healing after 3 to 6 months of appropriate treatment should raise the consideration of an atypical cause, even if the distribution and clinical appearance are classic for a common chronic wound.

Once a wound is deemed atypical, a tissue sample is critical to include histologic evaluation with special stains, tissue culture (for infectious causes), and immunofluorescence testing (for some inflammatory or immune-based causes).

EVIDENCE-BASED PRACTICE

Tissue samples are mandatory for atypical wounds because many of the unusual causes of wounds can resemble each other, making visual diagnosis alone difficult and risky.

Etiologies of atypical wounds

Some of the most commonly encountered etiologies for an atypical wound include inflammatory causes, infections, vasculopathies, metabolic and genetic causes, malignancies, and external causes. (See *Potential etiologies*

of atypical wounds.) However, a thorough medical history, including epidemiological exposure, family history, personal habits, and concomitant systemic diseases, along with a thorough physical examination in combination with histologic evaluation and laboratory testing, will provide critical information necessary for a correct diagnosis of an atypical wound.

Inflammatory causes

Among the most interesting—and probably more common—causes of atypical wounds are the inflammatory ulcers. Although a variety of inflammatory and immunologic diseases affect the skin, two relatively common causes of inflammatory ulcers are vasculitis and pyoderma gangrenosum.

Vasculitis

Vasculitis is defined as inflammation and necrosis of the blood vessels, which can ultimately result in end organ damage.[3] (See photographs in the color section, page C27.) Often idiopathic, vasculitis is a reaction pattern that may be triggered by certain reactants, among these are underlying infections, malignancy, medications, and connective tissue diseases. (See *Potential etiologies of vas-*

Potential etiologies of vasculitis

Although not all-inclusive, the most common causes of vasculitis are listed below.

Infections
- *Streptococcus spp.*
- *Mycobacterium tuberculosis*
- *Staphylococcus spp.*
- *Mycobacterium leprae*
- Hepatitis viruses A, B, and C
- Herpes virus
- Influenza virus
- *Candida spp.*
- *Plasmodium spp.*
- Schistosomiasis

Medications
- Penicillin
- Sulfonamides
- Tamoxifen

- Streptomycin
- Oral contraceptives
- Thiazides

Chemicals
- Insecticides
- Petroleum products

Foods
- Milk
- Gluten

Connective tissue and other inflammatory diseases
- Systemic lupus erythematosus

- Dermatomyositis
- Sjogren's syndrome
- Rheumatoid arthritis
- Behçet's syndrome
- Cryoglobulinemia
- Scleroderma
- Primary biliary cirrhosis
- Human immunodeficiency virus infection

Malignancies
- Lymphomas
- Leukemias
- Multiple myeloma

culitis.) Clinically, vasculitis varies depending on the size of the underlying vessel affected. For example, lesions may include a reticulated erythema due to disease of the superficial cutaneous plexus, or may present as widespread purpura, necrosis, and ulceration due to disease in larger, deeper vessels. Patients may also have similar involvement of different end organs (such as the kidney, lung, central nervous system, and the GI tract).[4]

Circulating immune (antibody-antigen) complexes, which deposit in blood vessel walls, are the cause of many types of vasculitis.[5] Tissue biopsies will confirm the presence of vasculitis if performed early, and biopsies of perilesional skin may detect the type of immunoglobulin involved in the process. Biopsies performed later in the course of lesion development may fail to reveal immunoreactants as inflammatory cells, and their byproducts will degrade immunoglobulins. Tissue culture may aid by determining if the vasculitis is due to an infectious process. Once a diagnosis is confirmed histologically, evalua-

tion of other organ systems and an attempt to determine the eliciting factor is mandated.

If identified—and if possible—the causative agent should be addressed. Additionally, treatment of the vasculitis is based on the extent of the disease. (See *Diagnostic tests for vasculitis,* page 394.) Mild disease that's limited to the skin can be treated with only supportive care, for example, leg elevation and dressings. Treatments with limited adverse effects, such as colchicine, dapsone, antihistamines, or nonsteroidal anti-inflammatory agents, may also be used. If skin disease is extensive or systemic involvement is present, more aggressive treatment including systemic steroids, anti-inflammatory agents, or immunosuppressants may be needed.[6] (See *Vasculitis treatment options,* page 395.)

Pyoderma gangrenosum

The term *pyoderma gangrenosum* is actually neither infectious nor gangrenous. Rather, it's an inflammatory process of unknown etiology that leads to painful skin ulcers. Pyoderma gangrenosum is characterized by the appearance of one or more chronic ulcerations with violaceous undermined borders.[7] (See photographs in the color section, page C26.) It mainly affects adults and its usual course is that of recurring, destructive ulcers, which begin as pustules and resolve with cribriform scars. Several clinical variants of pyoderma gangrenosum have been described including ulcerative, pustular, bullous, vegetative, and peristomal types.

PRACTICE POINT

Because a diagnostic test to confirm pyoderma gangrenosum doesn't exist and a number of other conditions may resemble it clinically, a correct diagnosis relies on the clinical presentation and exclusion of other causes.

It's important for the clinician to search for underlying diseases when a diagnosis of pyoderma gangrenosum is rendered because it is associated with other conditions in up to 75% of patients.[8] (See *Systemic diseases associated with pyoderma gangrenosum*, page 396.) Among these are inflammatory bowel disease, arthritis (seropositive and seronegative), monoclonal gammopathies, and other hematologic disorders and malignancies. Pyoderma grangrenosum lesions can occur around the stoma in persons with inflammatory bowel disease.[9] (See photographs in the color section, page C26.)

The mechanism by which pyoderma gangrenosum lesions develops is unknown; however, it's believed that pathergy (the development of lesions in areas of trauma) plays a role. In susceptible people, even minimal trauma to the skin can result in the production of pyoderma gangrenosum lesions, such as pustules or ulcers.

Curative treatment doesn't exist. The course of pyoderma gangrenosum waxes and wanes; however, corticosteroids are usually helpful.[10] For limited or mild disease, topical or intralesional steroids may be used. For more severe or widespread disease, systemic steroids can be used, although their adverse effects limit long-term use. A variety of systemic therapies can be used including antibiotics with anti-inflammatory properties or systemic steroids. Immunosuppressant or anti-inflammatory agents may also be useful; for example, cyclosporine also appears quite effective in treating this disorder. (See *Pyoderma gangrenosum treatment options*, page 397.) Infliximab (Remicade), a monoclonal antibody to tumor necrosis factor alpha, has been reported to be useful.[11] Infliximab is FDA-approved to treat Crohn's disease and rheumatoid arthritis. A randomized study evaluating the efficacy of different treatment modalities for pyoderma gangrenosum hasn't been done.

Infectious causes

Infectious causes of atypical wounds may be due to a variety of different organisms, some of which aren't commonly encountered in the United States. For example, atypical mycobacteria (other than leprosy and tuberculosis) and fungi (other than dermatophytes and candida) infections are occasionally detected upon diagnostic testing. Infection caused by *Vibrio vulnificus* may be responsible for lower leg ulcers in geographic areas where there's warm salt water.

Atypical mycobacterial infection

Atypical mycobacteria are ubiquitous in the environment and weren't generally viewed as human pathogens until the 1950s, when several cases of disease caused by these organisms were reported.[12] Cutaneous infection usually results from exogenous inoculation, and predisposing factors include a history of preceding trauma, immunosuppression, or chronic disease. While *Mycobacteria marinum* is the most common agent of skin infection by atypical mycobacteria,[13] many others have been reported in recent decades. (See Mycobacteria *species that cause skin ulcers,* page 398.) The cutaneous lesions vary depending on the causative agent, and may present as granulomas, small superficial ulcers, sinus tracts, or large ulcerated lesions localized in exposed areas. (See Hansen's disease photograph in the color section, page C26.)

Histologically, mycobacterial infections present as granulomas and abscesses that are difficult to distinguish from those of leprosy and cutaneous tuberculosis. Diagnosis will invariably depend on tissue culture or more recent techniques, such as polymerase chain reaction and gene rearrangement studies.

The appropriate therapy will depend on the causative agent because susceptibility to antibiotics varies. In some cases, simple excision of the cutaneous lesions or a combination of excision and chemotherapy often is most beneficial to the patient.

Buruli ulcer

Buruli ulcer is a health problem in the tropical areas of many emerging countries. Since 1980, Buruli ulcer, has emerged as an important cause of human suffering. It was first encountered in 1897 when Sir Albert Cook described large ulcers in Uganda. In 1940, MacCallum identified an organism similar to *M. ulcerans* in an ulcer of a 15-year-old in Bainsdale, Australia. Large ulcers were then

Vasculitis treatment options

Extent of disease	Treatment options
Mild	• Leg elevation • Compression dressings • Antihistamines • Nonsteroidal anti-inflammatory drugs • Anti-inflammatory antibiotics • Topical steroids • Support stockings • Dapsone • Colchicine • Potassium iodide
Extensive or systemic	• Dapsone • Systemic steroids • Stanozolol • Cyclophosphamide • Methotrexate • Azathioprine • Cyclosporin • Plasmapheresis • Mycophenolate mofetil • Tacrolimus • Other anti-inflammatory or immunosuppressant drugs

observed along the Nile River in the Buruli county of Uganda in 1961, hence the name of the disease. Buruli ulcer is caused by *M. ulcerans*, from the family of bacteria which causes tuberculosis and leprosy.

The World Health Organization (WHO) has defined Buruli ulcer as an infectious disease of the skin and subcutaneous tissue characterized by painless nodules, papule, plaque, or edema evolving into a painless ulcer with undermined edges and edema. Progression of the disease is associated with extensive sloughing and massive ulceration particularly over joints and may lead to contractures. Significant areas of the torso, face, or an entire limb may be involved. Limb cases often require amputation (See photograph in the color section, page C27.)[14]

During the course of this disease, extensive cutaneous ulcers occur as it progresses from

Systemic diseases associated with pyoderma gangrenosum

No diagnostic test exists to confirm the presence of pyoderma gangrenosum. In addition, pyoderma gangrenosum is typically associated with other conditions.[8] Reported associations are listed below.

Inflammatory bowel disease
- Ulcerative colitis
- Regional enteritis
- Crohn's disease

Arthritis
- Seronegative arthritis
- Rheumatoid arthritis
- Osteoarthritis
- Psoriatic arthritis

Hematologic abnormalities
- Myeloid leukemia
- Hairy cell leukemia
- Myelofibrosis
- Myeloid metaplasia
- Immunoglobulin A monoclonal gammopathy
- Polycythemia rubra, polycythemia vera
- Paroxysmal nocturnal hemoglobinuria
- Myeloma
- Lymphoma

Immunologic abnormalities
- Systemic lupus erythematosus
- Complement deficiency
- Hypogammaglobulinemia
- Hyperimmunoglobulin E syndrome
- Acquired immunodeficiency syndrome

of life who suffers with this disease.[14,15] (See photograph in the color section, page C27.)

The majority of those suffering from Buruli ulcer are younger than age 15. Early diagnosis is key to treating this disease. Early diagnosis, while the disease is in the nodular stage, allows curative surgical resection to minimize late complications.[14,15] Treatment can also include antituberculous drugs (rifampicin) and aminoglycosides. In more extensive cases, wide excision and grafting are often recommended, however limited excision followed by small islet grafts may be successful. Aminoglycosides are also be helpful in preventing the extensive ulcers, contractures, edema, and other late sequelae of this devastating disease.[14,15]

Healing is often slow and is associated with significant functional incapacity due to contractures and amputation. Treatment is complicated by the resistance of the organism to most medical regimens due to the ability of the organism to suppress the immune system of the host. Disease progression is directly related to a decrease in the level of interferon-Á, a Th1 cytokine, as well as a concomitant increase in Th2 cytokine interleukin-10.[14] Buruli ulcer has been clearly identified as an immunodeficiency disease. Reversing the deficiency of interferon-Á and/or decreasing the interleukin-10 level has been identified as a novel therapeutic target for interventional development.

The disease, its treatment, and the resulting disabilities are a significant burden to patients, their families, and their society. In some countries such as Ghana, patients and families are reluctant to seek treatment due to lack of money or misunderstanding that treatment can prevent amputation.[15] Educational sessions for clinicians to recognize Buruli ulcer early as well as changing patient, family, and societal resistance to seeking early treatment, have met with success and the number of late cases of this disease has declined in Ghana.[14,15]

Deep fungal infections
Deep fungal infections of the skin can be divided into subcutaneous and systemic mycosis. The subcutaneous mycoses result from traumatic implantation of the etiologic agent into the subcutaneous tissue, development of

the early, more treatable, nodular form to the ulcerative form that can result in the loss of skin and soft tissue. Although it's rarely fatal, the extensive disabilities and disfigurement have a profound impact on a patient's quality localized disease, and eventual lymphatic spread. In rare instances, hematogenous dissemination can occur, especially in immunocompromised hosts. As may occur with sporotrichosis or chromomycosis, ulcers from deep fungal infections are found worldwide and can present in a wide variety of clinical settings.[16,17]

Systemic mycoses are the result of systemic penetration of pathogenic fungi, the lungs being the most common port of entry. These infections are restricted to the geographic areas where the fungi occur, especially tropical countries such as Central and South America. After an initial pulmonary infection, the fungi can spread hematogenously or via lymphatic vessels to other organs, including the skin. A decrease in immunity will lead to expression of the fungal infection, as is commonly observed in patients infected with human immunodeficiency virus (HIV).

PRACTICE POINT

A thorough patient history assists in allowing a clinician to consider a diagnosis of systemic mycoses because of the limited area in which the causative fungi occur.

Pyoderma gangrenosum treatment options

Type of treatment	Treatment options
Topical	• Topical steroids • Topical tacrolimus • Nicotine patch • Intralesional steroids
Systemic	• Steroids • Antibiotics (dapsone and minocycline) • Cyclosporin • Clofazamine • Azathioprine • Methotrexate • Chlorambucil • Cyclophosphamide • Thalidomide • Tacrolimus • Mycophenalate • Mofetil • Intravenous immunoglobulin • Plasmapheresis • Infliximab

Sporotrichosis

Sporotrichosis is a subacute or chronic fungal infection caused by the fungus *Sporothrix schenckii*. Occurring as a consequence of traumatic implantation of the fungus into the skin, it's often associated with lymphangitis. Less commonly, inhalation of the conidia can lead to pulmonary infection and subsequently spread to the bones, eyes, central nervous system, and viscera. Systemic disease is seen in individuals with impaired immunity, such as alcoholic and HIV-infected patients.[18]

S. schenckii, a saprophyte in the environment, has been isolated in a variety of plants and other fauna, as well as animals (bites or scratches from animals, such as armadillos and cats). Individuals whose professional or leisure activities expose them to the environment are at greater risk of acquiring the infection. Sporotrichosis is treated with systemic medications, including saturated solution of potassium iodide, itraconazole, fluconazole,

terbinafine, and amphotericin B. Topically applied heat may also be used because the organism grows at low temperatures.

EVIDENCE-BASED PRACTICE

Because it's difficult to distinguish the presence of sporotrichosis directly from host tissues, culture on Sabouraud dextrose agar medium should be performed.[17,18]

Chromoblastomycosis

Chromoblastomycosis is a subcutaneous mycosis caused by several pigmented fungi including *Fonsecaea pedrosoi*, *Fonsecaea compacta*, *Phialophora verrucosae*, *Cladosporium carinii*, and *Rhinocladiella aquaspera*. These fungi are acquired through inoculation of the causative agents in the skin, after

Mycobacteria species that cause skin ulcers

Mycobacterium species	Clinical manifestations	Diagnosis	Treatment
M. marinum	• Swimming pool granuloma	Tissue culture	• Antituberculous drugs
M. ulcerans	• Subcutaneous nodule • Deep ulcers	Tissue culture	• Surgical excision
M. scrofulaceum	• Cervical lymphadenitis • Fistulae	Tissue culture	• Surgical excision
M. avium-intracellulare	• Small ulcers with erythematous borders	Tissue culture	• Surgical excision • Chemotherapy
M. kansaii	• Crusted ulcerations	Tissue culture	• Antituberculous drugs • Minocycline
M. chelonei	• Painful nodules and abscesses • Surgical wound infection	Tissue culture	• Erythromycin • Tobramycin • Amikacin • Doxycycline
M. fortuitum	• Painful nodules and abscesses • Surgical wound infection	Tissue culture	• Amikacin • Doxycycline • Ciprofloxacin • Sulfamethoxazole

which infection mycosis develops at the site of inoculation. These microorganisms can be found in soil throughout the world; however, the disease is most common in tropical and subtropical climates, with the majority of cases seen in South America.[19]

Primarily affecting men ages 30 to 50, the principal lesion is a slow-growing papule that eventuates into a verrucous nodule. Exposed areas are involved with extremities being affected in 95% of the cases, especially the lower limbs.[20] The surface of the lesion may be covered by scales or may be ulcerated with serosanguineous crusts. Black dots can be often observed; these dots are rich in fungi and represent the site of transepidermal elimination of necrotic tissue.

Diagnostic examinations should include scrapings from the lesion with potassium hydroxide 20%; tissue samples should be obtained from biopsies for tissue culture and histology.

The disease tends to be chronic and difficult to treat, and may lead to lymphedema and elephantiasis. Ulcerated and cicatricial lesions have been reported to develop into carcinoma. Small lesions can be cured by surgical excision; however, chronic lesions are often resistant to treatment.

Systemic antifungal agents, such as ketoconazole, itraconazole, terbinafine, and amphotericin B, have been used, alone or in combination, with variable results.[21,22] Itraconazole is perhaps the most effective. Cryosurgery has also been used alone and in combination with itraconazole. Local heat therapy and flucytosine can also be effective therapeutic modalities.

Paracoccidioidomycosis

Paracoccidioidomycosis (South American blastomycosis) is a chronic, infectious disease caused by the fungus *Paracoccidioides brasiliensis*, a saprophyte of soil and decaying vegetation found in tropical and subtropical climates. Infection occurs via a respiratory route with occasional dissemination to other organs, including the skin. Patients present with painful ulcerative lesions of the mouth, face or, less frequently, the extremities. Involvement of regional lymphatics is characteristic.[23]

Diagnosis can be established by isolation and identification of the etiologic agent with a culture. Treatment includes amphotericin B and the azoles derivatives, such as itraconazole and ketoconazole.

Mycetoma

Mycetoma is a chronic infection of the skin and subcutaneous tissues characterized by local edema, sinus tract formation, and the presence of grains—hard concretions representing colonies of the etiologic agent. It occurs worldwide, but most commonly in tropical and subtropical regions. The most common agent in Central and South America is *Nocardia brasiliensis*, which is found in soil.[24] This agent is rarely found in the United States but when it does occur, *Pseudallescheria boydii* is the most commonly isolated agent.

Men ages 20 to 40 are most frequently affected. After trauma, a slow-growing, painless nodule develops, which may discharge purulent material and grains. Neighboring lesions may interconnect with each other, giving rise to the sinus tracts that are characteristic of the disease.

Diagnosis can be established based on clinical findings; additional examinations may include biopsy and tissue culture. On ultrasonographic evaluation, the mycetoma grains, capsules, and the resulting inflammatory granulomas have characteristic appearances.[25] Treatment is difficult. Surgical excision, commonly in combination with chemotherapy, may be effective. Sulfonamides, tetracycline, erythromycin, rifampin, oral azoles, and amphotericin B may be used[26,27] depending on sensitivities of the etiologic agent.

Vibrio vulnificus infection

Vibrio vulnificus, a bacteria, is found widely in Atlantic Coast waters and raw shellfish.[28] It produces extracellular proteolytic and elastolytic enzymes and collagenases that favor tissue invasiveness. Wound infection with *V. vulnificus* occurs when contaminated seawater enters the body through a break in the epidermal barrier, commonly during fishing or water sport activities. Pustular lesions, lymphangitis, lymphadenitis, and cellulitis may ensue; in some cases, rapid progression to myositis and skin necrosis follows. Treatment of *V. vulnificus* wound infections consists of antibiotics, such as tetracycline and an aminoglycoside, and wound care.[29]

Primary septicemia from *V. vulnificus* occurs 24 to 48 hours after the ingestion of raw oysters, especially in patients with hepatic cirrhosis, diabetes, renal failure, or immunosuppression. Clinically, fever and hypotension may be present, along with the development of bullous cellulitis and necrotic skin ulcers.

Necrotizing fasciitis

Necrotizing fasciitis (NF) is an uncommon but life-threatening soft tissue infection characterized by rapidly spreading inflammation and necrosis of the skin, subcutaneous fat, and fascia.[30] (See photograph in the color section, page C28.) Rapid, early intervention may prevent morbidity and mortality; however, left untreated, the mortality rate may reach over 70%.

The incidence of necrotizing fasciitis has been reported to be 0.40 cases per 100,000 population.[31] Although it's rare, certain conditions can predispose patients to developing the disease, including immunocompromised states such as diabetes mellitus, acquired immunodeficiency syndrome (AIDS), and malignancy[32] as well as trauma, such as burns, lacerations, or minor trauma. (See *Conditions leading to necrotizing fasciitis,* page 400.)

Necrotizing fasciitis is categorized as type 1 or type 2 depending on which organisms are cultured. Type 1 necrotizing fasciitis is caused by a polymicrobial infection from aerobic and anaerobic bacteria such as *Clostridium* and *Bacteroides* species. Type 2 necrotizing fasciitis consists of group A *Streptococcus* (*S. pyogenes*) with or without a coexisting *Staphylococcal* infection.

Necrotizing fasciitis can affect any area of the body, but it most commonly occurs on the extremities. Involvement of the genitalia

Conditions leading to necrotizing fasciitis

The conditions listed below place patients at risk for necrotizing fasciitis.[33]
- Age 50 and older
- Alcoholism
- Anal fissure
- Atherosclerosis
- Diabetes mellitus
- Diverticulum
- Hemorrhoids
- Hypertension
- Immunosuppression
- Intravenous drug use
- Malignancy
- Malnutrition
- Obesity
- Renal failure
- Surgery
- Trauma
- Urethral tear

is referred to as Fournier's gangrene and usually results from a polymicrobial infection. There is a higher mortality rate when the head, neck, chest, and abdomen are involved because those areas tend to be refractory and, as such, are more difficult to treat.

Early on, patients generally present with a clinical picture similar to cellulitis. As with less aggressive cases of cellulitis, redness and edema can be seen at the site, with a spreading, diffuse inflammatory reaction that blends into the surrounding tissue. The overlying skin is shiny and tense without any clear lines of demarcation. However, patient complaints of severe pain are usually out of proportion to the clinical lesion. This characteristic clue of necrotizing fasciitis may be the only hint of a deeper, more aggressive infection. It's critical to be alert for this sign because the earlier the diagnosis is made, the earlier treatment can be instituted and the better the chance of survival exists.

Over time, frank cutaneous gangrene may extend beyond the skin and into the subcutaneous fat and fascial planes below. Separation of the necrotic tissue along the fascial planes with suppuration may occur.

Myonecrosis develops in the underlying muscle. Lymphadenitis, lymphangitis, crepitation, and venous thrombosis are seen less often.

Metastatic abscesses have been reported in the liver, lung, spleen, brain, and pericardium, but are rare. In addition to cutaneous manifestations of necrotizing fasciitis, there are systemic findings as well and with progression of disease. Patients will usually appear toxic with high fever, chills, and constitutional symptoms. In fulminant cases, multiorgan system failure occurs.

Vasculopathies

A heterogeneous group of disorders are classified under this category. Vasculopathy is characterized by occlusion of small vessels within the skin due to thrombi or emboli, which leads to tissue hypoxia and the clinical manifestations of purpura, livedo reticularis, and painful ulcers. Cryofibrinogenemia, monoclonal cryoglobulinemia, and antiphospholipid antibody syndrome are among the causes that commonly present as atypical skin ulcerations of the lower extremities.

Cryofibrinogenemia

Cryofibrinogenemia occurs as a primary (idiopathic) disorder or in association with underlying diseases, such as infectious processes, malignancy, or collagen, vascular, or thromboembolic disease. The clinical presentation is painful cutaneous ulcerations located on the leg and foot; these lesions are usually unresponsive to treatment. Other cutaneous findings include livedo reticularis (a netlike erythema), purpura, ecchymoses, and gangrene. (See photograph in the color section, page C27.) The pathogenesis of the lesions is related to the in vivo occlusion of small blood vessels initiated in the distal extremities by the abnormal precipitate. This hypothesis is corroborated by the pathology findings of cryofibrinogen, consisting of thrombi within superficial dermal vessels due in part to protein deposition. Cryofibrinogen is a circulating complex of fibrin, fibrinogen, and fibronectin along with albumin, cold-insoluble globulin, and factor VIII. The complex is soluble at 98.6° F (37° C) but forms a cryoprecipitate at 39.2° F (4° C).[34] Additionally, this complex can be made to clot with thrombin. The mechanism by which cryofibrinogen is produced isn't well-understood.

Treatment is symptomatic or, in secondary disease, directed to the underlying cause.[35] Agents which lyse fibrin thrombi are helpful. Stanozolol, streptokinase, and streptodornase have been used with success.

Cryoglobulinemia

Cryoglobulinemia occurs when deposits of cryoglobulins lead to the formulation of thrombi in medium and small vessel walls.[36] Three types of cryoglobulins have been identified; type I or monoclonal cryoglobulinemia may be seen in patients with malignant diseases, such as myeloma, or benign lymphoproliferative conditions, such as Waldenström's macroglobulinemia. This classically leads to thrombotic phenomena but can clinically resemble vasculitis. Type II, or mixed, cryoglobulinemia combines polyclonal and a monoclonal immunoglobulin; this type of cryoglobulinemia is seen less often in association with malignancies and is more often associated with infectious or inflammatory diseases. Type III is comprised of only polyclonal immunoglobulin and is most commonly associated with hepatitis C infection and the monoclonal component is immunoglobulin (Ig) M kappa. Both type II and III cryoglobulinemia cause vasculitis, which can lead to skin ulcers.[37] Other skin manifestations include acral cyanosis, Raynaud's phenomenon, livedo reticularis, altered pigmentation of involved skin, and palpable purpura, which may progress to blistering and frank ulceration. Some patients may have systemic manifestations, such as arthritis, peripheral neuropathy, and glomerulonephritis. Diagnosis is based on skin biopsies, which show either vasculopathy or vasculitis, and subsequent detection of cryoglobulin by electrophoresis.

PRACTICE POINT

Evaluate the patient with vasculitis for type II or III cryoglobulinemia; these conditions can cause vasculopathy.

Treatment should be directed at the underlying cause when cryoglobulinemia is associated with hepatitis C. Interferon alpha-2b is used to treat hepatitis C and may result in resolution of the associated cryoglobulinemia. Plasmapheresis alone or in combination with prednisone or immunosuppressive drugs (cyclophosphamide or chlorambucil [Leukeran] has also been used to treat cryoglobulinemia.[38,39]

Antiphospholipid antibody syndrome

Antiphospholipid antibody syndrome is characterized by elevated titers of antiphospholipid antibodies in association with venous or arterial thrombosis, recurrent fetal loss, and thrombocytopenia. Antiphospholipid antibodies are immunoglobulins (IgG, IgM, or both). The lupus anticoagulant, anticardiolipin antibodies, and Venereal Disease Research Laboratories (VDRL) test (false positive) are all antiphospholipid antibodies and any or all may be present as part of the syndrome.[40,41] Antiphospholipid antibody syndrome may present as primary disease or may be secondary to an underlying autoimmune disease such as systemic lupus erythematosus (seen in about 50% of cases). The syndrome has also been associated with malignancy and infectious states. The exact pathogenic mechanism of antiphospholipid antibody syndrome remains unknown.

The clinical hallmark of this disease is the presence of livedo reticularis. Arterial and venous thrombosis may elicit a variety of skin lesions, including ulcerations (most commonly), superficial thrombophlebitis, and cutaneous infarcts. Any organ system can be affected. Placental vessel thrombosis and ischemia can result in miscarriage precipitated by placental insufficiency. The proposed mechanism responsible for this event is a reduction of annexin V (a cell-surface protein with anticoagulant properties) on the trophoblast cells promoting a procoagulant state that leads to thrombosis at the maternal-fetal interface, and subsequent damage to the placenta and eventual fetal loss.[42] Treatment includes the use of aspirin, warfarin, and prednisone, but response isn't uniform.

Metabolic disorders

Metabolic diseases are uncommon causes of chronic wounds. One condition, called calciphylaxis, is commonly seen in a subset of patients undergoing chronic hemodialysis who developed secondary hyperparathyroidism.[43] This leads to deposition of calcium within soft tissue and the vasculature and, eventually, tissue death.

Calciphylaxis

Calciphylaxis is a rare, often fatal condition, characterized clinically by progressive cutaneous necrosis, which frequently occurs in patients with end-stage renal disease. Many eliciting factors have been suggested but the most common linking phenomenon is the development of secondary hyperparathyroidism.[43,44] Secondary hyperparathyroidism causes elevated calcium-phosphate product and development of vascular, cutaneous, and subcutaneous calcification that, in turn, leads to tissue death. Calciphylaxis typically develops after beginning dialysis and is seen in approximately 1% of patients with chronic renal failure and 4.1% of patients receiving hemodialysis.[45] The prognosis for patients who develop calciphylaxis is grim, with an estimated 5-year survival rate of less than 50%.[46] In addition to skin involvement, the pathophysiologic process may also occur within internal organs which, along with sepsis from infected skin wounds, is a major cause of morbidity and mortality.

The cutaneous manifestations begin as red or violaceous mottled plaques, in a livedo reticularis-like pattern. This signifies a vascular pattern and these early ischemic lesions often progress to gangrenous, ill-defined, black plaques. With time, the plaques ulcerate and become tender; indurated ulcers can lead to auto-amputation. The ulcers of calciphylaxis are usually bilateral and symmetric, and may extend deep into muscle. Vesicles frequently appear at the periphery of the ulcers. (See photographs in the color section, page C28.)

It's believed that patients develop this condition as a result of a hypersensitivity reaction.[43,47-49] In certain circumstances, a patient may be sensitized by a specific agent, such as parathyroid hormone, hyperphosphatemia, or hypercalcemia, among other sensitizing agents. Once a patient is sensitized, the hypersensitivity reaction is induced in response to a challenging agent, such as systemic steroids, infusion of albumin, iron dextran, immunosuppression, or trauma. The hypersensitivity reaction leads to the development of calcinosis, inflammation, and sclerosis associated with calciphylaxis.

Diagnosis can usually be based on clinical findings. Although vascular processes may present similarly, laboratory evaluation looking for the presence of an elevated calcium, phosphate, or calcium x phosphate product confirms calciphylaxis. An elevated intact parathyroid hormone level along with radiographic evidence and confirmatory histology also help confirm a diagnosis. Calcification of the intima and media of small- and medium-sized vessels in the dermis and subcutaneous tissue are characteristic of calciphylaxis. Radiographic findings include pipe stem calcifications due to the calcium deposits outlining the vessels in these patients.

As secondary infections may have tragic sequelae, treatment of infected ulcers is critical. Swab and tissue cultures from the wound may aid in guiding antibiotic therapy.

The treatments used for patients with calciphylaxis can be divided into either medical or surgical therapies[43-49] and are often used in tandem. (See *Calciphylaxis treatment options*.)

Malignancies

Malignancies may present either as wounds (see photographs in the color section) or developing from wounds. Nonmelanoma skin cancer, lymphomas, and sarcomas may ulcerate as they outgrow their blood supply. Alternatively, chronic wounds may develop into a malignancy, most commonly squamous cell carcinoma. This phenomenon is termed *Marjolin's ulcer* after the author who first described cells from an edge of a chronic wound that have undergone malignant change—an occurrence that can be seen in up to 2% of chronic wounds.[50] A similar phenomenon may also occur in scars, burn wounds, sinus tracts, chronic osteomyelitis, and even vaccination sites.

The precise mechanism of malignant degeneration in chronic wounds isn't known, although several theories have been proposed.[51-53] In addition to squamous cell carcinoma, basal cell carcinomas and other neoplasms, such as Kaposi's sarcoma and lymphoma, have also been found in chronic wounds.

Early identification of malignancy, typically via biopsy of suspected lesions, is critical. Treatment of biopsy-confirmed neoplasia includes excision with margins; amputation of the affected limb may be necessary in some cases. Mohs surgery (to ensure complete removal of the primary lesion) has been used successfully to treat malignancy arising from chronic osteomyelitis.[50]

External causes

External causes of atypical wounds include spider bites, chemical injury, chronic radiation exposure, trauma, and factitial ulcers.[54] A thorough patient history is the most valuable tool in determining the etiologic agent in ulcers caused by external factors.

Spider bites

At least 50 spider species in the United States have been implicated in causing significant medical conditions; however, the *Loxosceles* (brown recluse or violin spider) and the *Latrodectus* (black widow) species are the most well-known to cause skin necrosis and ulcers in the Americas.

Loxoscelism

The bite of *L. reclusae* is usually painless and often goes unnoticed; however, 10% of patients will experience progression to more significant wounds.[55] In these patients, enlargement of the bite site occurs within 6 to 12 hours, with associated pain and general symptoms, such as fever, malaise, headaches, and arthralgias. As the disease progresses, a pustule, blister, or large plaque forms at the bite site. These wounds may present as a deep purple plaque surrounded by a clear halo (vasoconstriction) and surrounding erythema—the so-called red, white, and blue sign.

With bites occurring in areas of greater fat content, such as the abdomen, buttocks, and thighs, necrosis develops more frequently. When the eschar is shed, an ulcer may result. Healing of the ulcer is generally very slow and may take up to 6 months.

The differential diagnosis includes foreign body reaction, infections, trauma, vasculitis, and pyoderma gangrenosum. Treatment consists of cooling the bite site, elevation (if possi-

---

Calciphylaxis treatment options

Medical treatment options
- Phosphate binders
- Decreased calcium in dialysate
- Antibiotics
- Low phosphate diet
- Calcitriol
- Diphosphonates
- Avoidance of challenging agents
- Avoidance of systemic steroids
- Hyperbaric oxygen
- Anticoagulation
- Cyclosporine
- Stanozolol

Surgical treatment options
- Parathyroidectomy
- Wound care and debridement
- Amputation
- Renal transplantation
- Skin grafting using either autologous or tissue engineered skin

---

ble), and analgesics. The use of systemic steroids may prevent the enlargement of the necrotic areas. Dapsone has also been recommended at a dose of 100 mg per day in adults.

Latrodectism

The black widow spider, or *Latrodectus mutans,* is easily recognized by a bright red hour-glass on the abdomen. The painless bite is followed by severe pain, swelling, and tenderness at the site where the bite occurred. Systemic symptoms, such as headaches and abdominal pain, may follow but they subside in 1 to 3 days. Treatment includes local ice, calcium gluconate, and the administration of specific antivenin. Black widow bites are rarely fatal; death may occur in children, those with comorbidities, or elderly people.

Chemical burns

A variety of chemical products are capable of producing skin wounds.[56] Cutaneous injury caused by caustic chemicals progresses continually after the initial exposure and, if not properly cared for, may produce painful ulcers that are difficult to heal. The lesions caused by alkalis are usually more severe than those caused by acids; however, the severity of the burn is determined by the mode of action and concentration of the chemical as well as the duration of contact before treatment is initiated.[56] Prolonged irrigation with water for 30 minutes or more is the most important initial treatment, followed by standard burn care.

Certain chemicals possess unique properties that require special additional therapy, such as hydrofluoric acid (application of 25% magnesium sulfate), chromic acid (excision of the affected area), and phenol (application of polyethylene glycol mixed with alcohol 2:1).[54]

Radiation dermatitis

After exposure to ionizing radiation exceeding 10 Gy, local skin reactions characterized by mild erythema, edema, and pruritus may occur.[57] This acute radiation dermatitis usually begins 2 to 7 days after exposure, peaks within 2 weeks, and gradually subsides. With exposure to higher doses, intense erythema with vesiculation, erosion, and superficial ulceration may ensue. Postinflammatory pigmentary abnormalities, telangiectasia, and atrophy are common.

Excision of the affected area and hyperbaric oxygen have been suggested as possible treatment options.

Factitial dermatitis

The term factitial dermatitis denotes a self-imposed injury. The clinical appearance of these ulcers is usually particular, with sharp or linear edges in an area of easy access such as the extremities, abdomen, and anterior chest. (See photograph in the color section, page C29.)

The care includes evaluation and treatment of underlying psychological diseases and limitation of accessibility to the wound, such as placing a dressing or cast over the wound.

Drug-induced causes
Coumadin necrosis

Coumadin (warfarin)-induced skin necrosis is a rare complication of anticoagulant treatment. The incidence of this complication has been estimated to occur between 1:100 and 1:10,000 of patients treated with anticoagulants. Coumadin skin necrosis occurs almost exclusively between the 1st and 10th day after beginning anticoagulation, in association with the administration of a large initial loading dose of the drug. Although the precise nature of the disease is still unknown, advances in knowledge about protein C, protein S, and antithrombin III anticoagulant pathways have led to a better understanding of the mechanisms involved in pathogenesis.[58,59]

Postpartum women have a unique risk due to reduced levels of free protein S during the antepartum and immediate postpartum periods.[60] Manifestations range from ecchymoses and purpura, hemorrhagic necrosis, and maculopapular, vesicular urticarial eruptions to purple toes.

Wounds are painful and usually evolve into full-thickness skin necrosis within a few days. Differential diagnosis between warfarin-induced skin necrosis and necrotizing fasciitis, gangrene and other causes of skin necrosis may be difficult.[61]

Local wound care can be conservative, but may include debridement and grafting, depending on the extensiveness of the wound. Previously uncomplicated courses of warfarin therapy don't obviate the possibility of skin necrosis with future warfarin administrations. Initiation of low-dose warfarin with heparin can reduce the likelihood of this disorder.

Extravasation

Solutions of calcium, potassium, bicarbonate, hypertonic dextrose, cardiac drugs, chemotherapeutic drugs, cytotoxic drugs, and antibiotics can lead to extravasation injury. Tissue loss can evolve into extensive wounds. Local wound care with debridement and eventual skin grafting is usually required for extensive skin and tissue loss. (See photographs in the color section, C30.)

Wounds with less tissue loss can be managed conservatively with the same outcome.[62] Because many extravasation injuries occur on the hands, scar management and return of function remains a problem. Proper administration through the correct needle size (small), vein size (large), and dilution of the medication is best. Infusion should be performed as slowly as possible to allow adequate dilution into the blood. Any complaints of pain during infusion warrant immediate cessation of the solution, assessment of the I.V. site, and adherence to treatment protocols for extravasation as deemed necessary. Calcium gluconate is less likely to extravasate and should be used instead of calcium chloride for the management of low serum levels, especially those levels that aren't life-threatening. Because many of these cases may elicit external review and sometimes legal review, documentation is crucial to determine what care was given prior to, and after, the medication was given. Nurses need to be especially vigilant when administering medications prone to extravasation.

Summary

Treating the underlying cause, when possible, is the initial step in caring for patients with atypical wounds. Anti-infective agents may be used for infectious ulcers, malignancies may require surgical removal, and anti-inflammatory agents may be used for inflammatory ulcers. In addition, the use of a moist healing environment, compression dressings (in the absence of arterial insufficiency) for leg lesions, off-loading areas at risk for prolonged pressure, and maximizing patients' nutritional status are essential.

Despite these measures, healing is often slow in patients with atypical wounds. Prolonged healing leads to increased morbidity and decreased quality of life as well as an increase in direct and indirect costs of care. Adjunctive therapies are often used, aimed at both increasing the number of patients who will heal (effectiveness of therapy) and the speed at which they heal (cost-effectiveness of therapy).

Show what you know

1. Which of the following is the most important reason to recognize a wound as atypical?

   A. The wound may be contagious.
   B. Treatment varies based on etiology.
   C. Standard wound healing therapies don't apply.
   D. To bill correctly.

ANSWER: B. It's critical to recognize when a wound is caused by an etiology other than prolonged pressure, neuropathy, or abnormal vascular supply, so that appropriate measures may be undertaken to make a correct diagnosis and provide appropriate therapy. Although an infectious agent that's contagious may be a cause of an atypical ulcer, this isn't common. Although oftentimes specific therapies for atypical wounds exist, these are usually coupled with principles of good wound care, such as compression, off loading, moist wound healing, and others. Billing for medical therapies is based on Evaluation and Management Codes as opposed to CPT codes.

2. Which of the following may be performed on tissue biopsies of wounds?

   A. Histology
   B. Culture
   C. Immunofluorescence
   D. All of the above

ANSWER: D. As a variety of etiologies cause atypical wounds, a variety of techniques are used to confirm these etiologies. Histology is critical for diagnosing inflammatory, malignant, and infectious causes. Biopsies for tissue culture aid in diagnosing infectious causes and biopsies for immunofluorescence will aid in diagnosing some inflammatory and autoimmune diseases.

3. Which of the following shouldn't typically be debrided?

   A. Diabetic foot ulcer
   B. Ulcers due to infectious causes
   C. Pyoderma gangrenosum ulcers
   D. Ulcers due to vasculitis

ANSWER: C. In susceptible people, even minimal trauma to the skin can result in the production of pyoderma gangrenosum lesions, such as pustules and ulcers. This phenomenon is called *pathergy*. Therefore, debridement of an ulcer secondary to pyoderma gangrenosum may lead to severe worsening of the ulcer.

4. Sporotrichosis is a fungal infection caused by:

   A. *Sporothrix schenckii*
   B. *Mycobacterium ulcerans*
   C. *Fonsecaea pedrosoi*
   D. *M. marinum*

ANSWER: A. *Sporothrix schenckii* causes sporotrichosis. *M. ulcerans* and *M. marinum* are species of mycobacteria. *Fonsecaea pedrosoi* is a pigment fungi related to chromoblastomycosis.

5. *Cryofibrinogenemia is classified as a:*

A. mycobacterium.
B. pyoderma gangrenosum.
C. vasculopathy.
D. metabolic disease.

ANSWER: C. Cryofibrinogenemia is a painful cutaneous ulceration classified as a vasculopathy. Mycobacterium is a bacteria. Pyoderma gangrenosum is an inflammatory ulcer, and metabolic disease is an uncommon cause of chronic wounds.

6. *Which type of wound is a rare, often fatal condition characterized by progressive cutaneous necrosis that occurs in patients with end stage renal disease?*

A. Calciphylaxis
B. Vasculopathy
C. Radiation dermatitis
D. Chemical burn

ANSWER: A. Calciphylaxis is the correct answer. Vasculopathy, radiation dermatitis, and chemical burns are all other types of atypical wounds.

7. *Factitial dermatitis is a:*

A. rare condition.
B. self-imposed injury.
C. red rash.
D. dry, scaly scab.

ANSWER: B. Factitial dermatitis is a self-imposed injury usually found in easily accessible areas such as the extremities, abdomen, and anterior chest. The other options are incorrect.

References

1. Phillips, T.J., and Dover, J.S. "Leg Ulcers," *Journal of the American Academy of Dermatology* 25(6 Pt 1):65-87, December 1991.
2. Falabella, A., and Falanga, V. "Uncommon Causes of Ulcers," *Clinics in Plastic Surgery* 25(3):467-79, July 1998.
3. Lotti, T., et al. "Cutaneous Small-Vessel Vasculitis," *Journal of the American Academy of Dermatology* 39(5 Pt 1):667-87, November 1998.
4. Gibson, L.E. "Cutaneous Vasculitis: Approach to Diagnosis and Systemic Associations," *Mayo Clinic Proceedings* 65(2):221-29, February 1990.
5. Jennette, J.C., and Falk, R.J. "Small-vessel Vasculitis," *New England Journal of Medicine* 337(21):1512-23, November 20, 1997.
6. Scott, D.G., and Watts, R.A. "Systemic Vasculitis: Epidemiology, Classification and Environmental Factors," *Annals of Rheumatic Disease* 59(3):161-63, March 2000.
7. von den Driesch, P. "Pyoderma Gangrenosum: A Report of 44 Cases with Follow-Up," *British Journal of Dermatology* 137(6):1000-1005, December 1997.
8. Callen, J.P. "Pyoderma Gangrenosum," *Lancet* 351(9102):581-85, February 1998.
9. Park, H.H. "Case study: Caring for a Patient with Peristomal Pyoderma Gangrenosum," *JWCET* 24(3):29-31, July/September 2004.
10. Powell, F.C., and Collins, S. "Pyoderma Gangrenosum," *Clinics in Dermatology* 18(3):283-93, May-June 2000.
11. Geren, S.M., et al. "Infliximab: A Treatment Option for Ulcerative Pyoderma Gangrenosum," *Wounds* 15(2): 49-53, May 2003.
12. Groves R. "Unusual Cutaneous Mycobacterial Diseases," *Clinics in Dermatology* 13(3):257-63, May-June 1995.
13. Hautmann, G., and Lotti, T. "Atypical Mycobacterial Infections of the Skin," *Dermatologic Clinics* 12(4):657-68, October 1994.
14. Kwyer, T.A., and Ampadu, E. "Buruli Ulcers: An Emerging Health Problem in Ghana," *Advances in Skin and Wound Care* 19(9):479-86, Nov-Dec 2006.
15. Ampadu, E., Kwyer, T.A., Otcher, Y. Buruli Ulcer: Picture of an emerging health challenge and the response in Ghana. JWCET 26(4):30-36, 2006.
16. Rivitti, E.A., Aoki, V. "Deep Fungal Infections in Tropical Countries," *Clinics in Dermatology* 17(2):171-90, March-April 1999.
17. Kauffman, C.A. "Sporotrichosis," *Clinical Infectious Disease* 29(2): 231-236, August 1999.
18. Davis, B.A. "Sporotrichosis," *Dermatologic Clinics* 14(1):69-76, January 1996.
19. Bonifaz, A., et al. "Treatment of Chromoblastomycosis with Itraconazole, Cryosurgery, and a Combination of Both," *International Journal of Dermatology* 36(7):542-47, July 1997.
20. Guerriero, C., et al. "A Case of Chromoblastomycosis due to Phialophora Verrucosa Responding to Treatment with Itraconazole," *European Journal of Dermatology* 8(3): 167-68, April-May 1998.
21. Tanuma, H., et al. "Case Report. A Case of chromoblastomycosis Effectively Treated with Terbinafine. Characteristics of Chromoblastomycosis in the Kitasato Region, Japan," *Mycoses* 43(1-2): 79-83, 2000.
22. Kumarasinghe, S.P., and Kumarasinghe, M.P. "Itraconazole Pulse Therapy in Chromoblastomycosis," *European Journal of Dermatology* 10(3):220-22, April-May 2000.
23. Bernard, G., and Duarte, A.J. "Paracoccidioidomycosis: A Model for Evaluation of the Effects of Human Immunodeficiency Virus Infection on the Natural History of Endemic Tropical Diseases," *Clinical Infectious Disease* 31(4):1032-39, October 2000.
24. Salinas-Carmona, L.C. "Nocardia Brasiliensis: From Microbe to Human and Experimental Infections," *Microbes and Infection* 2(11):1373-81, September 2000.
25. Fahal, A.H., et al. "Ultrasonographic Imaging of Mycetoma," *British Journal of Surgery* 84(8): 1120-22, August 1997.
26. Young, B.A., et al. "Mycetoma," *Journal of the American Podiatric Medical Association* 90(2): 81-84, February 2000.
27. Boiron, P., et al. "Nocardia, Nocardiosis and Mycetoma," *Medical Mycology* 36(S1):26-37, 1998.
28. Kumamoto, K.S., and Vukich, D.J. "Clinical Infections of Vibrio Vulnificus: A Case Report and Review of Literature," *Journal of Emergency Medicine* 16(1):61-66, January-February 1998.

29. Serrano-Jaen, L., and Vega-Lopez, F. "Fulminating Septicaemia Caused by Vibrio Vulnificus," *British Journal of Dermatology* 142(2):386-87, February 2000.

30. Trent, J.T., and Kirsner, R.S. "Diagnosing Necrotizing Fasciitis," *Adv Skin Wound Care* 15: (3) 135-38, May-June, 2002.

31. Kotrappa, K.S., et al. "Necrotizing Fasciitis," *Am Fam Phys* 53:1691–96, 1996.

32. Gannon, T. "Dermatologic Emergencies," *Postgrad Med* 96:67–82, 1994.

33. Ault, M.J., et al. "Rapid Identification of Group A Streptococcus as a cause of Necrotizing Fasciitis," *Annals of Emergency Medicine* 28(2):227-30, August 1996.

34. Brungger, A., et al. "Cryofibrinogenemic Purpura," *Archives of Dermatological Research* 279(suppl):S24-S29, 1987.

35. Falanga, V., et al. "Stanozolol in Treatment of Leg Ulcers due to Cryofibrinogenaemia," *Lancet* 338(8763):347-48, August 1991.

36. Piette, W.W. "Hematologic Associations of Leg Ulcers," *Clinics in Dermatology* 8(3-4):66-85, July-December 1990.

37. Rallis, T.M., et al. "Leg Ulcers and Purple Nail Beds. Essential Mixed Cryoglobulinemia," *Archives of Dermatology* 131(3):342-46, March 1995.

38. Yancey Jr., W.B., et al. "Cryoglobulins in a Patient with SLE, Livedo Reticularis, and Elevated Level of Anticardiolipin Anti-bodies," *American Journal of Medicine* 88(6):699, June 1990.

39. Karlsberg, P.L., et al. "Cutaneous Vasculitis and Rheumatoid Factor Positivity as Presenting Signs of Hepatitis C Virus-induced Mixed Cryoglobulinemia," *Archives of Dermatology* 131(10):1119-23, October 1995.

40. Smith, K.J., et al. "Cutaneous Histopathologic Findings in Antiphospholipid Anti-body Syndrome," *Archives of Dermatology* 1990(9):126, 1176-83, September 1990.

41. Selva, A., et al. "Pyoderma-gangrenosum-like Ulcers Associated with Lupus Anticoagulant," *Dermatology* (2):189, 182-84, 1994.

42. Rote, N.S. "Antiphospholipid Antibodies, Annexin V, and Pregnancy Loss," *New England Journal of Medicine* 337(22):1630-31, November 27, 1997.

43. Smiley, C.M., et al. "Calciphylaxis in Moderate Renal Insufficiency: Changing Disease Concepts," *American Journal of Nephrology* 20(4):324-28, July-August 2000.

44. Roe, S.M., et al. "Calciphylaxis: Early Recognition and Management," *The American Surgeon* 60(2):81-86, February 1994.

45. Kim, Y.J., et al. "Calciphylaxis in a Patient with End-Stage Renal Disease," *Journal of Dermatology* 28(5):272-75, May 2001.

46. Budisavljevic, M.N., et al. "Calciphylaxis in Chronic Renal Failure," *Journal of the American Society of Nephrology* 7(7):978-82, July 1996.

47. Kang, A.S., et al. "Is Calciphylaxis Best Treated Surgically or Medically?" *Surgery* 128(6):967-72, December 2000.

48. Oh, D.H., et al. "Five Cases of Calciphylaxis and a Review of the Literature," *Journal of the American Academy of Dermatology* 40(6 Pt 1):979-87, June 1999.

49. Hafner, J., et al. "Uremic Small-Artery Disease with Medical Calcification and Intimal Hyperplasia (So-called Calciphylaxis): A Complication of Chronic Renal Failure and Benefit from Parathyroidectomy," *Journal of the American Academy of Dermatology* 33(6):954-62, December 1995.

50. Chang, A., et al. "Squamous Cell Carcinoma Arising in a Nonhealing Wound and Osteomyelitis Treated with Mohs Micrographic Surgery: A Case Study," *Ostomy Wound Management* 44(4):26-30, April 1998.

51. Fishman, J.R.A., and Parker, M.G. "Malignancy and Chronic Wounds: Marjolin's Ulcer," *Journal of Burn Care Rehabilitation* 12(3):218-23, May-June 1991.

52. Lautenschlager, S., and Eichmann, A. "Differential Diagnosis of Leg Ulcers," *Current Problems in Dermatology* 27:259-70, 1999.

53. Natarajan, S., et al. "A Non-healing Ulcer Associated with Malignant Lymphoma," *Journal of Wound Care* 9(1):45-46, January 2000.

54. Newcomer, V.D., and Young Jr., E.M. "Unique Wounds and Wound Emergencies," *Dermatologic Clinics* 11(4):715-27, October 1993.

55. Smith, D.B., et al. "Brown Recluse Spider Bite: A Case Study," *Journal of Wound, Ostomy Continence Nursing* 24(3):137-43, May 1997.

56. Bates, N. "Acid and Alkali Injury," *Emergency Nursing* 7(8):21-26, December-January 2000.

57. Caccialanza, M., et al. "Results and Side Effects of Dermatologic Radiotherapy: A Retrospective Study of Irradiated Cutaneous Epithelial Neoplasms," *Journal of the American Academy of Dermatology* 41(4):589-94, October 1999.

58. Porock, D., et al. "Management of Radiation Skin Reactions: Literature Review and Clinical Application," *Plastic Surgical Nursing* 19(4):185-90, April 1999.

59. Sallah, S., et al. "Recurrent Warfarin-induced Skin Necrosis in Kindreds with Protein S Deficiency," *Hemostasis* 28(1):25-30, 1998.

60. Cheng, A., Scheinfeld, N.S., et al. "Warfarin Skin Necrosis in a Postpartum Woman with Protein S Deficiency," *Obstetrics and Gynecology* 90(4 Pt 2): 671-72, 1997.

61. Chan, Y.C., Valenti, D., Mansfield, A.O., Stansby, G. "Warfarin Induced Skin Necrosis," *British Journal of Surgery* 87 (3):266-72, 2000.

62. Kumar, R.J., Pegg, S.P., Kimble, R.M. "Management of Extravasation Injuries," *Australia and New Zealand Journal of Surgery* 71(5):285-89, 2001.

CHAPTER 20

Wounds in special populations

After completing this chapter, you'll be able to:

- identify the unique risk factors for pressure ulcer development in the critically ill patient

- describe risk assessment tools and methods appropriate for use with the critically ill patient

- list special considerations for pressure ulcer treatment in the critically ill patient

- describe successful strategies for reducing the incidence of pressure ulcers in the patient who has a spinal cord injury

- identify risk factors of pressure ulcers in the patient with a spinal cord injury

- discuss the major health complications of a spinal cord injury

- describe the impact of highly active antiretroviral therapy (HAART) on the prevalence of skin disorders in the patient with human immunodeficiency virus (HIV) or acquired immunodeficiency syndrome (AIDS)

- describe six common infectious skin disorders and two common noninfectious skin disorders in the patient with HIV or AIDS that results in altered skin integrity

- discuss two of the neoplastic skin disorders seen in the patient with HIV or AIDS

- identify pediatric pressure ulcer risk assessment tools

- describe factors placing neonates and children at risk for pressure ulcers

- discuss the disparities between the neonatal and pediatric patient and the adult patient that may lead to potential problems in skin and wound care

- identify skin problems commonly found in the bariatric patient

- discuss unique risk factors and pressure ulcer prevention strategies for the bariatric patient.

Intensive care population

Janet E. Cuddigan, PhD, RN, CWCN, CCCN

Pressure ulcer incidence and prevalence

Pressure ulcer incidence is higher in patients in the intensive care unit (ICU) than in patients in other units. Studies have reported the incidence of pressure ulcers in ICU patients as:

- 40% in 22 patients on intra-aortic balloon pumps[1]
- 30.6% in 36 trauma patients[2]
- 20% (stage I through IV) and 15% (stage II through IV) in 40 medical ICU patients[3]
- 14% in 57 surgical ICU patients on ventilators or experiencing hemodynamic instability[4]
- 12% in 136 medical, surgical, and respiratory ICU patients[5]
- 12.4% (stage II or greater ulcers) in 186 patients in a neurologic ICU[6]
- 8% (stage II and greater ulcers) in 412 surgical ICU patients[7]
- 8% in 110 patients randomly assigned to one of three support surfaces.[8]

Similar pressure ulcer incidence rates have been found in pediatric ICU (PICU) patients. In a multisite study of 322 PICU patients, the incidence was 27%.[9] These patients tend to develop pressure ulcers on the occiput more often than adult patients due to the higher proportion of body weight in the head.[9,10] In addition, high frequency oscillation ventilation is used more frequently in pediatric than in adult patients, often creating friction and shear injuries to the head.[11]

Risk factors

All too often, the critically ill patient survives a life-threatening illness with the aid of advanced technology, yet faces weeks or months of additional treatment for a painful, disfiguring, and potentially preventable complication—a pressure ulcer. The intensive care population encompasses a broad range of physiologically unstable patients.

The key component of a pressure ulcer prevention program for an ICU patient is an initial risk assessment to identify the specific level and type of risk the patient faces. Frequent follow-up assessments are also essential for prevention. If pressure ulcers develop, you should supplement aggressive treatment with continued preventive measures, including frequent reassessment.

Risk assessment tools

There is an ongoing debate in the research literature and clinical arena regarding the most valid and reliable method of evaluating pressure ulcer risk status in the critically ill patient. Options include standard risk assessment tools (for example, Braden Scale,[12] Norton Scale,[13] Waterlow Scale[14]), risk assessment tools designed specifically for the critically ill patient (for example, Jackson-Cubbin Scale for adults[15] and Braden Q for pediatrics[16]), individual risk factors unique to the critically ill patient (for example, hemodynamic instability, poor oxygenation, use of vasopressors), or professional judgment. The answer to this debate is "all of the above."

Standardized risk assessment tools such as the Braden Scale still provide a good general screening tool for risk status in the critically ill patient. They also help focus our preventive interventions on the type and level of risk (for example, mobility, nutrition, and moisture). In a prospective study of 186 neurological ICU patients, the Braden Scale was a better predictor of pressure ulcers than any other factor, except low body mass index on admission.[6] With a cutoff score of 16, all patients developing stage II or greater pressure ulcers were considered at risk; however, the false-positive rate was 81.9%. The high false-positive rate may be due to over-prediction by the Braden Scale, or the fact that the staff may have succeeded in preventing pressure ulcers in some patients whose scores indicated risk. In the same study, a cutoff score of 13 more accurately predicted pressure ulcers, with a sensitivity of 91.4%, but a false-negative rate of 1.8%. Other authors have recommended different Braden Scale cutoff scores.[2,17] Clinical practice is moving away

Pressure ulcer risk factors in intensive care patients

Epidemiologic studies of critically ill patients show the following individual risk factors are associated with the development of pressure ulcers:

- being "too unstable to turn"[17] or "turned less often"[10]
- days in bed and days without nutrition[6]
- longer length of stay[6,12]
- low albumin levels[12]
- low body mass index on admission[5]
- use of vasoconstrictive agents.[18]

Many of these risk factors can be included under the more general categories of the Braden Scale. For example, "too unstable to turn" could fit into the Braden subscale of mobility. None of these individual risk factors carry enough "statistical weight" to be included in a risk assessment scale; however, keep them in mind as you're assessing the unique risks of critically ill patients.

from using the total Braden Scale score as a basis for intervention and toward risk-based prevention programs that focus on moderating or eliminating the specific type of risk identified by subscale scores. Subscale scores also provide information about the degree of risk, so we can modify the intensity of interventions accordingly.

How do risk assessment tools specifically designed for the critically ill patient measure up? Several investigators have developed risk assessment scales specific to the intensive care population.[7,15,18-22] These tools show varying levels of accuracy, yet none have undergone the degree of validation testing of the Braden Scale. The most thoroughly tested of the "designer tools" is the Jackson-Cubbin Pressure Ulcer Risk Calculator. When compared with the Braden Scale in 112 critically ill patients, the Jackson-Cubbin Scale resulted

in better specificity (61% vs. 26%), but worse sensitivity (89% vs. 97%).[23] In other words, the Jackson-Cubbin Scale did a better job of predicting who did not get pressure ulcers, and a less effective job of predicting those who did get pressure ulcers.

Several studies correlate higher Acute Physiological Assessment and Chronic Health Evaluation (APACHE) II or III scores among intensive care patients with pressure ulcer development.[5,19,24] The APACHE scale is based on physiologic factors, age, and chronic health conditions. It's predictive of patient mortality, so it isn't surprising that the scale that predicts the death of a patient would also predict the tissue death associated with pressure ulcers.

Are there individual risk factors for pressure ulcers that are unique to the critical care population and highly predictive of pressure ulcer development.? Research by deLaat and colleagues[25] identified over 50 risk factors from epidemiologic studies and concluded that "no discriminatory risk factor for pressure ulcer development could be identified in the critically ill population.[25] (See *Pressure ulcer risk factors in intensive care patients*.)

Several authors have looked for the "one or two additional risk factors" that would make the Braden Scale more predictive of pressure ulcer development in the critically ill patient, yet none have developed a tool that has clinical utility and predictive validity. The most validated is Quigley and Curley's study of PICU patients. They adapted the descriptions in the Braden Scale for the pediatric population and added a tissue perfusion and oxygenation subscale. Recent findings demonstrate high predictive validity for PICU patients, however the tissue perfusion and oxygenation subscale has not been tested in adult populations.[9]

Risk assessment depends on a finely integrated combination of risk assessment tools, such as the Braden Scale to screen for type and level of risk, and knowledge of population specific risk factors from the research literature and clinical judgment. To develop a successful preventive plan, each risk factor or an abnormal Braden subscore should be addressed comprehensively, given the patient's physiologic condition. Risk assessment should be conducted daily and reassessed with major changes in the patient's condition.

Risk-based prevention

Although allocating resources according to the overall level of risk estimated by a total Braden Scale score is useful, a risk-based prevention program should be based on each patient's unique level and type of risk. Target your interventions to address low subscale scores. For example, if mobility and activity subscores are low (1 or 2) and moisture subscores are high (4), focus your interventions on mobility and activity issues. The following discussion focuses on the unique needs of the critically ill patient within the common categories of risk including mobility, activity, and nutrition, among others.

Mobility

The critically ill patient's level of mobility must be taken into consideration when assessing pressure ulcer risk. Although the standard of care recommends repositioning high-risk patients every 2 hours, a study of 74 ICU patients indicated that only 2.7% of the patients had a change in body position every 2 hours.[26] If the patient's condition prevents position changes, provide a bed that allows additional pressure redistribution. If the patient can't be turned completely due to hemodynamic instability, small shifts in position may be effective as an adjunct to more complete position changes.[27] Too frequently, the memory of a patient desaturating or becoming hypotensive during turning prevents us from resuming a turning schedule. Reassess the patient to determine when you <u>can</u> resume turning. Starting with slower, more gradual turns may allow the patient time to compensate for hemodynamic instability related to turning. Measures to restore hemodynamic stability and oxygenation will of course support a return to mobility sooner. Decreased mobility may also result from paralytics, sedation, coma, or spinal instability.

PRACTICE POINT

Use caution when turning a patient.

Is he lying on any tubes or medical devices? Are endotracheal tubes putting pressure on the lips or mouth? Check these points before you turn him.

Patients in respiratory distress may be placed in the prone position to improve partial pressure of arterial oxygen to fraction of inspired oxygen ratios. However, prone positioning creates a whole new set of pressure points, including the chin, jaw, breasts, anterior ribs, pelvic bones, genitalia (for males), anterior knees, and toes. Ensure that pressure is offloaded in these areas. Using pressure-redistributing mattresses and "bridging" to offload pressure points may be helpful. There are several special prone positioning devices that are commercially available. Be aware that significant facial edema may develop in a patient while in the prone position. Without proper oral care, skin around the mouth and cheeks may become macerated from saliva. Assess the patient for tubes, devices, or positioning strategies that may increase pressure in this position. Patients in respiratory distress may also be placed on rotation beds to improve pulmonary status. Make sure that the patient is secure in the bed and friction and shear injuries don't occur with rotation. Monitor the patient through at least one complete turning cycle to assess for friction and shear problems, as well as crimping of tubes (especially endotracheal) during rotation.

Bed selection

Selecting the optimal bed can be vital in the care of a critically ill patient. It may be cost-effective to have pressure-redistributing mattresses on all beds in an ICU if patient acuity and pressure ulcer incidence tend to be high.[28-30] The cost-benefit ratio may vary according to the overall patient acuity in your unit. The decision to order a bed with such features as alternating pressure, low-air-loss, or fluidized air, should be triggered by low scores on the Braden mobility-activity subscales or in the presence of conditions, such as pharmacologic paralysis and sedation. Patient needs including moisture and temperature control should also be considered. An analysis of randomized controlled trials published prior to 2004 suggested that high specification foam may be more effective than regular mattresses for moderate to high risk patients and low-air-loss beds may reduce ulcers in ICU patients.[31,32]

PRACTICE POINT

Don't counteract the pressure-redistributing effects of a specialized bed by using extra layers of sheets and underpads. Also don't use padding because it increases pressure. However, you should:

• use incontinence pads recommended by the bed manufacturer for patients who need moisture management
• make sure that any powered specialty bed is turned on and adjusted for maximum pressure redistribution for each individual patient.

Remember, specialty beds don't replace turning and positioning, nor do they adequately relieve heel pressure.

Positioning

Patient positioning is another need to be considered with the critically ill patient. Although the sacrum and the coccyx are the most frequent sites of pressure ulcers in these patients, heels are a close second and the incidence of heel ulcers is increasing. Therefore, vigilant protection of the heels in the critically ill patient is essential.[33] Your patient assessment should include findings that alert you to vascular insufficiency (pulses, [palpated or Doppler], capillary refill time, color, warmth, shiny hairless skin, ankle-brachial pressure index, toe pressure, pulse wave-form analysis, and vascular studies). Patients in shock experience constricted vessels in their extremities, accentuating the problem. Devices such as Rooke boots may keep the heels warm (supporting perfusion) and protected, but they don't relieve pressure. Likewise, cloth heel protectors may decrease the risk of skin injury from friction, but not relieve pressure. A number of commercial heel protectors are designed to relieve heel pressure by "suspending" the heel. Correct placement is essential to prevent additional

rubbing or pressure. Remove heel protectors regularly to inspect the skin. Placing a pillow or bath blanket under the calves to elevate the heels is an effective technique in patients who aren't agitated. Remember, heels are the one area where you can truly relieve pressure.

Proper positioning can also help the patient with a critical respiratory condition. There is convincing research evidence that a 45-degree backrest elevation reduces the incidence of ventilator-associated pneumonia. Head-of-bed elevation is also recommended for patients at high risk for aspiration, even if not mechanically ventilated.[34] Placing a patient with respiratory difficulty in an elevated position is a tried-and-true method of facilitating breathing, yet all of these essential interventions may increase sacral injury from shear as the patient slides down in bed. Placing pillows under the patient's arms may help support him in the upright position and may also improve respiratory excursion.

Activity

The patient's level of activity needs to be taken into consideration. Getting a critically ill patient into a chair—even a stretch or Cadillac chair—can be challenging due to the potential problems with postural hypotension, oxygenation, coordination of multiple tubes and invasive lines, and dependence on ventilators. Some bed manufacturers make beds that adjust to a sitting position, which may be an effective alternative for improving early activity. Regardless of these devices, the patient should progress to sitting in a chair.

PRACTICE POINT

If you can get the patient into a chair, don't forget a seat cushion. A 3" to 4" (7.5 to 10 cm) thick foam cushion is usually adequate. In a study involving interface pressure measurement, sheepskin and gel cushions were found to have little pressure-reducing effect.[35]

In another study involving interface pressure measurement in healthy volunteers, the seating position with the lowest interface pressure was the sitting back (seat tilted) posture with lower legs on a rest. If the seat can't be tilted back, an upright seating posture with feet on the ground is preferable.[36] Check for slouching and reposition the patient as needed. Periodically adjust his position (for example, with liftoffs or mechanical adjustments of the head-of-bed elevation) and don't leave him in the chair for more than 1 hour at a time. When the patient has returned to bed, check his skin carefully for areas of redness.

Sensory perception

Reduced sensory perception can significantly increase a patient's risk of pressure ulcers. Patients scoring low on the sensory perception subscale include those with spinal cord injuries, head trauma, pharmacological paralysis, heavy sedation, and coma. Carlson's[5] Braden Scale validation study of 136 critically ill patients found the sensory perception subscale to be the most predictive of pressure ulcer risk. Patients with a low sensory score may not feel pressure-induced discomfort and may not be able to change position. As long as the patient lacks this ability, the nursing staff must assume the responsibility for anticipating pressure-induced discomfort and ensuring routine repositioning and pressure redistribution. Special attention should be paid to checking under the various medical devices (such as splints, tubes, and oxygen masks) for proper fit and signs of pressure-induced injury.

Moisture

Moisture can put the critically ill patient at risk for pressure ulcers. Numerous sources in the critically ill patient, the most obvious being fecal and urinary incontinence, can produce moisture. Typical measures for preventing it include correcting incontinence (when possible), using pads or briefs that wick moisture away from the skin, using moisture barrier creams, frequent changing and cleaning, and assessing skin for maceration and yeast infections.

Don't underestimate other sources of moisture damage that may macerate skin and increase the risk of pressure ulcers. For example, wound drainage may be excessive and require absorptive dressings, such as foams and alginates. Critically ill patients may exhibit massive, generalized edema. Small injuries such as skin tears may lead to leakage of large amounts of exudates and serum proteins, particularly in patients with low serum albumin levels. Use absorptive dressings and pads to wick moisture away from the skin. Skin protectants may be appropriate for some patients.

Nutrition

Poor nutrition is another risk factor for pressure ulcer development in the critically ill patient.[7] Initiate oral or enteral feeding as soon as possible. If these methods of feeding aren't feasible, weigh the risks and benefits of total parenteral nutrition. Recommend a dietary consult within 48 hours of admission if the patient's Braden nutrition subscale score is 3 or less. Even if nutritional supplementation is provided, be aware that it may be inadequate to meet the increased metabolic needs of a critically ill patient despite your best efforts.

Friction and shear

The factors of friction and shear must also be considered as pressure ulcer risk factors in the critically ill patient. Friction injury may occur with agitation or with insufficient help with turning. Shear injury in the sacrum is a problem when the patient slides down in the bed or chair. Make sure you have enough help when turning and positioning. Use lift sheets and slide boards. When the patient is sitting in a chair or in bed, place pillows under his arms to support his weight and lessen the chance of shear injury.

Skin assessment

Total skin assessment should be performed on every shift with precise documentation of all breaks in skin integrity. The Agency for Health Care Policy and Research (AHCPR), now called the Agency for Health Care Research and Quality (AHRQ), guidelines recommend that pressure ulcers be assessed and measured weekly. Pressure ulcers may deteriorate more rapidly in the medically unstable, critically ill patient, therefore he should be assessed more frequently.

PRACTICE POINT

Pressure ulcers can be a source of sepsis in a critically ill, immunocompromised patient.

Damage related to medical devices

Be aware of unusual sites of pressure injury, such as under medical devices (casts, splints, external pelvic fixators, pins, traction devices, or heel lifters). Bilevel Positive Airway Pressure (bi-PAP) masks, indwelling catheter tugging, and endotracheal tubes—common sources of pressure injury in the intensive care environment—can also be easily overlooked as a potential site for pressure ulcer development. Check anterior surfaces for the patient who has been placed in a supine position.

Pressure injuries can occur internally from tracheostomy and endotracheal tubes; use the minimal occlusive volume to prevent tracheal damage. Assess the intubated patient's oral cavity and lips with a flashlight by shifting his position slightly without disrupting the tube's level. Tape or commercial tube tamers may be used. Likewise, inspect the site of tracheostomy stoma; excessive exudate around the tracheostomy stoma can cause skin breakdown. Consider more absorptive dressings, such as foam or alginates, under tracheostomy tubes with a lot of mucus and drainage rather than a low absorptive split-gauze dressing. Whenever you can, avoid using rigid equipment on the critically ill patient; for example, switch to a soft cervical collar when possible.

PRACTICE POINT

Always provide thorough oral care for the intubated patient to prevent pressure-related wounds.

Deep tissue injury

The exact nature of deep tissue injury (DTI) is still being investigated.[37] (See chapter 13, Pressure ulcers, for more information). Be careful when assessing early DTIs, which can be mistaken for stage I pressure ulcers. (See DTI photograph in the color section, page C17.) For example, a patient who develops a deep purple area on his buttocks following a sustained period of hypotension and immobility might not have a stage I pressure ulcer, even if the skin is intact. Such a wound is consistent with deep-tissue damage, which will become apparent as dead superficial tissues slough off. The area should be offloaded to prevent further damage; it should also be reassessed frequently, with the expectation that the wound may continue to show signs of deterioration.

Summary

Pressure ulcers are more common in the critically ill patient. Prevention is certainly more challenging. However, with a special eye for the unique needs of the critically ill patient, pressure ulcer incidence can be reduced in this high-risk population.

Spinal cord injury population

Susan L. Garber, MA, OTR, FAOTA, FACRM

Spinal cord injury incidence and prevalence

Between 183,000 and 230,000 people in the United States have spinal cord injuries and approximately 11,000 new cases are reported every year.[38] The veteran population comprises 22% of the spinal cord injury population.[39] The National Spinal Cord Injury Database documents five major categories of etiology:

- motor vehicle crashes (44.5%)
- falls (18%)
- acts of violence (17%)

- recreational sporting activities (13%)
- causes that don't fit into any of these categories (8%).[40]

A spinal cord injury occurs most frequently in males ages 16 to 30 (55%).[38] Although the average age is 32 and the most frequently occurring age at injury is 19; the median age is 25. More than 82% of the patients in the spinal cord injury database are male. Among patients injured since 1990, 59% are White, 28% are Black, 8% are Hispanic, 2% are Asian, 0.4% are American Indian ethnicity, 0.5% are of unknown ethnicity, and 2.5% are unclassified.[38] Almost half of the spinal cord injury population had completed high school at the time of injury. Given the young age at onset of injury, more than half are single. Although most are employed at the time of injury, more than 14% are unemployed.[40]

The patient with a spinal cord injury is subject to various complications. For instance, pulmonary complications are the most common cause of death during both the acute and chronic phases after a spinal cord injury.[41] Other potential complications arising soon after injury—some of which may become lifelong problems—include pressure ulcers, urinary tract infections, osteoporosis, fractures, and heterotopic ossification.

Additionally, pressure ulcers are among the most common long-term secondary medical complications found at annual follow-up visits.[42] As such, they are a serious, costly, and potentially life-threatening complication of a spinal cord injury. Clinical observations and research studies have confirmed staggering costs and human suffering, including a profound negative impact on the patient's general physical health, socialization, financial status, and body image, compounded by a loss of independence and control.[43]

Reliable and current data on the incidence and prevalence of pressure ulcers in the patient with a spinal cord injury has been difficult to obtain, primarily because limitations of the methods used prevent standardization of the statistics. These limitations include the use of different classification systems to stage pressure ulcers, the inability to compare varied populations (for example, acute or chronic spinal cord injury) presenting with or developing pressure ulcers, and the use of different methods of obtaining data (such as direct observation or retrospective chart review).[44]

Scope of the problem

Some available data reflect the scope of the problem; the database of the Spinal Cord Injury Model Systems is one of the most reliable. The National Institute on Disability and Rehabilitation Research sponsors the Model Systems Program, a federal extramural grant program of selected research and demonstration sites. Model System sites provide exemplary, state-of-the-art care from the time of injury through acute medical care, comprehensive rehabilitation, and long-term follow-up and health maintenance services. An individual can be included in the database only if he was admitted to a system facility within 24 hours of trauma. As far back as 1981,[45] the Model System database included statistics on pressure ulcers in patients with spinal cord injuries. According to the 1998 National Spinal Cord Injury Statistical Center Annual Report, 34% of patients admitted to a Model System facility within 24 hours of a spinal cord injury developed at least one pressure ulcer during acute care or rehabilitation.[46] On follow-up, 15% had a pressure ulcer at their first annual examination, 20% at year 5, 23% at year 10, 24% at year 15, and 29% at year 20. These numbers are based on 4,065 patients of whom 2,971 developed pressure ulcers. Other investigators have reported prevalence rates that ranged from 17% to 33% in populations of patients with spinal cord injuries residing in the community.[45,47,48]

High rates of pressure ulcer recurrence also have been reported, with rates ranging from 21% to 79% regardless of treatment.[49-51] A number of epidemiologic studies have found that 36% to 50% of all patients with spinal cord injuries who develop pressure ulcers will develop a recurrence within the first year after initial healing.[47,48,51-53] Niazi and colleagues[51] reported a recurrence rate of 35% regardless of the type of treatment (medical or surgical). Holmes et al[54] found that 55% of their sample, most of which had a history of severe previous ulcers, experienced recurrence within 2 years after surgical repair. In a 20-year study in Canada (1976 to 1996), Schryvers and colleagues[49] found recurrence rates of 31% at the same site for severe ulcers, requiring surgery in 168 patients with spinal cord injuries. Goodman et al[50] observed a recurrence or new ulcer development rate of 79% within a 1- to 6-year follow-up time frame.

The financial burden of pressure ulcers is undoubtedly immense, although estimates of the cost of preventing and treating pressure ulcers in the patient with a spinal cord injury are not readily available. Miller and DeLozier[55] reported that the total cost of treating stage II, III, and IV pressure ulcers in hospitals, nursing homes, and home care was approximately $1.335 billion per year. One could extrapolate from these data the financial implications of pressure ulcers for the patient with a spinal cord injury. However, the financial burden of pressure ulcers doesn't begin to reflect the personal and social costs experienced by the patient and his family. These include loss of independence and self-esteem; time away from work, school, or family; and, ultimately, diminished quality of life.

Risk factors

There are more than 200 risk factors for the development of pressure ulcers reported in the literature. Most of the risk factors were derived from studying elderly nursing home residents. However, many of the risk factors for these patients differ from those experienced by patients with spinal cord injuries. Immobility increases the risk of pressure ulcer development in both populations; unlike nursing home residents, however, patients with spinal cord injuries typically oversee or direct their own daily care and are expected to take primary responsibility for pressure ulcer prevention. The literature is often contradictory regarding the effects of a particular risk factor or set of factors potentially responsible for the development of pressure ulcers. These contradictions occur due to the limitations imposed by the variables among studies. Different populations (for example, acute or chronic spinal cord injury), inadequate sample sizes, different ways of standardizing the dependent measures, and poor or uncontrolled study designs all add confusion to the interpretation of study results.[56-57]

Despite these limitations, a number of pressure ulcer risk factors specific to the patient with a spinal cord injury have been identified and described in the literature. Byrne and Salzberg's[56] study (1996) summarized the major pressure ulcer risk factors for the patient with a spinal cord injury as:
- severity of the spinal cord injury (immobility, completeness of the spinal cord injury, urinary incontinence, and severe spasticity)
- preexisting conditions (advanced age, smoking, lung and cardiac disease, diabetes and renal disease, and impaired cognition)
- residence in a nursing home
- nutrition (malnutrition and anemia).

The Consortium for Spinal Cord Medicine Clinical Practice Guidelines (Pressure Ulcer Prevention and Treatment Following Spinal Cord Injury)[44] categorized pressure ulcer risk factors in a spinal cord injury as:
- demographic factors (age, gender, ethnicity, marital status, and education)
- physical or medical and spinal cord injury-related factors (level and completeness of the spinal cord injury; activity and mobility; bladder, bowel and moisture control; and comorbidities, such as diabetes and spasticity)
- psychological and social factors (psychological distress, financial problems, cognition, substance abuse, adherence, and health beliefs and practices).[44]

As far back as 1979, Anderson and Andberg[58] identified psychological factors associated with the development of pressure ulcers, including the patient's unwillingness to take responsibility in skin care, low self-esteem, and dissatisfaction with life activities. Gordon and colleagues[59] also found poor social adjustment in the patient with a spinal cord injury and a pressure ulcer.

The recurrence of pressure ulcers in the patient with a spinal cord injury has been associated with gender (male), age (younger), ethnicity (Black), unemployment, residence in a nursing home, and previous pressure ulcer surgery.[51,60,61] Most of the literature describing recurrence following surgery focuses on

PATIENT TEACHING

Preventing pressure ulcers at home

Patients with spinal cord injuries are at risk for developing pressure ulcers even after they leave your care. Teach the patient and his family the following strategies to help him prevent pressure ulcers after he has returned home.

- Perform daily visual and tactile skin inspection.
- Maintain good personal hygiene.
- Perform frequent turning and repositioning, including frequent weight shifts.
- Use support surfaces for the bed and wheelchair.
- Maintain adequate nutrition.

---

surgical techniques.[62-65] Investigators have reported recurrence rates of 11% to 29% in cases with postoperative complications and 6% to 61% in cases without postoperative complications.[61,66-68] Of these investigators, Relander and Palmer[67] recommended that social factors be studied to determine the causes of pressure ulcer recurrence after surgical repair and suggested that the patient who doesn't display the appropriate knowledge regarding pressure ulcer prevention should be counseled before consideration for surgery. Disa and colleagues[61] reported that high recurrence rates among patients with traumatic paraplegia were associated with substance abuse and the absence of an adequate social support system; they suggested developing more effective educational programs for both patients and caregivers. In other studies by Mandrekas and Mastorakos,[68] Baek et al,[69] and Rubayi et al,[70] investigators reported that inadequate patient education with regard to pressure ulcer prevention contributed to the recurrence rates.

PRACTICE POINT

Innovative educational programs are needed to provide patients with spinal cord injuries with information and the motivation necessary to regain some measure of control over their lives.

Risk-based prevention

The patient with a spinal cord injury is at risk for the development of pressure ulcers from the moment of injury. Prolonged immobilization during the hours and days immediately after injury significantly increases the risk. Pressure reduction strategies to protect vulnerable anatomical areas of the body should be implemented soon after emergency medical intervention and spinal stabilization.

PRACTICE POINT

Pressure ulcer development is a lifelong concern for the patient with a spinal cord injury.

Preventing pressure ulcers is a major component of both informal and formal educational sessions during rehabilitation. A regimen of preventive strategies is developed for each patient and includes information and instructions that are given to the patient and his family following a spinal cord injury.[71] (See *Preventing pressure ulcers at home.*)

Printed materials or videotapes are frequently used to augment the educational sessions, some of which may go with the patient when he is discharged. Because most patient education programs are hospital-based, little is known about what information the patient retains, which behaviors or activities are practiced routinely, and the compatibility of the patient's lifestyles with prevention strategies. In the 1970s and 1980s, a number of spinal cord injury centers established comprehensive pressure ulcer prevention education programs.[72-74] Both inpatient and outpatient programs advocated multidisciplinary, coordinated, structured, and wide-ranging approaches to prevention. Some of these programs serve as models for practice today.[75]

Skin assessment

The patient with a spinal cord injury and a pressure ulcer should undergo two assessment phases. The first phase is a comprehensive evaluation and examination, including:
- complete patient history
- physical examination
- laboratory tests
- assessment of psychological health, behavior, and cognitive status
- information on social and financial resources and the availability and utilization of personal care assistance
- assessment of positioning, posture, and related equipment.[44]

The second phase of assessment consists of a detailed description of the pressure ulcer itself and surrounding tissues, including the following factors:
- anatomical location and general appearance
- size in terms of length, width, depth, and wound area
- stage or severity
- exudate
- odor
- necrosis
- undermining
- sinus tracts
- infection
- granulation and epithelialization
- wound margins and surrounding tissue.[44]

Photographs can also be useful in these assessments.

PRACTICE POINT

Patients with darkly pigmented skin are particularly vulnerable to undetected pressure ulcers. Although areas of damaged skin appear darker than the surrounding skin, tactile information must be used in addition to visual data when assessing patients with darker skin. The skin may be taut and shiny, indurated, and warm to the touch. Color changes may range from purple to blue. Remember, pressure-damaged dark skin doesn't blanch when compressed.[76]

Treatment

Prevention and treatment are inextricably linked across the continuum of care for the patient with a pressure ulcer.[77] During rehabilitation following a spinal cord injury, the patient is exposed to a great deal of information about the major physiological changes that have occurred as well as how to prevent or manage the potential secondary complications, such as pressure ulcers and urinary tract infections. Unfortunately, much of this information isn't absorbed during this early posttraumatic phase, resulting in episodes of potentially life-threatening conditions once the patient returns to his home and community. Coupled with non-retention of information is today's significant decrease in length of stay that makes structured education sessions during hospitalization almost impossible. The treatment of pressure ulcers is a complex process, based on a number of patient- and pressure ulcer-related factors.

Nonsurgical treatment

Nonsurgical treatment for pressure ulcers is a multistep process. The elements of a comprehensive treatment plan include cleaning, debridement, applying dressings, and assessing the need for (and appropriateness of) new technologies aimed at wound healing. As mentioned, education, in the form of printed materials or discussions with health care professionals, is intended to prevent recurrence in the patient with a spinal cord injury.

Surgical treatment

Stage III and IV pressure ulcers are frequently treated surgically in the patient with a spinal cord injury. The goals of surgical closure include:

- preventing protein loss through the wound
- reducing risk of progressive osteomyelitis and sepsis
- preventing renal failure
- reducing costly and lengthy hospitalization
- improving hygiene and appearance
- expediting time to healing.[44,78,79]

The surgical process includes:
- excision of the ulcer and surrounding scar, underlying bursa, and soft-tissue calcification removal of underlying necrotic or infected bone
- filling dead space with fascia or muscle flaps
- improving vascularity and distribution of pressure over bony prominences
- resurfacing the area with a large flap so that the suture line is away from areas of direct pressure
- providing a flap that leaves options for future surgeries.[78-79]

Preoperatively, the rehabilitation and surgical teams coordinate their efforts to control local wound infection, improve and maintain nutrition, regulate the bowels, control spasms and contractures, and address comorbid conditions. Previous pressure ulcer surgery, smoking, urinary tract infection, and heterotopic ossification could affect surgical outcomes.[44]

New surgical techniques for pressure ulcers have been developed and are being used to improve surgical outcomes. More recently, new surgical techniques to repair pressure ulcers are being evaluated.[80-84] However, reports of long-term follow-up of the status of the skin and recurrence have been limited. One study by Lee[80] used a new wound closure technique and followed patients for 102 days after which 18 of 21 (86%) wounds in 13 patients remained closed. Sorensen and colleagues[85] suggested that thorough preoperative debridement, patient compliance, control of comorbidities, professional postoperative support, and sufficient pressure relief were essential if surgical success is to be achieved.

Other studies reveal the protective mechanisms against pressure ulcer recurrence. For example, Krause and Broderick[86] reported that 13% of their sample of 633 subjects had recurring pressure ulcers of one or more per year. Their study suggested that lifestyle, exercise, and diet were protective mechanisms against pressure ulcer recurrence. Chen and colleagues[87] studied the effects of age, time period (1994 to 2002 vs. 1984 to 1993), and SCI duration. These investigators found that although during the first 10 years of a person's spinal cord injury (SCI), pressure ulcer risk was relatively stable, there was a significant trend toward increasing pressure ulcer prevalence between 10 and 15 years post-injury. Factors associated with pressure ulcers included age (elderly), gender (male), race (African American) marital status (single), education (less than high school), unemployment, completeness of injury, residing in a nursing home, and history of pressure ulcers and rehospitalization.

EVIDENCE-BASED PRACTICE

Postsurgical care includes keeping the surgical site pressure-free, using specialty beds to maximize pressure reduction, mobilizing the patient progressively, and providing patient and family education.[44]

Support surfaces

Support surfaces are devices or systems intended to reduce the interface pressure between a patient and his bed or wheelchair.[77] Support surfaces don't heal pressure ulcers; rather, they are prescribed by a clinician and incorporated into a comprehensive pressure ulcer prevention and management program. Static or dynamic mattresses, mattress overlays, or specialty beds may be used at various times to reduce the patient's risk of developing pressure ulcers. Materials, such as foams and gels, used alone or in combination, and elements, such as air and water, also used alone or in combination, are being used across patient-care and home environments. Wheelchair cushions and seating systems of various materials and designs are intended to

Support surface pros and cons

This chart presents the major categories of support surfaces with their advantages and disadvantages.

Major types	Common applications	Advantages	Disadvantages
Static support surface	• Pressure ulcer prevention • Individual may be kept off pressure ulcer	• Reduces interface pressure • Is cost-effective when properly matched to individual • Does not consume power	• May result in shearing • Moisture and heat build up
Alternating pressure surface	• Individual who requires more pressure reduction than a static mattress	• Relieves pressure intermittently	• Intermittent elevated pressure • Moisture retention possible
Low air-loss surface	• Individual who has more than 1 turning surface impaired due to multiple pelvic pressure ulcers or other factors	• Reduces interface pressure • Manages moisture and heat	• Shear reduction depends on design; possible noise • Complicated activities of daily living maneuvers and transfers
Air-fluidized bed	• Postoperative flap surgery • Deterioration of multiple pelvic pressure ulcers	• Reduces interface pressure below capillary closing pressure • Manages moisture	• Most expensive • Vulnerable to respiratory or dehydration problems • Premature drying of moist dressings • Significant electric energy requirement • Noise • Limited ability to elevate head of the bed

Adapted with permission from the Paralyzed Veterans of America (PVA). *Prevention and Treatment of Pressure Ulcers Following Traumatic Spinal Cord Injury: A Clinical Practice Guideline for Health-Care Professionals.* Washington, D.C.: Paralyzed Veterans of America; 56-57, 2000.[44]

reduce pressure and maximize balance and stability when a patient is in a wheelchair. (See *Support surface pros and cons.*)

PRACTICE POINT

No single product meets every patient's needs, or all the needs of a single patient. Use your experience and your judgment in concert with objective selection of products to match the device to the patient.

New interventions

A number of adjunctive therapies have been reported in the literature with varying degrees of success in treating pressure ulcers in the patient with a SPI, including:

- electrical stimulation
- ultraviolet and laser therapy
- normothermia
- hyperbaric oxygen and ultrasound
- subatmospheric pressure therapy (vacuum-assisted closure)
- nonantibiotic drugs
- topical agents
- skin equivalents
- growth factors.

Among these, only electrical stimulation has enough reported scientific evidence supporting it to justify its use as a treatment for pressure ulcers in the patient with a SPI.[88,89]

Summary

Although SCI research has increased tremendously in recent years, designing and conducting randomized, controlled trials that are capable of producing compelling observational evidence on which to base management of pressure ulcers has been lacking. Despite advances in pressure ulcer treatment, little scientific evidence points the way to preventing pressure ulcers in the SCI population. Research efforts should focus on prospective studies to prevent recurrence that include long-term follow-up programs that promote self-management.

HIV/AIDS population

Carl A. Kirton, MA, RN, ACRN, APRN,BC

Skin alteration in HIV and AIDS patients

The skin is the most commonly affected organ in patients infected with human immunodeficiency virus (HIV). In fact, in the early 1980s it was the identification of an unusual skin lesion in young homosexual men that prompted the search for the virus that causes acquired immunodeficiency syndrome (AIDS). A broad range of infectious and noninfectious skin lesions may develop during both the asymptomatic and symptomatic course of the disease. Alteration in the skin is often the first manifestation of an impaired immune system and may be a sign or symptom of a serious opportunistic infection. Skin alterations can also indicate advancing disease.

Several points regarding HIV, skin disease, and its treatments are noteworthy. Lesions that are common in the non–HIV-infected adult population may present atypically in HIV-infected persons. In addition, skin disorders often aren't responsive to the usual treatments, may be present for longer than expected, and may develop into chronic, disfiguring disorders. Skin lesions may also be the precursor of a life-threatening illness.

> **PRACTICE POINT**
>
> Prompt and accurate investigation of skin lesions in the HIV-infected patient is essential and often warrants collaboration with an HIV specialist.

The effective combination of several antiretroviral drugs to suppress viral replication with consequent repletion of the CD4-positive (CD4+) lymphocyte count is often known as highly active antiretroviral therapy (HAART). HAART-based regimens and drugs that prevent or treat opportunistic infections have contributed to a significant decline in HIV-associated morbidity and mortality. Some skin disorders also decreased in incidence with HAART, including Kaposi's sarcoma, eosinophilic folliculitis, molluscum contagiosum, bacillary angiomatosis, and condylomata acuminate. It has been estimated in one study that HAART has reduced the total number of HIV patients with skin problems by 40%.[90] Although HAART and regimens that treat opportunistic infections have improved the quality of life for patients infected with HIV, adverse reactions to drugs have increased. Such severe adverse reactions are much more frequent in HIV-infected patients with very low CD4+ lymphocyte counts (usually < 50 cells/mm^3). It's estimated that adverse drug reactions in HIV-infected adults have increased from 8% to 23%.[90] Drugs often associated with adverse effects include sulfonamides, co-trimoxazole, and tuberculostatics as well as many of the antiretrovirals.

Infectious skin disorders

The immunocompromised status of patients with HIV or AIDS puts them at greater risk for infectious bacterial or viral skin disorders, such as herpes virus, cytomegalovirus, human papillomavirus, molluscum contagiosum, *Staphylococcus* and *Streptococcus,* and bacillary angiomatosis.

Herpes virus

Breakouts of grouped blister-like lesions typically caused by the common herpes virus are easily recognized and common in patients with HIV at all stages of the disease. Herpes zoster may occur either early or late in the course of HIV-induced immunosuppression, and may be the first clinical clue to suggest undiagnosed HIV infection. Herpes infection may occur on the oral and genital mucosa as well as the perianal region. Lesions typically manifest as painful, grouped vesicles on an erythematous base that rupture and become crusted. History and clinical presentation are often all that's necessary to establish the disorder; therefore, confirmatory tests, such as the Tzanck smear preparation, biopsy, or viral culture are rarely necessary. In patients with advanced HIV, a herpetic infection may develop into chronic ulcers and fissures with a substantial degree of edema.

Herpes zoster occurs with higher frequency among HIV-seropositive patients than among those who are seronegative. A longitudinal study demonstrated an incidence of 29.4 cases of herpes zoster per 1,000 person-years among HIV-seropositive patients, as compared with 2.0 cases per 1,000 person-years among HIV-seronegative controls.[91] Uncomplicated zoster outbreaks should be treated for 10 days with either acyclovir (Zovirax), famciclovir (Famvir), or valacyclovir (Valtrex). Painful atrophic scars, persistent ulcerations, and acyclovir-resistant chronic verrucous lesions may also develop. (See *Herpes virus teaching tips.*)

PRACTICE POINT

Healing of herpetic lesions is usually complete in less than 2 weeks. If they haven't healed within 3 to 4 weeks, the patient may have a drug-resistant virus. Acyclovir-resistant cases of varicella-zoster virus or herpes simplex virus infection require treatment with I.V. foscarnet (Foscavir).

PRACTICE POINT

A patient with herpes zoster involving V1, the ophthalmic division of the trigeminal nerve, should be referred to an ophthalmologist immediately due to the risk of corneal ulceration. Signs or symptoms of this condition, such as painful vesicular lesions on the tip of the nose or lid margins, should be considered an ocular emergency.

Cytomegalovirus

Up to 90% of patients with AIDS develop acute, active cytomegalovirus (CMV) infection at some point during their illness.[92] When the skin is involved, cytomegalovirus may cause a number of different clinical manifestations including ulcers, verrucous lesions, and palpable purpuric papules. CMV commonly affects the GI tract in advanced disease and patients often develop perianal ulcerations. It's treated with hospitalization for infusion of I.V. ganciclovir (Cytovene), foscarnet (Foscavir), or cidofovir (Vistide).

PRACTICE POINT

Ulcers are commonly secondarily colonized with CMV and many patients have combined herpes simplex and CMV infections.

Human papillomavirus infections

The most common skin complaint of HIV-positive patients is warts caused by the human papillomavirus. It has been shown that immune deficiency is associated with increased frequency of human papillomavirus infections, suggesting that the emergence of human papillomavirus is modulated by the patient's immune status.

Dull-colored papules erupt anywhere on the skin, including the anal mucous membrane, vagina, scrotum, penis, and mouth. Their appearance, size, and number vary with the site. Warts can range in size from less than 1 mm to 2 cm "cauliflower lesions." Treatment, although effective, rarely eradicates human papillomavirus entirely. Destructive measures—such as the application of topical chemicals (for example, salicylic or trichloroacetic acid), cryotherapy with liquid nitrogen, and ablative surgery—are standard measures used for common verrucae (warts). Condyloma acuminata can be treated by using podophyllin resin 10% to 50% in tincture of benzoin, 3% cidofovir ointment, intralesional interferon-alpha, liquid nitrogen cryotherapy, electrodesiccation and curettage, or carbon dioxide laser.

PATIENT TEACHING

Imiquimod (Aldara) 5% if often pre-scribed to prevent recurrence. Instruct the patient to apply to his warts at night 3 times per week for up to 16 weeks.

PATIENT TEACHING

Recent evidence in the literature and anecdotal evidence from patient reports suggest that the application of duct tape is successful at removing warts however this strategy has not been formally tested in HIV-infected patients.[93]

Plantar verrucae are generally treated with topical 40% salicylic acid plaster applied daily, with paring of hyperkeratotic areas, although intralesional bleomycin and liquid nitrogen therapy have also been used. Verruca plana and filiform verrucae are commonly treated with topical tretinoin alone or in combination with 5-flurouracil. Light electrodessication and liquid nitrogen application may be used as an adjunct therapy. Verrucous carcinoma requires excisional surgery. (See *Postprocedure care for HPV infection,* page 424.)

Molluscum contagiosum

Molluscum contagiosum is a benign, usually asymptomatic viral skin infection caused by the poxvirus that causes no systemic manifestations. The diagnosis can usually be made from the characteristic appearance of dome-shaped, umbilicated translucent papules that may develop on any cutaneous site, especially the genital areas and the face. In the patient with AIDS, lesions may become widespread, disfiguring, and resistant to treatment. The prevalence of molluscum contagiosum in the patient with AIDS is 5% to 18%.[95] Treatment is generally by destructive measures including cryotherapy or curettage. (See *Molluscum contagiosum teaching tips,* page 425.)

Staphylococcus or *Streptococcus*

In general, most bacterial infections are caused by *Staphylococcus* and *Streptococcus* organisms and are commonly encountered in immunocompetent patients. Primary bacterial lesions manifest as vesicles, papules, and

PATIENT TEACHING
Postprocedure care for HPV infection

Lesions associated with human papillomavirus (HPV) typically require either chemical or surgical excision following treatment of the viral cause.

Postprocedure patient teaching should include the following.

- Medication usually isn't needed after removal of lesions. Topical anesthetic ointments may be used to minimize discomfort. Sitz baths may aid resolution when large areas are treated; silver sulfadiazine (Silvadene) ointment or antibiotic ointment may not only be soothing, but may also reduce the possibility of superficial infection. No dressing is required, but some patients may request a sanitary napkin for treated genital lesions. Ice packs are helpful.
- Cryonecrosed lesions will progress from erythema to edema, and then will turn black. The lesions will disappear within a few days, and healing should be complete in 7 to 8 days. For chemically cauterized lesions, the healing process is usually less than 1 week.
- Treated areas should be washed and dried gently each day of the healing process. Postcryotherapy management is similar to a superficial partial thickness burn.
- Counsel the patient to report excessive discomfort or any signs of infection.[94]

pustules, and are often pruritic. It's the pruritic feature that often leads the patient to scratching, subsequently resulting in a break in the epithelial surface followed by excoriation of the lesion. Some lesions (such as impetigo) may contain purulent fluid. Diffusely red, warm, tender areas in the skin suggest soft-tissue cellulitis or a deep-seated infected wound. Treatment with dicloxacillin, cephalexin, or ciprofloxacin is indicated in bacterial infections. Wounds caused by bacterial infections should be assessed regularly and treated accordingly. (See chapter 7, Wound bioburden.)

Bacillary angiomatosis

Bacillary angiomatosis is a bacterial infection caused by organisms of the genus *Bartonella* (formerly *Rochalimaea*), specifically *B. quintana* and *B. henselae*. These cutaneous vascular lesions are characteristically small reddish to purple papules that are tender to touch. Lesions may ulcerate and then be covered by a crust. Complicated bacillary angiomatosis infections occur when the lesion is located deep in the subcutis, extending to involve soft tissue and bone. Infection with bacillary angiomatosis leads to systemic involvement. Biopsy and special staining is often necessary to definitively identify the organism. Treatment with erythromycin or doxycycline provides a prompt response. (See *Bacillary angiomatosis teaching tips,* page 426.)

 PRACTICE POINT

With the advent of HAART, bacillary angiomatosis infections are rarely seen. These infections may mimic Kaposi's sarcoma, which should therefore remain the differential diagnosis until the actual causative agent is identified.

Noninfectious skin disorders

The immunocompromised status of patients with HIV and AIDS also puts them at greater risk for noninfectious skin disorders.[97]

PATIENT TEACHING
Molluscum contagiosum teaching tips

- Molluscum contagiosum can be transmitted through direct contact.
- The lesions are prone to autoinoculation, and in male patients, shaving the beard area has been reported to cause particularly severe infections, with lesions encompassing the entire face.
- Cryonecrosed lesions will progress from erythema to edema, and then will turn black. The lesions will disappear within a few days, and healing should be complete in 7 to 8 days.
- For chemically cauterized lesions, the healing process is usually less than 1 week.

Prurigo nodularis

Prurigo nodularis (PN) ("itchy bumps") has been reported to be increasing in incidence in patients with HIV infection. Generally, these lesions are a sign of advanced HIV disease, and typically appear in individuals with CD4 cell counts of less than 50 and are commonly found in darkly pigmented individuals. These lesions are also commonly seen in patients that are co-infected with HIV and hepatitis C. There is a tendency for symmetrical distribution on the extensor surfaces of the limbs; however, the trunk may be involved. The face and palms are seldom affected although no part of the body is exempt.[98]

The exact cause of this pruritic eruption is unknown. There is uncertainty as to whether prurigo nodularis is a primary cutaneous disease or whether it's a pathologic reaction secondary to pruritus and scratching provoked by a separate cause. In the patient with hepatitis C it's thought that the circulating immune complexes are deposited into the skin triggering the response.

Patients with prurigo nodularis are consumed with relief from itching, which is not relieved by antihistamines. Because of this obsession with relief, breaks and tears in the skin often occur with subsequent abscesses, ulcers, folliculitis, or cellulitis.

Topical or intralesional glucocorticoids are the treatment of choice. Other topical treatments, such as topical vitamin D3 and topical capsaicin, have also been reported to be ef-

fective. Oral treatments, such as cyclosporin and thalidomide, have been shown to improve both the appearance of the skin and pruritus.

Cutaneous drug eruptions

Cutaneous drug-induced eruptions are common manifestations of drug hypersensitivity in HIV-infected patients. Bactrim (trimethoprim-sulfamethoxazole), the most effective drug in the prevention and treatment of *Pneumocystis carinii* pneumonia, is known for causing cutaneous eruption in patients with HIV infection. For trimethoprim sulfamethoxazole (TMP/SMX), the rate of cutaneous eruption is 20% to 80% in people with HIV infection, compared with 1% to 3% in persons without HIV infection, possibly due to altered drug metabolism, decreased glutathione levels, or both.[99]

 PRACTICE POINT

Approximately 50% to 60% of HIV-positive patients have been shown to develop a cutaneous eruption from Bactrim. A Bactrim drug eruption is characterized by widely disseminated spread eruptions of fine pink to red macules and papules involving the trunk and extremities.

In its severe form, Stevens-Johnson syndrome and toxic epidermal necrolysis may

PATIENT TEACHING
Bacillary angiomatosis teaching tips

The most common reservoirs for the bacilli that cause bacillary angiomatosis are domestic cats and cat fleas. Clients with AIDS should avoid rough play with cats and situations in which scratches from cats are likely to occur. Cats shouldn't be allowed to lick open wounds or cuts. All cats should be treated for fleas, or other flea control measures should be followed.[96]

also develop. Stevens-Johnson syndrome is characterized by fever, widespread blisters of the skin, and mucous membranes of the eye, mouth, or genitalia. Toxic epidermal necrolysis is a more serious manifestation, which involves widespread areas of the skin with confluent bullae that can lead to loss of skin in massive sheets.

PRACTICE POINT

Toxic epidermal necrolysis may lead to secondary infection with sepsis, volume depletion, and high output cardiac failure as a consequence of widespread denudation of the skin. Patients who develop toxic epidermal necrolysis must be treated aggressively in an acute care setting.

PRACTICE POINT

Because Bactrim is the most effective drug in the prevention and treatment of *Pneumocystis carinii pneumonia*, it's advised that the patient with cutaneous reactions be desensitized in a controlled setting (such as a hospital or clinic).

Neoplastic disorders

Patients with HIV and AIDS are at risk for a variety of neoplastic disorders [97]

Lymphoma

Although lymphomas generally start in the lymph nodes or collections of lymphatic tissue in organs, such as the stomach or intestines, the skin may also be affected. Non-Hodgkin's lymphoma usually manifests as pink to purplish papules or nodules. Deeply seated soft-tissue involvement may expand superficially, forming dome-shaped nodules that often ulcerate. Cutaneous Hodgkin's disease appears similar to non-Hodgkin's lymphoma. The diagnosis is made by the identification of atypical cells having a Reed-Sternberg-like morphology. Treatments include methotrexate, prednisone, bleomycin, adriamycin, cyclophosphamide, and vincristine.

Kaposi's sarcoma

Kaposi's sarcoma is a vascular neoplastic disorder. Prior to the use of HAART, Kaposi's sarcoma was the most common skin disorder seen in men who have sex with men with AIDS. The pathogenesis of Kaposi's sarcoma has now been identified as a Human herpes virus type 8. This virus is transmitted sexually, which, in part, explains the epidemiology of Kaposi's sarcoma predominantly in men who have sex with the male population.

Clinically, Kaposi's sarcoma skin lesions may be pink, red, brown, or purple macules, patches, plaques, nodules, or tumors and can appear almost anywhere on the body, including the mucous membranes. The appearance of many cutaneous lesions typically predicts visceral organ involvement. When pressure-bearing areas such as the base of the spine are involved, lesions often ulcerate. When tumors involve the lymphatics, marked edema may develop leading to diffuse swollen areas of the skin and subsequent breaks in the skin.

Diagnosis of Kaposi's sarcoma is usually based on the finding of purplish skin lesions. Biopsy is rarely necessary, but may be performed because bacillary angiomatosis mimics the lesions. HAART is considered the first-line treatment for Kaposi's sarcoma lesions, and when CD4 cells improve, lesions tend to regress. Other treatments include liquid nitrogen cryotherapy for small cutaneous lesions; radiation treatment and electron-beam therapy are used in selected cases. Radiotherapy is effective for painful lesions of the palms and soles. Intralesional injections of vinblastine sulfate at biweekly intervals are also effective, especially if the patient has only a few small lesions; however, the injections are painful. With more advanced disease, systemic therapy with interferon and liposomally encapsulated doxorubicin and daunorubicin are effective agents.

Summary

Skin disorders are common in patients with HIV and AIDS. Accurate identification of skin lesions is critical so appropriate treatment can be implemented. Consultation with an HIV or AIDS clinician is helpful in the comprehensive care of these patients.

Neonatal and pediatric populations

Mona Mylene Baharestani, PhD, ANP, CWOCN, FCCWS, FAPWCA

Pressure ulcer prevalence and incidence

Pressure ulcer prevalence rates as high as 27% have been reported in pediatric intensive care units (PICU) and 20% in neonatal intensive care units (NICU), with the majority of these ulcers occurring within 2 days of admission.[100-104] Among hospitalized children in non-critical areas variable prevalence rates of 0.47% to 13% have been cited.[105,106] These rates dramatically increase in children with spinal cord injuries (22% to 55%)[107] and myelomeningocele (37% to 97%).[108,109]

Incidence rates among hospitalized non-critical children range from 0.29% to 6%,[105,110] while PICU incidence rates range from 3.4% to 27%.[100,104] (See *PICU pressure ulcer incidence,* page 428.) Reports of pressure ulcer incidence in the NICU range from 19% to 23%.[102,111]

Financial impact

For example, in a 4-year longitudinal study, the skin status of children with spina bifida and spinal cord injuries were tracked at the Children's Hospital Medical Center of Akron.[112] Of the 4,533 hospital days studied, 994 (22%) were attributed to pressure ulceration at a cost of over $1.3 million.[112]

Anatomical distribution

The occiput is the most common anatomical site for pressure ulcer formation in patients from birth to age 3, as the head comprises a disproportionately higher percentage of their total body weight.[111,113] When supine, it's the occiput that is the primary pressure point with the greatest interface pressure.[114,115] In older children, similar to adults, the sacrum and heels are the most common sites for pressure ulceration. Among children with myelomeningocele, pressure ulcers are most frequently seen over the gibbus, ischial region, and perineum.[108]

PRACTICE POINT

The occiput is the most common site for pressure ulcers in children from birth to age 3.

Complications

Pressure ulcer formation in neonatal and pediatric populations can result in increased

PICU pressure ulcer incidence

This chart shows incidence rates of pressure ulcers in the pediatric intensive care unit (PICU) by study investigator and year.

Investigator	Year	Incidence
Neidig et al[113]	1989	16.9% (pre-guideline) 4.8% (post-guideline
Zollo et al[153]	1996	26%
Willock[154]	2000	15.6%
Curley et al[104]	2003	27%
McLane et al[100]	2004	3.4%
Bahrestani et al[102]	2004 2005	20% (pre-guideline) 5.8% (post-guideline)

morbidity, mortality, infection, sepsis, osteomyelitis, pain, scarring alopecia altered body image, grief, anxiety, depression, social isolation, and increased parental and family stress.[112,116-119]

Risk factors

Pressure ulcer development has traditionally been viewed as uncommon among neonatal and pediatric populations given the presumed relative ease of repositioning and frequency of movement. But, as survival rates among critical and chronically ill premature neonates and children improve through technological advances, so too does risk increase for pressure ulcer formation. Premature neonates with edematous, dry skin, attenuated rete ridges, little-to-no subcutaneous tissue, and immature organ systems are especially susceptible to the deleterious effects of pressure and shear forces.[120-123] Their anatomically immature skin is further challenged by multiple negative physiological responses to repositioning. In fact, repositioning of premature neonates can result in agitation, apnea, bradycardia, emesis, airway obstruction, tachycardia, and slower oxygenation recovery time than any other form of handling. Consequently, pro-

longed periods of immobilization may be maintained, especially among those on extracorporeal membrane oxygenation (ECMO) and high frequency oscillatory ventilation (HFOV).[124-126]

Medical equipment or devices

Pressure exerted on the soft tissue from monitoring and respiratory equipment also greatly increases the risk for ulcer formation in this highly vulnerable population. In fact, Willock and colleagues found that 50% of neonatal and pediatric pressure ulcers were directly associated with equipment pressing on the skin.[127] (See *Common devices that cause pressure ulcers in neonates and children.*) High risk for ala, caudal septal, columnar, and nasal bridge pressure ulceration, secondary to nasal prong and mask continuous positive air pressure (CPAP), is of concern in all NICUs.[128-129] Preventive measures, such as hourly prong or mask repositioning with skin assessments and use of protective hydrocolloid or silicone dressings, often prevent the occurrence of these devastating ulcers.[129]

Interestingly, in a retrospective cohort study of 64 NICU patients by Schmidt and colleagues, univariate analyses revealed that while more patients on HFOV developed pressure ulcers than those on conventional ventilation (53% vs.12.5%), multivariate and life-table analyses found PICU length of stay (LOS) to be statistically more significant, not ventilator type.[130] Among proned children with acute respiratory distress syndrome (ARDS) increased risk of pressure ulcer development on the chin, chest, shoulders, knees, iliac crests, sternum, pretibial crests, ears, and corners of the mouth have been reported.[101]

In a case-controlled study of 118 PICU patients by McCord and colleagues, edema, PICU LOS greater than 96 hours, increased positive expiratory pressure (PEEP), weight loss, and not turning the patient or using a specialty bed in turn mode were all identified as risk factors for pressure ulcer development.[131] Neidig and others, found that in pediatric open heart surgery patients, turning was not initiated postoperatively until hemodynamic and respiratory stability were achieved, as turning was not viewed as a priority.[113] Furthermore, positioning of the head was often limited by internal and external jugular catheters, head and neck edema, and air leakage around endotracheal tubes with movement.[113]

Paralysis

Paralysis has been shown to be a risk factor for pressure ulcers in children in several studies.[107,108,132] In an attempt to obtain a more comprehensive understanding of pressure ulcer development among children and adolescents with spinal cord injuries (SCIs), a retrospective study was undertaken at the Chicago Shriners Hospitals for Children.[107] Seventy-eight patients were enrolled who sustained a SCI at age 12 or younger. Of these 78 children, 43 (55%) developed at least one pressure ulcer, for a group total of 155 ulcers.[107] The risk factors identified were: complete injuries, presence of scoliosis, and paraplegia. Those with paraplegia were more likely to have ulcers than those with tetraplegia and especially if the child was younger than age 12.[107]

Common devices that cause pressure ulcers in neonates and children

- Arm boards
- Endotracheal tubes
- Head dressings and hats
- Improperly worn or fitted orthotics
- Nasal prongs and continuous positive airway pressure (CPAP) masks
- Nasogastric or orogastric tubes
- Outgrown wheelchair or cushion
- Plaster casts
- Tracheal plates or ties
- Transcutaneous oxygen tension ($tcPO_2$) probes

Other risk factors

In a longitudinal study spanning over two decades at the Children's Orthopedic Hospital & University of Washington's Birth Defects Clinic, morbidity and risk factors associated with skin breakdown in patients with myelomeningocele were analyzed by Okamoto.[108] Among the 227 patients who developed pressure ulcers, high paraplegia, high sensory impairment, mental retardation, large head size, kyphosis or kyphoscoliosis, chronic fecal or urinary soiling, and an abnormal upper extremity neurologic examination were all implicated.[108] Okamoto, also noted that rates of pressure ulcer formation increased with age, until the children were 10 or 11, at which time occurrence leveled off at 20% to 25%.[108]

In a retrospective, exploratory study by Samaniego of 69 pediatric outpatients with a primary diagnosis of myelodysplasia, paralysis, insensate areas, high activity, and immobility were all identified as pressure ulcer risk factors.[132]

Lack of caregiver knowledge regarding risk factors and effective pressure ulcer prevention measures are also critical factors impacting patient risk.[110] In fact, the beliefs held by many clinicians is that pressure ulcers are 'inevitable', 'irrelevant' or 'simply not a

Neonatal and pediatric pressure ulcer risk assessment tools

This chart lists several studies that established pressure ulcer risk assessment tools in neonatal and pediatric patients.

Author	Tool	Based on	N
Barnes[156]	Barnes	Literature review	None
Bedi[136]	Bedi	Adult Waterlow	None
Cockett[140]	Cockett	Literature review	None
Garvin[137]	Garvin	Not specified	None
Huffiness and Logsdon[111]	NSRAS	Adult Braden	32
Oding and Patterson[115]	Pattold Pressure Scoring System	Literature review Key components for maintaining skin	None
Pickersgil[135]	Derbyshire	Medley and Adult Waterlow	None
Quicley and Curley[134]	Braden Q	Adult Braden Expert panel	322
Waterlow[141]	Pediatric Waterflow	Pediatric pressure ulcer risk factor identification and incidence study (Waterlow)	302
Willock[138,139]	Glamorgan	Literature review Expert panel Pediatric pressure ulcer risk factors study (Willock)	336

problem in the neonatal and pediatric population' are in themselves risk factors.[133-135]

Risk assessment tools

Currently there are nine published pediatric pressure ulcer risk assessment scales[111,115,134-138,140-141] (See *Neonatal and pediatric pressure ulcer risk assessment tools.*)[142-145] (See also *Neonatal and pediatric skin condition scales,* pages 432 and 433.) However, the only pediatric pressure ulcer risk assessment scales for which there is published sensitivity and specificity data are the Braden Q,[134] Neonatal Skin Risk Assessment Scale (NSARS),[111] and Glamorgan.[138]

Both the Braden Q[134] and NSARS[111] were modeled after the adult Braden Scale for predicting pressure ulcer risk. In developing the Braden Q scale, Quigley and Curley adapted the six subscales descriptions for the pediatric population and added a tissue perfusion and oxygenation subscale.[104,134] In a multisite prospective study of 322 PICU patients, which excluded children with intracardiac shunting or unrepaired congenital heart disease, the Braden Q was found to be 88% sensitive and 58% specific at a cut-off score of 16.[104] The Braden Q is recommended for those age 21 days through age 8. For children older than age 8, Quigley and Curley suggest that the Braden Scale be utilized.[104]

Setting	Age	Sensitivity	Specificity
Pediatric acute care	Not specified	Not performed	Not performed
PICU Progressive care unit	Neonate > age 12	Not performed	None
PICU	Not specified	Not performed	None
PICU	Not specified	Not performed	None
NICU	26 to 40 weeks' gestation	83%	81%
PICU	Not specified	None	None
Not stated	Not specified	No	None
PICU	21 days to age 8	88% (Modified version 92%)	58% (Modified version 59%)
Pediatric acute care	Neonate to age 12	None	None
Pediatric acute care	Birth to age 18	98.4%	67.5%

NSARS measures six subscales pertinent to neonates.[111] The subscales are based on validity testing among 32 NICU patients and demonstrated a sensitivity of 83% and a specificity of 81%.[111] The Glamorgan Scale[138] is comprised of 11 statistically significant pediatric risk factors that include:
- inability to move without great difficulty or deterioration in condition
- inability to change position without assistance/inability to control body movement
- some mobility, but reduced for age
- equipment, objects, or hard surface pressing or rubbing on skin
- significant anemia (Hb < 9g/dl)
- persistent pyrexia (temperature > 99.5° F [37.5° C] for more than 12 hours)
- poor peripheral perfusion
- inadequate nutrition
- low serum albumin (< 3.5g/dl)
- weight < 10th percentile
- incontinence (if inappropriate for age).

These risk factors were identified through literature review, clinical experts, and Willock's own study data, which examined the characteristics of 61 hospitalized patients with pressure ulcers and 271 patients with no ulcerations.[138,139,146] At a cut-off score of 15, the Glamorgan Scale is 98.4% sensitive and 67.4% specific.[138]

PRACTICE POINT

Use a pressure ulcer risk assessment scale designed for pediatric patients.

Neonatal and pediatric skin condition scales

This chart lists various studies about neonatal and pediatric skin condition scales.

Author	Tool	Based on	N
Lund & Osbourne[143]	Neonatal Skin Condition Scale	AWHONN & NANN Neonatal Skin Care Guidelines[56]	1,006
McGurk[144]	Northampton Neonatal Skin Assessment Tool	Northampton General Hospital Skin Integrity Pressure Ulcer Standards	None
McGurk[144]	Northampton Children's Skin Assessment Tool	Northampton General Hospital Skin Integrity Pressure Ulcer Standards	None
Perez-Woods and Malloy[145]	Loyola University Neonatal Skin Assessment Scale (LUNSAS)	Literature review Panel of experts	None
Suddaby and Collegue[142]	Starkid Skin Scale	Braden Q	347

Pressure redistribution products

Although children are typically placed on support surfaces designed for adults, the clinical efficacy and safety of this practice raises serious concerns.[137,147] Low-air-loss-beds designed for adults do not have the numerical option to accommodate for the height and weight of an infant or small child.[100] Children and infants often sink in and between cushions.[100] When adult specialty beds are placed in the turn mode, the occiput of small children pivots on the same pressure point, potentially increasing shear and friction and not redistributing pressure.[131] If a low-air-loss bed or alternating overlay is clinically indicated, only those that are age appropriate, clinically efficacious, and safe should be used in accordance with manufacturer's recommendations. Products currently available in these categories are the Nimbus® Pediatric System (Huntleigh Healthcare LLC, Eatontown, NJ), an alternating overlay for patients weighing between 13 and 55 lb and the Pedia-dyne® (KCI, Inc., San Antonio,

TX), a low-air-loss bed for patients weighing 15 to 60 lb.

According to the findings of Solis and colleagues, pressure redistribution devices effective for children are statistically different than those used for adults.[114] In their study of 13 healthy children ages 10 weeks to age 13.5, the highest interface pressure readings were noted under the occiput (average 59 mm Hg.).[114] In older, larger children ages 10 to 14, the highest pressures were in the sacral area.[114] Convoluted foam (2" to 4" thick) was effective in decreasing these interface pressures.[114] Similarly, in a 2002 pilot study at Texas Children's Hospital by McLane and colleagues, of 54 healthy children, the highest interface readings were on the occiput from infancy to age 6, and occiput, coccyx, and heels in ages 6 to 18.[148] For children younger than age 2, use of the Delta Foam overlay (Span America, Greenville, SC) resulted in the lowest interface occiput pressures.[148] For children older than age 2 the Delta Foam overlay and use of a Gel-E Donut pillow (Children's Medical Venture, Norwell, MA)

Setting	Age	Sensitivity	Specificity	Inter-rater Reliability
NICU, Special Care Unit, Well baby nursery	Birth to 28 days of age	None specified	None specified	65.9% to 89%
Not stated	Not stated	None specified	None specified	None specified
Not stated	Not stated	None specified	None specified	None specified
NICU	Neonates	None specified	None specified	90%
Pediatric acute care	PICU med-surg oncology adolescents	17.5%	99%	85%

significantly lowered occipital pressure and provided similar pressure redistribution to the Efica low-air-loss bed (HillRom Inc., Batesville, IN).[148]

PRACTICE POINT

Because children are not "small adults" they should not be placed on adult support surfaces but instead on pressure redistribution products specifically designed for their specialized loading needs.

Selection of appropriate support surfaces and positioning devices is adjunctive to manual offloading of pressure, as is medically feasible. In an examination of children undergoing cardiovascular surgery, Neidig and colleagues reported a 3.4-fold decrease in occipital pressure ulcer incidence after institution of 1.5" foam cushions under all patients heads in the operating room, followed by at least every 2 hour postoperative head repositioning in the PICU.[113]

Given that upwards of 50% of pressure ulcers are related to pressure from equipment and devices,[127] it's important to perform frequent skin assessments and to rotate blood pressure cuffs and transcutaneous oxygen tension ($tcPO_2$) probes and provide sufficient padding under tracheostomy plates, nasal prongs and CPAP masks, arm boards, plaster casts, and traction boots. Proper fitting of orthotics, wheelchairs, and wheelchair cushions as children grow must also be ensured. Beds and cribs should be inspected to ensure that no tubing, leads, hard toys, nor syringe caps are inadvertently left under the patient's skin.[127] Tapes securing nasogastric and orogastric tubes, head dressings, and hats should be gently removed and the skin assessed, for pressure injuries.

PRACTICE POINT

Because almost half of pressure ulcers in children occur from tubes and devices, checking the skin beneath them to prevent breakdown is critical.

Nutritional considerations

Malnutrition affects 15% to 20% of patients admitted to the PICU.[149] The systemic and immunological ramifications of malnutrition on this compromised population further limits their tissue tolerance to pressure, friction, and shear, especially as third spacing occurs. It's essential that the protein, caloric, and hydration needs of neonates and children be addressed as part of a comprehensive pressure ulcer prevention and treatment plan.

Topical management

When selecting a topical agent for use in the neonatal and pediatric population, it is critical to consider: the patient's age and degree of integumentary maturity, skin condition, product adherence, potential for skin sensitization, impact of product absorption and need for avoidance of products containing dyes, fragrances, and preservatives.[150] Knowledge of product safety and manufacturer's recommendations in the neonatal and pediatric population is essential.

Normal saline and sterile water are commonly used for wound cleaning in this population. Amorphous and sheet, preservative-free hydrogels and hydrofibers are utilized for pressure ulcer treatment, while thin hydrocolloids, foams, thin films, and silicone-based dressings may be used in both prevention and treatment. If the ulcer is necrotic and wound closure is the goal of treatment, then an appropriate method of debridement (surgical or autolytic) should be performed. (See chapter 8, Wound debridement.) Although there are anecdotal case reports of topical enzymes having been used in the neonatal and pediatric populations, manufacturer recommendations are only for those over age 18; safety data for those younger does not exist.

PRACTICE POINT

Before using a topical agent, check with the manufacturer to see if it's safe to use on the skin or wound of a pediatric patient.

In the treatment of extensive, full-thickness pressure ulcers, negative pressure wound therapy as delivered by the V.A.C.® (KCI, Inc., San Antonio, TX) may be utilized to achieve wound closure or as a bridge to surgical closure. In the presence of osteomyelitis, the need for appropriate systemic antibiotics must be addressed.

Patient education

Education regarding pressure ulcer risk factors and effective prevention and treatment measures is essential for school nurses, teachers, teacher's aides, professional and lay caregivers, as well as for children and their families at high risk. Integral to pediatric education is the recognition of each child's uniqueness, the developmental characteristics of each age group, and the psychological and psychosocial factors that they face.[104,127]

Parents of high-risk infants should be taught to perform skin assessments during bathing, diaper changes, and catheterization. They should be warned of the risk of ulcer formation over the knees, ankles, and feet when crawling begins.[107] During the toddler and preschool-aged phase, children can be taught how to perform skin checks on their doll or teddy bear and then on themselves.[107] School-aged children with upper extremity abilities, should be taught 'liftoffs' with the use of mirrors to check the buttocks, and how to ensure that their wheelchair cushion is functioning properly.[107] Written educational materials, alarm clocks or watches as reminders for 'liftoffs,' and rewards for assuming self-care are beneficial.[107] Parents should maintain a safety-net role in their child's care, as they begin to relinquish control.[107] Educating teenagers is best provided on a one-on-one basis with respect for their privacy.[107] Educational materials that are concise and focused on their tasks are best received.[107] Watches with automatic alarms to serve as a reminder for 'liftoffs' are of benefit during this developmental stage as well.[107] Graphic images of pressure ulcers and discussion of the possible need for hospitalizations and surgery and time away from friends and social events will assist in emphasizing the importance of prevention.[107]

PRACTICE POINT

The pressure ulcer prevention teaching plan should be specific to the child's age, developmental level, and individual characteristics.

Summary

Based on available pressure ulcer prevalence and incidence data, neonates and children are at risk for developing pressure ulcers.[152] Support surfaces and topical products manufactured for adults may not be suitable for use in neonates and children as the clinical efficacy and safety are unknown.

The development of much needed neonatal and pediatric focused pressure ulcer clinical practice guidelines and educational programs must address the immature integument of the premature neonate with potential for absorptive toxicity, disparities in weight distribution, and the physiological and psychological uniqueness of this population, while acknowledging the basic tenets found in adult models.

Bariatric patient population

Janet Cuddigan, PhD, RN, CWCN, CCCN

An important health care concern

The National Center for Health Statistics reports that 30% of American adults are obese—over 60 million people.[157] Health care facilities specializing in bariatric surgeries have been aware of the need for appropriate equipment and special skin care protocols for this population for years.[158-160] Facilities without bariatric specialty services are challenged to meet the needs of an ever-increasing bariatric population. Failure to address the needs of this patient population may even put the health care facility at legal risk.[160]

Classifying the bariatric patient

What makes a person bariatric? This category can be based on amount of body weight compared to height, as well as where the person's weight is located on their body. The National Heart, Lung, and Blood Institute (NHLBI) provides the following classifications for obesity based on body mass index (BMI).[161,162]

- Overweight = BMI 25 to 29.9
- Class I obesity = BMI 30.0 to 34.9
- Class II obesity = BMI 35.0 to 39.9
- Class III (extreme) obesity = BMI greater than 40
- BMI = body weight in kilograms/body height in meters squared.

The distribution of body weight should also be assessed. Health risks (and skin care needs) vary between those with "apple-shaped" versus "pear-shaped" physiques. (See *Identifying body shapes*, page 436.) The "waist-to-hip circumference ratio" is often used to describe these differences. The patient with an apple-shaped physique has a greater waist-to-hip ratio and greater risk of cardiovascular disease. The pear-shaped individual has a lower ratio, but may need special chairs and commodes to accommodate a larger hip size.[159]

Meeting patient needs

With the ever-increasing rates of obesity, all health care facilities need to have bariatric skin care protocols in place and "ready access" to beds, chairs, commodes, walkers, and other equipment appropriate for bariatric patients. Advanced preparation of protocols and equipment is essential to meet the needs of these patients. Morbidly obese patients frequently have significant health care problems, such as hypertension, type 2 diabetes, coronary artery disease, stroke, gallbladder disease, osteoarthritis, sleep apnea, respiratory problems, and increased risk for certain cancers.[163] Despite these risks, bariatric patients may delay medical treatment out of fear or embarrassment. Ask yourself these questions as you develop your institutional readiness:

- Is your facility prepared to handle the special needs of these patients as they enter the emergency department?
- Is your staff prepared to provide safe respectful care of the patient while avoiding injuries to either patient or staff members?

Bariatric patients have many needs. For example, a prospective study of 31 patients following Roux-en-Y anastomoses bypass

Identifying body shapes

The waist-to-hip ratio (WHR) is often used to describe the differences between the two types of body shapes: apple-shaped and pear-shaped (as shown in these illustrations). The apple-shaped physique is associated with hypertension.

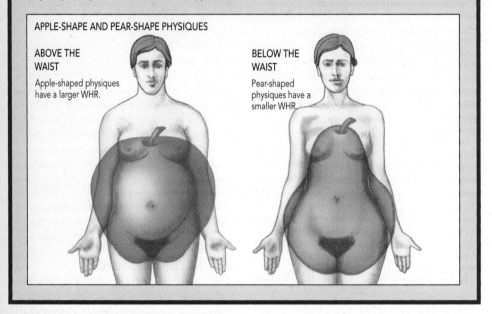

APPLE-SHAPE AND PEAR-SHAPE PHYSIQUES

ABOVE THE
WAIST

Apple-shaped physiques
have a larger WHR.

BELOW THE
WAIST

Pear-shaped
physiques have a
smaller WHR.

surgery that measured knowledge of incision care as well as discharge concerns found increased patient fear with lower levels of knowledge.[164] A comprehensive discussion of special bariatric needs is beyond the scope of this chapter. Discharge and educational needs of postsurgical procedure bariatric patients are summarized in Pieper, Sieggreen, et al (2006).[165] The focus of our discussion will be on skin assessment and care with the goal of maintaining skin integrity.

Skin assessment

A complete skin assessment is the first step in any skin care protocol. A cursory assessment of the skin is not sufficient. Breasts, pannus, and other areas of high adiposity should be gently lifted to inspect all skin surfaces particularly the skin folds. When examining the skin you may find certain benign conditions that more commonly occur in obese individuals. These include:

• Acanthosis nigricans—hyperpigmented (often brown) irregular plaques in skin folds (especially axilla and back of the neck). The plaques often feel like velvet when touched, but may eventually become rougher in texture. Although acanthosis nigricans is usually a benign condition, changes that may indicate malignancy (for example, bleeding or inflammation) should be referred to the primary care provider for follow up. This condition is associated with obesity, but also with other systemic diseases, such as hyperinsulinemia and cancer. A 12% ammonium lactate cream applied 2 times per day may improve the condition.[166]

• Skin tags—common in obese patients and usually benign. They may be surgically removed for cosmetic reasons.[166]

• Androgen effects—adipose tissue synthesizes testosterone. Obese female patients may show male-pattern baldness, excessive hair growth in other areas, and acne.[166]

• Stretch marks (striae distensae)—from stretching of connective tissue, collagen rupture, and dermal scarring.[166]

• Plantar hyperkeratosis—excessive weight on the feet leads to thickening of the weight-bearing surfaces on the soles. Treatment includes weight loss and orthotic shoe inserts to protect bony prominences from breakdown.[166]

More serious skin problems are often found during the initial assessment of obese patients, such as cellulitis, skin infections, lymphedema, hemosiderosis and other skin changes associated with venous insufficiency of the lower extremities; venous ulcers; infection, seroma, poor healing, or dehiscence of surgical wounds; intertrigo; and pressure ulcers.[166,167] Many of these conditions are covered in other chapters of this book. Here we will give special consideration to prevention and treatment of intertrigo and pressure ulcers as they relate to bariatric patients.

Intertrigo

Intertrigo is inflammation of the skin folds.[168] The inflammatory changes are often in mirror images where one skin surface touches another. Intertrigo or intertriginous dermatitis are actually fairly broad terms that cover a variety of skin disorders found between the folds of the skin. Although this condition can be found in any patient, obese patients are at higher risk because multiple large skin folds create conditions ideal for inflammation and infection. These conditions include moisture (as perspiration is trapped under skin folds creating maceration), pressure of large skin folds on underlying skin creating areas of pressure induced injury, friction (as one skin surface moves across another), shear with movement resulting in fissures at the base of the skin fold, physical challenges in maintaining hygiene, and the warm, dark, moist conditions that favor growth of yeast and fungal infections. Secondary bacterial skin infections may also develop and progression to cellulitis is certainly a risk if not treated. (See photographs in the color section, page C32.)

Intertrigo can develop in any skin fold, but is most common under the breasts, abdominal skin folds (pannus), axillae, submaxillary area, and groin or perineum. Obese patients may report a history of skin irritation under skin folds. Their risks of recurrence often increases once hospitalized due to confounding factors, such as bed rest, immobility, fever, and use of such medications as antibiotics and steroids.

Preventing intertrigo

Prevention of intertrigo is a key component of any bariatric skin care protocol. Preventive interventions focus on keeping the skin clean, dry, and well supported, and minimizing the effects of moisture, pressure, friction, and shear. Use a gentle soap or no-rinse skin cleaner for bathing.[166] Pat skin dry with a soft cloth. Moisture accumulation between skin folds is an ongoing problem between bathing. Soft absorbent pads, such as soft linen, ABD, or non-occlusive high-air-flow incontinence pads, can be placed between skin folds to offload pressure, absorb moisture, and lessen friction and shear with movement. Some facilities have had success with a new product, called InterDry, designed to be placed in the skin folds of bariatric patients (shown below in place).

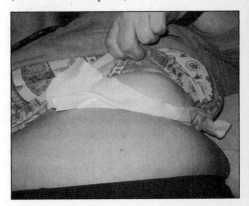

A properly fitted non-synthetic brassiere may also help achieve these goals in large-breasted women. Any material placed between skin folds should be changed frequently.

When repositioning bariatric patients in bed, make sure that the pannus is well supported with a pillow and separate the legs with a pillow between the knees to make sure there is adequate airflow to skin fold areas. Low-air-loss beds may help dry moist areas, however, a less expensive alternative is placing air tubing under the sheets to circulate air.

Some authors recommend the use of cornstarch, talc, moisture barriers, and prophylactic antifungal powders and creams.[166,169] Powders often cake creating more skin damage when removed. Moisture barriers are most effective when placed on skin subjected to external sources of moisture, such as urine, feces, and wound drainage. Products containing dimethicone may reduce friction. There is no evidence to support the use of prophylactic antifungal agents. At the first signs of Candida intertrigo, topical antifungals should be started.

Treating intertrigo

A wide variety of products have been used to treat intertigo,[169] however, the most effective treatments are based on an analysis of the underlying etiology. Candida should be treated with topical antifungal products; systemic antifungal agents such as fluconazole may be necessary in severe cases. Likewise, bacterial infections of the skin may be treated with topical antibiotics, but should be treated with systemic antibiotics if not improving or if progressing to cellulitis. Topical and systemic steroids may be useful in cases of atopic or contact dermatitis.[168]

Unfortunately, intertrigo may continue to plague obese patients even after weight loss. Panniculectomy and other forms of recontouring surgery may be necessary to remove excessive skin folds after weight loss has been achieved.[170]

Pressure ulcers
Prevention

Pressure ulcer prevention has been discussed in chapter 13, Pressure ulcers. This discussion focuses on the unique risk factors and needs of the bariatric patient in preventing pressure ulcers.

Unique risk factors

There are several factors that increase pressure ulcer risk in the bariatric patient. Adipose tissue is not well vascularized, and

therefore, more susceptible to the ischemic effects of pressure. Pressure mapping studies indicate that pressure is distributed somewhat differently in obese patients. In patients of normal weight, high-pressure areas in the supine position are predominantly over bony prominences (for example, the head, sacrum, and heels). In the obese patient, a large amount of weight-induced force is distributed over the entire supine surface. Pressures may be high over bony prominences, but high-pressure areas are also seen in traditionally soft tissue areas such as the buttocks. Even though the surface area is larger in an obese patient, there is still often greater tissue weight than normal on traditionally soft tissue areas. (See *Pressure distribution*.)

Risk assessment
Standard risk assessment tools such as the Braden Scale are still important as a general screening tool for pressure ulcer risk status. However, you should delve more deeply into each subscale when caring for an obese patient. Consider the following questions when planning care for your bariatric patients:
• If on bed rest, what positioning strategies will improve respiration, without increasing shear risk?
• Can pillows be placed under the arms to prevent sliding and shear? Would a trapeze over the bed help with patient mobility?
• Is the bed wide enough for the patient to turn?
• Even though the patient may appear overweight, is their nutritional status really adequate?
• If moisture from incontinence is an issue, could it be improved by providing a bariatric bedside commode or walker to ambulate to the bathroom?
• Because stress incontinence is frequently a problem in obese patients due to greater weight on the pelvic floor, are you also creating a functional incontinence because you have not provided the appropriate toileting equipment?

Bariatric equipment
In order to meet the individualized needs of your bariatric patients, a full range of bariatric support equipment must be used including bariatric chairs, commodes, toilets,

Pressure distribution

High pressure areas more focused in areas of bony prominence in patients with a lower body mass index (BMI). A more diffuse pattern of high pressure distribution is evident in the patient with a higher BMI.
High pressure areas occur over soft tissue areas as well as bony prominences.

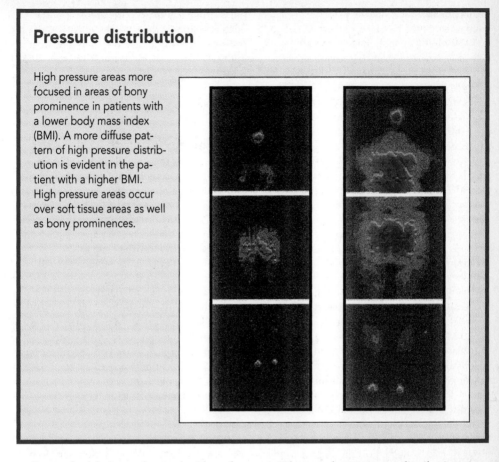

walkers, wheelchairs, and canes besides, of course, the correct size bed. Proper equipment should be made available well in advance of the patient's arrival. Both rental and purchase arrangements are available from a wide variety of manufacturers.

When selecting a bariatric bed, some basic criteria should be considered. Determining this criteria includes asking yourself these questions:

- Is the bed wide enough?
- Can the patient turn in the bed?
- What is the weight capacity for the bed?
- Even if the usual weight capacity of the bed is appropriate for your patient's weight, does your patient "bottom out" or leave indentations in the bed over areas of higher weight distributions? (Remember the discussion about apple-shaped versus pear-shaped physiques.)

- What are the pressure redistribution capacities of the bed?
- Is a trapeze (or other supportive structure) available so that the patient can assist with turning?
- Does the bed have a turn assist mode?
- Does the bed have features to assist with moisture control if indicated?
- Is the bed designed for easy patient egress that will help facilitate remobilization?

Staff concerns
Equipment characteristics and safety features are of equal concern for the staff. Can staff transport the patient in the bed? Can the bed fit through the doors of the hospital? Can the bed be easily steered? Are bariatric-size lifts and air transfer mattresses available? Have the staff been properly trained to use bariatric equipment to ensure both staff and patient safety?

Repositioning

Repositioning the bariatric patient is both an art, as well as a science. Routine turning should be accomplished by a team of trained caregivers and in a manner that preserves the patient's dignity. When possible, enlist the patient's help in turning. Patients and their families often have very useful suggestions for achieving and maintaining mobility despite challenges.

When repositioning bariatric patients in bed, several strategies are particularly important. When repositioning every 2 hours, be sure to "offload" bony prominences the patient has been lying on. Rather than repositioning pillows under the patient's shoulders and hips, you should turn the patient off bony prominences. This may take several people or use of turn assist devices to accomplish without creating friction or shear injuries. Without adequate assistance, you are more likely to drag rather than lift the patient. Grabbing and pulling on a patient may also cause skin tears. Small shifts in body weight may be effective based on the research of Oertwich.[171] However, small shifts are intended as an adjunct, not a replacement, to regular repositioning in high-risk patients.

Offloading heels

Heels should be floated off the surface of the bed with pillows under the calf or positioning devices. Examine the unique anatomy of your patient's lower extremities. Patients with large calves may be naturally suspending their heels off the surface of the bed. Feel under the heel and leg to note any high-pressure areas that can be relieved with properly placed pillows that redistribute weight. When using heel-positioning devices, make sure they are properly sized for your patient and can be applied without creating high-pressure areas under straps or other areas of the device.

Pannus care

The pannus or "abdominal apron" and other areas of adipose tissue are suspended by gravity when the patient is standing. While on bed rest, these tissues create pressure on the underlying skin. Place pillows or soft folded bath blankets under the pannus and other skin folds to keep the area dry and offload pressure. If the patient has any tubes or other medical devices, make sure they are not under the weight of the pannus or other skin folds. An object as simple as a pillow between the legs can help prevent damage from a Foley catheter.

Ulcer locations and characteristics

Pressure ulcers that do develop in obese patients often have slightly different characteristics. They develop over bony prominences, but also over other areas of high tissue pressure such as the buttocks. Bilateral hip ulcers are often commonly seen in patients placed in chairs too narrow for their hip size.[159] Bariatric patients seem to be at higher risk for pressure damage related to medical devices (such as tubes, oxygen tubing, endotracheal tubes, oximetry probes, and tight narrow tracheostomy ties). Many of these pressure ulcers can be prevented with proper selection of bariatric-sized equipment, proper application of equipment, and frequent inspection of the skin under the equipment for high-pressure areas or tissue damage.

Deep tissue injury

There is some clinical speculation that deep tissue injury (DTI) may also be more common in obese patients. Deep pressure may predispose the patient to deep injury. When assessing the skin of bariatric patients, check carefully for subtle signs of DTI, such as slight discoloration of the skin, and changes in skin temperature and texture. If DTI is suspected, offload the affected area in an attempt to reduce pressure and salvage any tissue that is injured, but not ischemic.

Summary

Strategies based on expert opinion, patient and family experience, and the limited published scientific evidence of the bariatric patient population have been presented. Little research has been conducted on appropriate skin care and pressure ulcer prevention in this population. Research has been cited when available, yet much remains to be done.

Conclusion: Special populations

With the vast variety of special patient populations, proper consideration and care are paramount in the treatment of skin conditions, particularly pressure ulcers. In the intensive care setting, some pressure ulcers may be unavoidable. Vigilant monitoring is necessary to find and treat these ulcers as soon as they develop. Remember, pressure ulcers may be a source of sepsis in an already compromised patient. Assess the patient and determine his, and his family's, wishes, and adapt your goals accordingly. Aggressive treatment may be necessary to minimize tissue damage and relieve pain. Some patients may be too physiologically unstable for interventions such as turning. In such cases the priority is saving the patient, sometimes at the expense of the skin.

The patient with a spinal cord injury faces a lifelong risk for the development of pressure ulcers. Although mostly preventable, pressure ulcers are a deterrent to achieving rehabilitation goals, may contribute to a loss of independence, and interfere with the pursuit of educational, vocational, and leisure activities after a spinal cord injury. It's now possible to identify patients with a spinal cord injury at highest risk for pressure ulcers so that effective prevention strategies can be incorporated into their lifestyles.

In HIV and AIDS patients, skin disorders are common. Accurate identification of skin lesions is critical so appropriate treatment can be implemented. Consultation with an HIV or AIDS clinician is helpful in the comprehensive care of these patients.

Neonates and children face unique problems from the development of pressure ulcers. Because support surfaces and topical products are mostly manufactured for adults, they are not suitable for use in this population. Therefore, neonates and children require skin care specific to their needs.

Finally, proactive planning, preparation, proper equipment, interdisciplinary teamwork, and sensitivity are important hallmarks in providing appropriate care to bariatric patients.

Show what you know

1. Risk assessment for pressure ulcer development in the critically ill patient should include:

   A. a validated screening tool.
   B. assessment of unique risk factors common in intensive care unit (ICU).
   C. professional judgment.
   D. all of the above.

ANSWER: D. Critically ill patients are at extremely high risk for pressure ulcers. A combination of approaches should be used in appraising risk.

2. A risk-based prevention program for pressure ulcers in the ICU should be based on each subscale of a risk assessment tool.

   A. True
   B. False

ANSWER: A. Each critically ill patient has a unique level and type of risk. Each subscale should be addressed separately with appropriate interventions.

3. All of the following are major risk factors for pressure ulcer development in the spinal cord injury population except:

   A. preexisting conditions.
   B. severity of the spinal cord injury.
   C. gender.
   D. nutrition.

ANSWER: C. Gender isn't a risk factor for pressure ulcer development. Preexisting conditions, severity of the spinal cord injury, and nutrition are all major risk factors for pressure ulcer development.

4. The most commonly occurring complication of a spinal cord injury is:

   A. fracture.
   B. urinary tract infection.
   C. pressure ulcer development.
   D. osteoporosis.

ANSWER: B. Urinary tract infection is the most commonly occurring complication of a spinal cord injury. Pressure ulcer development is second. Fractures and osteoporosis are also other complications that may occur.

5. Highly active antiretroviral therapy (HAART) has impacted skin disorders in patients with human immunodeficiency virus (HIV) in which one of the following ways:

A. Adverse effects of HAART have led to an increase in the number of skin disorders seen in the patient infected with HIV.
B. There has been a decrease in the incidence of skin disorders seen in the patient with HIV.
C. There has been an increase in the number of noninfectious skin disorders in the patient with HIV.
D. Viral infections are the only skin disorders affected by HAART.

ANSWER: B. HAART-based regimens have contributed to a significant decrease in HIV-associated morbidity and mortality, including many of the cutaneous manifestations of HIV infection. The other options are incorrect.

6. *Patients with prurigo nodularis and HIV should be screened for which one of the following disorders?*

A. *Pneumocystis carinii* pneumonia
B. Syphilis
C. Thyroid disease
D. Hepatitis C

ANSWER: D. Prurigo nodularis is often seen in patients with hepatitis C as a result of the extrahepatic manifestation of liver disease. The other disorders are incorrect.

7. *What percentage of pressure ulcers in children are caused by medical equipment or devices?*

A. None
B. 25%
C. 50%
D. 75%

ANSWER: C. Studies support that about 50% of pressure ulcers in children occur under medical devices.

8. *Which one of the following is a pressure ulcer risk assessment scale that can be used for a 5-year-old child?*

A. Braden Scale
B. Waterlow Scale
C. Starkid Skin Scale
D. Glamorgan Scale

ANSWER: D. The Glamorgan Scale is correct. The Braden scale is not designed for adults but can be used for children older than age 8. The Braden scale is *not* the same as the Braden Q Scale, which can be used for young pediatric patients. The Waterlow Scale is for adults; however, the Waterlow Pediatric Scale could be used for a 5-year-old child. The Starkid Skin scale is used to assess skin condition and not pressure ulcer risk. Remember: *Skin assessment is not the same as pressure ulcer risk assessment.*

9. *Acanthosis nigricans is always a benign condition and there is no treatment.*

A. True
B. False

ANSWER: B. Acanthosis nigricans is usually benign but occasionally undergoes malignant changes. Ammonium lactate cream may improve the condition.

10. *Proper positioning for the bariatric patient confined to bed includes:*

A. using small shifts in body weight to replace turning.
B. keeping the head of the bed flat at all times to prevent shear.
C. avoiding pillows between the legs.
D. supporting the pannus and other large skin folds.

ANSWER: D. The pannus and other skin folds should be supported. "Offload" turns are necessary; small shifts may be an adjunct but do not replace turning. The head of the bed may need to be elevated for proper respiration; supporting the arms with pillows will lessen the chance of sliding and sacral shear. Pillows should be placed between the legs to provide air and pressure redistribution and avoid compression and pressure damage to a Foley catheter.

References

1. Jesurum, J., et al. "Balloons, Beds, and Breakdown: Effects of Low-air-loss Therapy on the Development of Pressure Ulcers in Cardiovascular Surgical Patients with Intra-aortic Balloon Pump Support," *Critical Care Nursing Clinics of North America* 8(4):423-40, December 1996.
2. Baldwin, K.M., and Ziegler, S.M. "Pressure Ulcer Risk Following Critical Traumatic Injury," *Advances in Wound Care* 11(4):168-73, July-August 1998.
3. Pender, L.R., and Frazier, S.K. "The Relationship between Dermal Pressure Ulcers, Oxygenation and Perfusion in Mechanically Ventilated Patients," *Intensive Critical Care Nursing* 21(1):29-38, 2005.
4. Sideranko, S., et al. "Effects of Position and Mattress Overlay on Sacral and Heel Pressures in a Clinical Population," *Research in Nursing & Health* 15(4):245-51, August 1992.
5. Carlson, E.V., et al. "Predicting the Risk of Pressure Ulcers in Critically Ill Patients," *American Journal of Critical Care* 8(4):262-69, July 1999.
6. Fife, C., et al. "Incidence of Pressure Ulcers in a Neurologic Critical Care Unit," *Critical Care Medicine* 29(2):283-90, February 2001.
7. Eachempati, S.R., et al. "Factors Influencing the Development of Decubitus Ulcers in Critically Ill Surgical Patients," *Critical Care Medicine* 29(9):1678-82, September 2001.
8. Ooka, M., et al. "Evaluation of Three Types of Support Surfaces for Preventing Pressure Ulcers in Patients in a Surgical Critical Care Unit," *Journal of Wound Ostomy Continence Nursing* 22(6):271-79, November 1995.
9. Curley, M.A., et al. "Predicting Pressure Ulcer Risk in Pediatric Patients: The Braden Q Scale," *Nursing Research* 51(1): 22-33, January-February 2003.
10. Willock, J., et al. "Pressure Sores in Children—the Acute Hospital Perspective," *Journal of Tissue Viability* 10(2):59-62, April 2000.

11. Schmidt, J.E., et al. "Skin Breakdown in Children and High Frequency Oscillatory Ventilation," *Archives of Physical Medicine and Rehabilitation* 79:1565-69, 1998.

12. Braden, B.J., and Bergstrom, N.A. "Clinical Utility of the Braden Scale for Predicting Pressure Sore Risk," *Decubitus* 2(3):44-51, July-August1989.

13. Norton, D., et al. *An Investigation of Geriatric Nursing Problems in Hospital.* London: National Corporation for the Care of Old People, 1992.

14. Waterlow, J. "Pressure Sores: A risk Assessment Card," *Nursing Times* 81(48):49-55, 1985.

15. Jackson, C. "The Revised Jackson/Cubbin Pressure Area Risk Calculator," *Intensive Critical Care Nursing* 15(3):169-75, June 1999.

16. Quigley, S.M, and Curly, M.A.Q. "Skin Integrity in the Pediatric Population: Preventing and Managing Pressure Ulcers," *JSPN* 1(1):7-18, 1996.

17. Lewicki, L.J., et al. "Sensitivity and Specificity of the Braden Scale in the Cardiac Surgical Population," *Journal of Wound Ostomy Continence Nursing* 27(1):36-41, January 2000.

18. Batson, S., et al. "The Development of a Pressure Area Scoring System for Critically Ill Patients: A Pilot Study," *Intensive Critical Care Nursing* 9(3):146-51, September 1993.

19. Inman, K.J., et al. "Clinical Utility and Cost-effectiveness of an Air Suspension Bed in the Prevention of Pressure Ulcers," *JAMA* 269(9):1139-43, March 3, 1993.

20. Jiricka, M.K., et al. "Pressure Ulcer Risk Factors in a Critical Care Unit Population," *American Journal of Critical Care* 4(5):361-67, September 1995.

21. Lowery, M.T. "A Pressure Sore Risk Calculator for Critical Care Patients: 'The Sunderland Experience'," *Intensive Critical Care Nursing* 11(6):344-53, December 1995.

22. Weststrate, J.T., et al. "The Clinical Relevance of the Waterlow Pressure Sore Risk Scale in the Critical Care Unit," *Critical Care Medicine* 24(8):815-20, August 1998.

23. Seongsook, J., et al. "Validity of Pressure Ulcer Risk Assessment Scales; Cubbin and Jackson, Braden and Douglas Scale," *International Journal of Nursing Studies* 41(2):199-204, February 2004.

24. Theaker, C., et al. "Risk Factors for Pressure Sores in the Critically Ill," *Anesthesia* 55(3):221-24, March 2000.

25. deLaat, E.H.E.W., et al. "Epidemiology, Risk and Prevention of Pressure Ulcers in Critically Ill patients: a literature review." *Journal of Wound Care* 15(6):269-75, June 2006.

26. Krishnagopalan, S., Johnson, E.W., Low, L.L., and Kaufman, L.J. "Body Positioning of Intensive Care Patients: Clinical Practice versus Standards," *Critical Care Medicine* 30(11): 2588-92, 2002.

27. Oertwich, P.A., et al. "The Effects of Small Shifts in Body Weight on Blood Flow and Interface Pressure," *Research in Nursing & Health* 18(6):481-88, December 1995.

28. Hibbert, C.L., et al. "Cost Considerations for the Use of Low-air-loss Bed Therapy in Adult Critical Care," *Intensive Critical Care Nursing* 15(3):154-62, June 1999.

29. Inman, K.J., et al. "Pressure Ulcer Prevention: A Randomized Controlled Trial of Two Risk-directed Strategies for Patient Surface Assignment," *Advances in Wound Care* 12(2):72-80, March 1999.

30. Jastremski, C.A. "Pressure Relief Bedding to Prevent Pressure Ulcer Development in Critical Care," *Journal of Critical Care* 17(2):122-25, June 2002.

31. Cullum, N., et al. "Beds, Mattresses and Cushions for Pressure Sore Prevention and Treatment," (Cochrane Review). In: *The Cochrane Library,* Issue 1. Chichester, UK, John Wiley & Sons, Ltd., 2004.

32. Reddy, M., et al. "Preventing Pressure Ulcers: A Systematic Review," *JAMA* 296(8):974-84, August 23-30, 2006.

33. Burdette-Taylor, S.R., and Kass, J. "Heel Ulcers in Critical Care Units: A Major Pressure Problem," *Critical Care Nursing Quarterly* 25(2):41-53, August 2002.

34. Grap, M.J., and Munro, C.L. "Quality Improvement in Backrest Elevation: Improving Outcomes in Critical Care," *AACN Clinical Issues* 16(2):133-39, 2005.

35. Defloor, T., and Grypdonck, M.H. "Do Pressure Relief Cushions Really Relieve Pressure?" *Western Journal of Nursing Research* 22(3):335-50, April 2000.

36. Defloor, T., and Grypdonck, M.H. "Sitting Posture and Prevention of Pressure Ulcers," *Applied Nursing Research* 12(3):136-42, August 1999.

37. Black, J.M., and the National Pressure Ulcer Advisory Panel. "Moving Toward Consensus on Deep Tissue Injury and Pressure Ulcer Staging," *Advances in Skin and Wound Care* 18(8):415-16, 418, 420-21, October 2005.

38. National Spinal Cord Injury Statistical Center, Birmingham, Alabama. "Spinal Cord Injury: Facts and Figures at a Glance," *Journal of Spinal Cord Medicine* 25(2):139-40, Summer 2002.

39. Lasfargues, J.E., et al. "A Model for Estimating Spinal Cord Injury Prevalence in the United States," *Paraplegia* 33(2):62-8, February 1995.

40. Go, B.K., et al. "The Epidemiology of Spinal Cord Injury," in Stover, S.L., et al., eds. *Spinal Cord Injury-Clinical Outcomes from the Model Systems.* Gaithersburg, Md.: Aspen Publishers, Inc., 1995.

41. Ragnarsson, K.T., et al. "Management of Pulmonary, Cardiovascular, and Metabolic Conditions after Spinal Cord Injury," in Stover, S.L., et al., eds., *Spinal Cord Injury-Clinical Outcomes from the Model Systems.* Gaithersburg, Md.: Aspen Publishers, Inc., 1995.

42. McKinley, W.O., et al. "Long-term Medical Complications after Traumatic Spinal Cord Injury: A Regional Model Systems Analysis," *Archives of Physical Medicine Rehabilitation* 80(11):1402-10, November 1999.

43. Langemo, D.K., et al. "The Lived Experience of Having a Pressure Ulcer: A Qualitative Analysis," *Advances in Skin & Wound Care* 13(5):225-35, September-October 2000.

44. Garber S.L., et al. "Prevention and Treatment of Pressure Ulcers Following Traumatic Spinal Cord Injury: A Clinical Practice Guideline for Health-Care Professionals," *Consortium for Spinal Cord Medicine Clinical Practice Guidelines.* Washington, D.C.: Paralyzed Veterans of America, 2000.

45. Young, J.S., and Burns, P.E. "Pressure Sores and the Spinal Cord Injured: Part II," *Spinal Cord Injury Digest* 3:11-26, 48, 1981.

46. Yarkony, G.M., and Heinemann, A.W. "Pressure Ulcers," in Stover, S.L., et al., eds., *Spinal Cord Injury: Clinical Outcomes from the Model Systems.* Gaithersburg, Md.: Aspen Publishers, 1995.

47. Fuhrer, M.J., et al. "Pressure Ulcers in Community-resident Persons with Spinal Cord Injury: Prevalence and Risk Factors," *Archives of Physical*

Medicine Rehabilitation 74(11):1172-77, November 1993.

48. Carlson, C.E., et al. "Incidence and Correlates of Pressure Ulcer Development after Spinal Cord Injury," *Journal of Rehabilitation Nursing Research* 1(1):34-40, 1992.

49. Schryvers, O.I., et al. "Surgical Treatment of Pressure Ulcers: A 20-year Experience," *Archives of Physical Medicine Rehabilitation* 81(12):1556-1562, December 2000.

50. Goodman, C.M., et al. "Evaluation of Results and Treatment Variables for Pressure Ulcers in 48 Veteran Spinal Cord-injured Patients," *Annals of Plastic Surgery* 43(6):572-74, June 1999.

51. Niazi, Z.B., et al. "Recurrence of Initial Pressure Ulcer in Persons with Spinal Cord Injuries," *Advances in Wound Care* 10(3):38-42, May-June 1997.

52. Goldstein, B. "Neurogenic Skin and Pressure Ulcers," in Hammond, M.C., ed., *Medical Care of Persons with Spinal Cord Injury*. Washington, D.C.: DVA Employee Education System and Government Printing Office, 1998.

53. Salzberg, C.A., et al. "Predicting and Preventing Pressure Ulcers in Adults with Paralysis," *Advances in Wound Care* 11(5):237-46, September 1998.

54. Holmes, S.A., et al. "Preventing Recurrent Pressure Ulcers After Myocutaneous Flap in Persons with Spinal Cord Injury," in preparation for submission to *Archives of Physical Medicine and Rehabilitation*.

55. Miller, H., and DeLozier, J. "Cost Implications," in Bergstrom, N., and Cuddigan, J., eds., *Treating Pressure Ulcers: Guideline Technical Report*, Vol II, No. 15, Rockville, Md.: U.S. Department of Health and Human Services, Public Health Service, Agency for Health Care Policy and Research. Publication 96-N015, 1994.

56. Byrne, D.W., and Salzberg, C.A. "Major Risk Factors for Pressure Ulcers in the Spinal Cord Disabled: A Literature Review," *Spinal Cord* 34(5):255-63, May 1996.

57. Rintala, D.H. "Quality-of-life Considerations," *Advances in Wound Care* 8(4):71-83, July-August 1995.

58. Anderson, T.P., and Andberg, M.M. "Psychosocial Factors Associated with Pressure Sores," *Archives of Physical Medicine Rehabilitation* 60(8):341-46, August 1979.

59. Gordon, W.A., et al. "The Relationship between Pressure Sores and Psychosocial Adjustment in Persons with Spinal Cord Injury," *Rehabilitation Psychology* 27:185-91, 1982.

60. Yasenchak, P.A., et al. "Variables Related to Severe Pressure Sore Recurrence," [Abstract]. Orlando: Annual Meeting of the American Spinal Injury Association (ASIA), 1990.

61. Disa, J.J., et al. "Efficacy of Operative Cure in Pressure Sore Patients," *Plastic Reconstructive Surgery* 89(2):272-78, February 1992.

62. Scheflan, M. "Surgical Methods for Managing Ischial Pressure Wounds," *Annals of Plastic Surgery* 3(3):238-47, March 1982.

63. Romm, S., et al. "Pressure Sores: State of the Art," *Texas Medicine* 78(4):52-60, 62, April 1982.

64. Pers, M. "Plastic Surgery for Pressure Sores," *Paraplegia* 25(3):275-78, June 1987.

65. Buntine, J.A., and Johnstone, B.R. "The Contributions of Plastic Surgery to Care of the Spinal Cord Injured Patient," *Paraplegia* 26(2):87-93, April 1988.

66. Hentz, V.R. "Management of Pressure Sores in a Specialty Center—A Reappraisal," *Plastic Reconstructive Surgery* 64(4):683-91, October 1979.

67. Relander, M., and Palmer, B. "Recurrence of Surgically Treated Pressure Sores," *Scandinavian Journal of Plastic Reconstructive Surgery* 2(1):89-92, 1988.

68. Mandrekas, A.D., and Mastorakos, D.P. "Management of Decubitus Ulcers by Musculocutaneous Flaps: A Five-year Experience," *Annals of Plastic Surgery* 28(2):167-74, February 1992.

69. Baek, S., et al. "The Gluteus Maximus Myocutaneous Flap in the Management of Pressure Sores," *Annals of Plastic Surgery* 5(6):471-76, December 1980.

70. Rubayi, S., et al. "Proximal Femoral Resection and Myocutaneous Flap for Treatment of Pressure Ulcers in Spinal Cord Injury Patients," *Annals of Plastic Surgery* 27(2):132-37, August 1991.

71. Garber, S.L., et al. "A Structured Educational Model to Improve Pressure Ulcer Prevention Knowledge in Veterans with Spinal Cord Dysfunction," *Journal of Rehabilitation Research and Development* 39(5):575-88, September-October 2002.

72. Andberg, M.M., et al. "Improving Skin Care through Patient and Family Training," Topics in Clinical Nursing 5(2):45-54, July 1983.

73. Krouskop, T.A., et al. "The Effectiveness of Preventive Management in Reducing the Occurrence of Pressure Sores," Journal of Rehabilitation R&D 20(1):7483, July 1983.

74. King, R.B., et al., eds. "The Skin," in *Rehabilitation Guide*. Chicago: The Rehabilitation Institute of Chicago, 1977.

75. Bergstrom, N., et al. "Pressure Ulcers in Adults: Prediction and Prevention," Guideline Report No. 3. Rockville, Md.: U.S. Department of Health and Human Services, Public Health Service, Agency for Health Care Policy and Research. AHCPR Publication No. 93-0013, May 1992.

76. Bennett, M.A. "Report of the Task Force on the Implications for Darkly Pigmented Intact Skin in the Prediction and Prevention of Pressure Ulcers," *Advances in Wound Care* 8(6):34-35, November-December 1995.

77. Bergstrom, N., et al. "Treatment of Pressure Ulcers," Guideline Report No. 15. Rockville, Md.: US Department of Health and Human Services, Public Health Service, Agency for Health Care Policy and Research. AHCPR Publication No. 96-N014, December 1994.

78. Netscher, D., et al. "Surgical Repair of Pressure Ulcers," *Plastic Surgery Nursing* 16:225-33, 239, Winter 1996.

79. Clamon, J., and Netscher, D.T. "General Principles of Flap Reconstruction: Goals for Aesthetic and Functional Outcome," Plastic Surgery Nursing 14:9-14, Spring 1994.

80. Lee, E.T. "A New Wound Closure Achieving and Maintaining Device Using Serial Tightening of Loop Suture and Its Clinical Applications in 15 Consecutive Patients for Up to 102 Days," *Ann Plastic Surg* 53(5):436-41, 2004.

81. Akyurek, M., et al. "A New Flap Design: Neural-island Flap. *Plast Reconstr Surg* 114(6):1467-77, 2004.

82. Ichioka, S., et al. "Triple Coverage of Ischial Ulcers with Adipofascial Turnover and Fasciocutaneous Flaps," *Plast Reconstr Surg* 114(4):901-905, 2004.

83. Ichioka, S., et al. "Regenerative Surgery for Sacral Pressure Ulcers Using Collagen Matrix Substitute Dermis (Artificial Dermis)," *Ann Plast Surg* 54(4):383-89, 2003.

84. Lin, M.T., et al. "Tensor Fasciae Latae Combined with Tangentially Split Vastus Lateralis Musculocutaneous Flap for the Reconstruction of Pressure Sores," *Ann Plast Surg* 53(4):343-47, October 2004.

85. Sorensen, J.L., et al. "Surgical Treatment of Pressure Ulcers," *Am J Surg* 188 (suppl 1A):42-51, 2004.

86. Krause, J.S., and Broderick, L. "Patterns of Recurrent Pressure Ulcers after Spinal Cord Injury: Identification of Risk and Protective Factors 5 or More Years after Onset," *Arch Phys Med Rehabil* 85(8)1257-264, 2004.

87. Chen, Y., et al. "Pressure Ulcer Prevalence in People with Spinal Cord Injury: Age-period-duration Effects," *Arch Phys Med Rehabil* 86:1208-13, 2005.

88. Baker, L., et al. "Effect of Electrical Stimulation Waveform on Healing of Ulcers in Human Beings with Spinal Cord Injury," *Wound Repair and Regeneration* 4(1):21-28, January-February 1996.

89. Wood, J.M., et al. "A Multicenter Study on the Use of Pulsed Low-intensity Direct Current for Healing Chronic Stage II and III Decubitus Ulcers," *Archives of Dermatology* 129(8):999-1009, August 1993.

90. Calista, D., et al. "Changing Morbidity of Cutaneous Diseases in Patients with HIV after the Introduction of Highly Active Antiretroviral Therapy Including a Protease Inhibitor," *Am J Clin Dermatol* 3:59-62, 2002.

91. Buchbinder, S.P., et al. "Herpes Zoster and Human Immunodeficiency Virus Infection," *Journal of Infectious Disease* 166(5):1153-1156, November 1992.

92. Klatt, E.C., and Shibata, D. "Cytomegalovirus Infection in the Acquired Immunodeficiency Syndrome," *Archives of Pathology and Laboratory Medicine* 112(5):540-44, May 1988.

93. Focht, D.R. III, et al. "The Efficacy of Duct Tape vs Cryotherapy in the Treatment of Verruca Vulgaris (The Common Wart)," *Arch Pediatr Adolesc Med* 156, 971-74, 2002.

94. Apgar, S.A., and Pfenninger, J.L. "Treatment of Vulvar, Perianal, Vaginal, Penile and Urethral Condyloma Acuminata," in Pfenninger, J.L. and Fowler, G.C (eds). *Procedures for Primary Care Physicians,* 1st ed. St. Louis: Mosby-Year Book, Inc, 1994.

95. Czelusta, A., et al. "An Overview of Sexually Transmitted Diseases. Part III. Sexually Transmitted Diseases in HIV-Infected Patients," *Journal of the American Academy of Dermatology* 43(3):409-32, September 2000.

96. Zwolsi, K., and Talotta, D. "Bacterial Infections," in Kirton, C. *Handbook of HIV/AIDS Nursing.* St. Louis: Mosby-Year Book, Inc, 2001.

97. Goldstein, B., et al. "Correlation of Skin Disorders with CD4 Lymphocyte Counts in Patients with HIV/AIDS," *Journal of the American Academy of Dermatology* 36(2, pt. 1): 262-64, February 1997.

98. Lee, M.R., and Shumack, S. "Prurigo Nodularis: A Review," Australasian Journal of Dermatology 46(4):211-18, 2005.

99. Farrell, J., et al. "Characterization of Sulfamethoxazole and Sulfamethoxazole Metabolite-specific T-cell Responses in Animals and Humans," *J Pharmacol Exp Ther* 306:229-37, 2003.

100. McLane, K.M., et al. "The 2003 National Pediatric Pressure Ulcer and Skin Breakdown Prevalence Survey," *JWOCN* 31(4):168-78, 2004.

101. Curley, M.A.Q., et al. "Predicting Pressure Ulcer Risk in Pediatric Patients: The Braden Q Scale," *Nursing Research* 52(1):22-31, 2003.

102. Baharestani, M., et al. "A Neonatal & Pediatric Evidence-linked Pressure Ulcer & Skin Care Performance Improvement Initiative," Poster abstract presented at the Symposium on Advanced Wound Care and Medical Research Forum on Wound Repair, April 21-24, 2005, San Diego, Calif., 2005.

103. Curley, M.A.. "Prone Positioning of Patients with Acute Respiratory Distress Syndrome: A Systematic Review," *American Journal of Critical Care* 8(6):397-405, November1999.

104. Curley, M.A., et al. "Pressure Ulcers in Pediatric Intensive Care: Incidence & Associated Factors," *Pediatric Critical Care Medicine* 4(3):284-90, 2003.

105. Baldwin, K. "Incidence and Prevalence of Pressure Ulcers in Children," *Advances in Skin & Wound Care* 15:121-24, 2002.

106. Groeneveld, A., et al. "The Prevalence of Pressure Ulcers in a Tertiary Care Pediatric and Adult Hospital," *JWOCN* 31(3):108-20, 2004.

107. Hickey, K., et al. "Pressure Ulcers in Pediatric Spinal Cord Injury," *Topics in Spinal Cord Injury Rehabilitation* 6(suppl):85-90, 2000.

108. Okamoto, G.N., et al. "Skin Breakdown in Patients with Myelomeningocele," *Arch Phys Med & Rehab* 64:20-23, 1983.

109. Thompson, H., et al. "The Recurrent Neutrotrophic Buttock Ulcer in the Myelomeningocele Paraplegic: A Sensate Flap Solution," *Plast & Reconstr Surg* 108(5):1192-96, 2001.

110. Waterlow, J. "Pressure Sore Risk Assessment in Children," *Paediatric Nursing* 9(6):21-24, 1997.

111. Huffiness, B., Lodgson, M.C. "The Neonatal Skin Risk Assessment Scale for Predicting Skin Breakdown in Neonates," *Issues Comprehensive Nurs* 20:103-14, 1997.

112. Pallija, G., et al. "Skin Care of the Pediatric Patient," *J of Pediatric Nursing* 14(2):80-87, 1999.

113. Neidig, J.R.E., Kleiber, C., Oppliger, R.A. "Risk Factors Associated with Pressure Ulcers in the Pediatric Patient Following Open-heart Surgery," *Prog Cardiovascular Nurs* 4(3):99-106, 1989.

114. Solis, I., et al. "Supine Interface Pressure in Children," *Arch Phys Med Rehabil* 69:524-26, 1988.

115. Olding, L., Patterson, J. "Growing Concern," *Nursing Times* 94(38):74-79, 1998.

116. Brook, I. "Microbiological Studies of Decubitus Ulcers in Children," *J of Pediatric Surg* 26(2):207-209, 1991.

117. Gershan, L.A. "Scarring Alopecia in Neonates as a Consequence of Hypoxaemia-hypoperfusion," *Arch Dis Child* 68:591-93, 1993.

118. Kumar, K.A., Kumar, E. "A Pressure Sore in an Infant," *J of Wound Care* 2(3):145-146, 1993.

119. Kozierowski, L. "Treatment of Sacral Pressure Ulcers in an Adolescent with Hodgkin's Disease," *JWOCN* 23(5):244-47, 1996.

120. Eichenfield, L.F., Hardaway, C.A. "Neonatal Dermatology," *Current Opinion in Pediatrics* 11(5):471-78, 1999.

121. Campbell, J.M., Banta-Wright, S.A. "Neonatal Skin Disorders: A Review of Selected Dermatological Abnormalities," *J Perinat Nurs* 14(1):63-83, 2000.

122. Siegfried, E.C. "Neonatal Skin and Skin Care," *Pediatric Dermatology* 16(3):437-46, 1998.

123. Malloy, M.B., Perez-Woods, R.C. "Neonatal Skin Care: Prevention of Skin Breakdown," *Pediatric Nursing* 17(1):41-48, 1991.

124. Jetlefsen, L. "Postcranial Moulding," *Neonatal Network* 5(7):44, 1987.

125. Norris, S., Campbell, L.A., Brenkert, S. "Nursing Procedures and Alterations in Transcutaneous Oxygen Tension in Premature Infants," *Nursing Research* 31(6):330-35, 1982.

126. Long, J.G., et al. "Excessive Handling as a Cause of Hypoxemia," *Pediatrics* 65(2):203-207, 1980.

127. Willock, J., Harris, C., Harrison, J., Poole, C. "Identifying the Characteristics of Children with Pressure Ulcers," *Nurs Times* 101(11):40-43, November 2005.

128. Friedman, J. "Plastic Surgical Problems in the Neonatal Intensive Care Unit," *Clinics in Plastic Surgery* 25(4):599-617, 1998.

129. Smith, Z.K. "Adapting a Soft Silicone Dressing to Enhance Infant Outcomes," *OWM* 52(4):30-32, April 2006.

130. Schmidt, J.E., et al. "Skin Breakdown in Children and High Frequency Oscillatory Ventilation, *Arch Phys Med Rehab* 79:1565-69, 1998.

131. McCord, S., McElvain, V., Sachdeva, R, Schwartz, P., Jefferson, L.S. "Risk Factors Associated with Pressure Ulcers in the Pediatric Intensive Care Unit," *JWOCN* 31(4):179-83, July-August 2004.

132. Samaniego, I.A. "A Sore Spot in Pediatrics: Risk Factors for Pressure Ulcers," *Pediatric Nursing* 29(4):278-82, 2003.

133. Storm, K., Lund, J.T. "Skin Care of Preterm Infants: Strategies to Minimize Potential Damage," *J of Neonatal Nursing* 5(2):13-15, 1999.

134. Quigley, S.M., Curly, M.A.Q. "Skin Integrity in the Pediatric Population: Preventing and Managing Pressure Ulcers," *JSPN* 1(1):7-18, 1996.

135. Pickersgill, J. "Taking the Pressure Off," *Paediatric Nursing* 9(8):25-27, 1997.

136. Bedi, A. "A Tool to Fill the Gap-developing a Wound Risk Assessment Chart for Children," *Professional Nurse* 9(2):112-20, 1993.

137. Garvin, G. "Wound and Skin Care for the PICU," *Crit Care Nurs Q* 20(1):62-71, 1997.

138. Willock, J., Anthony, D., Baharestani, M. "An Examination of the Inter-rater Reliability of the Glamorgan Pressure Ulcer Risk Assessment Scale," 2006. (Manuscript submitted).

139. Willock, J., Anthony, D., Baharestani, M. "Regression Analysis to Compare the Glamorgan, Braden Q and Garvin Paediatric Pressure Ulcer Risk Assessment Scales," 2006 (Manuscript submitted).

140. Cockett, A. "Paediatric Pressure Sore Risk Assessment," *Tissue Viability Society* 8(1):30, 1998.

141. Waterlow, J. "Pressure Sores in Children: Risk Assessment," *Paediatric Nursing* 10(4):22-23, 1998.

142. Suddaby, E.C., et al. "Skin Breakdown in Acute Care Pediatrics," *Pediatric Nursing* 31(2):132-48, 2005.

143. Lund, C.H., Osborne, J.W. "Validity and Reliability of the Neonatal Skin Condition Score," *JOGNN* 33(3):320-27, 2003.

144. McGurk, V., et al. "Skin Integrity Assessment in Neonates and Children," *Paediatric Nursing* 16(3):15-18, 2004.

145. Perez-Woods, R., Malloy, M.B. "Positioning and Skin Care of the Low-birth Weight Neonate," *NAACOGS Clin Issue Perinat Womens Health Nurs* 3(1):97-113, 1992.

146. Willock, J. "A Study to Identify Characteristics Associated with Pressure Injury in Children," *School of Care Sciences, University of Glamorgan*, Pontypridd, UK: The General Nursing Council for England and Wales Trust, 2003.

147. Law, J." Transair® Paediatric Mattress Replacement System Evaluation," *Br J Nurs* 11(5):343-46, 2002.

148. McLane, K.M., Krouskop, T.A., McCord, S., Fraley, J.K. "Comparison of Interface Pressures in the Pediatric Population among Various Support Surfaces," *JWOCN* 29(5):242-51, 2002.

149. Norris, M.K., Steinhorn, D.M. "Nutritional Management during Critical Illness in Infants and Children," *AACN Clin Issues Crit Care Nurs* 5(4):485-92, 1994.

150. Hoath, S., Narandren, V. "Adhesives and Emollients in the Preterm," *Seminars in Neonatology* 5:289-96, 2000.

151. Garvin, G. "Wound Healing in Pediatrics," *Nursing Clinics of North America* 25(1):181-192, 1990.

152. Baharestani, M., Ratliff, C., and the National Pressure Ulcer Advisory Panel (NPUAP). "Pressure Ulcers in Neonates and Children: An NPUAP White Paper. *Advances in Skin & Wound Care*. 2006 (Manuscript submitted).

153. Zollo, M.B., et al. "Altered Skin Integrity in Children Admitted to a Pediatric Intensive Care Unit," *J Nurs Care Qual* 11(2):62-7, 1996.

154. Willock, J., Hughes, J., et al. "Pressure Sores in Children: The Acute Hospital Perspective," *Tissue Viability Society* 10(2):59-62, 2000.

155. Association of Women's Health, Obstetric and Neonatal Nurses (AWHONN). Neonatal skin care. Evidence-based clinical practice guideline. Washington (DC): Association of Women's Health, Obstetric and Neonatal Nurses (AWHONN); 54, January 2001.

157. Barnes, S. "The Use of a Pressure Ulcer Risk Assessment Tool for Children," *Nurs Times Supp* 100(14):56-8, 2004.

157. Centers for Disease Control and Prevention, *Overweight and Obesity*. Atlanta: Centers for Disease Control and Prevention, 2006.

158. Gallagher, S.M. "Restructuring the Therapeutic Environment to Promote Care and Safety for Obese Patients," *J Wound Ostomy Continence Nursing* 26:292-97, 1999.

159. Gallagher, S. "Taking the Weight Off with Bariatric Surgery," *Nursing 2004* 34(3):58-64, 2004.

160. Gallagher, S. "The Challenges of Obesity and Skin Integrity," *Nursing Clinics of North America* 40(2):325-35, 2005.

161. Centers for Disease Control and Prevention, *Overweight and Obesity: Defining Overweight and Obesity*. Atlanta: Centers for Disease Control and Prevention, 2006.

162. NHLBI, *Clinical Guidelines on the Identification, Evaluation, and Treatment of Overweight and Obesity in Adults*, Washington, D.C.: National Heart Lung and Blood Institute, 262, 1998.

163. CMS, *Decision Memo for Bariatric Surgery for the Treatment of Morbid Obesity* (CAG-00250R). Washington, D.C.: Centers for Medicare & Medicaid Services, 2006.

164. Pieper, B., et al. "Bariatric Surgery: Patient Incision Care and Discharge Concerns," *Ostomy/Wound Management* 52(6):48-61, 2006.

165. Pieper, B., et al. "Discharge Information Needs of Patients after Surgery," *JWOCN* 33(3):281-90, 2006.

166. Hahler, B. "An Overview of Dermatological Conditions Commonly Associated with the Obese Patient," *Ostomy/Wound Management* 52(6):34, 2006.

167. Wilson, J.A. and Clark, J.J. "Obesity: Impediment to Postsurgical Wound Healing," *Advances In Skin & Wound Care,* 17(8):426-35, 2004.

168. Janniger, C.K., et al. "Intertrigo and Common Secondary Skin Infections," *American Family Physician,* 72(5):833-38, 2005.

169. Mistiaen, P., et al. "Preventing and Treating Intertrigo in the Large Skin Folds of Adults: A Literature Overview," *Dermatology Nursing* 16(1):43, 2004.

170. Gallagher, S. and Gates, J.L. "Obesity, Panniculitis, Panniculectomy, and Wound Care: Understanding the Challenges," *Journal of Wound, Ostomy, and Continence Nursing* 30(6):334-41, 2003.

171. Oertwich, P.A., A.M. Kindschuh, and Bergstrom, N. "The Effects of Small Shifts in Body weight on Blood Flow and Interface Pressure," *Res Nurs Health* 18(6):481-88, 1995.

CHAPTER 21

Palliative wound care

Diane K. Langemo, PhD, RN, FAAN

OBJECTIVES

After completing this chapter, you'll be able to:

- define palliative wound care
- delineate palliative wound treatment
- delineate treatment for a fungating wound
- delineate treatment for a radiation wound.

Defining palliative wound care

Palliative care is focused on holistically supporting the individual for comfort rather than cure, or healing of the wound, while improving the quality of living and dying. In 1990, the World Health Organization (WHO) defined palliative care as care that affirms life and views death and dying as part of a normal process that neither speeds nor delays death, provides relief from pain and other symptoms, and offers support to the patient and family.[1] Further, a 2002 National Consensus Project identified palliative care as an organized and highly structured system that focuses care on promoting the greatest comfort for and dignity of the patient (www.nationalconsensusproject.org)[2] and is best delivered by a multidisciplinary team.[3] (See chapter 1, Quality of life and ethical issues.) In response to these national efforts, 22.2% of hospitals in the United States adopted palliative care programs by 2004.[4] However, in spite of these national level studies and the growth in palliative care programs, public policies have focused very little on palliation.

Although the usual care plan involves healing a wound, for individuals at the end of life (with a nonhealing wound,) palliative wound care may be desired and most appropriate. While often overlooked as the largest organ of the body, the skin can fail along with the other organs.[5] It's illogical to expect the skin to heal concomitant with the failure of other vital organ systems.[5,6] And most individuals, if not all, at the end of their lives are at risk for developing a pressure ulcer.[7]

However, with education and teaching, which should include a thorough question and answer session between the patient and family and physician and other health care professionals, the goal of care should then be established. The decision to move a patient from a curative to a palliative treatment plan requires that the clinician has determined that the wound is ultimately nonhealing (rather than undertreated), and that it indeed is the patient's desire to do so.[8,9]

Extent of the problem

Estimates are that by the year 2030, 20% of the United States population will be age 65 or older[10] and over 157 million Americans will suffer from chronic illnesses.[11] Given this demographic shift, a significant increase must be expected in the number of frail, elderly patients for whom cure may not be the goal. Overall, little information is available on wounds at the end of life.[12] Currently, however, wounds affect more than one-third of the nearly 1 million hospice patients in the United States, as well as many more patients at the end of life who are not under hospice care.[12] Although standard wound care with a curative focus averages $1,600 per patient per month,[13] the $118 per diem for a hospice patient's total care falls far short of that needed to heal a wound.[14]

Less than 20 studies on pressure ulcer prevalence and incidence in end-of-life patients appear in the literature and, of those that do, most report on subjects with a cancer diagnosis. Little evidence on the prevalence and incidence of end-of-life wounds is available.[15] Reported prevalence rates vary between 13%[16] and 47%,[17,18,19] and incidence rates vary from 8%[3] to 17%.[16-21] In a home hospice study, Reifsnyder and Hoplamazian[22] found a 15% to 27% prevalence of pressure ulcers in a population with a 72-year mean age where the primary diagnosis was cancer. The primary comorbidity was cognitive-related disorders with dementia being the primary risk factor.

In a cross-sectional study of 383 hospice patients, 35% had skin wounds and, of these, 50% were pressure ulcers. The same author did a case-series analysis of 192 consecutive patients referred for wound consultation. The mean age was 82 years, 67% were female, and the subjects had multiple comorbidities, with dementia being the primary disorder. The researcher found that 40% of the wounds were pressure ulcers, with the primary location on the sacrum, followed by the heel, foot, and leg.[6] In both populations, pressure ulcers were almost exclusively stage III and IV, with concomitant necrosis and gangrene.[6] Tippett concluded that "wounds at the end of life are a problem of tragic proportion for the nearly 1 million hospice patients and millions of other frail, elderly persons living with chronic disease."[6]

Skin care needs of the palliative care patient

End-of-life patients have a diminished hunger and thirst mechanism, leading to dehydration, decreased oral intake, and impaired metabolism. Dehydration impairs skin turgor, leaving tissue vulnerable to new breakdown. A decrease in protein intake leads to protein wasting and malnutrition. In addition, albumin provides colloid oncotic pressure to hold liquid in the vascular system. When oncotic pressure is decreased, fluid leaves the vascular system and goes to interstitial spaces causing tissue edema, lowered blood pressure, and impaired blood flow. Impaired oxygenation also slows healing, due to decreased hemoglobin levels, impaired gas exchange, and decreased blood pressure.[23]

Patients at the end of life are particularly at risk for skin breakdown, due in large part to an impaired immune system. The goal of palliative care is to optimize quality of life through control of physical symptoms and attention to the patient's psychosocial needs. Preventing skin breakdown, as well as treating it, go a long way to meeting palliative care goals. Skin breakdown can be prevented and treated through risk appraisal and assessment, meticulous skin care, good positioning, reducing friction and shear, using support surfaces, supporting nutrition and hydration, and managing moisture.

End-of-life wound care focuses on:

- pain
- odor
- exudate
- bleeding
- self-image
- dignity
- quality of life.

Patient and wound assessment

It's essential to perform a complete head-to-toe assessment of the end-of-life patient, including physical and psychosocial health and overall quality of life. The assessment should establish both risk for and presence or absence of skin breakdown. The Pressure Sore Risk Assessment Scale for Palliative Care[18] was developed for use on the individual at or near the end of life. The seven subscales include sensation, mobility, moisture, activity in bed, nutrition and weight change, skin condition, and friction and shear. Scores can range from 7 to 28. A score of 12 and under indicates low risk; 13 to 17, medium risk; 18 to 21 high risk; and 22 and over, very high risk. Risk assessment can be done weekly or with significant changes in condition. (See *Hunters Hill Marie Curie Centre Pressure Ulcer Risk Assessment,* pages 452 and 453.)

Wounds or ulcers in end-of-life patients are often chronic in nature, as healing is significantly impaired due to physical condition and existing comorbidities. A chronic pressure ulcer has a well-defined border with surrounding nonblanchable erythema. When induration is present, it can extend outward from the wound edges. Many chronic wounds have rolled under edges that impede healing and wound closure. Rolled under edges occur when the wound bed is dry. In response, the wound attempts to preserve what little moisture is present and epithelialization is slowed, leaving the wound bed uncovered. Most wounds have drainage and chronic wound drainage contains destructive enzymes, as well as fibroblasts that are less effective at produc-

ing collagen to heal the wound.[24] (See chapter 5, Acute and chronic wound healing.)

Maintenance of skin integrity

Careful attention to skin care in the end-of-life patient is exceedingly important, as a feeling of cleanliness can enhance an overall sense of comfort and well being and address any odor problems that might be present. A low pH skin cleanser is useful along with a moisture barrier to minimize the effects of excess moisture. Excess moisture can cause skin maceration, which interferes with the ability of the skin to withstand friction, shear, and pressure, thus making it vulnerable to injury.[27] Therefore, gently cleanse the skin, paying attention to the sacrum, elbows, and heels, which are prone to friction and pressure injury.[25-26] Avoid massage over a reddened area as it can further damage tissue with already impaired perfusion.[27] A gentle overall body massage is often appreciated in an individual at the end of life, unless contraindicated.

Incontinence is of particular importance with palliative care patients because of the risk for skin injury and breakdown. When incontinence is present, primary goals are to enhance comfort, prevent and manage skin breakdown, and control odor. Feces are a chemical irritant to the skin, and their removal adds the element of a mechanical irritant, so gentleness is important.

Impaired mobility and repositioning

Any individual at the end of life experiences prolonged periods of inactivity or immobility, contributing to the occurrence of tissue ischemia from prolonged pressure.[28] Particularly vulnerable to pressure from inactivity are the heels, sacrum, and elbows. Suspending the heels over a pillow while supporting the entire length of the leg or using heel protectors is helpful in decreasing heel pressure.[27] A general guideline is to ensure that an individual in bed is turned every 2 hours. However, repositioning is challenging for a patient who's hemodynamically unstable, has a great deal of pain, is nauseous or is vomiting, or is unable to lay on one side or on the back.[21] Individual choices must be made after explaining the rationale for this intervention. (See chapter 11, Pressure redistribution.)

PRACTICE POINT

Individualize the patient's turning and positioning schedule based on his pain tolerance and comfort level.

Friction and shear

To protect the buttocks and sacral areas, use a lift sheet or an overhead trapeze.[25,26,28,29] Protect the sacral area or other bony prominences with a transparent film or hydrocolloid to minimize friction.[30] Many individuals at the end of life have impaired ventilation and require the head of the bed to be raised. However, it's recommended to maintain the head of the bed at the lowest elevation possible—preferably 30 degrees or lower—to minimize friction and shear to the sacrum and buttocks.[27] A pressure-redistributing mattress overlay or a specialty bed may also be helpful.[27] (See chapter 11, Pressure redistribution: Seating, positioning, and support surfaces.)

Support surfaces

Use a surface that redistributes weight over a larger area, thereby minimizing tissue pressures, particularly over bony prominences.[27] These surfaces are helpful for both the bed and the chair.

Nutrition and hydration

As the body systems are shutting down in the individual at the end of life, the food and fluid requirements generally decrease as well. Lessening of oral intake can occur weeks to months before death.[31] Poor nutrition in these individuals has been demonstrated in several studies.[32-34] Nutritional and hydration status can be further impaired, as the individual with a draining wound can lose large amounts of fluids and proteins in the exudate. At the end of life, the swallow reflex is decreased also, impairing food and fluid intake and leaving the individual vulnerable to aspiration. Helping the family and loved ones

to understand this end-of-life process can relieve their anxiety and stress. (See chapter 10, Nutrition and wound care.)

Palliative wound treatment

The goals of palliative wound care differ little from those of curative wound care, aside from the goal of healing. Palliative care is the primary focus when it becomes apparent that the wound has failed to progress or when the patient's clinical condition deteriorates to a point where aggressive measures are no longer appropriate. This can be particularly true in "nursing home residents with flexion contractures, cognitive impairment, and limited quality of life."[35] When it becomes apparent that the patient's life would not be significantly better from a quality-of-life standpoint, wound stabilization and palliation become the focus of care and include controlling pain, choosing appropriate dressings, managing infection, and protecting the periwound area.

Pain management

Both prevention and treatment of skin breakdown can be uncomfortable for individuals at the end of life. The majority of patients with a pressure ulcer experience moderate to severe pain, especially during dressing changes and wound bed treatments, and the pain can be acute or chronic.[36,37]

According to Rook, pain is anything the patient says it is,[38] accounting for the widely variant ways a patient can experience pain.

Pain in a wound can be caused by the tumor pressing on nerves and blood vessels or exposure of dermis.[39] Pain in wounds often arises from painful procedures including cleansing and dressing removal, particularly if the dressing is dry and adherent.[40] Given that an individual at or near the end of their life has a wound that likely will not heal, the wound and wound pain are chronic in nature. Chronic pain is pain that is persistent and can occur even when the wound is not being manipulated.[41] Concomitant acute

(Text continues on page 454.)

Hunters Hill Marie Curie Centre
Pressure Ulcer Risk Assessment

Patient's Name _____   Patient ID No. _____

SENSORY PERCEPTION
Ability to respond meaning-fully to discomfort related to pressure

1 No impairment
Communicates discomfort clearly

2 Slightly Limited
Responds to verbal commands but cannot always communicate discomfort or has sensory impairment in 1 or 2 extremities

---

MOISTURE
Degree of skin exposure to moisture/fecal matter

1 Rarely Moist
Skin rarely moist

2 Occasionally moist
Skin occasionally moist, extra linen required once per day approximately

---

MOBILITY
Ability to mobilize when out of bed

1 Walks frequently
Walks around bed at least once every 2 hours and outside room at least twice a day

2 Walks Occasionally
Walks occasionally during day for short distances but may require assistance

---

ACTIVITY
Ability to change body and limb position when in bed or chair

1 No limitation
Able to change position frequently and unaided

2 Slightly Limited
Makes slight but frequent changes in body or extremity position

---

SKIN CONDITION
Observed condition of skin in areas exposed to pressure

1 Skin condition good
Skin appearance good, no evidence of edema, discoloration, etc.

2 Fragile skin
Skin thin, fragile, dry, flaky, or edematous (e.g., due to age, steroids, edema, inflammation, or lymphedema)

NUTRITION/WEIGHT
Food intake or weight change pattern

1 Satisfactory
Food intake very good OR No significant weight change in last 6 months

2 Marginally adequate
Weight appears normal
Food intake slightly restricted

FRICTION/SHEAR
Presence of friction/shear

1 No apparent friction/shear
Can lift body or limb completely without sliding when moving in bed or chair

2 Occasional friction/shear
Occasionally slides down bed or chair or drags body or limbs—due to position and poor muscle strength or fatigue

---

| Low | 12 and under | Medium | 13 to 17 |
| High | 18 to 21 | Very High | 22 and over |

Date of Admission _____   Date of first assessment _____

		Date	Date	Date	Date
3 Very Limited Responds only to painful stimuli (i.e., moans or is restless or sensory impairment over half of body surface) (e.g., spinal cord compression)	**4 Severely impaired** Unresponsive due to impaired consciousness or analgesia/sedation or sensory impairment over most of body surface				
3 Very Moist Skin often but not always moist Linen changed at least once per shift	**4 Constantly Moist** Skin constantly moist with perspiration, urine, or lymphorrhea or in contact with fecal matter				
3 Chairfast Ability to walk severely limited Must be assisted into chair or wheelchair Spends more than 16 hours in chair or bed	**4 Completely Immobile** Spends all day in bed or chair—in excess of 20 hours (e.g., due to unconsciousness, pain, dyspnea, fatigue)				
3 Very Limited Only able to make occasional slight changes in body or limb position—usually requires assistance	**4 Immobile** Unable to change body or limb position due to - pain, sedation dyspnea, edema, conscious level, etc.				
3 Skin marks easily Skin easily marked by support surface	**4 Skin integrity broken** Skin surface altered (e.g., due to incontinence dermatitis, pressure damage, wound, or skin condition)				
3 Probably inadequate Significantly underweight or overweight OR Poor food intake	**4 Nutritional status very poor/severe cachexia** Nutritional status unsatisfactory due to cachexia, obesity, or minimal intake				
3 Frequent sliding Frequently slides down bed or chair Patient unable to lift limb or body without dragging (e.g, due to weakness)	**4 Almost constant friction/shear** Continually slides down bed or chair OR Severe lymphedema, spasticity or agitation results in almost constant friction				
	TOTAL SCORE				
	SUPPORT SURFACE				

pain can occur with dressing changes, treatments, and additional trauma to the area.

Assessment of pain is now mandatory based on the 2000 Joint Commission on Accreditation of Healthcare Organizations (JCAHO)[42] accreditation guidelines. Pain, in fact, is now called the fifth vital sign. The new Centers for Medicare and Medicaid Services Guidelines Tag 309 on quality of life also mandate the assessment of pain in long-term care.[43] Every individual with a pressure ulcer must be assessed for pain that emanates either from the ulcer itself or related to care of the ulcer. Even though an individual is incapable of expressing pain, they can still be experiencing pain. (See "Pain assessment" in chapter 12, Pain management and wounds.)

Ascertain the goals and desires of both the patient and family related to care, including pain control. Management of wound pain is based on a balance of appropriate wound care, medication as needed, and conservative measures.[2] Analgesics should be prescribed based on the WHO guidelines for control of cancer pain and within local prescribing parameters and guidelines.[1] Premedication for breakthrough pain prior to treatments and dressing changes is also recommended.

Keep the patient informed of what will be done and when it will be done and what the patient can do to help alleviate or minimize the pain and anxiety. Complementary therapies, such as relaxation, distraction, visualization, or music, may also calm an anxious patient.[49,50]

A mild to moderate opioid, such as 1 mg morphine or diamorphine mixed with 1 mg of a hydrogel,[47,48] or nonopioid medication can be used, as can a topical that contains a local anesthetic agent (for example, one with lidocaine, such as EMLA cream, Lidoderm, or Regencare).[48,51,53] One hospital solely dedicated to caring for palliative patients has developed a unique mixture of Balmex and lidocaine 2.75%, which may be applied topically to painful and odorous wounds. They have reported success with this strategy.[54] Wound treatment pain can also be minimized by using minimal mechanical force for cleansing (4 to 15 psi irrigation force); using warmed products, such as normal saline or gauze pads[46];and avoiding antiseptic and cytotoxic agents.[27,55]

PRACTICE POINT

Premedicating the patient with pain medication 20 to 30 minutes prior to changing the dressing should be a standard of care for patients with palliative wounds.

Wound dressings

When possible, select a dressing that can remain in place for several days; however, this isn't always possible when a large amount of exudate is present. A dressing that protects periwound skin is also desirable, as is one that protects the wound from incontinence. Wet-to-dry dressings meet few of these goals.[56] As a rule, nonadherent dressings are best. When minimal or no drainage is present, a transparent, hydrocolloid, hydrogel, or composite dressing works well. When exudate is moderate, one could choose a hydrogel, hydrocolloid, foam, composite, or calcium alginate dressing. In the presence of heavy exudate, a composite, foam, or calcium alginate dressing could be used.[56] Moist wound care needs to be observed to prevent exposure of delicate nerve endings,[44] as dry, desiccated wound beds and dressings are nearly always painful.[45]

Wound colonization and infection

All chronic wounds are colonized with bacteria. Although fairly healthy individuals can tolerate this colonization, individuals near or at the end of life are less able to tolerate the bacteria. Classic signs of infection include redness, warmth, odor, edema, drainage longer than 5 days and viscous in nature or yellow or green in color, and, sometimes, confusion. Bacteremia can also occur and, when it does, is often caused by anaerobes and gram-negative bacteria (for example, *Staphylococcus aureus, Bacteroides fragilis*).[24]

Odor

Tissues deprived of oxygen and nutrients become devitalized and nonviable.[57] Necrotic material appears in the wound as the bacteria colonize, creating an odor, which varies depending on the bacteria present. Nonviable tissue eventually serves as a culture medium to support bacterial growth and inhibit leukocyte phagocytosis of bacteria.[57] Anaerobic bacteria are usually present in necrotic material, thrive in the absence of oxygen, and can bury deeper within the wound. Anaerobic bacteria[45] also have a stronger, more offensive odor that can be particularly distressing to the patient. The wound appearance becomes black and leathery with exposure to air or yellow/gray when exposed to moisture, which occurs over varying lengths of time depending on the underlying disorder.[45]

Nonsurgical (autolytic or enzymatic) debriding is recommended due to the tendency for bleeding and "seeding" of malignant cells in fungating and radiation wounds.[45,58] Topical metronidazole has also been used successfully to control odor.[59,60] Activated charcoal dressings are effective in quickly controlling odor[61] as are occlusive dressings and doing frequent dressing changes.[62] Room deodorizers are also helpful. Sugar paste and honey are once again being used for their antibacterial and debriding properties.[63,65] The high sugar content produces a hyperosmotic wound environment to inhibit bacterial growth and assist in debridement.[63,65]

PRACTICE POINT

Odor control is vital for enhancing the quality of life for patients with palliative wounds.

Exudate

All bacteria produce exudate, and the exudate color and odor vary according to the causative organism.[45] For example, green exudate generally indicates gram-negative, aerobic bacteria, which respond well to silver found in many dressings now on the market.[45]

Protection of the periwound area

Periwound skin protection is crucial because exudate can exacerbate skin damage,[66] as it

is liquid, sometimes caustic, and can cause maceration, breakdown, and itching.[55,67] Dressings that appropriately control exudate and don't unnecessarily increase wetness or dryness are recommended, such as an alginate, hydrofiber, foam, or nonadherent, with a secondary absorbent pad.[45,68,69] Be sure to change dressings when saturated, as heavy or overly saturated dressings can cause wound bed pain and irritate periwound skin. Alternatively, if exudate is minimal, a low absorbency dressing, such as a hydrocolloid or semi-permeable film, is recommended.[40] A barrier film around the periwound area is helpful in controlling damage from moisture.

Fungating wounds

Fungating wounds occur when the skin and its supporting blood and lymph vessels are infiltrated by a local tumor or from metastatic spread from a primary tumor.[72,73] It's reported that approximately 5% to 10% of patients with metastatic cancer will develop a fungating wound.[74] The incidence in elderly individuals over age 70 is higher.[70,75] Although these wounds often develop during the last months of life, they also can be present for years.[62]

The term fungating refers to a malignant process of both ulcerating and proliferative growth through direct invasion.[76,77] An ulcerating wound will produce a crater-like wound, whereas a lesion with a predominantly proliferative growth pattern often develops into a nodular "fungus" or "cauliflower" appearing lesion.[68,78] Mixed appearing lesions can also develop.[79,80] Skin tumors tend to become ulcerated as the skin is a bacterially contaminated surface.[81]

PRACTICE POINT

Families, support persons, and caregivers may need emotional support when viewing patients with fungating wounds.

When left untreated, a fungating wound can extend and cause extensive damage at the wound site through a combination of proliferative growth, loss of vascularity, and ulceration.[68] Although these wounds can occur

Common radiation wound skin reactions

- Flaking or peeling (dry desquamation)
- Erythema
- Alteration in pigmentation
- Hair loss
- Loss of perspiration or sebaceous excretion
- Changes in superficial blood vessels
- Edema
- Ulceration (moist desquamation)
- Scarring

Source: Smith, S. *Skin care following radiation therapy. The Clinician's Notebook.* Carrington Laboratories, Inc. Newsletter;1(3):1-3. Available at: http://www.woundcare.org/ newsvol2 n2./ar3.htm. Accessed February 21, 2006.

many places on the body, the breast is the most common site (62%).[44] The anatomical location makes it challenging to address these wounds, in addition to the fact that the surrounding tissue is delicate.

Even though the percent of cancer patients who develop a fungating wound is small, the complications and personal distress can be significant.[82] The wound appearance itself can be disturbing.[62] Yet, it is often the symptoms of the wound that cause the most distress, as the patient may have to cope with the additional problems of bleeding, exudate, odor, infection,[83,84] or pain, which is a constant reminder to patients of their progressive and incurable disease process.[82]

Fungating wounds rarely heal,[85] thus management is centered on symptom control, promotion of comfort, and maintenance or improvement of quality of life.[74,82] Assessment and management by the nurse and physician in particular, as well as other health care providers, is most challenging.[86] Therefore, excellent interdisciplinary care and patient-caregiver communication is essential.

Care of fungating wounds

Nonsurgical (autolytic or enzymatic) debridement is recommended due to the tendency for bleeding and "seeding" of malignant cells.[45,58] Fungating lesions are friable and predisposed to bleeding. Hemorrhage due to erosion of blood vessels is the most common emergency seen in fungating wounds and can also be related to the decreased platelet function within the tumor.[70] Blood vessels can become eroded from the tumor cells itself or secondary to necrosis or sloughing of tissues after radiotherapy.[71] To minimize bleeding, use nonadherent dressings, maintain a moist wound bed, and clean by gentle irrigation rather than swabbing.[69] Dry dressings can cause bleeding when they adhere to the wound bed and should be avoided.[45] An alginate dressing has a high seaweed content and exchanges sodium ions for calcium ions in the wound bed, thus encouraging the clotting cascade. Alginates must be used with caution in fragile tumors as they can also cause bleeding.[47] Hemostatic surgical sponges can also be used and left in place for a time.[62]

Radiation wounds

Radiation therapy targets a high-energy X-ray beam to an area of treatment. The target area is usually a tumor, the area surrounding the tumor, or an area where a tumor has been surgically removed. While each treatment is designed to target tissue at a particular depth, the tissues overlying the site can be affected as well.[87]

Radiation-related skin changes or ulcerations can occur in soft tissues during the course of therapy, immediately after the therapy, or a long time following the therapy.[87] Skin problems can also be noted in individuals who underwent treatments years ago prior to the technological improvements in the radiation machines. The skin reactions seen are generally specific to the area that was irradiated, and the inflammation can occur almost immediately.[88] Acute erythematous wounds result from the dilated blood vessels in the irradiated area. The ulceration may be large and may initially present as a draining sinus.[89]

Oncology Nursing Society classification for skin reactions[92]

0	None
1	Faint erythema or dry desquamation
2	Moderate to brisk erythema or patchy moist desquamation, most confined to skin folds and creases; or moderate edema
3	Confluent moist desquamation ≥1.5 cm diameter and not confined to skin folds; pitting edema
4	Skin necrosis or ulceration of full-thickness dermis; may include bleeding not induced by minor trauma or abrasion

Adapted from Oncology Nursing Society. *Radiation Therapy Patient Care Record: A Tool for Documenting Nursing Care*. Pittsburgh: ONS, 2002, with permission of the publisher.

The more common skin reactions include skin that flakes or peels, redness, changes in pigmentation, loss of hair, decreased or absent perspiration, superficial blood vessel changes, edema, ulceration, and scarring.[90,91] (See *Common radiation wound skin reactions*.)

At the cellular level, changes can be reflected at the site by poor healing. Healing is impeded related to atrophy of the epidermis and epidermal accessory structures, microvascular occlusions, exuberant connective tissue, decreased fibroblast reproduction, and significant amounts of cellular damage.[89,90]

Most radiation-related lesions are superficial. In 1994, the Oncology Nursing Society created a classification system for radiation ulcers. This system was refined in 2002. The five-level classification system ranges from "0" or no skin problem within a radiation field to "4" or skin necrosis or ulceration of full-thickness dermis.[92] (See *Oncology Nursing Society classification for skin reactions*.)

Treatment of a radiation-induced skin lesion is essentially like other types of wounds. Any tissue within a radiation field must be considered at high risk for potential breakdown and should be kept clean, appropriately moistened, and protected from potential injury. Skin can also be protected by avoiding restrictive clothing, adhesives, harsh chemicals, heat or sunlight, and trauma. Should a minor skin reaction, such as erythema or dry desquamation occur, the same guidelines apply, along with using a topical hydrogel or obtaining an order for a steroid cream.[90] Moist desquamation is also treated in the manner as above, with the addition of a nonadherent or foam dressing to manage the wound environment. It's important to cover the wound to prevent evaporation of fluid, to control pain, and reduce risk of infection.[88]

Severe ulceration or necrosis needs to be treated as an open wound, using moist wound healing principles.[90] However, it's important to first rule out a new malignancy in the area.[88] Skin grafting or growth factor application may be required.[92] As a consequence of the vascular changes and resultant hypoxia, irradiated tissues have a decreased ability to fight infection. Avoiding or controlling infection is important, and antibiotics are best delivered topically.[89] The vascular changes and hypoxia also are responsible for pain being present in these ulcerations.[89] These wounds are typically difficult to manage and slow to heal. In all instances, systemic support is necessary to enhance the patient's healing potential to minimize further trauma to the wound site.

Summary

While cure is not always realistic, it's possible to provide compassionate and symptom-relieving care for patients who have palliative wounds. This includes balancing the management of local wound symptoms, such as pain, odor, exudate, and bleeding, while preserving patient dignity, self-esteem, and maximizing quality of life. Few randomized clinical trials or other research studies exist in the area of palliative wound care. However, there is a consensus document from the international palliative wound care initiative that looks at managing these wounds across the life continuum.[93] Continued study is needed to more clearly understand when a palliative care goal is appropriate. A comprehensive palliative wound care program needs to be developed in clinical agencies that work with these patients. The interdisciplinary team would include the physician, nurses, wound care specialists, dietitian, chaplain services, social services, and pain and hospice consultants.[35] Palliative care units are increasing in number, particularly for patients who are chronically, but not terminally, ill.[94] Wounds treated appropriately, even when the goal is not healing, can markedly improve in 50% of the cases, even on a hospice unit.[6]

Show what you know

1. Which of the following defines palliative care?

    A. An organized and highly structured system to deliver care focused on promoting the greatest comfort and dignity of the patient.
    B. Care that affirms life yet strives to deliver highly organized care to an individual that is focused on regaining a former health state.
    C. A care delivery system focused on wound healing and elimination of symptoms.
    D. Care that is delivered at home by loved ones without the involvement of health care providers.

ANSWER: A. Palliative care is focused on holistically supporting an individual for comfort rather than care or healing of a wound, while improving both the quality of living and dying. Palliative care affirms life and views death as part of a normal process and is implemented to neither delay nor speed death. Palliative care provides relief from pain and other symptoms, yet is not focused on the complete elimination of these symptoms.

2. Which of the following situations would constitute palliative wound care?

    A. Wet-to-dry dressing changes every 4 hours around the clock
    B. Calcium alginate dressings used on a necrotic appearing wound with minimal exudate
    C. Silver impregnated dressings used on a wound with little evidence of inflammation and essentially no evidence of infection
    D. A hydrogel dressing placed on a wound every 3 days and as needed

ANSWER: D. A hydrogel dressing that is placed on a wound every 3 days and as needed is recommended in a palliative patient with a wound, as the hydrogel provides for a moist wound environment, which is soothing and comforting to the patient. It assists in protecting the periwound skin from maceration and is nonadherent, which is desirable. A silver-impregnated or calcium alginate dressing is not necessary unless there is heavy exudate or signs of infection or moderate to severe inflammation. Wet-to-dry dressings that are changed every 4 hours could likely contribute to periwound maceration and would be painful if changed every 4 hours.

3. Which one of the following orders should the clinician question in caring for a fungating wound?

    A. Using nonadherent dressings
    B. Using cold saline when irrigating the wound
    C. Using a mixture of morphine with amorphous hydrogel
    D. Using music and other relaxation techniques when providing care

ANSWER: B. Warm rather than cold saline is recommended when irrigating wounds in palliative care patients. Answers A, C, and D are appropriate management strategies.

4. A patient with a grade 3 ONS classification of skin reaction would require which one the following interventions:

    A. None, skin is normal
    B. Frequent application of skin moisturizer
    C. Use of a protective skin barrier
    D. Enzymatic debridement ointment three times per day

ANSWER: C. The skin is moist and desquamated, so it needs protection from injury caused by the edema and wetness. Answer A is incorrect because the skin is compromised and needs care. Answer B is incorrect as the skin is too moist already. Answer D is incorrect as debridement is not indicated. In addition, debridement agents do not need to be applied as frequently as three times per day.

References

1. World Health Organization. *Cancer Pain Relief*, 2nd ed. Geneva: WHO, 1996.

2. National Institutes of Health. *Improving End-of-Life Care. State-of-the-Science Conference Statement.* Bethesda, Md.: NIH, December 6-8, 2004.

3. Alvarez, O., et al. "Chronic Wounds: Palliative Management for the Frail Population," *Wounds* 2002:14(8 Suppl):1-27.

4. Morgan L. "Palliative Care Programs Surging Trend in U.S. Hospitals," *Public Health News* (online) December 13, 2005. Available at: http://www.medicalnewstoday.com/medicalnews.php?newsid=34875. Accessed March 2, 2006.

5. Langemo, D.K., and Brown, G. "Skin Fails Too: Acute, Chronic, and End-Stage Skin Failure," *Advances in Skin & Wound Care* 19(4):206-11, 2006.

6. Tippett, A.W. "Wounds at the End of Life," *Wounds* 17(4):91-98, 2005a.

7. van Rijswijk, L., and Lyder, C.M. "Pressure Ulcer Prevention and Care: Implementing the Revised Guidance to Surveyors for Long-Term Care Facilities," *Ostomy/Wound Management* 4(Suppl):7-19, 2005.

8. Weissman, D.E. *End-of-Life Cares Eases Pain and Prepares Patient for Death.* Health Link, Medical College of Wisconsin 2003. Available at: http://healthlink.mcw.edu/article/100171698.html. Accessed February 21, 2006.

9. Langemo, D.K. "When the Goal is Palliative Care," *Advances in Skin & Wound Care* 19(2):148, 150-54.

10. Rice, K.N., et al. "Factors Influencing Models of End-of-Life Care in Nursing Homes: Results of a Survey of Nursing Home Administrators," *Journal of Palliative Medicine* 7(5):668-75, 2004.

11. Covinsky, K.E, et al. "The Last 2 Years of Life: Functional Trajectories of Frail Older People," *Journal of the American Geriatric Society* 51(4):492-98, 2003.

12. Tippett, A.W. "Wounds at the End of Life," *Journal of Palliative Medicine* 8(1):243, 2005b.

13. Southwest Missouri State University. "Four-Day Wound Management Workshop," Warrensburg, Mo., September 2001.

14. National Hospice and Palliative Care Organization. *NHPCO Facts and Figures.* Available at http://nhpco.org/i4a/pages/index.cfm?pageid=3383. Accessed February 23, 2006.

15. Schim, S.M., and Cullen, B. "Wound Care at End of Life," *Nursing Clinics of North America* 40(2):281-94, 2005.

16. Hanson, D., et al. "The Prevalence and Incidence of Pressure Ulcers in the Hospice Setting: Analysis of Two Methodologies," *American Journal of Hospice Palliative Care* 8(5):18-22, 1991.

17. Galvin, J. "An Audit of Pressure Ulcer Incidence in a Palliative Care Setting," *International Journal of Palliative Nursing* 8(5):214-21, 2002.

18. Chaplin, J. "Pressure Sore Risk Assessment in Palliative Care," *Journal of Tissue Viability* 10(1):27-31, 2000.

19. Bale, S., et al. "Pressure Sore Prevalence in a Hospice," *Journal of Wound Care* 4(10):465-66, 1995.

20. Olson, K., et al. "Preventing Pressure Sores in Oncology Patients," *Clinical Nursing Research* 7(2):207-24, 1998.

21. Hatcliffe, S., and Dawe, R. "Monitoring Pressure Sores in a Palliative Care Setting," *International Journal of Palliative Nursing* 2(4):182-86, 1995.

22. Reifsnyder, J., and Hoplamazian, L. "Incidence and Prevalence of Pressure Ulcers in Hospice," *Journal of Palliative Medicine* 8(1):244, 2005.

23. Sussman, C. "Wound Healing Biology and Chronic Wound Healing," in *Wound Care: A Collaborative Practice Manual for Physical Therapists and Nurses.* Edited by Sussman, C., and Bates-Jensen, B. Gaithersburg, Md.: Aspen Pubs., 1998.

24. Maklebust, J., and Sieggreen, M. *Pressure Ulcers: Guidelines for Prevention and Management*, 3rd ed. Philadelphia: Lippincott Williams, & Wilkins, 2001.

25. Chaplin, J., and McGill, M. "Pressure Sore Prevention," *Palliative Care Today* 8(3):38-39, 1999.

26. Dealey, C. *The Care of Wounds.* Oxford: Blackwell, 1999.

27. Wound, Ostomy, Continence Nurses Society. *Guideline for Prevention and Management of Pressure Ulcers.* Glenview, Ill.: WOCN, 2003.

28. Horn, S.D., et al. "The National Pressure Ulcer Long-term Care Study: Pressure Ulcer Development in Long-Term Care Residents," *Journal of the American Geriatric Society* 52(3):359-67, 2004.

29. Peerless, J., et al. "Skin Complications in the Intensive Care Unit," *Clinics in Chest Medicine* 20(2):453-67, 1999.

30. European Pressure Ulcer Advisory Panel. *Pressure Ulcer Prevention Guidelines.* Oxford: EPUAP, 1998.

31. End-of-Life Nursing Education Consortium (EL-NEC). *Training Program: Faculty Guide.* Washington, D.C.: American Association of College of Nursing and City of Hope National Medical Center, 2002.

32. Bergstrom, N., and Braden, B. "A Prospective Study of Pressure Sore Risk Among Institutionalized Elderly," *Journal of the American Geriatric Society* 40(8):747-58, 1992.

33. Berlowitz, D.R., and Wilking, S.V. "Risk Factors for Pressure Sores: A Comparison of Cross-Sectional and Cohort-Derived Data," *Journal of the American Geriatric Society* 37:1043-1059, 1989.

34. Pinchovsky-Devin, G., and Kaminski, M.V. "Correlation of Pressure Sores and Nutritional Status," *Journal of the American Geriatric Society* 34:435-40, 1986.

35. Ennis, W.J., and Meneses, P. "Palliative Care and Wound Care: 2 Emerging Fields with Similar Needs for Outcome Data," *Wounds* 17(4):99-104, 2005.

36. Dallam, L., et al. "Pain Management and Wounds," in *Wound Care Essentials: Practice Principles.* Edited by Baranoski, S. and Ayello, E.A. Philadelphia: Lippincott Williams & Wilkins, 2002.

37. Pasero, C.L. "Procedural Pain Management," *American Journal of Nursing* 98(7):18-20, 1998.

38. McCaffrey, M., and Pasero, C. "Pain: Clinical Manual, 2nd ed. St. Louis: Mosby, 1999.

39. Manning, M.P. "Metastasis to Skin," *Seminars in Oncology Nursing* 14(3):240-43, 1998.

40. Jones, M., et al. "Dressing Wounds," *Nursing Standard* 12(39):47-52; quiz 55-56, 1998.

41. Krasner, D. "The Chronic Wound Pain Experience: A Conceptual Model," *Ostomy/Wound Management* 41(3):20-29, 1995.

42. Joint Commission on Accreditation of Healthcare Organizations. *Improving the Quality of Pain Management Through Measurement and Action.* Oak Brook, Ill.: JCAHO, March 2003.

43. Centers for Medicare & Medicaid Services. CMS Manual System, Publication 100-07S. State Operations, Provider Certification. Department of Health and Human Services, November 12, 2004.

44. Hallett, A. "Fungating Wounds," *Wound Care Society Education Leaflet.* Huntingdon, U.K.: Wound Care Society, 1993

45. Hampton, S. "Managing Symptoms of Fungating Wounds," *Journal of Cancer Nursing* 20(1):21-28, 2006.

46. Hollingworth, H. "Wound Care—Less Pain, More Gain," *Nursing Times* 93(46):89-91, 1997.

47. Grocott, P. "Controlling Bleeding in Fragile Fungating Tumors," *Journal of Wound Care* 7(7):342, 1998.

48. Twillman, R.K., et al. "Treatment of Painful Skin Ulcers with Topical Opioids," *Journal of Pain Symptom Management* 17(4):39-42, 1997.

49. Ryman, L., and Rankin-Box, D. "Relaxation and Visualization," in *The Nurse's Handbook of Complementary Therapies,* 2nd ed. Edited by Rankin-Box, J. London: Balliere Tindall, 2001.

50. Downing, J. "Pain in the Patient with Cancer," *Nursing Times Clinical Monographs* London: NT Books, 1999.

51. Smith, N.K., et al. "Non-Drug Measures for Painful Procedures," *American Journal of Nursing* 97(8):18-20, 1997.

52. Chaplin, J. "Wound Management in Palliative Care," *Nursing Standard* 19(1):39-42, 2004.

53. Briggs, M., and Nelson, E.A. "Topical Agents or Dressings for Pain in Venous Leg Ulcers," Oxford: The Cochrane Library, 2001.

54. Kalinski, C. "Palliative Strategies in the Care of Tumors and Chronic Wounds," Symposium on Advanced Wound Care April 30-May 3 2006, San Antonio, Texas.

55. Agency for Health Care Policy and Research. Treatment of Pressure Ulcers. Clinical Practice Guideline No. 15, publication No. 95-0652. Rockville, Md.: U.S. Department of Health and Human Services, Public Health Service, 1994.

56. Baranoski, S., and Ayello, E.A. "Wound Treatment Options," in *Wound Care Essentials: Practice Principles.* Edited by Baranoski, S., and Ayello, E.A. Philadelphia: Lippincott, Williams, & Wilkins, 2003.

57. Slavin J. "Wound Healing: Pathophysiology," *Surgery* 17(4):I-V, April 1999.

58. Grocott, P. "Palliative Management of Fungating Malignant Wounds," *Journal of Community Nursing* (online) 14(3):2000. Available at: *http://www.jcn.co.uk/ backiss.asp?YearNum= 2000&MonthNum=03&ArticleID=221* Accessed February 21, 2006.

59. Gilchrest, B. "Wound Infection," in *Wound Management Theory and Practice.* Edited by Miller, M., and Glover, D. London: Nursing Times Books, 1999.

60. Cutting, K. *Wounds and Infection Education Leaflet.* Huntingdon U.K.: Wound Care Society, 1998.

61. Williams, C. "Clinisorb Activated Charcoal Dressing for Odour Control," *British Journal of Nursing* 8(15):1016-1019, 1999.

62. Naylor, W. *World Wide Wounds: Part 1: Symptom Control in the Management of Fungating Wounds.* Available at: *http://www.worldwidewounds.com/ 2002/march/Naylor/Symptom-Control-Fungating-Wounds.* Accessed February 20, 2006.

63. Cooper, R., and Molan, P. "The Use of Honey as an Antiseptic in Managing *Pseudomonas* Infection," *Journal of Wound Care* 8(4):161-64, 1999.

64. Edwards, J. "Wound Management (2): Managing Malodorous Wound," *Journal of Community Nursing* (online) 14(4):2000. Available at: *http://www.jcn.co.uk/backiss.asp?YearNum=2000 &MonthNum=04&ArticleID=136.* Accessed February 21, 2006.

65. Molan, P.C. "The Role of Honey in the Management of Wounds," *Journal of Wound Care* 8(8):415-18, 1999.

66. Cameron, J., and Powell, S. "Contact Kept to a Minimum," *Nursing Times Wound Care Supplement* 92:39:84-86, 1996.

67. Bergstrom, N., et al. *Pressure Ulcers in Adults: Prediction and Prevention.* Clinical Practice Guideline No. 3, Rockville, Md.: U.S. Department of Health and Human Services, Public Health Service, Agency for Health Care Policy and Research Publication. No. 93-0047, 1992.

68. Grocott, P. "The Management of Fungating Malignant Wounds," *Journal of Wound Care* 5:232-34, 1999.

69. Pudner, R. "The Management of Patients with Fungating or Malignant Wounds," *Journal of Community Nursing* (online) 12(9):1998. Available at: *http://www.jcn.co. uk/backiss.asp?YearNum= 1998&MonthNum=09&ArticleID=82.* Accessed February 21, 2006.

70. Haisfield-Wolfe, M.E., and Rund, C. "Malignant Cutaneous Wounds: A Management Protocol," *Ostomy/Wound Management* 43(1):56-60, 62, 64-66, 1997.

71. Beare, P.G., and Myers, J.L. *Adult Health Nursing,* 3rd ed. St. Louis: CV Mosby, 1998.

72. Hastings, D. "Basing Care on Research," *Nursing Times* 89(13):70-76, 1993.

73. McMurray, V. "Managing Patients with Fungating Malignant Wounds," *Nursing Times* 99:55-57, 2003.

74. Dowsett, C. "Malignant Fungating Wounds: Assessment and Management," *British Journal of Community Nursing* 8:394-400, 2002.

75. Ivetic, O., and Lyne, P.A. "Fungating and Ulcerating Malignant Lesions: A Review of the Literature," *Journal of Advanced Nursing* 15(1):83-88, 1990.

76. Mortimer, P.S. "Management of Skin Problems: Medical Aspects," in *Oxford Textbook of Palliative Medicine,* 2nd ed. Edited by Doyle, D., et al. Oxford: Oxford University Press, 1998.

77. Englund, F. "Wound Management in Palliative Care," *RCN Contact* 2-3, Winter 1993.

78. Collier, M. "The Assessment of Patients with Malignant Fungating Wounds—A Holistic Approach: Part 1," *Nursing Times* 93(440):(Suppl)1-4, 1997.

79. Carville, K. "Caring for Cancerous Wound in the Community," *Journal of Wound Care* 4(2):66-68, 1995.

80. Young, T. "The Challenge of Managing Fungating Wounds," *Community Nurse* 3(9):41-44, 1997.

81. Majno, G., and Joris, I. *Cells, Tissues, and Disease: Principles of General Pathology.* Oxford: Blackwell Science, 1996.

82. Naylor, W. "Using a New Foam Dressing in the Care of Fungating Wounds," *British Journal of Nursing* 10(Suppl 6):S24-30, 2001.

83. Piggin, C. "Malodourous Fungating Wounds: Uncertain Concepts Underlying the Management

of Social Isolation," *International Journal of Palliative Nursing* 5:216-21, 2003.

84. Schiech, L. "Malignancy Cutaneous Wounds," *Clinical Journal of Oncology Nursing* 5:305-309, 2002.

85. Bird, C. "Managing Malignant Fungating Wounds," *Professional Nurse* 15(4):253-256, 2000.

86. Laverty, D. "Fungating Wounds: Informing Practice Through Knowledge/Theory," *Brit J Nurs* 12(Suppl 15):S29-40, 2003.

87. Bryant, R. "Skin Pathology," in *Acute and Chronic Wounds: Nursing Management.* Edited by Bryant, N. New York: Mosby Year Book, 1992.

88. Black, J.M., and Black, S.B. "Complex Wounds," in *Wound Care Essentials: Practice Principles.* Edited by Baranoski, S., and Ayello, E.A. Philadelphia: Lippincott Williams & Wilkins, 2003.

89. Williams, H.D. *Radiation ulcers.* Available at: *http://www.emedicine. com/plastic/topic 466.htm.* Accessed February 20, 2006.

90. Smith, S. *Skin Care Following Radiation Therapy. The Clinician's Notebook.* Carrington Laboratories, Inc. Newsletter;1(3):1-3. Available at: *http://www.woundcare.org/newsvol2n2./ ar3.htm.* Accessed February 21, 2006.

91. Rudolph, R. "Radiation Ulcer," in *Chronic Problem Wounds.* Edited by Rudolph, N., and Noe, N.M. Boston: Little, Brown & Co., 1983.

92. Mendelsohn, E., et al. "Wound Care After Radiation Therapy," *Advances in Skin & Wound Care* 15(5):216-224, 2002.

93. Ferris, F.D., et al. *Palliative Wound Care Managing Chronic Wounds Across Life's Continuum: A Consensus Statement from the International Palliative Wound Care Initiative,* 2004. Available at: *http://www.palliativewoundcare.info.* Accessed June 10, 2006.

94. Morrison, R.S. "Palliative Care Outcomes Research: The Next Steps," *Journal of Palliative Medicine* 8(1):13-15, 2005.

CHAPTER 22

Wound care: Where we were, where we are, where we're going

Elizabeth and Sharon

Where we were

It has been said that the "past is prologue." Indeed, it may come as no surprise that, historically, wound care was not seen as a specialty. Wound care seemed to suffer from lack of oversight, with no evidence of team effort or multidisciplinary focus. However, it has become increasingly clear that by revisiting our collective wound care history, we as clinicians can learn valuable information to put to use as we care today and plan for the future.

Dressing wounds has traditionally been a job for nurses. Some of the earliest pictures of nurses depict young women covering the wounds of soldiers with gauze dressings. And, for many years, that's all we did with wounds—passively cover them using strict sterile technique to keep out debris. An essential skill was learning how to use sterile forceps to pick up and handle gauze-dressing materials. Wet-to-dry dressings were the gold standard.

We believed that turning a patient and positioning him in a 90-degree angle would relieve pressure—some patients were even secured in that position for several hours! Massaging the area around a decubitus ulcer (what we now call a *pressure ulcer*) was a common intervention. We believed that a dry wound was a good wound. Heat lamps were occasionally positioned over the local wound area to assist in this "dry healing" method. Wounds were "painted," and even soaked, in povidone-iodine solution. Scabs were considered a positive sign. Many "home inventive" remedies were developed to put in the wound, and different parts of the country had their own local favorites: sugar and bourbon, sugar and povidone-iodine, grape jelly, honey, and antacids, to name a few. "We've always done it this way," or "It works" were the yardsticks we used, rather than evidence and research findings.

Wound assessment meant looking for green or yellowish fluid and odors that indicated the presence of infection. We used a swab culture inserted into the wound drainage to assess for infection.

Wound care practices were passive. We cleaned the wound, covered it, and waited patiently as the wound healed. And, because it was the expectation that chronic wounds would take months or even years to heal, the typical hospital stay was long. In the past, many patients' wounds closed and healed before they were even discharged.

Where we are

Bertolt Brecht once said "Because things are the way they are, things will not stay the way they are." We can apply this vision to the ever-changing world of wound care to determine where we currently are.

A wound care revolution with emphasis on a team approach has occurred over the last five decades. The 1960s discovery of moist wound healing, coupled with advancements in wound dressing materials, has dramatically changed wound care practices. We now understand that wound healing must take place in a moist environment so that epithelial cells can migrate from the wound edges to reepithelialize, or close, the wound. This process is likened to the cells' "leap-frogging." In a dry wound, these cells have to burrow down underneath the wound bed to find a moist area upon which to move in order to migrate forward.

This new understanding of the importance of moist wound healing based on wound physiology has required the development of new dressing materials. Film dressings and hydrocolloid dressings were among the first dressing materials able to maintain a moist wound-healing environment. With the advent of these new dressings, clinicians had to learn new application techniques and, more impor-

tantly, accurately pinpoint the clinical significance of wound fluid findings. In addition, the use of antimicrobial dressings has grown over the past few years, and it seems that the use of silver has been combined with many forms and types of dressings on the market today. And, the old concept of honey in healing has been revived in the form of new dressings using Menuka honey.

The practice of using the same dressing material for the entire wound healing time is no longer valid. Indeed, because wound characteristics change, so too should the choice of wound dressings. For example, a deep wound with a large amount of drainage requires a highly absorbent dressing, such as a hydrofiber, alginate, or foam. As the depth and amount of drainage decreases, a hydrogel, hydrocolloid, or film dressing might be used. Over the course of healing, the treatment plan will change as the wound fills with granulation tissue and epithelialization occurs.

Wound bed preparation continues to be an important foundation for tissue rebuilding. Adequate and continuous wound debridement is needed because it removes necrotic tissue, which is a barrier to migrating cells. Enzymatic agents (selective and nonselective chemicals), autolytic (moisture retentive dressings), mechanical (wet-dry dressings, whirlpool, and irrigation), and surgical/sharp as well as biological (maggot) therapy are the debridement options from which clinicians can select the best method of clearing the wound bed of dead tissue and preparing it for rebuilding of tissue. However, changes in reimbursement coverage regarding the number of debridements could have an effect on practice.

The way acute wounds are closed has also changed. Collagen sutures are occasionally used after cardiac catheterization, and staples have replaced sutures for closing some surgical incision wounds. Skin bonding materials are being used to "glue" wound edges back together.

Some of the solutions previously used to clean wounds (Dakin's solution, povidone-iodine, hydrogen peroxide, acetic acid) were found to kill the very fibroblast cells that were needed to allow granulation tissue repair. The pressure ulcer treatment guidelines of the Agency for Healthcare Research & Quality (AHRQ, formerly the Agency for Healthcare Policy & Research, or AHCPR) provide recommendations about which solutions are harmful and which are appropriate to use in wound care.

Our advanced understanding of wounds has also caused a revision of our view of what's "normal" in a healing wound. Clinicians needed to learn to discriminate between the normal collection of fluid under newer dressings and "pus." Similarly, we've revised our view about wound odors. Different odors occur as wound fluid interacts with different dressing materials—wounds being treated with alginate dressings, for example, may smell like "low tide."

The notion that all wounds are alike has also changed as we've learned that understanding of the wound's *etiology* is essential for appropriate care. Local wound care products as well as supportive care must be individualized for the particular wound. For example, a venous ulcer may require an absorptive dressing or a hydrogel, as well as necessary compression therapy. A variety of layered bandages beyond the classic 100-year-old treatment (Unna boot) are now being used. These new practices are serving to minimize edema and accelerate wound repair. Checking for ankle-brachial index (ABI) and pulses using a Doppler device has also become a standard step in the total assessment of a patient with a peripheral vascular ulcer.

Pressure redistribution as well as an appropriate dressing must be part of the care plan for pressure ulcers. Support surfaces available as cushions, overlays, replacement mattresses, and specialty beds now exist to assist in offloading of pressure. The very way in which we position patients has also changed. The AHRQ pressure ulcer treatment guidelines recommend a 30-degree angle rather than the old 90-degree position. Further, massaging the periwound area is no longer a recommended practice.

Wound culturing technique has also evolved. Quantitative bacterial cultures obtained from wound fluid or tissue are now considered the gold standard. However, if a facility can't do tissue cultures then the Levine swab technique should be employed.

Also per AHRQ pressure ulcer treatment guidelines, clean technique rather than sterile can now be used in chronic wounds.

Although there is a lag time in implementing study findings in practice, research and technology, do continue to advance the science of wound care. Research has demonstrated that acute and chronic wounds heal differently, necessitating a new approach to wound management. Bench scientists continue to add to our understanding of the biologic and molecular processes of wound healing. Wound healing options, such as negative pressure therapy are now used to interact in the wound healing process in highly exudative and difficult to heal wounds. Derived from a patient's own platelets or in drug form dispensed in a tube, growth factors are now used to aid in healing diabetic wounds. Research continues as to the combinations and quantities of growth factors, and when to use them, to best enhance wound healing. Yet another way technology is providing new options for wound management is in the use of bioengineered skin equivalents for healing chronic wounds. These skin equivalents are effective in accelerating the process of reepithelialization, in decreasing scar formation, and in accelerating the healing process of chronic wounds.

The number of therapies from which clinicians can choose to assist in healing wounds has also grown. Such therapies include electrical stimulation, ultrasound, and lasers and medicine therapy (HBO- hyperbaric oxygen). With this proliferation of various modalities and products available, clinicians are faced with deciding which treatment options to use and in what combination to best accelerate wound healing. Research continues into determining just what *are* the healing rates for the commonly seen chronic wounds—pressure ulcers, venous ulcers, and diabetic/neuropathic ulcers.

Thanks to the efforts of numerous individuals and organizations and agencies, awareness of pressure ulcers has come to the forefront. The role of prevention in wound care has taken on new meaning, which could be, in part, due to increased interest by regulatory bodies in skin injuries and pressure ulcers across care settings. The importance of skin care is also beginning to emerge as clinicians are being held accountable. Indeed, preventing pressure ulcers and protecting the skin are key patient safety initiatives especially as pay for performance is being pilot-tested in the United States.

Wound care is no longer the sole province of nurses; it's now a specialty practiced by physicians, podiatrists, nurses, physical therapists, and occupational therapists, to name a few. Multidisciplinary teams provide comprehensive care to patients with acute and chronic wounds in a variety of settings, including inpatient, outpatient, long-term care, and home-health settings. With the expansion in the number of professionals involved in wound healing, communication is more important than ever. In addition, centers and clinics specializing in wound care have been established across the country and abroad. However, in the United States, as the length of hospital stay has decreased, wound care has had to move even more aggressively to the outpatient setting.

Instruction in the form of continuing education courses, clinical symposia, and specialized programs is available to teach clinicians the essentials as well as the advanced knowledge of managing wounds in the twenty-first century. Some of this education is even available over the Internet. Specialized knowledge of wound care may be achieved through certification in wound care from the American Academy of Wound Management (AAWM) or the Wound, Ostomy, and Continence Nurses Society (WOCN).

Legal issues have also affected wound care. Lawsuits regarding lack of adequate wound management have become common. Are pressure ulcers avoidable? This question is still being debated in courtrooms around the country. Medical, nursing, and other health care experts are being used to argue for both the plaintiff and the defendant.

Regulatory and organizational guidelines support best practices. Health care facilities continue to struggle with the costs of health care. Long-term care facilities and home-care agencies are required to track and improve outcomes of care in wound patients. Outcome-based quality improvement has arrived in the acute care setting. Evidence based practice continues to be a challenge for all health care providers.

Where we're going

"The care of the future is mine" so says the motto of Hunter-College Bellevue School of Nursing. What will wound care look like in the future? Curricula in all health care disciplines will assure that graduates have the wound care essentials needed for future practitioners. Certification in wound care will be required for practice. Wound care may, one day, be approved by the American Medical Association as a medical speciality.

Wound care goals will change for some patient populations. For example, in acute care, minimally invasive surgeries will reduce the number of acute incision wounds that health care providers have been accustomed to seeing. We might see the day when nurses in home care are the only ones to see healed wounds and are the experts in scar management. Those working in acute care will never see a healed acute wound, because the patient will go home within a few hours or days of surgery. Laparoscopic incision sites may be the only wounds acute care providers have to treat.

Because people are living longer and many chronic illnesses lead to "skin failure," the idea that some wounds won't heal may become increasingly accurate. Patients who are dying may have wounds that can't or won't heal; for these patients, palliative wound care will replace wound closure as a goal. The idea of palliative wound care with emphasis on comfort and preventing wound deterioration rather than wound closure will require clinicians and regulatory partners to rethink wound care practices.

The standard hospital mattress will be a thing of the past. High-tech support surfaces, with special features we can't begin to imagine, will become the gold standard in health care.

As wound care continues to be patient focused, pain in wound care will take on more consideration. Less painful and less frequent wound cleaning and dressing change will replace present practice. The role of nitric oxide will become more prominent in wound care. Wound care products and treatments based on cell biology and gene therapy will be developed not just to assist in the wound healing process, but to accelerate the repair process. Wound chambers with specific antibiotic therapy may provide us with a better microenvironment in which to heal wounds. More collaboration between bench scientist and clinicians will help us to address the gaps in research regarding wound care practices. Our female diabetic patients will finally have the designer shoes that accommodate their foot deformities.

Technology will continue to make wound care practices easier, more efficient, and less time-consuming. Will reimbursement improve to keep up with the trends in technology? Telemedicine will be integrated into every health setting. Will regulatory agencies support the financial demands of this new patient care arena? Time will give us the answers to these questions.

Bonding with our patients will occur through a small monitor screen, not via the personal touch of the past. Handheld scanning devices will be used by health care providers to detect stage I pressure ulcers so that preventive measures can be implemented before the epidermis breaks down. Wound "dip sticks" will tell us the wound's pH and other characteristics and be linked to the right product to use. Just as our cars have climate control, wound products will adapt to form the appropriate environment for healing to occur. Clinicians will speak into a microphone device on their identification badges to document wound characteristics during dressing changes, and their documentation will automatically be processed to the patient's chart and the physician's office. Electronic signatures will be triggered by our fingerprints. The universal electronic medical record will be a reality. We may consult internationally through computers and telemedicine, making our health care system borderless.

All these developments may sound farfetched, but the discipline of wound care is evolving into higher, innovative technology that we can't conceive of. Quantum leaps—in the way we think about wounds and understand healing and in technologies—will occur among health care practitioners, patients, and caregivers. The future of wound care will undoubtedly be truly amazing. We look forward in future editions to seeing when and how many of our predictions become realities.

Index

INDEX

---

i refers to an illustration; t refers to a table; **boldface** indicates color pages.

i refers to an illustration; t refers to a table; **boldface** indicates color pages.

---

i refers to an illustration; t refers to a table; **boldface** indicates color pages.

---

i refers to an illustration; t refers to a table; **boldface** indicates color pages.

---

i refers to an illustration; t refers to a table; **boldface** indicates color pages.

---

i refers to an illustration; t refers to a table; **boldface** indicates color pages.

i refers to an illustration; t refers to a table; **boldface** indicates color pages.